Gloria Newton, APRN, FNP-BC

Gloria Newton, APRN, FNP-BC

Dermatology for Advanced Practice Clinicians

FIRST EDITION

Margaret A. Bobonich, DNP, FNP-C, DCNP, FAANP

Assistant Professor
Case Western Reserve University School of Medicine
and Frances Payne Bolton School of Nursing
Director, Dermatology NP Residency
Department of Dermatology
University Hospitals Case Medical Center
Cleveland, Ohio

Mary E. Nolen, MS, ANP-BC, DCNP

Director, Dermatology NP Fellowship
Lahey Hospital and Medical Center
Department of Dermatology
Burlington, Massachusetts

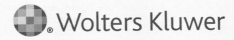

Philadelphia • Baltimore • New York • London
Buenos Aires • Hong Kong • Sydney • Tokyo

Acquisitions Editor: Shannon W. Magee
Product Development Editor: Maria M. McAvey
Developmental Editor: Lisa Marshall
Editorial Assistant: Zachary Shapiro
Production Project Manager: Cynthia Rudy
Design Coordinator: Teresa Mallon
Manufacturing Coordinator: Kathleen Brown
Senior Marketing Manager: Mark Wiragh
Prepress Vendor: S4Carlisle Publishing Services

9 8 7 6 5 4 3 2 1

Printed in China

Library of Congress Cataloging-in-Publication Data

Bobonich, Margaret A., author.
  Dermatology for advanced practice clinicians / Margaret A. Bobonich, Mary E. Nolen.
     p. ; cm.
  Includes bibliographical references and index.
  ISBN 978-1-4511-9197-4 (alk. paper)
  I. Nolen, Mary E., author.   II. Title.
  [DNLM: 1.   Skin Diseases.   WR 140]
  RL74
  616.5—dc23

2014023342

RRS1409

CONTRIBUTORS

Lakshi M. Aldredge, MSN, ANP-BC

Nurse Practitioner
Portland VA Medical Center
Portland, Oregon

Glen Blair, RN, MSN, ANP-C, DCNP

Associate Nurse Leader
Harvard Vanguard Medical Associates
West Roxbury, Massachusetts

Margaret A. Bobonich, DNP, FNP-C, DCNP, FAANP

Assistant Professor
Case Western Reserve University School of Medicine and
Frances Payne Bolton School of Nursing
Director, Dermatology NP Residency
Department of Dermatology
University Hospitals Case Medical Center
Cleveland, Ohio

Niki Bryn, APRN, GNP-BC, NP-C, DCNP

Nurse Practitioner
Dermatology and Skin Health
Dover, New Hampshire

Susan Busch, MSN, ANP-BC

Nurse Practitioner
Lahey Hospital and Medical Center
Department of Dermatology
Burlington, Massachusetts

Cathleen K. Case, MS, ANP, DCNP

Nurse Practitioner
Reliant Medical Group
Worcester and Leominster, Massachusetts

Janice T. Chussil, MSN, ANP-C, DCNP

Nurse Practitioner
Klein Dermatology & Associates
Portland, Oregon

Melissa E. Cyr, MSN, ANP-BC, FNP-BC

Nurse Practitioner
Lahey Hospital and Medical Center
Department of Dermatology
Burlington, Massachusetts

Pamela K. Fletcher, DNP, RN, FNP-BC, DCNP

Assistant Professor
Northern Kentucky University College of Health Professions
Highland Heights, Kentucky
UC Health Dermatology
Southgate, Kentucky

Victoria Garcia-Albea, MSN, PNP, DCNP

Nurse Practitioner
Mystic Valley Dermatology
Stoneham, Massachusetts
Lahey Hospital and Medical Center
Department of Dermatology
Burlington, Massachusetts

Victoria Griffin, RN, MSN, ANP-BC, DCNP

Nurse Practitioner
Harvard Vanguard Medical Associates
Wellesley, Massachusetts

Diane Hanna, MSN, DNP

Regional Medical Liaison
Celgene
Overland Park, Kansas
Director of Clinical Research and Nurse Practitioner
Modern Dermatology
Shawnee, Kansas

Linda Hansen-Rodier, MS, WHNP-BC

Nurse Practitioner
Northeast Dermatology
North Andover, Massachusetts

Kathleen E. Dunbar Haycraft, DNP, FNP/PNP-BC, DCNP, FAANP

Nurse Practitioner
Riverside Dermatology
Hannibal, Missouri

Dea J. Kent, MSN, RN, NP-C, CWOCN, DNP-C

Director of Quality Assurance, Long Term Care
Nursing Home Oversight, Community Health Network
Indianapolis, Indiana

Victoria Lazareth, MA, MSN, NP-C, DCNP

Nurse Practitioner
UMass Memorial Medical Center
Worcester, Massachusetts

Gail Batissa Lenahan, APRN, DCNP

Nurse Practitioner
Foundation Skin Surgery and Dermatology at Foundation
Medical Partners
Nashua, New Hampshire

Mary E. Nolen, MS, ANP-BC, DCNP

Director, Dermatology NP Fellowship
Lahey Hospital and Medical Center
Department of Dermatology
Burlington, Massachusetts

Kelly Noska, RN, MSN, ANP-BC
Nurse Practitioner
Lahey Hospital and Medical Center
Department of Dermatology
Burlington, Massachusetts

Katie Brouillard O'Brien, MSN, ANP-BC
Nurse Practitioner
Mystic Valley Dermatology
Stoneham, Massachusetts

Theodore D. Scott, RN, MSN, FNP-C, DCNP
Nurse Practitioner
Southern California Permanente Medical Group
San Marcos, California

Diane Solderitsch, MSN, FNP
Nurse Practitioner
University Hospitals Case Medical Center
Cleveland, Ohio

Dorothy Sullivan, MSN, APRN-BC, NP-C
Nurse Practitioner
Lahey Hospital and Medical Center
Department of Dermatology
Burlington, Massachusetts

Jane Tallent, ANP-BC
Nurse Practitioner
Harvard Vanguard Medical Associates
Medford and Somerville, Massachusetts

Susan J. Tofte, MS, BSN, FNP
Nurse Practitioner and Assistant Professor
Oregon Health & Science University
Portland, Oregon

Susan Thompson Voss, APRN, DNP, FNP-BC, DCNP
Nurse Practitioner
Riverside Dermatology
Hannibal, Missouri

PREFACE

"The eye sees only what the mind is prepared to comprehend."
. . . . Henri Bergson, French philosopher and educator

For centuries, educators have emphasized the importance of knowledge and its impact on how we view or interpret the world. This is particularly relevant as we proceed through the twenty-first century, with increasing demand for health care and limited access to specialties such as dermatology. As a result, primary care providers shoulder a significant burden for the care of patients with dermatologic complaints. Advanced practice clinicians (APCs) are uniquely positioned to help satisfy this growing demand, and will likely encounter one out of every three patients with a dermatologic complaint. For that reason, APCs are responsible to ensure that they have the knowledge and skills to develop competency in evaluating skin conditions.

For most of us, there was minimal education and clinical experience in dermatology during our master's programs. Acquiring this knowledge and clinical acumen is challenging, especially for those interested in pursuing a career in dermatology. We have seen, firsthand, the educational gaps that exist between APC education and practice, and have endeavored to develop structured, interprofessional post-master's education for dermatology NPs. So after years of teaching, mentoring, and lecturing health care professionals in both nursing and medicine, we set out to create a dermatology text dedicated to APCs.

The content of this book focuses on skin diseases that are high volume (most common conditions seen in practice); high morbidity (causing disability or high impact on the community); and high mortality (life- or limb-threatening). Our aim was to create a practical approach to learning dermatology that can impact clinical practice with an emphasis on recognition, diagnosis, management, and collaboration. This book outlines the essential dermatology knowledge and skills for APCs in primary care and provides a strong foundation for new clinicians specializing in dermatology.

The chapters have been designed in an orderly and user-friendly manner, offering tables, algorithms, and lists that we have found to be the most beneficial for the busy clinician. Common pitfalls, clinical pearls, and guidelines for referral and consultation are recommended on the basis of the scope of practice for our professions and specialty practice. Given the visual nature of dermatology specialty, more than 600 photographs are included to guide APCs to a prompt and accurate diagnosis—helping the mind understand what one's eyes are seeing.

It is our hope that this will become an everyday reference that will be your "go to" book for skin-related patient complaints. We encourage you to start at the beginning to master the basic concepts outlined in the first two chapters. Understanding the structure and function of the skin is key to distinguishing normal from abnormal, and for making clinicopathologic correlations. Algorithms can guide you from the primary morphology of a lesion to differential diagnosis groups with easy reference to chapter content.

This text is ideal for new and experienced APCs alike. Students can utilize this text to learn more about dermatology during their master's programs, enabling them to be more prepared to evaluate and treat patients with dermatologic complaints. A greater knowledge of dermatology gained through this user-friendly text can enhance your professionalism, decrease anxiety about treating patients with unknown rashes, and most importantly, produce better patient outcomes.

Enjoy!

Margaret A. Bobonich, DNP, FNP-C, DCNP, FAANP
Mary E. Nolen, MS, ANP-BC, DCNP

ACKNOWLEDGMENTS

I am extremely grateful for the wisdom and guidance of my mentors who believed in me and the role of an advanced practice clinician from the very beginning. Dr. Richard Johnson and the Harvard Community Health Plan provided the first opportunity for me to practice in an expanded role at a time when no one could have anticipated the significance of that decision. Dr. Samuel Moschella and Dr. Laurie Tolman have provided not only continuous encouragement, friendship, and support of my work but a professional and collaborative environment within which I could flourish.

Through the vision of Dr. Suzanne Olbricht and the cooperation and participation of the Lahey Clinic in Burlington, Massachusetts, we have been able to create a model for the postgraduate education of nurse practitioners in dermatology. The need for postgraduate residency training is now being recognized across the specialties, and I believe that it will help provide the much-needed continuing education of this important group of providers.

To Margaret, you were the true force behind this work and I thank you for your guidance in this process. Our combined clinical and academic abilities made us the consummate team (M&M)

I have the greatest respect for your knowledge, teaching abilities and style, and I am proud to be your colleague and friend.

It is because of you all that this book has been realized, and to each of you, I will be forever grateful.

My sincere apologies to family and friends for being so unavailable this past year.

Mary

To Dr. Kevin Cooper and Dr. Neil Korman, there are simply no words that can express my sincerest gratitude for sharing this journey with me and realizing the concept of true collaborative practice.

To Mary Nolen, you are the outstanding clinician, leader, and educator responsible for elevating the professionalism of APCs in dermatology. I am thankful to have had the opportunity to work with you in writing this book. You are my role model, mentor, and an amazing human being.

Most importantly, I thank my husband, Steve, whose love and tireless effort helped make this book a reality. I could not have done it without you. To my sons, Michael and Chase, you inspire me to be better. And finally, to my father and mentor, Hank, I love and miss you.

Margaret

We thank Dr. Thomas Habif for his support, encouragement, and willingness to share his wonderful photographs. We appreciate the hard work by our expert dermatology NP colleagues who contributed their valuable knowledge and experience to this book. To Lisa Marshall, Shannon Magee, Maria McAvey, and all of the staff at Wolters Kluwer, thank you for your patience and guidance through this creative but arduous publishing process.

M&M

CONTENTS

CHAPTER 1

Structure, Function, and Diagnostic Approach to Skin Disease

Margaret A. Bobonich

Primary and nondermatology specialty care clinicians see the majority of patients with skin complaints on a daily basis. While patients make appointments to see their provider for a physical or blood pressure management, they commonly add an *"Oh, by the way…"* skin complaint. In contrast, many patients call the office or central scheduling and cite their reason for seeking treatment as a "rash." This common, catch-all term reported by so many patients can leave the provider wondering what kind of eruption is really on the other side of the examination room door. Clinicians must be knowledgeable in evaluating skin lesions, which could range from skin cancer to a sexually transmitted infection.

Cutaneous lesions may represent more than just a skin disease and can be a manifestation of an underlying systemic process. Conversely, cutaneous conditions can cause systemic disease, dysfunction, and death. Psychosocial conditions can also be the cause or sequelae of skin conditions but are often negated. So in addition to maintaining competency in a primary specialty, clinicians need to acquire the essential knowledge and skills in dermatology—a daunting task given that there are almost 3,000 dermatology diagnoses.

The best approach for acquiring basic competency in the recognition and initial management of dermatologic disease (*dermatoses*) is to focus on conditions that are:

- *High volume*—the most common skin conditions seen in clinical practice;
- *High morbidity*—skin disease that is contagious or can impact quality of life or the community; and
- *High mortality*—life-threatening conditions that require prompt recognition.

This chapter outlines essential dermatology concepts, including anatomy and physiology, morphology of skin lesions and algorithmic approach for the assessment of *any* skin condition. This will enable clinicians to develop the knowledge and decision making skills for far more than the 50 most common skin conditions. Subsequent chapters provide a comprehensive review of hundreds of skin conditions that MUST be considered in a differential diagnosis, ensuring an accurate diagnosis and optimal patient outcome.

STRUCTURE AND FUNCTION

Understanding the normal structure and function of the skin enhances your ability to correlate clinical and histologic findings associated with skin lesions (Figure 1-1). The skin is not only the largest organ but also the most visible, allowing both patients and clinicians the opportunity to observe changes and symptoms.

The skin is complex and dynamic and provides a physical barrier against the environment; an innate and adaptive immunity that protects the body from pathogens; and thermoregulation. The skin is also responsible for vitamin D synthesis and protection from ultraviolet radiation on non-hair-bearing skin. It is a reservoir for medication administration and is a sensory organ (pain, pressure, itch, temperature,

touch). It comprises the epidermis, dermis, subcutaneous tissue, and adnexa or skin appendages and has regional variability in its thickness and structures. *Glabrous* skin does not have hair follicles or sebaceous glands, is located on the palms and soles, and is generally thick. In general, thin skin over the rest of the body houses a variable number of appendages, including the nails, hair, and sebaceous and sweat glands.

Epidermis

Commonly referred to as the "dead skin" layer, the epidermis is the locus of important structures and function (Figure 1-2). Cellular structures include keratinocytes, Langerhans cells, Merkel cells, and melanocytes. Nucleated *keratinocytes* differentiate as they ascend from the basal layer to the surface, filling with keratin and losing their nucleoproteins. *Langerhans cells* are intraepidermal macrophages responsible for phagocytosis of antigens and migration into the lymphatics and presentation to T cells. The immune function of the epidermis is paramount to our health. *Merkel cells* are believed to have a somatosensory function and are responsible for light touch and possible neuroendocrine function. *Melanocytes* synthesize the pigment which accounts for the variation in skin color among races. They are found in the dermis during fetal life and migrate to the basement membrane.

The layers (*strata*) of the epidermis are responsible for protecting the body from the environment as both a mechanical and chemical barrier. Each strata has unique characteristics and functions (Table 1-1). Flattened keratinocytes with a thickened cell membrane create the stratified layer (shingles on a roof) in the stratum corneum, which is not capable of metabolic activity. This cornified layer saturated in a lipid complex provides a virtually impermeable barrier and minimizes water loss. Thus, any defect or impaired function of this layer can lead to pathologic changes and disease.

Dermis

The dermis comprises fibroblasts, histiocytes, and mast cells, and is separated from the epidermis at the *basement membrane* (dermal–epidermal junction or DEJ). It adjoins with the *papillary dermis* (upper portion). Fibroblasts produce collagen (90% of the dermis), elastin, and ground substances, which comprise the majority of the dermis and are the supporting matrix of the skin (Figure 1-3). The dermis is also responsible for the continued immune response initiated in the epidermis by Langerhans cells, as well as neutrophils, lymphocytes, monocytes, and mast cells. Blood vessels, lymphatics, and sensory nerve endings for pain, itch, pressure, temperature, and touch are present. Arrector pili muscles in the dermis contract to make hair follicles stand up, creating the "goose bumps" effect. The *reticular dermis* (lower portion) joins with the subcutaneous or fat layer of the skin.

Subcutaneous Layer

The subcutaneous layer, also referred to as *fatty tissue* or *hypodermis*, comprises adipose cells and connective tissue, which varies in

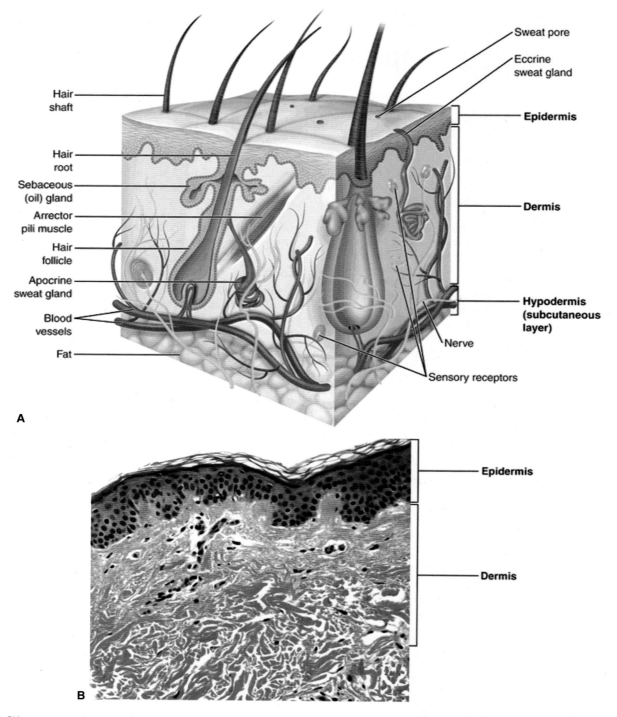

FIG. 1-1. Skin anatomy and histology. **A:** Anatomy of the skin. **B:** Corresponding photomicrograph of the skin showing the cellular distinction between the epidermis and dermis.

thickness according to the body location. The hypodermis provides a layer of protection for the body, thermoregulation, storage for metabolic energy, and mobility of the skin.

Adnexa

Adnexa or appendages of the skin include the hair, nails, and eccrine and apocrine glands. The structure of hair and nails is discussed in chapter 14.

Glands

Eccrine glands

Chiefly responsible for thermoregulation of the body, the *eccrine* or *sweat glands* are tubules that extend from the epidermis through the dermis and are triggered by thermal and emotional stimuli. Although they are diffusely spread over the body, most are located on the palms and soles, and can contribute to hyperhidrosis or

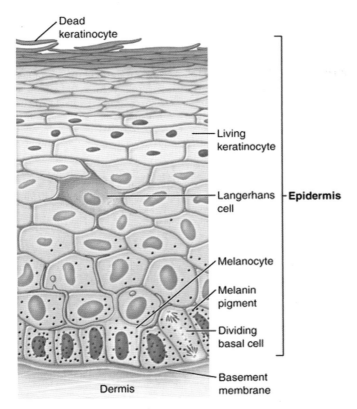

FIG. 1-2. Layers of the epidermis.

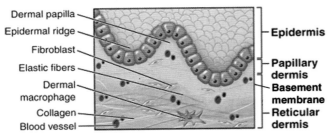

FIG. 1-3. Dermis.

hypohidrosis. Eccrine glands maintain an important electrolyte and moisture balance of the palms and soles.

Apocrine glands

Found only in the axillae, external auditory canal, eyelids, mons pubis, anogenital surface, and areola, *apocrine glands* secrete a minute amount of an oily substance that is odorless. The role of these glands is not clearly understood.

ASSESSMENT OF THE SKIN

Clinicians should elicit a good patient history and perform a proper skin examination in order to generate a complete differential diagnosis.

History

Practitioners are afforded very limited time to assess, diagnose, treat, and document patient care. The patient history is sometimes slighted in view of time spent on the physical examination or patient education. However, the importance of an appropriate history relative to the skin complaint should not be overlooked. The history should begin with the patient's general health and proceed with a focused or complete history relative to the skin complaint and presence of systemic symptoms (Box 1-1). Be aware that patients may be very cursory with details about their health history as they perceive that it is inconsequential to their skin condition. For example, a female seeking treatment for acne may fail to omit oral contraceptives on her medication list or her medical history of polycystic ovarian syndrome. Both can impact the clinician's ability to adequately assess, diagnose, and manage her skin condition.

Medications are one of the most significant aspects of a history, receive the least attention, and yet have the greatest risk of impacting the patient's skin condition. Medication history should not only include prescription drugs, but over-the-counter and illicit drugs, supplements, herbals, and "borrowed" medications. Chapter 17 provides tips on taking a medication history. The elderly and adolescents are known for sharing drugs and may be sheepish about admitting to it. NSAIDs are one of the most common causes of drug eruptions, but often omitted from their medication list. Oral contraceptives, which can have a significant impact on the skin, are commonly omitted from the patient's list of medications.

TABLE 1-1	Strata of the Epidermis	
STRATUM (LAYER)	**CHARACTERISTIC**	**FUNCTION**
Corneum	Brick and mortar layer Lipid matrix and barrier Antimicrobial peptides	Mechanical protection; limits transepidermal water loss; limits penetration of pathogens (bacterial, viral, and fungal) or allergens
Lucidium	Only on soles and palms	Protection
Granulosum	Keratin and fillagrin >80% of mass of epidermis	Profillagrin cleved into fillagrin, and loricin forming cornified envelop
Spinosum	Lamellar granules (containing ceramides) Langerhans cells	Found intracellularly in upper layer but migrate to corneum where most effect, responsible for lipid barrier function Defends against microbial pathogens
Basale	Cuboidal basal cells with nucleus and integrins Scattered melanocytes	Integrins responsible for adhesion to dermis Initiation of keratinocyte differentiation Migration upward to stratum corneum takes 2–4 wk

BOX 1-1	Complete History for the Assessment of Skin Lesions

Demographic Data
Age, sex, race—predilection in some diseases/conditions

Allergies
Drug, environmental, food (possible cross-reactivity)

Medications
See chapter 17 (if drug-related eruption is suspected)
Prescription, over-the-counter, birth control, herbal supplements, illegal drugs

Medical and Surgical History
Personal (birth history for children), including skin cancer
Family (hereditary disease association or genodermatoses)
Pregnancy or lactation

History of Lesion or Eruption
Onset, circumstances, and duration
Spread and/or course of the skin condition
Aggravating or relieving factors
Associated symptoms—itching, pain, drainage, blisters, or odor
Previous episodes, treatment and response
Impact on sleep, eating, social activities, work, and school

Social History
Occupation and hobbies
Sunscreen use, tanning behaviors, and UVR exposure
Alcohol intake and smoking
Exposures (infectious or environmental)
Sexual behavior and orientation
Travel
Living conditions or household (especially important for infectious diseases)
Family structure

Psychological History
Etiology or complication of skin conditions

Before concluding the history intake, it is recommended that clinicians inquire (an open-ended question) about any other specifics that the patient believes might be important about their skin condition. This invites communication and acknowledges the important role of the patient, family, and care givers in their patient-centered care. Patients may express grave concerns that their symptoms are similar to a disease discussed on a television talk show or health information discovered on an Internet search engine. Transparency in the patient's perception and expectations at the beginning of the office visit will enable the clinician to personalize care for a better patient experience.

Physical Examination

Physical examination of the skin is a skill that is developed through repeated and systematic evaluations of your patients. The extent of the examination is determined by the patient's symptoms and willingness to reveal their body. A complete skin examination is recommended for skin cancer screenings, with the patient completely disrobed and in a patient gown. It is also preferred for patients who come in with complaints of a skin eruption or those with systemic symptoms. In contrast, a focused examination from the waist up may be adequate for a chief complaint of acne that may require exposure of the back and chest. Clinicians should encourage patients to allow maximum visualization for a thorough examination while respecting their modesty and rights to limit their physical exposure.

A helpful guide is provided to aid in developing a systematic approach for a skin examination for either the entire body or regional areas (Box 1-2). It is not necessary to wear gloves for a skin examination, allowing the clinician to use touch to optimize their assessment. All providers should clean their hands prior to and after examining a patient. Patients, and our society in general, have become increasingly aware of infection control and appreciate seeing the clinician cleanse their hands while in their presence. Yet, universal precautions should always be observed when preforming cutaneous procedures, exposed to body fluids, or examining skin that is not intact. They should also be worn when infection is suspected or touching the anogenital area and then immediately discarded.

Diagnostics

While the history and physical examination are the foundation for developing differential diagnosis, diagnostic tests may be necessary to rule out disease or support a definitive diagnosis. Each chapter in this text identifies recommended tests relative to the disease, and chapter 24 describes common procedures in detail. In-office diagnostic tools that can easily be used by nondermatology clinicians include the Wood's light, KOH, or mineral prep. Diagnostic tests such as patch testing or tools such as dermoscopy should be reserved for dermatology clinicians trained in application and indications for practice.

One of the most important diagnostics used in the evaluation of cutaneous lesions is histopathology. Clinicians trained to perform shave and punch biopsies can send specimens for hematoxylin and eosin (H&E) staining, which provides microscopic analysis and reports on the pathologic changes in the skin. When indicated, immunohistology on patient tissue or sera utilizes various immunostaining techniques with light microscopy to identify antibodies. This is especially helpful in cutaneous manifestations with autoimmune diseases and is discussed in further detail in those chapters.

Clinicians should learn to competently interpret histopathology reports to ensure that clinicopathologic correlation exists, especially in inflammatory skin conditions. When there are questions regarding the report or interpretation, the clinician should discuss the biopsy with the pathologist. Most dermatology specialists send tissue biopsies to *dermatopathologists* who are specialty trained and board certified in dermatology with a fellowship in dermatopathology. They can provide a superior histologic analysis and opinion about possible diagnoses, especially when the clinician provides pertinent history, clinical findings, and their list of differential diagnoses.

ASSESSMENT OF SKIN LESIONS

Clinicians simply cannot know about every dermatosis, but they can develop assessment skills that will be the key to a timely and accurate diagnosis. Skin lesions can be described in a variety of ways and categorized by morphology, distribution, configuration, and arrangement. While some experienced dermatologists may use various approaches to diagnosis, these authors suggest that nondermatology and less experienced dermatology providers develop an algorithmic approach to diagnosis based on morphology of the primary lesion.

Morphology

The characteristics or structure of a skin lesion is referred to as *morphology*. Once the clinician has identified the morphology of the *primary* lesion or eruption, they can generate a differential diagnoses.

BOX 1-2 | **Complete Skin Examination**

How to Perform a Skin Examination

The two most important aspects of a complete skin examination are exposure and lighting.

Patient must be properly gowned so that each part of the body can be visualized.

Extra lighting may be needed for examination rooms without windows.

Always encourage the patient to undress completely; no peek-a-boo examinations!

Develop a systematic approach and use it for every skin examination.

Begin with the patient seated in front of you and slightly lower.

Gently use your fingers to glide across the skin—your touch can identify lesions and comfort the patient.

Scalp

Part the hair in various sections to visualize the scalp.

Look for papules, nodules, redness, scale, pustules, and scarring.

Hair and Nails

Note hair color, pattern, and texture (see chapter 14).

Look for hair thinning or loss and patterns; note the presence/absence of follicles.

Observe nails and periungual areas for discoloration, thickening, dystrophy, debris, or signs of infection.

Pigmented lesions can be found in unsuspecting places like beneath the nail.

Face

Get an overall view of the face.

Note the presence of scars and evidence of photodamage.

Look for redness, scaling, papules, pustules, comedones, skin tags, milia, keratoses, and pigmentation.

Mouth

Look for any brown or red spots on the lips.

Dryness and scale on the lips in the elderly may be caused by photodamage.

Chapped lips in children or adolescents may be contact dermatitis.

Examine the mouth for lesions on the palate, buccal mucosa, and tongue.

Patients on isotretinoin may have extreme dryness of facial skin and mucus membranes.

Eyes

Examine the inner and outer canthi, orbital area, and lid margins for papules.

Note scale, erythema, or plaques in the brows or lids.

Check for erythema, erosions, or drainage of the conjunctiva.

Ears

Look for scale or lesions on the helix

Examine posterior earlobes for keloids and postauricular sulcus for redness and scale

Check conchal bowl for open comedones, hyperpigmented plaques, scale, and scarring

Nose

Look and feel the bridge, sides, creases, and nasal rims

Note telangiectasias, ulcerations, and abnormal pigmentation

Dilated blood vessels may signify sun exposure and possibly rosacea

Look for papules, pustules, and rhinophyma

Neck

Note the color, texture and distribution, especially anterior and lateral aspect, and inferior chin (photoprotected areas)

Trunk

Visualize the trunk with the patient sitting, standing, or lying down

Be sure to examine the buttocks, hips, and perianal area

If patients defer an examination of their genitals, inquire about new lesions or changes

Check the often forgotten umbilicus for psoriasis, nevi, and melanoma

Arms and Hands

Inspect arms separately and raise to inspect the axilla and lateral trunk

Look for discoloration or depigmentation in the axillae

The antecubital fossa is a classic location for atopic eczema, whereas psoriasis and rheumatoid nodules favor the elbows.

Examine the dorsal and palmar surfaces of the hands, the fingers, and interdigital areas

Legs and Feet

Examine the legs individually and thoroughly

Socks must be removed, to examine the feet, toes, and interdigital spaces

Don't forget the plantar surface, which is a common place for pigmented lesions

Lymphadenopathy

Note occipital, posterior, and anterior cervical nodes with scalp lesions and infections

Check for regional and supraclavicular lymphadenopathy, as well as hepatosplenomegaly, in patients with a history of melanoma or squamous cell carcinoma

---

Use all the tools available to assess the "ABCDE" of melanoma. If in doubt, ask for help or refer to a dermatology specialist.

Often, dermatology textbooks and online resources use a morphology-based approach to categorize diseases. Therefore, clinicians who lack the ability to correctly identify the morphology of the primary lesion must resort to fanning through the color atlas of dermatologic conditions, hoping that they will see a similar lesion or rash.

Primary lesions

The morphology of a *primary skin lesion* can provide important information about the depth of the process and the location of the pathology, that is, the epidermis, dermis, and/or subcutaneous tissue. A thorough understanding of the structure and function of the skin will then allow the clinician to envision the underlying pathologic process and assist in making the clinicopathologic correlation. Flat lesions often represent disease located in the epidermis, while raised lesions usually involve the dermis and/or subcutis. All clinicians should be able to identify these basic morphological types that provide the foundation for the assessment and diagnosis of any skin condition (Figure 1-4).

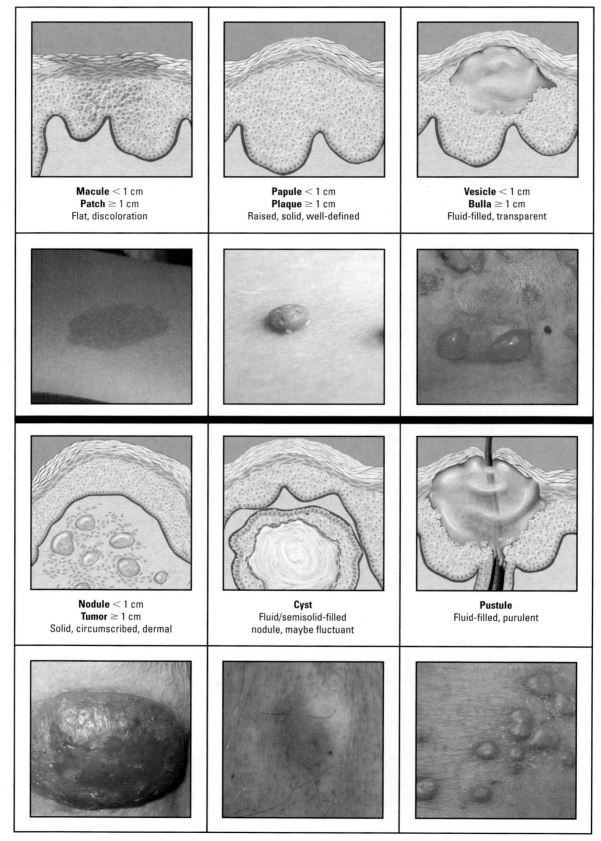

Macule < 1 cm
Patch ≥ 1 cm
Flat, discoloration

Papule < 1 cm
Plaque ≥ 1 cm
Raised, solid, well-defined

Vesicle < 1 cm
Bulla ≥ 1 cm
Fluid-filled, transparent

Nodule < 1 cm
Tumor ≥ 1 cm
Solid, circumscribed, dermal

Cyst
Fluid/semisolid-filled
nodule, maybe fluctuant

Pustule
Fluid-filled, purulent

FIG. 1-4. Morphology of *primary* lesions.

Secondary lesions

Secondary changes (scale, ulceration, lichenification, etc.) in the primary lesion can occur as the result of external factors, the process of healing, or complications from treatment (crusts, atrophy, purpura, scar, etc.). The characteristics of the *secondary skin lesions* provide further description (an adjective) about the primary lesion (noun). There are many descriptors, but several are commonly used in everyday practice (Figure 1-5).

Characteristics

The *configuration* of a lesion describes the shape, which can provide valuable clues. Annular plaques are characteristic of tinea and granuloma annulare. The *arrangement* is the location of lesions relative to each other. Lesions can be solitary, satellite (set apart from the body of the eruption), or clustered. While a red cherry angioma is typically a solitary lesion, the eruption of vesicles and pustules in herpes zoster is usually clustered and follows dermatomal arrangement.

Distribution

When observed, the *distribution* of skin lesions can provide valuable diagnostic clues. Lesions may be generalized or localized, or may favor particular areas of the body such as the interdigital spaces, acral areas, or mucous membranes. Many cutaneous and systemic diseases have hallmark clinical presentations based on the distribution of lesions (Figure 1-6). For example, lesions on the palms are characteristic of conditions like erythema multiforme, dyshidrotic eczema, secondary syphilis, and palmar-plantar psoriasis. Chronic scaly and erythematous patches or plaques on the extensor aspects of the extremities would favor a diagnosis of psoriasis compared to atopic dermatitis that usually affects the flexural surfaces. Care should be taken to note lesions involving the hair, nails, and mucous membrane which can be unique for some diseases. And lastly, the clinician should remember that the distribution of the lesions may change as a skin eruption progresses. Drug rashes typically start on the trunk and spread to the extremities (centrifugal). In contrast, erythema multiforme starts on the hands and feet, and advances to the trunk (centripetal).

Color

For most clinicians, the color of lesions is given little consideration and usually categorized as red or brown. But next time, take a closer look and use tangential lighting. Colors can provide insight into the underlying pathophysiology of the lesion. Red, purple, and blue lesions usually have a vascular etiology. Yellow and orange colors are typically the result of lipid, chemical, or protein deposition. Brown, black, and blue colors are associated with melanin or hemosiderin. White lesions can be associated with a lack of pigment and a "flesh-color" lesion refers to the patient's natural skin color.

Associated Symptoms

Symptoms such as pruritus, pain, and burning can be helpful in discerning a diagnosis. For example, pruritus is a classic symptom in urticaria compared to the burning sensation associated with angioedema. Other lesion symptoms reported may include tenderness, drainage, and odor. Clinicians should always be alert to systemic symptoms that may have proceeded or accompanied the cutaneous lesions. This should prompt a complete review of systems and detailed physical examination. Most importantly, patients presenting with red flag symptoms warrant *immediate* referral for further evaluation and management. Red flag signs and symptoms are febrile patients with a rash; altered levels of consciousness; facial edema or angioedema; purpura; oral or ocular mucosal ulcerations; bullae with mucosal involvement; chest pain or dyspnea; positive Nikolsky sign; and erythroderma (>80% body with erythema).

MORPHOLOGY-BASED APPROACH TO DIFFERENTIAL DIAGNOSIS

The foundation for a diagnosis of any skin lesion begins with a thorough history and physical examination. We suggest that the morphology of the primary lesion provide the first step in a systematic approach for generating a differential diagnosis. After the primary morphology is identified, the clinician can incorporate other lesion characteristics and associated findings to narrow the differential to arrive at the correct diagnosis.

Use of algorithms can be helpful (Figures 1-7 and 1-8). **Algorithms are intended as adjunctive tools accompanied by critical thinking.** Once the category of dermatoses is identified, key characteristics such as distribution, associated symptoms, and diagnostics studies are used to rule out or support the final diagnosis. Tables 1-2 to 1-5 provide abbreviated lists of differential diagnoses, including the most common skin conditions seen in primary care. More extensive lists of differential diagnosis can be found online, manuals, or tools such as Habif's Differential Diagnosis Deck (2012).

Ultimately, success with diagnostic tools like these algorithms requires routine use, good clinical judgment, and individualized patient care. Yet there are always uncommon diseases and atypical presentation that will challenge even the most experienced dermatology clinician. When the clinician is perplexed by the lesion or eruption, he or she should always consult with another experienced colleague or dermatology specialist.

CLINICAL PEARLS

- When there is a change in the surface of the skin, it usually indicates an epidermal process.
- Always perform a punch technique for the biopsy of any inflammatory lesion.
- Vesicles can be from an immune response or infectious process. Pustules are most often associated with infection.
- Consider the possibility of immunosuppression in patients with chronic or recurrent skin infections or atypical presentations.
- Pathologic processes occurring deep in the dermis or subcutaneous can leave the surface of the skin smooth but result in larger plaques that are not as circumscribed (wheals/hives compared to angioedema).
- Be aware of some of the *great mimickers* of skin disease: lupus erythematosus, tuberculosis (mycobacterium), cutaneous T-cell lymphoma, secondary syphilis, sarcoidosis, and amelanotic melanoma.
- Diffuse eruptions involving large BSA can overwhelm the clinician. *Always* start with the basics: the morphology of the primary lesion.

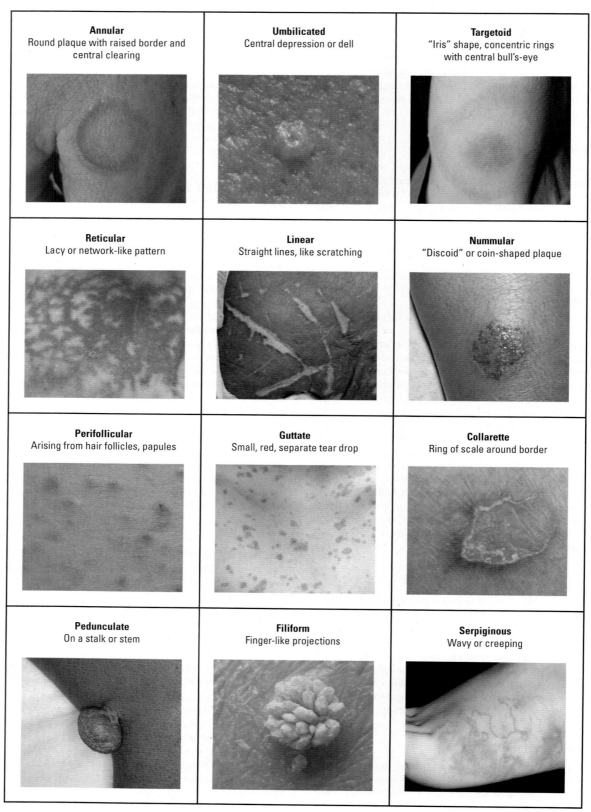

Annular
Round plaque with raised border and central clearing

Umbilicated
Central depression or dell

Targetoid
"Iris" shape, concentric rings with central bull's-eye

Reticular
Lacy or network-like pattern

Linear
Straight lines, like scratching

Nummular
"Discoid" or coin-shaped plaque

Perifollicular
Arising from hair follicles, papules

Guttate
Small, red, separate tear drop

Collarette
Ring of scale around border

Pedunculate
On a stalk or stem

Filiform
Finger-like projections

Serpiginous
Wavy or creeping

FIG. 1-5. Common characteristics of skin lesions.

Desquamation
Shedding or peeling of epidermis

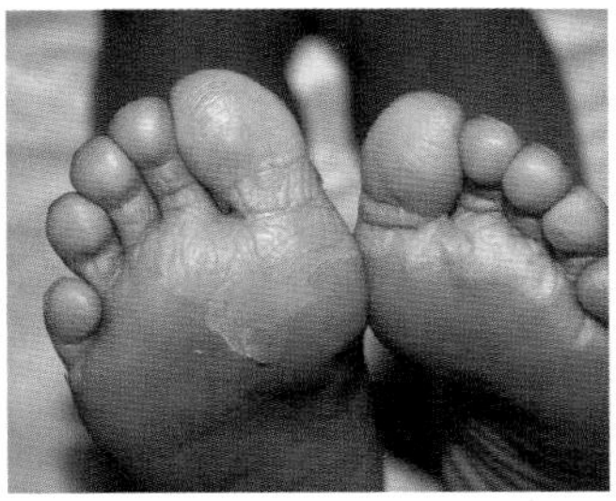

Crust
Dried serum, often
honey-color exudate

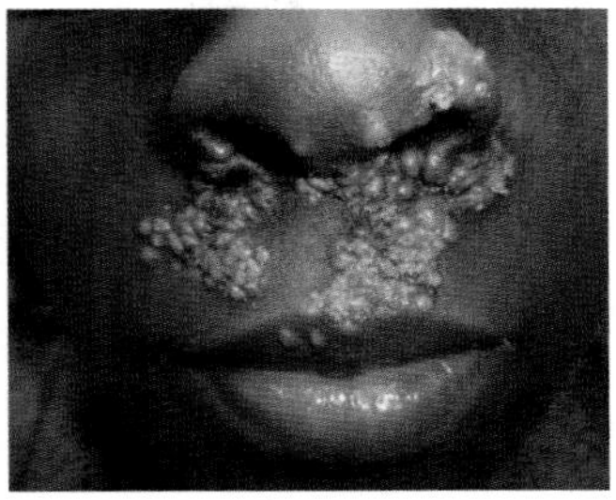

Morbilliform
Small macules, measles-like
appearance, usually red

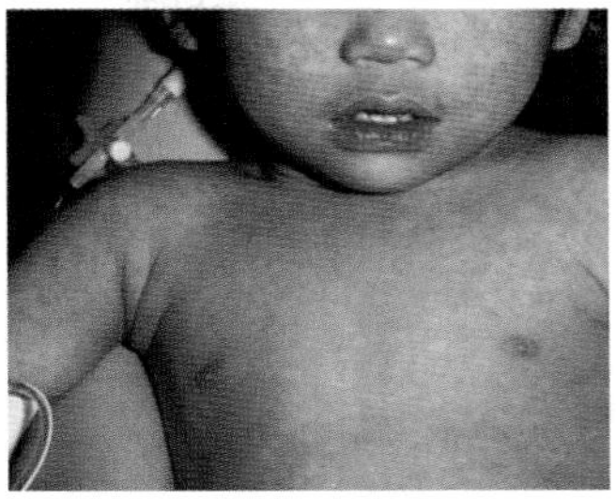

Wheal or Hives
Circumscribed, flat-topped plaques
lasting < 24 hr

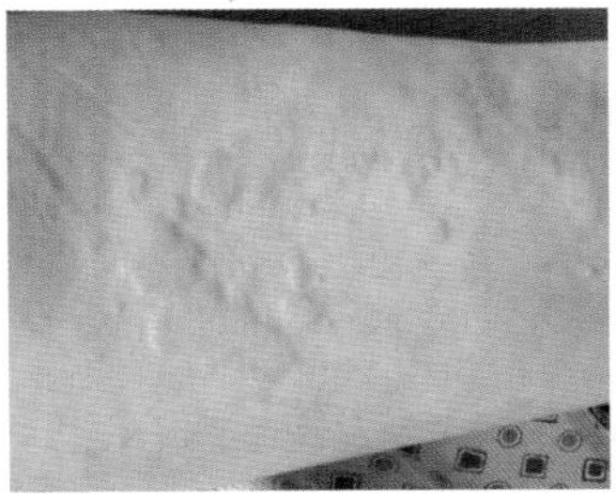

Angioedema
Edema in the dermis and cutis,
not well circumscribed

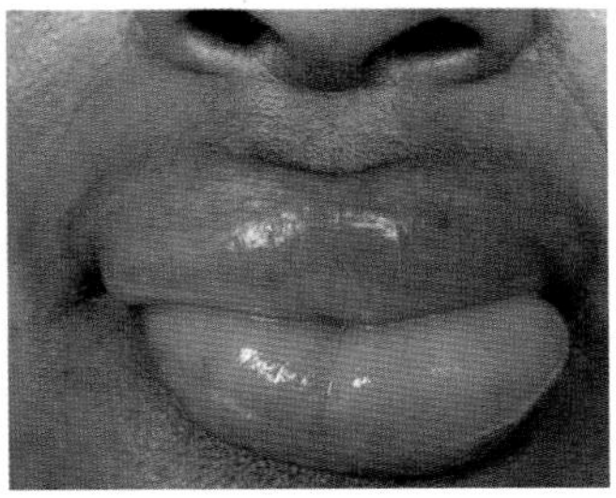

Fissure
Deep tears through the epidermis
and into dermis

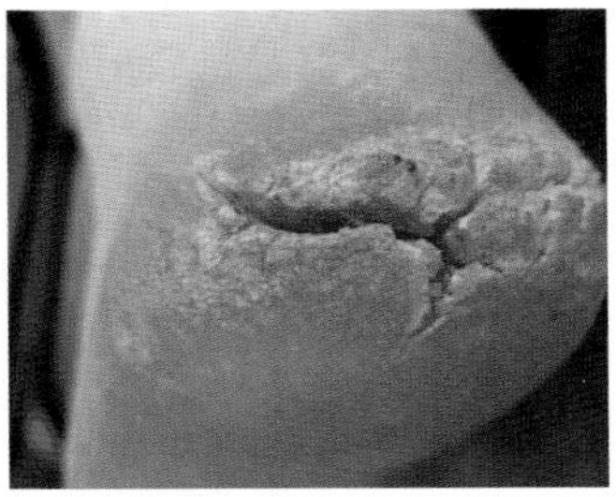

Ulceration
Focal loss of epidermis and dermis

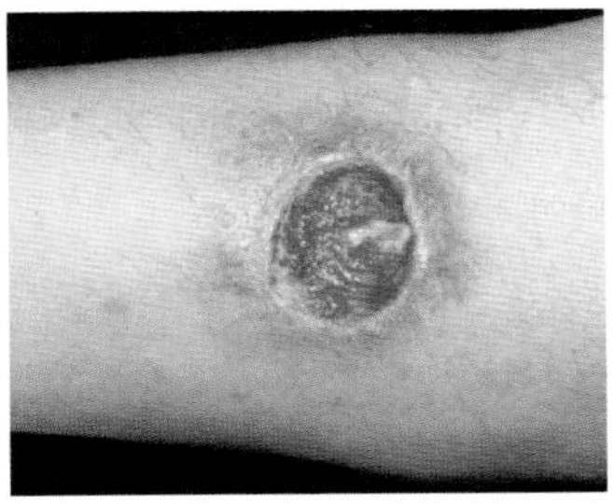

Excoriation
Neurotic type, irregular shape

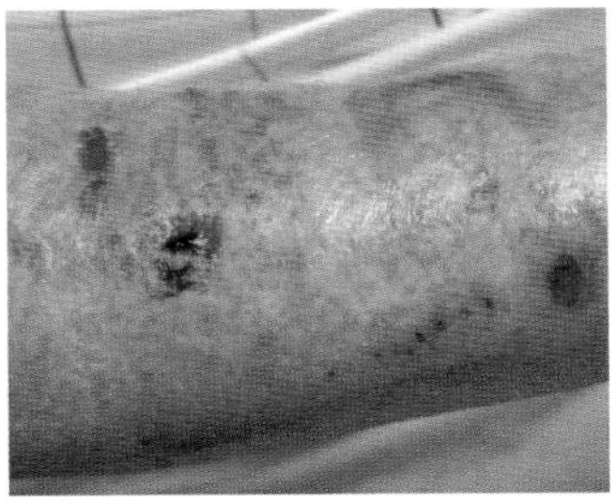

Excoriation
Linear wounds from scratching

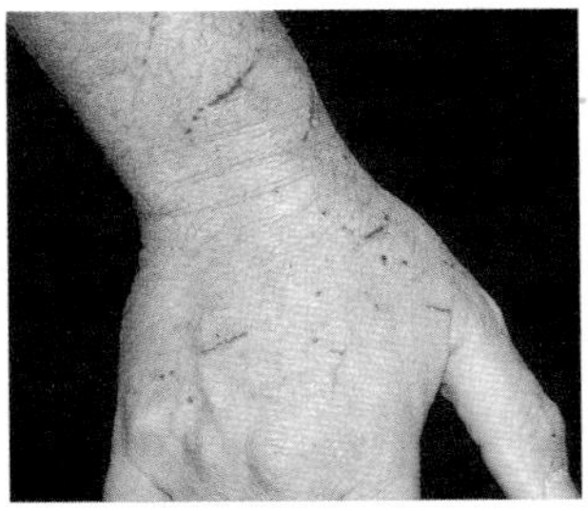

Purpura
Palpable and nonpalpable
extravasation of blood into tissues

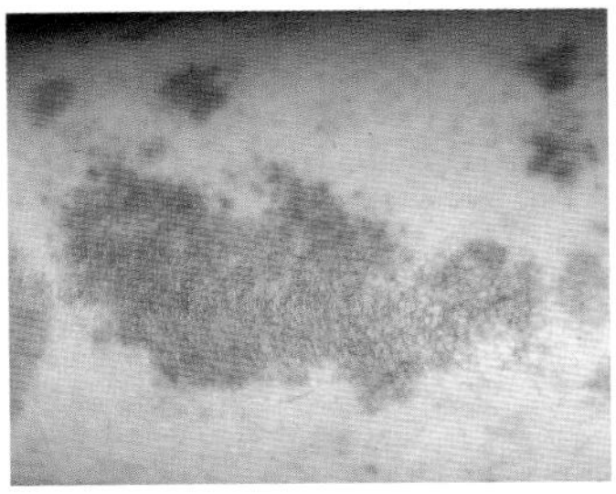

Petechiae
Nonpalpable, extravasation of
blood into tissues, <3 mm

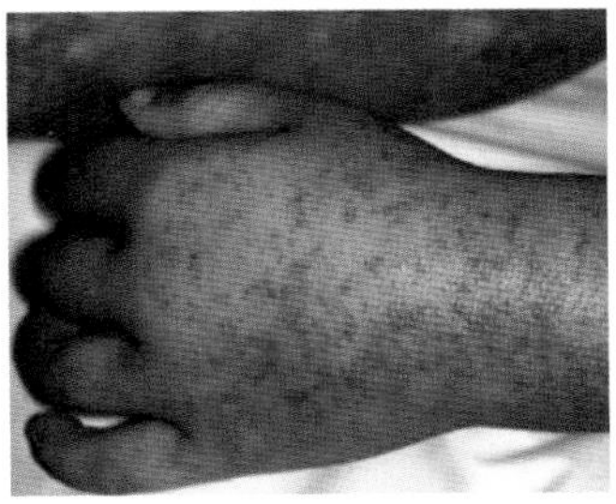

Lichenification
Thickened, exaggerated lines

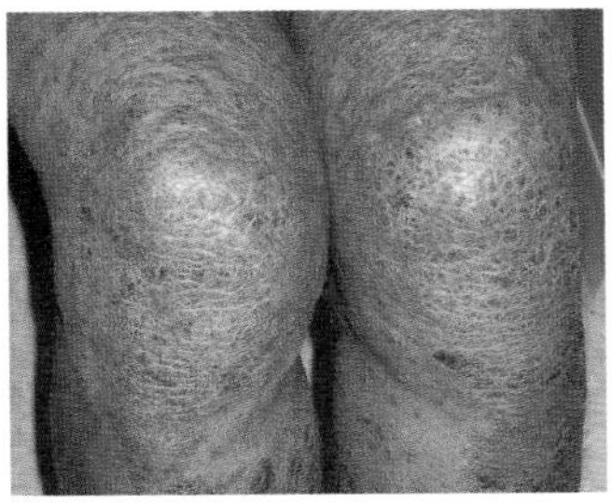

FIG. 1-5. Common characteristics of skin lesions *(continued)*

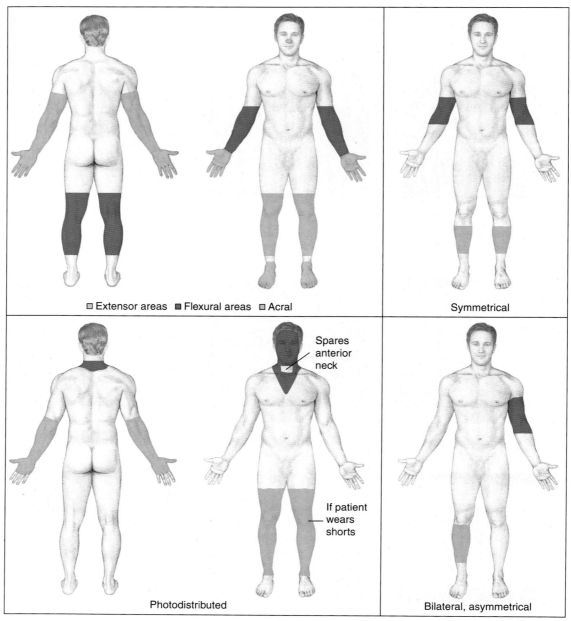

□ Extensor areas ■ Flexural areas □ Acral

Symmetrical

Photodistributed

Spares anterior neck

If patient wears shorts

Bilateral, asymmetrical

FIG. 1-6. DISTRIBUTION OF LESIONS. Bilateral, present on both sides of the body. **Symmetrical**, same location on both sides. **Zosteriform/herpetiform**, along one or more dermatomes, unilateral. **Acral**, ears, nose, feet/soles, hands/palms. **Seborrheic**, hair-bearing, and sebaceous glands; scalp, forehead, moustache/beard, and chest. **Diffuse/generalized**, scattered over large area; localized, specific to one particular area.

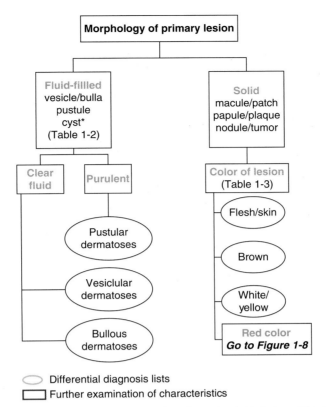

FIG. 1-7. Morphology-based approach to diagnosis of skin lesions. *Semi-solid material and often nodular.

TABLE 1-2	Fluid-Filled Dermatoses	
VESICLES (<1 CM)	**BULLAE (≥1 CM)**	**PUSTULAR**
Dyshidrotic eczema	Bullous impetigo	Acne vulgaris
Herpes simplex	Bullous tinea	Rosacea
Impetigo	Trauma/thermal	Drug-induced pustular acne
Varicella/zoster	Bullous erythema multiforme	Folliculitis–bacterial, candidiasis, pityrosporum
Tinea pedis	SSSS	
Scabies	SJS/TEN	Scabies
Contact dermatitis	Autoimmune blistering disease	Pustular psoriasis (especially palmar-plantar)
Hand-foot-and-mouth disease	Bullous drug eruption	Perioral dermatitis
Polymorphic light eruption	Lichen planus	Subcorneal pustulosis
Grover disease	Porphyria cutanea tarda	
Arthropod assaults	Diabetic bullae	
Erythema multiforme		
Dermatitis herpetiformis		
Id reaction		

SSSS, Staphylococcal scalded skin syndrome
SJS/TEN, Stevens–Johnson syndrome/toxic epidermal necrolysis.

TABLE 1-3	Lesions with Color	
FLESH COLOR	**BROWN**	**WHITE**
Rough	Freckles	Pityriasis alba
Skin tags	Skin tags	Idiopathic guttate hypomelanosis
Verruca	Lentigines	Tinea versicolor
Open comedones	Nevi (intradermal, compound, junctional)	Ash leaf macule
Actinic keratosis		Milia
Corns/callus	Seborrheic keratosis	Keratosis pilaris
Epidermal nevus	Tinea versicolor (pinkish)	Postinflammatory hypopigmentation
Smooth	Postinflammatory hyperpigmentation	Nevus anemicus
Molluscum contagiosum	Erythrasma	Morpheaform basal cell carcinoma
Basal cell carcinoma	Dermatofibroma	Vitiligo
Verruca/HPV	Café au lait	Piebaldism
Epidermoid cysts	Mongolian spot	Lichen sclerosus et atrophicus
Lipomas	Melanoma	Morphea
Keloids/ hypertrophic scar	Pigmented basal cell	Tuberous sclerosis
Granuloma annulare	Dysplastic nevus	*Yellow*
Neurofibromas	Congenital nevus	Xanthelasma
Pearly penile papules	Fixed drug eruption (purple)	Sebaceous hyperplasia
Adnexal tumors	Becker nevus	Necrobiosis lipoidica
		Morphea

HPV, human papilloma virus.

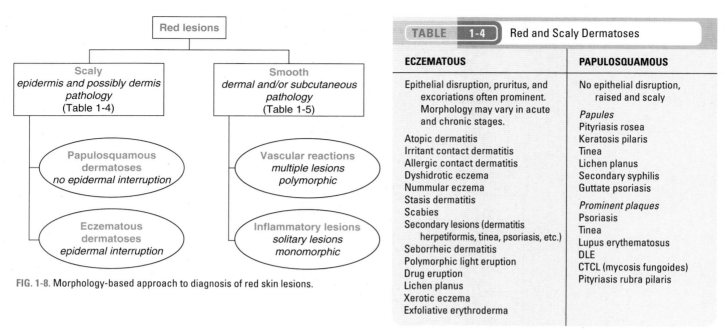

FIG. 1-8. Morphology-based approach to diagnosis of red skin lesions.

TABLE 1-4	Red and Scaly Dermatoses	
ECZEMATOUS	**PAPULOSQUAMOUS**
Epithelial disruption, pruritus, and excoriations often prominent. Morphology may vary in acute and chronic stages.	No epithelial disruption, raised and scaly
Atopic dermatitis	*Papules*
Irritant contact dermatitis	Pityriasis rosea
Allergic contact dermatitis	Keratosis pilaris
Dyshidrotic eczema	Tinea
Nummular eczema	Lichen planus
Stasis dermatitis	Secondary syphilis
Scabies	Guttate psoriasis
Secondary lesions (dermatitis herpetiformis, tinea, psoriasis, etc.)	*Prominent plaques*
Seborrheic dermatitis	Psoriasis
Polymorphic light eruption	Tinea
Drug eruption	Lupus erythematosus
Lichen planus	DLE
Xerotic eczema	CTCL (mycosis fungoides)
Exfoliative erythroderma	Pityriasis rubra pilaris

CtCL, cutaneous T-cell lymphoma: DLE, Discoid lupus erythematosus.

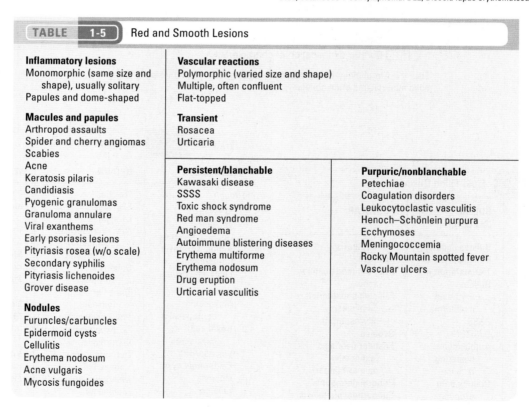

TABLE 1-5	Red and Smooth Lesions		
Inflammatory lesions Monomorphic (same size and shape), usually solitary Papules and dome-shaped	**Vascular reactions** Polymorphic (varied size and shape) Multiple, often confluent Flat-topped		
Macules and papules Arthropod assaults Spider and cherry angiomas Scabies Acne Keratosis pilaris Candidiasis Pyogenic granulomas Granuloma annulare Viral exanthems Early psoriasis lesions Pityriasis rosea (w/o scale) Secondary syphilis Pityriasis lichenoides Grover disease	**Transient** Rosacea Urticaria		
	Persistent/blanchable Kawasaki disease SSSS Toxic shock syndrome Red man syndrome Angioedema Autoimmune blistering diseases Erythema multiforme Erythema nodosum Drug eruption Urticarial vasculitis		**Purpuric/nonblanchable** Petechiae Coagulation disorders Leukocytoclastic vasculitis Henoch–Schönlein purpura Ecchymoses Meningococcemia Rocky Mountain spotted fever Vascular ulcers
Nodules Furuncles/carbuncles Epidermoid cysts Cellulitis Erythema nodosum Acne vulgaris Mycosis fungoides			

READINGS

Ackerman, A. B. (1975). Structure and function of the skin. Section I. Development, morphology and physiology. In S. L. Moschella, D. M. Pillsbury, & H. J. Hurley (Eds.), *Dermatology*. Philadelphia, PA: Saunders.

Bolognia, J. L., Jorizzo, J. L., & Schaffer, J. Y. (2012). *Dermatology*. Philadelphia, PA: Elsevier.

Calonje, E., Brenn, T., & Lazar, A. (2012). *McKee's pathology of the skin* (4th ed.). St. Louis, MO: Elsevier.

Habif, T. P. (2012). *Dermatology DDX deck* (2nd ed.). St. Louis, MO: Mosby.

Habif, T. P. (2009). *Clinical dermatology* (5th ed.). St. Louis, MO: Mosby.

Lynch, P. J. (1994). *Dermatology* (3rd ed.). Baltimore, MD: Williams & Wilkins.

CHAPTER 2

Corticosteroids and Topical Therapies

Susan Busch and Gail Batissa Lenahan

The skin is a large and complex organ that performs multiple functions allowing us to maintain a state of homogeneity. As a barrier, it protects against chemicals, microorganisms, ultraviolet radiation (UVR), and the loss of bodily fluids. It is a nutritive organ supplied by a network of superficial vessels that nourish and repair the skin. Constant vasodilation and constriction of blood vessels, along with the cooling response of sweat glands, accomplishes temperature regulation.

These functions can alter the moisture content in the skin and subsequently affect the penetration and efficacy of topical preparations. Percutaneous absorption (PCA) of topical treatments also varies depending on the thickness of the skin on different areas of the body. For instance, eyelid, antecubital, axillae, and genital skin are very thin and medication is quickly absorbed. The skin of the palms, soles, knees, and elbows is thicker, decreasing the rate of the absorption of medications applied. The presence or absence of occlusion also affects product permeability, rate, and potency of medications used.

This chapter will explore various topical formulations and the most appropriate use of each in the treatment of common dermatologic conditions. Sunscreens and their proper use will be presented, and an overview of botanical products will be outlined.

Systemic agents, specifically corticosteroids, are often used in dermatology, and we will review their optimum indications and usage. At times, oral agents may seem to be a more convenient option; however, topical therapies are often the better choice. With the correct usage of topical corticosteroid (TCS) therapies, side effects will be minimized.

SKIN HEALTH

Patients often ask about proper skin care. They are besieged with advertisements about the best and latest "miracle cream" and often believe that cost is equated with efficacy. For some, it is merely a factor of cosmesis, but many seek help because of uncomfortable and sometimes disfiguring skin conditions. Providing accurate information regarding product ingredients will help patients make better, more informed choices when faced with the myriad of options.

Cleansing

Everyone can benefit from a good skin care regimen. Recommendations regarding bathing and hand washing vary depending on a person's age, activity, environment, culture, and skin condition. Cleansing the skin too often can contribute to worsening of certain skin conditions such as acne and eczema. The use of antibacterial soaps, abrasive materials, and gadgets are not necessary, and can be harmful to the skin by contributing to antibiotic resistance, irritation, or allergic reactions.

Environment

Protecting the skin from all types of weather is important. Sun, wind, cold, and humidity can hinder the skin's protective function. In dryer climates, moisturizers should be applied within minutes of bathing to help prevent water evaporation and skin cracking, which can predispose patients with certain skin conditions to infection. Oil-free and noncomedogenic products are recommended for the skin of the face, while thicker moisturizers and those containing urea or lactic acid are more effective in treating hyperkeratotic skin commonly seen on the feet. Lactic acid, an α-hydroxy acid, is useful for softening dry, thick skin. This ingredient can also cause skin irritation and should not be used on delicate or inflamed skin.

In very cold climates, dry air from heating systems enhances water evaporation and contributes to the overall dryness of the skin. In humid climates, light-weight breathable clothing can help skin to remain dry. In all climates, sunscreen should be applied to exposed areas in the morning and reapplied every 2 hours when staying in the sun.

Healthy lifestyles also help maintain a person's youthful skin appearance. Incorporating regular exercise, maintaining a proper diet, minimizing alcohol intake, and avoiding smoking and excessive stress are key factors in protecting the skin from aging prematurely.

Irritants and Allergens

Individuals with sensitive skin should choose products less likely to include common allergens such as fragrances, dyes, lanolin, propylene glycol, and parabens. If there is a suspected allergy, referral to a dermatologist can help the patient identify the allergens through patch testing (see chapter 3). Furthermore, dermatologists can provide patients with lists of personal hygiene products (a "safe" list) that they should avoid and those that are free of specific allergens. Patients are still warned to check the ingredient list of all products; even those on the safe list can change ingredients without any notice. Otherwise, primary care clinicians can provide some general guidance on widely available moisturizers that are free of the most common allergens (Table 2-1). Patients should be warned that the label "hypoallergenic" does not mean that the product does not contain common sensitizers. This is a marketing claim used by manufacturers and is not standardized or monitored. It only means that the product may cause fewer allergic reactions or has lower amounts of common sensitizers compared to other brands.

Yet not all dermatitis is caused by allergens. Frequent hand washing with soap and water is sometimes necessary, but can aggravate skin that is already affected by dermatitis. Hand dermatitis may be due to allergens in cleansers or irritation from the harsh chemical ingredients that can damage the epidermis and trigger inflammation. Water itself is the most common irritant in hand dermatitis and

TABLE 2-1	Brand-Name Products Free of the Most Common Allergens*
CATEGORY	**PRODUCT†**
Wipes	7th Generation Free & Clear Baby Wipes
Cleansers	Aveeno Baby Cleanser Moisturizing Wash Eucerin Skin Calming Dry Skin Body Wash Free & Clear Liquid Cleanser for Sensitive Skin Vanicream Gentle Facial Cleanser VML Hypoallergenics Essence Skin-Saving Clear & Natural Soap Spring Cleaning Purifying Facial Wash for Oily Skin
Moisturizers	Aveeno Eczema Therapy Moisturizing Cream Baby Eczema Therapy Moisturizing Cream Cetaphil Oil Control Moisturizer SPF Eucerin Professional Repair for Extremely Dry Skin Lotion Vaniply Ointment for Sensitive Skin VML Hypoallergenics Red Better Daily Therapy Moisturizer
Lubricants	Fragrance- and preservative-free: Aquaphor Fragrance-, lanolin-, and preservative-free: white petrolatum or petroleum jelly

*Formaldehyde, fragrance (including botanicals), paraben mix/parabens, and propylene glycol.

†Retailers may sell old formulations of the brand. Manufacturers may change the formulation at any time and without warning or notice to consumers.

is often seen in health care workers. The use of a mild cleanser or a gel sanitizer made with at least 60% alcohol provides a less drying alternative. Alcohol gel sanitizers can prevent cracking and drying of the skin and should be used only on intact skin when hands are not visibly soiled.

TOPICAL THERAPIES

Moisturizers

Throughout this text, we will discuss skin conditions which involve, among other factors, a loss of the skin's barrier function. When the skin is dry, the epidermis cannot perform its protective function, allowing microbes and allergens easy access to stimulate inflammation and/or infection. To maintain hydration and proper barrier function, the skin should be cleansed daily with lukewarm water and dried with a patting motion (not rubbed vigorously) to preserve the oils in the skin. Within 3 minutes of a shower or bath, a moisturizer or emollient should be applied to the entire body. This helps to "seal" in the water and increase moisture in the stratum corneum.

Moisturizer is a term commonly used when referring to any topical that is applied to treat dry skin. Products that are actually *moisturizers* hydrate the skin by drawing water into the stratum corneum through the use of humectants such as urea, glycerin, lactic acid, or glycolic acid. *Emollients* soften the skin and can offer a protective barrier with a layer of oil or another occlusive agent. Products may have one or both properties, and selection of the topical is an individual preference based on texture, odor, and location of the application. Moisturizers are available as ointments, creams, and lotions. Ointments offer the most hydration and greatest barrier and are especially effective for thick, dry, and scaly areas.

Moisturizers are also used for cosmetic purposes and can be applied several times a day, particularly after hand washing. Many

contain sunscreen, fragrances, alcohol, preservatives, and other chemicals mentioned above that are known to cause contact dermatitis. Patients with allergies should be instructed to apply the best agent for their dry skin but to avoid known agents that can trigger contact dermatitis.

Wet Dressings

When skin integrity has been altered and the skin becomes weepy or wet, several wet dressing options are available over the counter. Aluminum acetate powder (Domebero) is a medication that can be mixed with water for its antiseptic and drying properties. Acetic acid solution can be prepared by adding a half cup of household white vinegar to a pint of water for its bactericidal quality. Patients should be instructed to soak clean facecloths in the liquid and wring them out before placing on the weeping rash. These hypertonic treatments are effective in drying blisters and are commonly used for severe sunburns, poison ivy rashes, or moist intertrigo, but must only be used until the wet aspect of the condition has resolved.

Application is recommended two to four times per day for no longer than 30 to 60 minutes. Cool temperature water is used to decrease inflammation, while lukewarm water may be used to stimulate circulation in an infectious process.

In the pediatric population, especially those children with atopic dermatitis, plain wet dressings are recommended to help with the itch. In these cases, an emollient or TCS ointment (if prescribed) is applied first, followed by plain-water-soaked gauze, and covered with dry dressings or cotton pajamas and left on overnight. Wet dressings should never be occluded with plastic wrap as this increases the risk for maceration and increases bacterial growth.

Bleach Baths

Bleach baths can also be used for patients who are at higher risk for superficial skin infections. Patients with atopic dermatitis or recurrent skin and soft tissue infections from methicillin-resistant staphylococcus aureus (MRSA) can benefit from sitting in a warm bleach bath once to twice weekly for 10 minutes to reduce the bacteria count on their skin, and reduce the itching experienced by these patients. The bath is made from one quarter of a cup of unscented household bleach in a full bathtub. This dilutes the bleach to avoid any harmful effects. The skin is then treated with an emollient immediately after exiting the bath.

Cosmetic Botanicals

Clinicians are often asked about skin care products, specifically those containing natural ingredients (Table 2-2). There is some evidence to suggest that botanical products may be useful, but the scientific data are lacking. For patients with sensitive skin, eczema, atopic dermatitis, inflammatory or pruritic conditions, products containing feverfew, colloidal oatmeal, or sunflower seed oil may provide some soothing relief. Patients with rosacea and pigmented lesions may benefit from products containing licorice root extract, which has skin lightening and anti-inflammatory properties.

Botanical extracts are being used with increased frequency in the cosmetic industry, and the future of antiaging products, in particular, appears to be promising. Today many cosmetic formulations are made of botanical extracts and may improve the health, texture, and integrity of the skin, hair, and nails. Botanicals are also being used in cleansers, moisturizers, and astringents. Therefore, it is important to have an understanding of the expected benefit of these products.

Table 2-2 includes a synopsis of the more popular botanical ingredients used in skin care products today, but does not represent

TABLE 2-2	Common Botanicals		
NAME	**ORIGIN**	**EFFECT**	**USE**
Aloe	Leaves of *Aloe vera*	Emollient, preventing infection	Eczema, wound care, ringworm, burns, insect bites
Arnica	Flowers of *Arnica montana*	Anti-inflammatory	Wound care, bruising, eczema, blisters (Avoid use on broken skin), acne, chapped lips
Calendula	Flowers of *Calendula officinalis* (pot marigold)	Antifungal, anti-inflammatory	Radiation induced burns, decubitus ulcers, bruising
Cayenne	Fruit of *Capsicum annuum*	Analgesic, warming stimulant	Neuropathic pain from shingles, massage oils, psoriasis
Chamomile	Dried flower heads and oil from *Matricaria chamomilla*	Antioxidant, antimicrobial, analgesic, anti-inflammatory	Wound care, burns
Chocolate	Seeds of *Theobroma cacao*	Antioxidant	Cocoa butter for chapped skin, burns, irritants
Dandelion	Leaves, flowers, or root of *Taraxacum officinale*	Anti-inflammatory, antioxidant, antibacterial, possible antitumor activity	Eczema, psoriasis, acne
Eucalyptus	Leaves, oil from *Eucalyptus globulus*	Antiseptic, astringent	Skin abscesses, minor wounds, bruises
Feverfew	Leaves, flowering tops of *Tanacetum parthenium*	Antioxidant, anti-inflammatory, anti-irritant, and anticancer properties. Orally, chewing leaves can cause ulceration and oral edema	Rosacea, antiaging, atopic dermatitis
Green Tea	Leaves, buds from *Camellia sinensis*	Anti-inflammatory, antioxidant	Healing wounds and photoprotection
Lavender	Flowers, essential oil from *Lavandula angustifolia*	Fragrance, antimicrobial, antianxiety	Fragrance, sleep inducer, sunburn, fungal infection, as rub form circulatory and rheumatic ailments
Lemongrass	Leaves, young stems, and oil of *Cymbopogon citratus*	Antiseptic, antibacterial, antifungal	Athlete's foot, ringworm
Licorice root extract*	Underground stem of *Glycyrrhiza glabra*	antioxidant, anti-inflammatory, antiviral and antimicrobial	Skin lightening, healing for herpes blisters, canker sores, sunburn, insect bites
Patchouli	Leaf, stem of *Pogostemon cablin*	Antibacterial, antifungal	Eczema, seborrhea, acne, eczema, mosquito repellent
Resveratrol	Skin and seeds of grapes, berries, peanuts, and other foods	antioxidant, anti-inflammatory, and antiproliferative agent	Antiaging, wrinkle reduction
Rosemary	Leaves, twigs from *Rosmarinus officinalis*	Anti-inflammatory, antioxidant, analgesic	Seborrhea, alopecia
Soy	Seeds from *Glycine max*	Antioxidant, anticarcinogenic, anti-inflammatory	Skin lightening, improve skin elasticity, moisturizer
Tea tree oil	Leaves from *Melaleuca alternifolia*	Antifungal, antimicrobial, anti-inflamamtory	Acne, onychomycosis, ringworm, dandruff eczema, insect bites
Witch hazel	Leaves, bark, twigs of *Hamamelis virginiana*	Astringent, antioxidant, anti-inflamamtory	Acne, contact dermatitis, bites, burns

*The oral form of licorice root extract can interact with angiotensin-converting enzyme inhibitors, aspirin, oral contraceptives, oral corticosteroids, diuretics, insulin, and stimulant laxatives.

Adapted from Foster, S., & Johnson, R. L. (2006). *Desk reference to nature's medicine*. Washington, DC: National Geographic Society.

all botanicals on the market and is not an endorsement. Patients with skin disorders should always use caution before using any new topical products, as they may include ingredients that can cause contact dermatitis. Providers can guide patients away from allergens included in these products that can initiate an irritant or an allergic response, no matter how "natural" the ingredients.

CORTICOSTEROIDS

Corticosteroids play a significant role in the treatment of dermatologic disorders. The fact that they can be used topically, intralesionally, and systemically provides the clinician numerous options for patient management. Corticosteroids are a synthetic derivative of the natural steroid, cortisol, which is produced by the adrenal cortex. There are two types of corticosteroids, glucocorticoids and mineralocorticoids. Glucocorticoids are the drugs most often used in dermatology and will be the focus of discussion in this chapter. In general, regardless of the method of administration, these drugs act as anti-inflammatory, immunosuppressive, and antiproliferative agents. When they are used topically, their vasoconstrictive properties determine their potency, and they are used to treat a wide range of disorders from acute allergic dermatitis to chronic immunobullous disorders. We will look more closely at these frequently used medications in the next two sections and will discuss their mode of administration, indications, and side effects and will make recommendations for use depending on the severity of the disorder.

Topical Corticosteroids

Many conditions seen in primary care and dermatology can be appropriately treated with a TCS. They penetrate the skin and work by decreasing the inflammatory pathways that cause the skin to become red and inflamed. Within days of use, however, the production of new skin cells is suppressed, creating the risk of atrophy and striae with long-term usage. The following factors can have an effect on treatment success and should be considered when prescribing any topical medication.

Percutaneous absorption

The ability of a topical medication to be effective is dependent on the transdermal delivery of the active ingredients from the stratum corneum of the epidermis to the underlying capillaries. There are many variables which can promote or impede PCA, including drug concentration, frequency of administration, occlusion, surface area involved, the vehicle, age and weight of patient, location on the body, and amount of time the topical is left on the skin. PCA is increased with hydrated (moist) skin, heat or elevated temperature, and the condition of skin barrier.

Vehicles

Topical agents are prepared in a variety of vehicles or bases that constitute the inactive portion of the medication, allowing the drug to be delivered into or through the skin (Table 2-3). Generic formulations of TCS may vary in the contents of the vehicle. Contact allergies may worsen if a generic product is substituted for a brand-name prescription. Vehicles can also alter the potency of the corticosteroid itself, which is why a drug may be class 1 in an ointment form but a different class in a cream or lotion vehicle. Additionally, consistency of the vehicle can be important.

Strength/frequency

A concentration of 1% indicates 1 g of drug will be contained in 100 g of the formulation. Efficacy of a topically applied drug is usually

TABLE 2-3		Vehicles for Topical Preparations
VEHICLE	**DEFINITION**	**PREFERENCES**
Solution	Homogenous mixture of two or more substances	Excellent for scalp/hair-bearing areas
Lotion	Liquid preparation, thicker than solution. Likely to contain oil, water, and/or alcohol	Lotions spread easily. Use in large areas
Cream	Thicker than lotion. Requires preservatives to extend shelf life Greater potential for allergic reactions	Use when skin is moist or exudative. Can be used in any area. Well tolerated
Ointment	Semisolid, mostly water-free. Petrolatum-based product. Spreads easily, penetrates better than creams	Choose when skin is dry or for increased penetration (thick skin). Messy in hairy areas
Gel	Aqueous, semisolid emulsion. Liquefies when in contact with skin	Great for hairy areas. Avoid on blistered skin, may sting
Foam	Liquid comprised of oil, solvents, and water packaged under pressure in aluminum cans	Great for scalp and thick plaques. Penetrates well without mess
Spray	Liquid dispensed through an aerosol container or atomizer	Helpful for hard to reach places. And scalp or hairy areas

not proportionate to the concentration. Doubling or halving the concentration often has a surprisingly modest effect on the response. Occlusion increases the penetration and ultimately the effectiveness of the product. Compounding of proprietary products with other ingredients may alter the stability of the drugs and should be done with caution if at all.

The common recommendation is to use the least potent TCS that is effective; however, using a TCS that is too weak may be ineffective and decrease compliance and patient confidence in the provider. Low-potency corticosteroid preparations can be used safely when needed on thinner skin. The common risks that apply to all TCS still exist when overused.

Ultrapotent or high-potency TCS should be used on a rotation schedule, with two or three daily applications for a 2-week period, followed by 1 or 2 weeks without TCS. Some clinicians advocate use of nonsteroidal agents or emollients during this break period. Paradoxically, stronger TCS (groups I and II) are commonly used in skin disorders such as lichen sclerosis and lichen planus that may involve mucosal skin without concern for atrophy.

Side effects

Common side effects with TCS or their vehicle's include contact dermatitis, acne-like eruptions, skin atrophy, hypopigmentation, telangiectasia, purpura, and striae, as well as ocular effects of increased intraocular pressure, cataract formation, and glaucoma. When using corticosteroids under occlusion, there is also a risk for folliculitis and maceration of the skin. In addition to patient education, providers can help reduce these risks by ordering only enough medication to achieve clearing. Refills may be given; however, follow-up appointments should be provided. Prescriptions given to poorly compliant patients should not be refilled indefinitely, and nonsteroidal alternatives may be a better option for some individuals.

Due to variability in generic formulations and the common addition of propylene glycol, a common allergen, allergic reactions from TCS can be a conundrum. If a corticosteroid allergy is suspected, desoximetasone ointment 0.05% is the treatment of choice until the allergen is confirmed. Referral to dermatology can identify specific allergens through patch testing with Thin-layer Rapid Use Epicutaneous Test (TRUE Test). This company has recently added tixocortol pivalate and budesonide, which can help identify TCS allergies. These products are widely used in dermatology and allergy practices. Testing for propylene glycol, however, requires a more comprehensive patch series such as the North American Series, which is usually provided only at larger academic or occupationally focused clinics. Any patient who is not improving on TCS should be reevaluated, and the provider should consider the following:

- Contact dermatitis due to the corticosteroid or preservative in the corticosteroid;
- Noncompliance;
- Tachyphylaxis (a decrease in the pharmacologic response after repeated administration of a topical agent); and
- Incorrect diagnosis: alternate diagnoses to consider include but are not limited to cutaneous T-cell lymphoma, drug reaction, or fungal infection.

Atrophy or thinning of the skin from the application of TCS can occur within a fairly short period of time with potentially permanent results. Atrophy can be manifested by fragile skin and stretch marks (Figure 2-1). Labeling on the tubes of TCS rather than on their outer boxes may help patients follow instructions on how much and where medications are to be applied, thereby reinforcing instructions given during the office visit.

Superficial staphylococcal folliculitis is a possible side effect of TCS, especially when using with occlusion. If noticed early, this can sometimes be reversed by drying out the skin with aluminum acetate compresses (i.e., Dombero); however, folliculitis often requires oral antibiotics to clear.

Adrenal suppression is a possible side effect of the stronger TCS, especially if used on a large surface area. This side effect is generally

TABLE 2-4	Estimated Amounts for Topical Medication		
LOCATION	PER APPLICATION, FTUs	AMOUNT FOR 2 WEEKS, ADULT (g)	
Entire face and neck	2.5	35	
One hand (both sides)	1	14	
One entire foot	2	28	
One arm (both sides)	3	42	
One leg	6	84	

Conversions: Adult: 30 g covers entire adult body in one application; children: ½ of the adult amount; infants (6–12 months): only ¼ of the adult amount; 1 FTU = 0.5 g per application.

FTU, fingertip unit.

reversible and frequently associated with long-term oral corticosteroid therapy.

Avascular necrosis (AVN) is another very rare side effect that can be caused by either topical or systemic corticosteroids. AVN has been documented with long-term use of TCS. Magnetic resonance imaging (MRI) of the hip may be ordered in the investigation of AVN symptoms, which include pain in the groin, hip, buttock, or knee that increases with activity and is relieved with rest.

Quantity

How much medication is needed to achieve the desired effect is always a question (Table 2-4). The fingertip unit (FTU) and rule of hand are two measurements used to determine how much product is needed and how much to prescribe. The FTU is the amount of topical medication that comes out of a tube with a 5 mm diameter and covers the area from the distal crease of the forefinger to the ventral aspect of an adult fingertip (Figure 2-2). For an adult, 2.5 FTU is needed to cover the entire neck and face. For a child (ages 1–5), one half of this amount would be needed to cover the same area. For an infant, quarter of the adult amount would be sufficient. One FTU

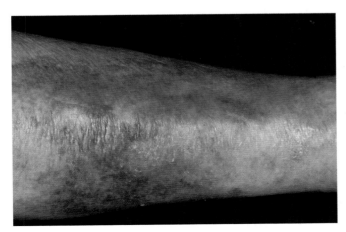

FIG. 2-1. Steroid atrophy.

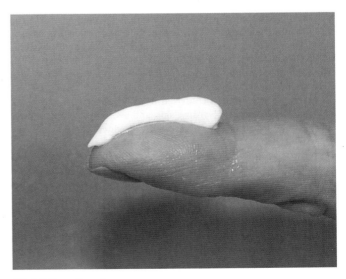

FIG. 2-2. Fingertip units.

weighs approximately 0.5 g. Therefore, an adult face and neck would require a 35-g tube of cream for a 2-week course of treatment.

The "rule of hand" describes the area to be treated. An area the size of four adult hands (including the digits) can be treated with 1 g of ointment or two FTU.

Occlusion

For increased penetration of very thick skin plaques or to treat a full body rash, occlusion may be used for a period of 2 hours twice daily. Medication is applied, and plastic wrap is used to cover the entire area where it is practical, such as an arm or leg. Alternatively, corticosteroid-impregnated tape such as Cordran Tape is available and useful for small, thickened areas. If the entire body surface is involved, a plastic suit, known as a sauna suit, can be worn for a few hours in the day after applying the corticosteroid to all areas. Occlusive plastic suits are inexpensive and can be found at most sporting goods stores.

Brand versus generic

Insurance companies often require that providers use generic in place of brand-name topical preparations. While generic products contain the same active ingredient, the product's vehicle often differs, altering the efficacy of the drug as well as contributing to the induction of contact dermatitis. The choice of a generic versus a brand-name drug is dependent on many patient-specific factors, but is often unfortunately determined by the insurance company's formulary.

Combination drugs

Commercially prepared TCS may be combined with drugs from a different class such as antifungal or antiyeast agents and are not generally recommended by dermatologist. They may provide some symptomatic relief, but may obscure the correct diagnosis. In addition, they can promote development of microbial resistance to antibiotics and may increase sensitization to ingredients. TCS have been successfully paired, however, with a vitamin D analog, calcipotriene (Dovonex, Vectical), in the treatment of psoriasis. Likewise, acne preparations are often combined, offer ease of use, and assist with the compliance of the younger patient.

Patient education and follow-up

The patient's ability and willingness to comprehend and comply with treatment recommendations can be influenced by a variety of factors, including the patient's relationship with their provider, the belief that the treatment will work, comprehension of directions provided, financial or time constraints, as well as the cosmetic elegance, or "feel" of the prescribed products. Patients are more likely to adhere to simple dosing schedules. It is helpful to provide them with clear verbal and written instructions.

Acne patients should be advised to avoid skin trauma by using minimal friction when cleansing skin and avoiding picking at their skin. When discussing topical retinoids, providers should refer to a "pea-sized" dab for the correct amount to apply to the face. Using the demonstration of a pea-sized emollient cream during an office visit may help patients better understand application instructions. For patients with psoriasis, demonstrating the application of emollients into thickened plaques can increase compliance and prescription efficacy. Recommending that all patients bring remaining tubes of products to their follow-up visits can help determine usage. Providers can consider creative options for patients to help them follow the agreed upon treatment plan. Smart phone features such as alarms and calendars can remind patients when to use their medications and return for follow-up appointments.

Systemic Corticosteroids

Many providers of dermatology services are extremely comfortable managing patients on TCS. It is instinctual to choose the proper dose, vehicle, and quantity for the patient. Those same practitioners, however, are far less comfortable when the patient requires additional and specifically systemic therapy. While there are numerous conditions which respond well to systemic corticosteroids and in fact may be essential, fear of side effects and rebound disease prevail. Oral administration usually takes preference over the intramuscular (IM) route although IM injection guarantees the proper dose and can be helpful if gastrointestinal side effects exist.

Systemic corticosteroids are classified as short, intermediate, and long acting. Prednisone, which is the corticosteroid of choice in dermatology, is an intermediate acting medication. Prednisone is actually the inactive form of the drug and must be converted to the active form, prednisolone, by the liver. It is generally given as a single daily, oral dose because it most closely approximates the body's natural diurnal variation. Divided doses are generally reserved for acute, life-threatening conditions and in general have an increased effect despite the same total daily dosage. In liver impaired patients, prednisolone is the drug of choice. The length of a treatment course depends entirely on the condition. In acute dermatoses such as contact dermatitis, a short 2- to 3-week tapering course or "burst" is suggested. In severe conditions which will require more than 4 weeks of treatment, an alternate day dosing schedule can be used. Once the skin condition has cleared, the dose will be carefully decreased in increments until the patient maintains improvement on a minimal dose.

Prednisone dosing

There are little data in the literature comparing or recommending the duration of therapy for corticosteroid use, and many practitioners are confused by the correct way to prescribe and taper the corticosteroids when needed. For example, when treating allergic contact dermatitis with oral corticosteroids, many experienced clinicians will treat with 40 to 60 mg per day for 2 weeks and will discontinue without taper. The risk involved with short-course therapy is rebound of the condition and not adrenal suppression. Some clinicians experienced in treating a widespread contact dermatitis for an adult prescribe prednisone 20 to 60 mg daily (depending on the extensiveness of rash and patient's weight) for 7 days followed by a tapering dose for an additional 7 to 14 days.

If the rash affects more than 20% of the body surface area, oral prednisone at a dose of 0.5 to 1 mg/kg/day for 7 days is given, then the dose may be reduced by 50% in the next 5 to 7 days and then tapered and discontinued over the following 2 weeks (Basow, 2013). See Box 2-1 for considerations in systemic corticosteroid selection and Table 2-5 for corticosteroid tapering suggestions.

BOX 2-1	Considerations for Systemic Corticosteroid Selection

Age and weight of patient
Comorbidities: diabetes mellitus, hypertension, peptic ulcer disease, osteoporosis
Systemic infections: fungal
Short term (2–3 weeks) versus long term (months)
Need for vitamin D and calcium supplementation
Biphosphonates if on oral corticosteroids for more than 4 weeks
Known hypersensitivities
Drug interactions
Frequency of dosing: b.i.d. dosing has a more potent effect than QD dosing but should only be used for acute therapy of life-threatening illness.

TABLE 2-5	Prednisone Taper Suggestions (Alternative to Medrol Pack)	
DURATION OF TAPER	**DOSE AND AMOUNT**	**PATIENT INSTRUCTIONS***
2 wk in decreasing daily doses	5-mg tabs, dispense #114	Day 1: Take 14 pills (70 mg), then decrease by 1 pill each day for 14 days
3 wk	10-mg tabs, dispense #70	Week 1: 6 tabs QAM Week 2: 3 tabs QAM Week 3: 1 tab QAM
4 wk (simplified)	10-mg tabs, dispense #70	Week 1: 4 tabs QAM Week 2: 3 tabs QAM Week 3: 2 tabs QAM Week 4: 1 tab QAM

Note: Calculations based on dosing 0.5–1 mg/kg for 150-lb (68 kg) adult.

*In addition to dosing, patient instructions should include: "To avoid recurrence of symptoms, do not stop taking pills without being instructed by your provider."

Side effects

Side effects associated with oral corticosteroid therapy are usually dose and duration dependent. Some preexisting conditions are associated with increased risk, including diabetes, hypertension, dyslipidemia, heart failure, cataracts or glaucoma, peptic ulcer disease, concurrent use of nonsteroidal anti-inflammatory drugs, presence of infection, low bone density, and osteoporosis.

Consider the patient's *risk of fracture* when prescribing oral prednisone. Bone loss is a serious, potential side effect of glucocorticoid therapy and needs to be monitored closely. To minimize bone loss, the following general principles should be kept in mind:

- The glucocorticoid dose and duration of therapy should be as low as possible.
- Topical therapy is preferred over systemic and should be used whenever possible.
- Weight-bearing exercises are recommended to prevent bone loss.
- Patients should avoid excess alcohol and smoking.

The American College of Rheumatology Task Force Osteoporosis Guidelines offer suggestions for patients taking any dose of glucocorticoids for greater than 3 months:

- Patients should maintain a total calcium intake of 1,200 mg per day and vitamin D intake of 800 IU per day through either diet and/or supplements.
- Bisphosphonates may be added based on the individual risks, which include gender, age, and fracture risk especially if the course of corticosteroids is intended for several months.
- Bone mineral density (BMD) testing is recommended at the initiation of glucocorticoid therapy and after 1 year for patients receiving any dose of glucocorticoids for greater than 3 months.

Avascular necrosis is a rare side effect that can be caused by either topical or systemic corticosteroids. As mentioned in the TCS section, a MRI scan may be ordered in the investigation of AVN symptoms. Patients should be advised that should signs and symptoms of AVN develop they should call their medical provider immediately.

Patient education and follow-up

When prescribing systemic corticosteroids, clinicians should educate patients for maximum outcomes and minimal side effects:

- Take prednisone with food.
- b.i.d. dosing will have a more potent effect than once per day dosing, but is not recommended for short-term treatment.
- Taking prednisone early in the morning helps diminish the possible side effects of hyperactivity or sleep disruption and decreases risk of adrenal suppression.
- Patients should be advised against stopping prednisone dosing abruptly and to continue medication until the entire taper course is complete to prevent rebound dermatitis.

All patients on long-term oral corticosteroids should be monitored for elevated blood sugar, hypertension, and weight gain after 1 month and then every 2 to 3 months. Complaints of eye pain, blurry vision, or halos may be indicative of increased intraocular pressures, and patient suffering from these complaints should be seen by an ophthalmologist. The provider should be most cautious in prescribing prednisone to patients who have the comorbidities of hypertension, diabetes, and obesity or to those who abuse alcohol or tobacco as these patients are already at high risk for developing infections, ulcers, and glaucoma. As long-term prednisone use is also associated with possible gastrointestinal perforation, an upper gastrointestinal series may be ordered if the patient has a history of peptic ulcer disease.

Patients who are on long-term prednisone therapy should be seen at least every 1 to 2 months for evaluation and more frequently if symptoms of possible complications arise. Close monitoring for possible side effects may be done in collaboration with the patient's dermatologist.

Special Considerations

Corticosteroids in pregnancy

Practitioners will inevitably encounter pregnant women in their practice and must be familiar with medication safety when providing care to this group of patients. Prescribing medication during pregnancy can be particularly challenging given the insufficient data and research on the safety of medications during this period. Some skin conditions of the pregnant woman require topical and systemic treatment. The Food and Drug Administration (FDA) pregnancy categories (Table 2-6) should always be considered.

Topical corticosteroids. During pregnancy, women are generally advised to avoid the TCS treatments that they have come to rely on during flares. In general, topical medications are often considered first-line therapy for most; however, there are times when systemic agents may be more appropriate.

The data on the effects of TCS used during pregnancy are limited; however, the current available data on the safety of mild-to-moderate TCS during pregnancy suggest a lack of association between their use by the mother and oral clefts, preterm delivery and fetal death as previously postulated. Therefore, the following recommendations for TCS use in the pregnant patient are as follows:

- Mild- to moderate-potency TCS should be preferred to more potent corticosteroids during pregnancy.
- Potent to very potent TCS should be used as second-line therapy for as short a time as possible.
- There is a small risk for fetal growth restriction when using potent/very potent TCS during pregnancy.
- There is a theoretically higher risk of adverse events with use of TCS when used in high-absorption areas such as eyelids, genitals, and flexures.

Systemic corticosteroids. There are limited data on the potential teratogenic effects on the fetus, mainly because of the ethical issues

TABLE 2-6	FDA Pregnancy Categories
CATEGORY	DEFINITION
A	Adequate and well-controlled studies have failed to demonstrate a risk to the fetus in the first trimester of pregnancy, and there is no evidence of risk in later trimesters.
B	Animal reproduction studies have failed to demonstrate a risk to the fetus, and there are no adequate and well-controlled studies in pregnant women.
C	Animal reproduction studies have shown an adverse effect on the fetus, and there are no adequate and well-controlled studies in humans, but potential benefits may warrant use of the drug in pregnant women despite potential risks.
D	There is positive evidence of human fetal risk based on adverse reaction data from investigational or marketing experience or studies in humans, but potential benefits may warrant use of the drug in pregnant women despite potential risks.
X	Studies in animals or humans have demonstrated fetal abnormalities, and/or there is positive evidence of human fetal risk based on adverse reaction data from investigational or marketing experience, and the risks involved in use of the drug in pregnant women clearly outweigh potential benefits.

involved in testing corticosteroids drugs in pregnancy. As mentioned previously, TCS are often considered the first line of therapy; however, when topical agents aren't enough, the provider and patient must weigh the risk versus benefit of oral agents.

With oral glucocorticosteroids, there is a potential for increased risk of premature rupture of the membranes (PROM) and intrauterine growth restriction. There may also be an increased risk of pregnancy-induced hypertension, gestational diabetes, osteoporosis, and infection. They should be avoided during the first trimester when the hard palate is forming. When necessary, the lowest effective dose should be used.

Glucocorticosteroids are excreted in breast milk, but their use during lactation is deemed compatible by the American Academy of Pediatrics (AAP) if justified by the potential benefit to the health of the mother. An alternative is to discard the breast milk for the first 4 hours following ingestion of a dose of prednisone >20 mg.

CLINICAL PEARLS

- Avoid prescribing Lotrisone for diaper dermatitis. The high potency TCS in this product is not FDA approved for children and is too strong for the diaper area. In addition, the antifungal is too weak to be effective.
- When prescribing a potent or ultrapotent corticosteroid, patients should not use more than one 45-g tube per week. Pharmacists will not usually refill ahead of time, so calculate correctly for best results.
- The popular and conveniently packaged Medrol dose pack (methylprednisolone) is an insufficient short-term remedy that tends to prolong patients' suffering due to rebound flaring.
- Mild- to moderate-strength TCS appear to be safe during pregnancy for short-term use. Avoid high-potency TCS if possible, especially during the first trimester. If high-potency corticosteroids are needed, as always, they should be used for the shortest amount of time.

ULTRAVIOLET LIGHT
Photobiology

In discussing the impact of the environment on skin health, UVR must be at the forefront to address the favorable benefits and negative impact of exposure. The basic concepts of photobiology are fundamental when assessing risks and benefits, and educating your patients (also see Chapter 23 Aging Skin). UV light is a form of radiation not visible to the human eye and is composed of three wavelengths: UVA, UVB, and UVC. These wavelengths differ primarily in the depth to which they penetrate the skin. The effects of UVB radiation can be immediate such as in sunburn or allergic skin reaction. UVA and UVB cause more long-term effects as in photoaging and skin cancer. UVC wavelengths are filtered by the ozone, do not reach the earth's surface and do not contribute to skin damage.

It is understood that the ozone layer around the earth is trapping less UVR than ever before and allowing more harmful light to penetrate the earth. This is especially important to think about when in high altitudes, as less ozone means less filtering of UV light, making one more susceptible to sun damage. According to statistics from the Denver Visitors Bureau, at 6,280 ft or approximately 1 mile above sea level, there is 25% less protection from UVR. Thin ozone linked with increased outdoor leisure activities puts the population at higher risk. Unfortunately, tanning is still considered fashionable and desired by many despite the fact that it is a primary cause of melanoma and nonmelanoma skin cancers.

UVR is measured in wavelengths. UVA accounts for 95% of the sun's UVR that reaches the earth and has two spectrums: UVA1 (340-400nm) and UVA2 (320-340nm). UVA1 has a longer wavelength and penetrates deeper in the dermis, resulting in greater biologic effect and DNA damage than UVA2. Interestingly, while UVA1 increases the risk for skin cancer and photoaging, it can also be utilized for therapeutic treatment of atopic dermatitis and other skin diseases. UVA rays also penetrate glass and clouds, increasing the risk for individuals who drive frequently for work or recreation and for those who do not use sunscreen as directed.

UVB rays are the middle-range wavelengths between 290 and 320 nm. They are found in combination with UVA in some tanning beds that contribute to the risk of this practice. Not only is UVB responsible for photoaging, sun tanning, and sunburns, it also causes ocular diseases such as cataracts, glaucoma, and macular degeneration. Paradoxically, specialized narrowband UVB is used in many dermatology settings to treat skin conditions such as psoriasis and can increase the risk of nonmelanoma skin cancers. Sun-protective measures are provided for eyes and noninvolved skin and are encouraged during all phototherapy treatments in dermatology offices.

UV Index

The UV Index (Figure 2-3) is a means of predicting the expected risk of overexposure to UVR from the sun. The National Weather Service calculates the UV Index forecast for most ZIP codes across the United States, and the Environmental Protection Agency (EPA) publishes this information. The UV Index is then accompanied by recommendations for sun protection and is a useful tool for planning sun-safe outdoor activities.

Ozone depletion, as well as seasonal and weather variations, causes different amounts of UVR to reach the earth at any given time. Taking these factors into account, the UV Index predicts the level of solar UVR and indicates the risk of overexposure on a scale from 0 (low) to 11 or more (extremely high). A special "UV alert" may be issued for a particular area, if the UV Index is forecast to be higher than normal.

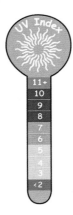

FIG. 2-3. The ultraviolet index forecasts the strength of the sun's harmful rays. The higher the number, the greater the chance of sun damage.

Sun Protection

Public education regarding skin cancers and the photodamaging effects of the sun has led to increased use of sunscreens in many populations. Australia is one country that has made great strides in educating the public about sun-protective measures. In 1980, it launched one of the most successful health campaigns in its history. The Slip Slop Slap Seek and Slide campaign is credited as playing a key role in the dramatic shift in sun protection attitudes and behaviors over the past two decades. Basal cell and squamous cell carcinomas have also decreased in Australia as well. Unfortunately, melanoma incidences continued to increase despite the attitude and behavioral change which may stress the importance of the multifactorial dimensions of UV sun exposure.

Sun avoidance during the hours of 10 a.m. and 4 p.m. is recommended. UVR is magnified by 85% when it is reflected off snow. Cloud cover only minimally decreases the intensity of the sun. Loose-fitting clothes and tightly woven fabrics in long pants and long shirts offer the best source of sun protection. Although we have made advances in educating patients regarding the use of sunscreen in the United States, more efforts are needed to encourage patients to use sun-protective clothing and sunglasses and to seek shade more often. Providing the public with outdoor tents in gathering places such as parks and beaches is one example of such an effort.

Sunscreen

Sunscreens are topical agents that lessen the effects of UV light by reflecting, scattering, or absorbing the light (Figure 2-4). Their efficacy is determined by their ability to protect against the erythema caused by both UVA and UVB. Sun-protective factor (SPF) is the unit of measure used to describe how well a sunscreen can protect the skin from the harmful effects of the sun. The SPF for each sunscreen is determined in a laboratory by comparing an individual's response to sun with and without sunscreen use. Dermatologists recommend patients choose sunscreen with an SPF of 30 or higher. The average adult should apply at least 2 tablespoons or a "shot glass full" on sun exposed areas of the body whenever outdoors for any length of time. Sunscreen should be reapplied every 2 hours or after sweating or swimming regardless of latitude.

On June 14, 2011, the U.S. FDA announced new requirements for sunscreens currently sold. Previously, there was no standard applied for SPF designation. Currently, the FDA requires the use of the term *broad spectrum* to be included on any sunscreen packaging which claims to prevent sun damage. This means that the product provides both UVA and UVB protection for the skin. Only broad-spectrum

Chemical sunscreens

Chemical sunscreens act to weaken ultraviolet radiation before it causes damage to DNA in the nuclei of skin cells. Chemical sunscreens absorb ultraviolet radiation within the

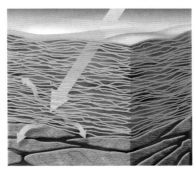

spaces between the skin cells, convert it into specific chemicals, and release the energy as insignificant amounts of heat. The higher the SPF rating of the chemical sunscreen, the longer it takes for sunlight to damage the skin.

Physical sunscreens

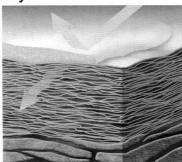

Physical sunscreens prevent ultraviolet radiation from entering the skin at all. Physical sunscreens form a thin film of inert metal particles (zinc oxide, etc.) that reflect back into the atmosphere.

FIG. 2-4. Illustration showing how sunscreens work.

sunscreens with an SPF value of 15 or higher can claim to reduce the risk of skin cancer and early skin aging if used as directed with other sun protection measures. Non-broad-spectrum sunscreens and broad-spectrum sunscreens with an SPF between 2 and 14 can only claim to help prevent sunburn.

Manufacturers cannot label sunscreens as *"waterproof"* or *"sweatproof,"* because these claims overstate their effectiveness. Water resistance claims on the front label must indicate whether the sunscreen remains effective for 40 minutes or 80 minutes while swimming or sweating, based on standard testing.

Sunscreens also cannot identify their products as *"sunblock"* (Figure 2-4) or claim to provide sun protection for more than 2 hours without reapplication. The product's label must not claim to provide protection immediately after application.

All sunscreens must include standard *"Drug Facts"* information on the back and/or side of the container. The FDA also mandates that sunscreen labels recommend reapplying sunscreen at least every 2 hours. (Cong. Rec., 2011)

Broad-spectrum sunscreens include at least one of the following ingredients: zinc oxide, titanium dioxide, avobenzone, or ecamsule to provide adequate UVA protection (Table 2-7). Helioplex is the name brand of a sunscreen stabilizer owned by Neutrogena. A stabilizer ensures the sunscreen ingredients are more photostable, preventing chemical breakdown when exposed to the sun. Only Loreal has the rights to the chemical ecamsule that is sold as Mexoryl sunscreen. Europe has several other sunscreen ingredients available that are not FDA approved.

TABLE 2-7	Sunscreen Ingredients		
INGREDIENT	**PROTECTION**		
	UVA1	UVA2	UVB
Physical agents			
Titanium dioxide	•		•
Zinc oxide	•		•
Chemical absorbers			
Aminobenzoic acid (PABA)			•
Butyl methoxydibenzoylmethane (Avobenzone)	•		
Dioxybenzone		•	•
Ecamsule (Mexoryl SX)		•	
Ethoxyethyl p-methoxycinnamate (cinoxate)			•
Homomenthyl salicylate (homosalate)	•		
Octyl methoxycinnamate (octinoxate)	•		
Oxybenzone	•	•	•
Octocrylene	•	•	•
Sulisonbenzone	•	•	•
Ethoxyethyl p-methoxycinnamate (cinoxate)			•

UVA, ultraviolet A; UVB, ultraviolet B.

Allergies to sunscreens

Practitioners often hear from patients that they are allergic to sunscreens. The most common reactions reported with the use of sunscreens are allergic contact dermatitis, photoallergic contact dermatitis, irritant contact dermatitis, and acne. There are two categories of sunscreens, "inorganic" or "physical" sunscreens, which include zinc oxide- and titanium dioxide-based products, and "organic" or "chemical" sunscreens, which include 15 different chemicals, including para-aminobenzoic acid (PABA) and benzophenones. PABA is no longer used in the manufacturing of most sunscreens today due to the incidence of allergic reactions. Oxybenzone, a type of benzophenone, is frequently used in sunscreens today and is now also known to cause contact dermatitis. Photoallergy has not been reported with the inorganic sunscreens; therefore, allergy-prone patients should be advised to choose these products. Examples of sunscreen brands that contain zinc and titanium dioxide as either the sole ingredient or main ingredient are Badger, Vanicream, Solbar zinc, Neutrogena Sensitive Skin, and Blue Lizard.

Sunscreen controversies

Oxybenzone, Retinyl Palmitate. Sunscreens have been approved by the FDA since 1978 and now cannot be sold without extensive testing. There has been controversy over several sunscreen ingredients, including both oxybenzone and retinyl palmitate. It has been claimed by some groups that oxybenzone accumulates in the body and can interfere with hormone levels. Other studies have demonstrated that no appreciable risk exists. Retinyl palmitate has been accused of causing free radicals, therefore increasing cancer risk. There are no published studies proving that sunscreen or their ingredients are toxic to humans or hazardous to human health.

Vitamin D. With improved sunscreens, there is now increased media attention and concern in the rise of vitamin D deficiencies resulting from sunscreen use. Much of this controversy is fueled by the very powerful tanning industry, who extols the benefits of tanning booths as a source of vitamin D. In fact, most individuals do not apply their sunscreen adequately or frequently enough to prevent sunburn or block the synthesis of vitamin D.

Given the risk of DNA damage to the skin and photocarcinogenesis from overexposure to UV light, it is advised that people focus on acquiring their daily recommendation of vitamin D from food or supplements. Vitamin D_3 (cholecalciferol/colecalciferol) is made by the body when UVB radiation interacts with 7-dehydrocholesterol that is present in skin. The amount of sun exposure required for this interaction is minimal, and can be satisfied by less than 15 minutes of exposing the face, hands, and neck during nonpeak hours daily. Vitamin D_3 is also found in some food products such as meat, oily fish, and fortified processed foods. It is also found as a dietary supplement. Vitamin D_3 is converted into its active form, calcitriol, by the kidneys and liver and helps form and maintain bone. Patients who are concerned about their vitamin D levels should discuss their options with their primary care provider.

Oral photoprotection

Polypodium leucotomos is the most studied form of oral photoprotection. Polypodium leucotomos is an extract from a fern grown in Central America. It has been shown to decrease erythema, DNA damage, UV-induced epidermal hyperproliferation, and mast cell infiltration in humans. However, one study suggested that Polypodium leucotomos only offered an SPF of 3, which is insufficient for most people. There may be a role for this oral product for patients with photosensitivity from lupus or other photoinduced conditions as a supplement to sunscreens. It should not to be used as a replacement for sun-protective clothing and sunscreen. This dietary supplement is sold as brand names Heliocare and FernCarePLE.

Clothing

Loose-fitting clothes and tightly woven fabrics in long pants and long sleeved shirts offer the best source of sun protection. A typical cotton T-shirt offers an SPF of about 5, and a wet T-shirt offers much less protection than a dry one. Darker colors may add a bit more protection than lighter ones. Hats with wide brims are highly recommended. Fashionable sun-protective clothing with the minimum standard ultraviolet protection factor (UPF) of 40 to 50+ is available by several companies such as Coolibar, Radicool Australia, Sunday Afternoons, Sun Precautions, Tilley Endurables, Tuga sun protective sunwear, and Wallaroo hat company.

Sunglasses

UV damage to the eyes is cumulative just as it is for the skin, so it is important to begin wearing sunglasses at an early age. Children's eyes are still developing and at higher risk for damage. Choose sunglasses that provide full protection against UV light. The coating used for UV protection is clear; so a tinted sunglass will not necessarily be more protective. Patients should look for a label or a sticker as follows:

- Lenses block 99% or 100% of UVB and UVA rays;
- Lenses meet ANSI Z80.3 blocking requirements. (This refers to standards set by The American National Standards Institute); and/or
- UV 400 protection (blocks light rays with wavelengths up to 400 nm, which means that your eyes are shielded from even the tiniest UV rays).

Sunless Tanning

There are no FDA regulations regarding sunless tanners and bronzers. These terms typically refer to products that provide a tanned appearance without exposure to the sun or other sources of UVR. The most common ingredient in sunless tanners is dihydroxyacetone (DHA), a color additive that darkens the skin by reacting with amino acids in the skin's surface. Bronzers are made from color additives approved by the FDA for cosmetic use. They stain the skin for a short time when applied and can be washed off with soap and water. DHA is being used commonly in salons and advertised as Spray Tan, but "misting" application has not been approved for use by the FDA. DHA is restricted to external application and should not be applied to the lips or any surface covered by mucous membranes. When using DHA containing products, it may be difficult to avoid exposure to the eyes, lips, or mucous membranes. Those who choose to use spray-tanning booths should then be sure to protect their eyes, lips, and mucous membranes from the spray.

CLINICAL PEARL

- Previously unseen seborrheic keratoses will become more visible as the keratotic cells absorb the sunless tanning chemical.

Tanning pills

Tanning pills contain canthaxanthin, a color additive similar to β-carotene, the substance that gives carrots their orange-like color. The FDA has approved some additives for coloring but they are not approved for use in tanning agents. Canthaxanthin, at high levels, can appear in the eyes as yellow crystals, which may cause injury and impair vision. There have also been reports of liver and skin problems.

Patient Education and Follow-up

It is important to teach patients that UVA and UVB light cause photoaging and is a known risk factor for melanoma, nonmelanoma skin cancers, and eye damage. UVR, from the sun and from tanning beds, is classified as a human carcinogen, according to the U.S. Department of Health and Human Services and the World Health Organization. Daily sunscreen application and UV-protective clothing and sunglass usage should be recommended to all patients. General UV protection advice should include the following (see Sun Safety tips for patients in Chapter 8):

- Emphasize choosing SPF 30 or greater.
- If acne prone, advise oil-free and noncomedogenic products. Most brand-name products marketed for the face are safe.
- Apply at least 20 minutes before exposure and reapply every 2 hours, or after swimming or excessive sweating.
- Sunscreens are not recommended for babies under 6 months of age as they have a larger body surface area and may absorb more active chemicals that are in sunscreens than is safe. Instead, emphasize sun avoidance and sun-protective clothing.
- Sunscreen spray should not be inhaled as the safety of the effects on mucous membranes and the lungs have not been determined. When sprayed, sunscreen may not afford adequate protection as much of the product escapes into the air.
- The expiration of sunscreens is 3 years after the purchase date. Discard before the expiration date if it has been exposed to extreme heat.
- Avoid tanning and tanning booths.
- Use extra caution near water, snow, and sand.
- Get vitamin D safely.

READINGS

Basow, D. S. (Ed.). (2013). *Management of Contact Dermatitis.* www.UpToDate

Berth-Jones, J. (Ed.). (2010). Topical therapy. *Rook's textbook of dermatology* (8th ed., pp. 73.1–73.52). Chichester, England: Wiley-Blackwell.

Chi, C., Wang, S., Mayon-White, R., & Wojnarowska, F. (2013, September 4). Pregnancy outcomes after maternal expsosure to topical corticosteroids; A UK population-based cohort study. *Journal of the American Medical Association,* E1–E7.

Craig, K., & Meadows, S. E. What is the best duration of steroid therapy for contact dermatitis (rhus)? *The Journal of Family Practice, 55,* 166–167.

Cong. Rec. (2011). FDA Sunscreen drug products for over the counter use.

DelRosso, J. Q., & Kircik, L. H. (2012, December). Not all topical corticosteroids are created equal! Optimizing therapeutic outcomes through better understanding of vehicle formulations, compound selection, and methods of application. *Journal of Drugs in Dermatology, 11,* 5–8.

FDA: FDA Sheds Light on Sunscreens. www.fda.gov/forconsumers/consumerupdates/ucm258416.htm

Ference, J. D., & Last, A. R. (2009, January 15). Choosing topical steroids. *American Family Physician, 79,* 135–140.

Gilchrest, B. (2008). Sun exposure and vitamin D sufficiency. *American Journal of Clinical Nutrition, 88*(suppl), 570S–577S.

Grossman, J. M., Gordon, R., Ranganath, V. K., Deal, C., Caplan, L., Chen, W., & Saag, K. G. (2010). Recommendations for the prevention and treatment of glucosteoid induced osteoporosis [Arthritis Care Res]. *American College of Rheumatology, 62,* 1515–1526.

Gupta, R., High, W. A., Butler, D., & Murase, J. E. (2013). Medicolegal aspects of prescribing dermatological medications in pregnancy. *Seminars in Cutaneous Medical Surgery, 32*(4), 209–216.

Habif, T. P. (2010). Topical therapy and topical corticosteroids. *In clinical dermatology. A color guide to diagnosis and therapy* (5th ed., pp. 75–90). China: Elsevier.

Kelly IV, J. D., & Wald, D. (2012). Femoral head avascular necrosis. *Medscape.* http://emedicine.medscape.com/article/86568-overview

Lebwohl, M., Heymann, W., Berth-Jones, J., & Coulson, I. (2006). *Treatment of skin desease. Comprehensie therapeutic strategies* (2nd ed.). London: Mosby.

Middelkamp-Hup, M. A., Pathak, M. A., Parrado, C., Goukassian, D., & Riuz-Diaz, F. (2004, December). Oral Polypodium leucotomas extract decreases ultraviolet induced damage of the human skin. *Journal of the American Academy of Dermatology, 51,* 910–918.

Romain, P. L. (Ed.). (2013). Use of anti-inflammatory and immunosuppressive drugs in rheumatic diseases during pregnancy and lactation. *UpToDate.* March 4, 2014.

Skin Cancer Foundation, Skin Cancer Prevention. www.skincancer.org/prevention/sun-protection/prevention-guidelines

Zirwas, M. (2012, December). Allergy to topical steroids. *Journal of Drugs in Dermatology, 11,* 9.

CHAPTER 3

Eczematous Disorders

Susan Tofte

Eczematous inflammation, commonly referred to as "eczema," is the most common of all inflammatory skin diseases. The term *eczema* actually comes from the Greek word "eczeo," which literally means to effervesce or boil over, and presents as a papulovesicular, weeping dermatitis. *Eczema* is a generic or general term used to describe a variety of eczemas, including nummular eczema, contact or irritant dermatitis, xerotic (asteatotic) eczema, dyshidrotic (pompholyx), dermatophytids (Ids), or seborrheic dermatitis. Atopic dermatitis (AD), although often incorrectly referred to as eczema, is a combination of eczema, asthma, and allergic rhinitis, known as the atopic triad.

In the most acute phase, eczema will appear intensely erythematous, often with vesicles which rupture, ooze, and become weepy. When secondary changes occur and eczema becomes less acute, erythema continues, but with increased scaling, excoriations, and sometimes fissures. Vesicles are usually dried at this stage. As eczema evolves into a chronic stage, the skin becomes lichenified with accentuated skin lines, the result of rubbing and scratching. Pruritus and evidence of scratching can be present at any stage, but is most intense during the acute stage when inflammation is more extreme. The skin barrier becomes more compromised with fissures and excoriations because of scratching, making it more susceptible to infection.

Histologic changes are similar in every stage of eczema, but vary depending on the degree of inflammation. Edema is most evident during the acute phase of eczema, revealing a high degree of spongiosis as well as larger numbers of lymphocytes. As eczema becomes chronic, histologic changes show more evidence of a thicker (lichenified) stratum corneum.

ATOPIC DERMATITIS

Many studies have been performed looking at the prevalence of AD in infants and children by using clinical evaluations, survey studies, and use of questionnaires coupled with clinical evaluation. These studies have been performed in Northern Europe, United States, and Japan, and prevalence of AD based on these studies is documented to be between 15% and 20% and is higher in children. Greater than 60% of AD cases develop during the first year of life; thus it is often referred to as a childhood disease. Although rare, it can present in adulthood. Research has shown that there is a strong concordance with monozygotic twins.

Quality of Life and Cost of Care

AD impacts not only the patient with the disease but impacts other family members, particularly parents who may find absences from work in order to stay home to care for their child affecting income and health benefits. Healthy siblings compete for attention and interface with parents, who find themselves consumed with the overwhelming task of caring for the child with AD. Research has suggested that caring for a child with type I diabetes mellitus is comparable to caring for a child with moderate-to-severe AD. Atopic dermatitis has more impact on the quality of life in childhood than any other childhood dermatoses with the exception of scabies. General pain and pruritus in any disease have a negative impact on the quality of life, but in AD when the pruritus is often intense and relentless, the negative burden is even greater, leading to disruptions in sleep, disruptions with play and recreational activities, as well as interference with normal social interactions and development. The economic impact of caring for a family member with AD has been compared to the cost of other chronic diseases such as emphysema or epilepsy. Within the past decade, the cost of care for AD was estimated to be over $ 300 million, with visits to the emergency room for acute extensive flares largely responsible for this cost.

Pathophysiology

AD is an inflammatory and xerotic skin disease. It is presumed that AD arises from genetic influence interfaced with environmental factors. There is a strong genetic association with epidermal barrier defects which encompass not only eczematous skin inflammation, but also allergic rhinitis (hay fever) and asthmatic influences. This trio, a combination of AD, asthma, and allergic rhinitis, is referred to as the "atopic triad." An overproduction of IgE and cytokines such as IL-4, IL-10, and IL-13 contribute to the inflammatory cascade of erythema, pruritus, and edema. Early age of onset, accompanied by respiratory allergy, and urban living may be predictors of more severe disease evolution. Very often children will outgrow the disease by the time they reach school age, but many continue to have the disease into adulthood where it may be localized to one area or region, such as the hands. This should be basic and fundamental, yet errors in bathing and moisturizing are the most common cause for persistent AD.

Epidermal Barrier Loss of Function

The ability for the skin barrier to absorb and hold water is essential in AD as well as in other xerotic skin diseases such as ichthyosis vulgaris. In the past 8 years, breakthrough research has uncovered filaggrin as a key protein in the normal skin barrier. Mutations of this essential protein for an intact skin barrier were found in the epidermis of patients with ichthyosis vulgaris as well as in patients with AD. These mutations represent a strong genetic predisposition for atopic eczema, asthma, and allergies.

Loss of filaggrin means a poorly formed stratum corneum and xerotic barrier that is prone to water loss and unable to protect the body. Xerosis leads to pruritus, which then promotes scratching and excoriations. As the skin barrier is further disrupted by prolonged itching and scratching, it becomes vulnerable to a host of potential infections and penetration of allergens that trigger IgE production.

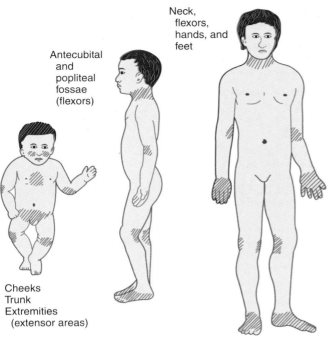

Antecubital and popliteal fossae (flexors)

Neck, flexors, hands, and feet

Cheeks
Trunk
Extremities (extensor areas)

FIG. 3-1. Distribution of atopic dermatitis at various ages. Children have involvement of their face and neck. The extensor aspects of extremities are affected in infants, whereas the flexural aspects are more affected in older children and adults. Atopic dermatitis usually spares the axillae and groin.

Clinical Presentation

The hallmark of AD is pruritus, which is often intense and relentless, disrupting every aspect of the patient's life. The course of AD tends to be chronic and relapsing. As an inflammatory skin disease, AD will present with varying degrees of erythema, inflammatory papules, which often coalesce to form eczematous plaques, as well as areas of weepy dermatitis. Often areas of involvement will evolve into scaly, xerotic plaques, and as the disease becomes chronic, lichenified changes are evident and indicative of extended periods of itching and scratching. Morphology and distribution vary with age (Figure 3-1). Typically in infants and very young children, AD will affect the face and extensor arms and legs (Figures 3-2 and 3-3A). The diaper region, where moisture tends to be retained, is often spared. In older

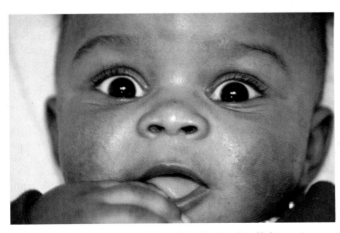

FIG. 3-2. Atopic dermatitis frequently affects the cheeks of infants.

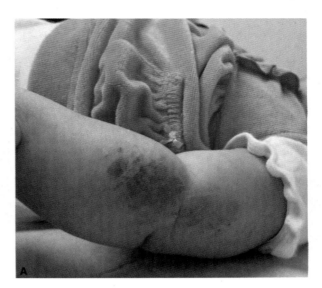

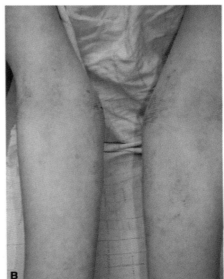

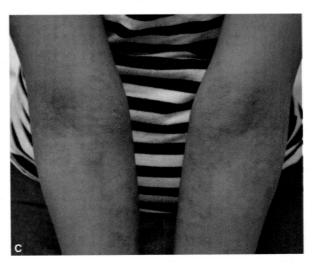

FIG. 3-3. A: Atopic dermatitis on the extensor forearms of an infant. This typically becomes more flexural, affecting the antecubital fossa as the child gets older. B: Typical distribution of atopic dermatitis in the antecubital fossa. C: AD on dark skin; it may be difficult to appreciate the erythema of scaly papules and plaques.

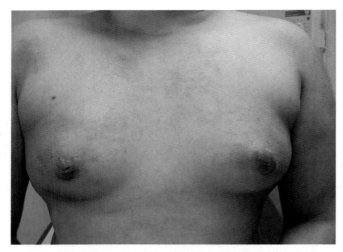

FIG. 3-4. Weepy nipple eczema on patient with atopic dermatitis.

children and adults, distribution favors flexural areas, including anterior neck, antecubital fossa, and popliteal space, and can affect the breasts, nipples, and trunk (Figures 3-3B 3-3C, and 3-4). The scalp, face, and eyelids can also be affected, and in general, the axillae and groin folds are spared at any age.

DIFFERENTIAL DIAGNOSIS Atopic dermatitis

- Tinea
- Psoriasis
- Nummular eczema
- Contact dermatitis
- Molluscum contagiosum dermatitis
- Seborrheic dermatitis
- Lichen simplex chronicus
- Cutaneous T cell lymphoma, mycosis fungoides type

Diagnostics

AD is a clinical diagnosis with common cutaneous features used to diagnose AD (Box 3-1). Additionally, the diagnoses can only be made after exclusion of differential diagnoses (above) with similar presentations. A KOH test can differentiate tinea from AD. Punch biopsy will identify psoriasis and other noneczematous dermatoses.

Management

Bathing and moisturizing

Patients are often misinformed about bathing and become confused with directions about when and how often to bathe. Bathing is beneficial; it hydrates the skin, allows for added penetration of topically applied therapies, and can help debride crusts and scaling. Generally 20 minutes in a bath is ample time for the skin to become hydrated and to absorb the maximum amount of water. Bathwater should be warm or cool (not hot), and patients should be ready to apply a moisturizer or topical corticosteroid (TCS) (never both on the same area) within 3 minutes of exiting the tub. Both moisturizers and TCS should be applied immediately after soaking hydration, when the stratum corneum is soft and supple and penetration of the treatments is maximized. In the most severe cases where skin involvement is extensive, wet wraps may be useful as a substitute for

BOX 3-1 | Clinical Criteria for a Diagnosis of Atopic Dermatitis

Essential features (both must be present)
Pruritus
Eczema (characteristic distribution and morphology)

Important features (support of the diagnosis of AD)
Early age of onset
Atopy (personal or family history, IgE reactivity)
Xerosis

Associated features (suggests the clinician consider the diagnosis of AD)
Nipple eczema
Facial pallor, white dermographism, delayed blanching response
Keratosis pilaris
Ichthyosis
Hyperlinear palms
Periocular (Dennie–Morgan lines) and/or perioral changes, cheilitis
Perifollicular accentuation
Lichenification/prurigo lesions

Adapted from Eichenfield, L.F., Hanifin, J.M., Luger, T.A., Stevens, S.R., & Pride, H.B. (2003). Consensus conference on pediatric atopic dermatitis. *Journal of the American Academy of Dermatology, 49*,1088–1095.

a soaking bath for a few days until the skin has begun to heal and getting into water is more comfortable.

Emollients

Once AD is adequately controlled, moisturizers on a regular, daily, or several-times-daily basis are essential to maintain control. Emollients are the cornerstone of maintenance therapy and prevention of relapse. Greasy or creamy emollients are always recommended, and some creamy emollients with a lipid concentration may provide an even more durable barrier than other water-based creams. Lotions tend to contain increased amounts of water and alcohol and, upon evaporation, may actually cause more dryness. A helpful hint when discussing with a patient is to remind them that creamy or greasy products are, with few exceptions, found in jars rather than in pump bottles. The skin barrier is important to the pathogenesis of AD, and many research trials are focused on perfecting skin barrier function in order to see better therapeutic outcomes with less need for medication.

Medications

Topical corticosteroids. TCS are the first-line therapy for AD and remain the most effective therapy for obtaining swift control of a flare. There are a myriad of choices, but generally a mid- to high-potency corticosteroid such as triamcinolone 0.1% ointment, fluocinonide 0.05% ointment or betamethasone 0.05% ointment will adequately treat a flare. Creams can be used if patients insist, but ointments are always preferred. Typically a mid-strength corticosteroid is applied twice daily for 3 to 5 days on the thinner skin areas (face, eyelids, neck, breasts, and buttocks) and twice daily for 7 full days on the trunk and extremities. For practical reasons and to avoid confusion, it is best to prescribe one-strength TCS for all areas involved and to eliminate the risk of mistakenly using a stronger corticosteroid in a thin-skinned area. A mid-strength TCS can safely be used 2 days per week for long-term control and to prevent relapse.

Calcineurin inhibitors. There are two nonsteroidal anti-inflammatory topical medications approved for use in AD, tacrolimus ointment (Protopic) and pimecrolimus cream (Elidel).

Applied to the skin, calcineurin inhibitors modulate the body's immune response in AD. Tacrolimus is available in two strengths 0.03%, which is approved for use in children aged 2 to 15 years, and 0.01%, which is approved for ages 15 years and older; and it is compounded in an ointment vehicle and prescribed for moderate-to-severe AD. Pimecrolimus is compounded in a cream vehicle with one strength and is prescribed for ages 2 and older with mild-to-moderate AD. Often calcineurin inhibitors are used for maintenance once the disease flare has been controlled with the use of a TCS first in the more acute stages of the flare. The cutaneous side effects of burning, itching, and stinging can be accentuated on flared skin and uncomfortable for patients, which may lead to noncompliance of the medication. Combination therapy of a mid-strength TCS 2 days per week and calcineurin inhibitors 5 days per week is a practical and effective plan to induce a remission, then for maintaining control of atopic disease.

In 2003, after both tacrolimus and pimecrolimus were approved by the Food and Drug Administration (FDA) for use in AD, a black-box warning was issued about the possible risk of cancer in both children and adults. The warning was based on sporadic spontaneous case reports of skin cancers in adults and lymphomas in children. To date there has been no statistical evidence linking development of cancer and the use of these topical agents, and short-term data on systemic side effects for both drugs are reassuring. Long-term safety data are ongoing. For this reason, the calcineurin inhibitors have been given the designation of second-line therapy, while TCS remain as first-line therapy for AD.

Antihistamines. Sedating antihistamines such as diphenhydramine or hydroxyzine can be helpful for their somnolent effect when taken at bedtime. They can help promote more restful sleep and help reduce scratching during the night and perhaps help to avoid children cosleeping with parents. Nonsedating antihistamines can be helpful for patients who suffer from allergic rhinitis, but should not be prescribed as an antipruritic treatment. Topical antihistamines are generally not recommended as they can be irritating to atopic skin and have the potential to cause allergic contact dermatitis (ACD).

Antibiotics. Oral antibiotics are needed to treat *Staphylococcus aureus* skin infections, which are commonly seen in patients with AD. Generally 5 days of cephalexin or dicloxacillin are adequate to treat a staph infection. Overuse of antibiotics potentially leads to methicillin-resistant *S. aureus* in AD patients and should be avoided. In patients who have frequent or recurring staph infections, addition of rifampin for 10 days or taking tetracycline for 30 days in conjunction with topical mupirocin may help halt the chronic nature of the infections. It is important for patients to recognize the signs of a skin infection and to know that it is often the reason for a flare, and if left untreated, their flare-up is likely to persist. Topical antibiotics such as polysporin or mupirocin can be used when the infection is localized and the skin is not flaring. If the patient develops recurrent skin infections, bleach baths can be helpful to decolonize the skin (one-quarter cup of bleach to a full tub for pediatric patients, one-half cup for adults). Culturing for sensitivities to rule out methicillin-resistant *S. aureus* is always advised if the patient does not to respond to standard antibiotic therapy.

Management of Severe and Extensive Disease

When flares are severe and extensive, oral corticosteroids may be necessary to regain control. Generally, a tapering dose of prednisone over the course of 6 days is adequate with the addition of a TCS at the end of the taper. In patients with recalcitrant disease, a course of cyclosporine (CSA) can be utilized. This is generally prescribed when intense topical therapy and/or courses of prednisone have not halted the AD flare. Baseline labs of chemistry panel, complete blood count, and urinalysis need to be obtained prior to starting this therapy and monitored monthly. Blood pressure is also monitored regularly. Due to the potential for renal toxicity and hypertension, it is not a therapy that can be used indefinitely, and after a 6-month course, transition to another therapy is warranted. Patients with known renal disease or uncontrolled hypertension should not take CSA. The starting dose of CSA when prescribed is usually at 5 mg/kg/day. This dose will quickly reduce both pruritus and inflammation and induce a remission, giving patients worn down by their disease a reprieve. After 6 months of therapy, transition to another therapy is usually indicated. Ultraviolet therapy or other systemic therapies, including methotrexate, azathioprine, mycophenolate mofetil, and interferon-γ, have shown varying levels of efficacy in AD patients.

Prognosis and Complications

It is important for AD patients to recognize possible extrinsic factors that may trigger a flare of their skin disease. Common trigger factors for AD flares are any type of infection, including viral, bacterial, fungal, and yeast infections (Figures 3-5A and B). Counseling patients to recognize signs of infection and treating quickly is important. Primary outbreaks of herpes simplex virus (HSV) can result in eczema herpeticum (Figure 3-5C). Treating HSV with acyclovir 400 mg t.i.d. for 1 week is adequate; however, treatment for eczema herpeticum should include zoster doses of antivirals. Checking for tinea when AD is flaring should be part of your physical exam. Checking toe web spaces, groin, and other intertriginous areas is important when looking for causes of a continued flare. Widespread fungal infections may need treatment with a systemic antifungal. Stress, dry climate, allergic reactions are also potential triggers. AD can severely impact a patient's (and their caregivers) quality of life and should be discussed with the patient. Abnormal pigmentation, lichenification, scars, striae, and secondary infections are complications from AD (Figure 3-5D).

Referral and Consultation

Severe AD patients require enormous amounts of clinic time to gain control of their disease. Psychological factors are often addressed, as are sleep, trigger factors, explanation of treatments, side effects, and detailed instructions regarding use of medications. An AD patient who becomes erythrodermic will need inpatient hospitalization. A referral to a dermatologic professional who specializes in atopic disease is appropriate. The National Eczema Association (NEA) is a nonprofit patient-centered organization for patients and their families. They offer a host of valuable educational information and support for families as well as for health care professionals.

Patient Education and Follow-up

AD patients require long periods of time and educational dialogue in order to understand the fundamentals of how to manage flares, then maintain control of the disease, and how to recognize signs of skin infections. Compliance to treatment plans is essential for maintenance once the skin disease is under control. Ideally a dermatology nurse will be involved in the teaching and demonstration of treatments, as this can be a time-consuming process that may not automatically be built into the providers' schedule. Studies have shown that nurse-led clinics help reduce the severity of AD outcomes in children and compliance increase up to 800%.

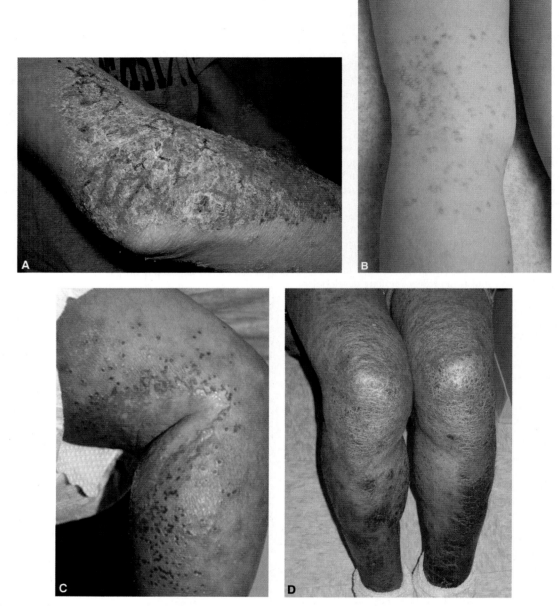

FIG. 3-5. A: Severe atopic dermatitis patient with staph impetiginization on upper extremity. **B:** Children with atopic dermatitis are at increased risk for molluscum contagiosum with the tendency to become widespread because of their tendency to scratch and spread the lesions. **C:** Eczema herpeticum featuring multiple eroded vesicles with umbilication and crusting overlying a patch of eczematous skin. **D:** Chronic scratching in AD can lead to alterations in pigmentation and lichenification.

NUMMULAR ECZEMA

Nummular eczema *(nummular or discoid dermatitis)* is a common and chronic skin disorder characterized by its annular or round, "coin shaped" lesions. Nummular eczema can, and often does, overlap with AD, stasis dermatitis, and asteatotic eczema. Males are more affected than females; and the age of onset is over 50 years for males but earlier for females around 30 years.

Pathophysiology

The pathogenesis of nummular eczema is not well understood. Some theorize that a microbial component plays a role, possibly due to bacterial colonization, although clear signs of infection are not always evident. It is also associated with contact sensitization (nickel, fragrances, chromates, balsam of Peru) and venous hypertension. It is evident that xerotic skin changes in elderly patients lend themselves to the development of cracking and fissuring of the stratum corneum in dry, cold winter weather and often progressing to nummular lesions. As the stratum corneum becomes increasingly compromised, it also becomes more damaged from scratching and manipulating due to the extreme pruritus and dryness, which is nearly always present in nummular eczema lesions. With the compromised skin barrier issue, various allergens now have a portal of entry through the skin, which may further aggravate the eczematous process.

Clinical Presentation

Nummular eczema is generally a very pruritic skin disease and follows a chronic course for many patients. A key and distinctive feature to keep in mind when evaluating a patient with nummular eczema is that unlike in AD, clinical signs of atopy and a history of atopy are not present in nummular eczema. The physical examination reveals erythematous annular plaques and sometimes thinner scaly patches, typically distributed on the upper and lower extremities (Figure 3-6). Males will show a predominance of involvement on the lower extremities and females more likely on the forearms and dorsal hands. Lesions are typically well-demarcated and start out as small papules that expand into larger plaques measuring between 1 and 3 cm. Acute plaques will be vesicular and weeping (Figure 3-7). However, a typical nummular eczema plaque eventually becomes lichenified and hyperkeratotic, demonstrating the chronicity of the lesions. Excoriations due to intense pruritus are nearly always evident in both acute and chronic lesions. Nummular eczema is often misdiagnosed as psoriasis or as a fungal infection by the primary care provider (PCP), because of the similarities in presentation since all of these skin diseases present with annular shaped skin lesions on initial presentation.

DIFFERENTIAL DIAGNOSIS Nummular eczema
• Tinea
• Psoriasis
• Contact dermatitis
• Psoriasis
• Lichen simplex chronicus
• Drug eruption
• Cutaneous T-cell lymphoma, plaque type

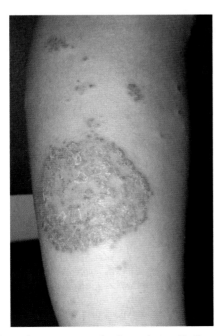

FIG. 3-6. Nummular eczema on the lower legs with the characteristic "coin-shaped," erythematous plaques.

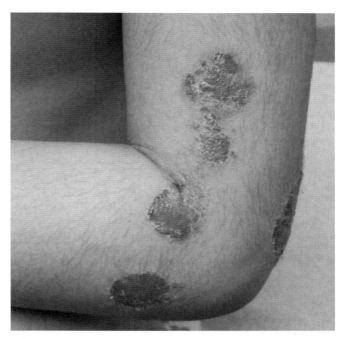

FIG. 3-7. Acute plaques of nummular eczema can be very vesicular and weepy erythematous, scaly annular "coin-shaped" lesions seen in nummular eczema.

Diagnostics

The diagnosis of nummular eczema is usually a clinical one. Bacterial cultures or KOH prep may be performed is infection is considered. A punch biopsy is not usually necessary and would yield nonspecific findings of spongiotic dermatitis that cannot differentiate it from other eczematous conditions. It would, however, help to exclude drug eruption, cutaneous T-cell lymphoma, psoriasis, and tinea. Patch testing may be recommended for severe or recalcitrant case.

Management

Nummular eczema generally requires a potent TCS such as clobetasol 0.05% ointment to provide adequate and effective treatment. An ointment rather than cream base is preferred, and application immediately after a shower, soaking bath, or wet compress is preferred. Sometimes occlusion of the lesions on the extremities for one week (at bedtime) will enhance penetration of the corticosteroid and accelerate healing. Occlusion of a plaque can be achieved by wrapping the extremity with plastic wrap after the application of the TCS. Cordran tape, an impregnated tape with flurandrenolide, can be applied directly to the lesion and left on for 12 hours.

Systemic corticosteroids may be needed in short bursts for the more severe and severely pruritic cases, but generally TCS are adequate to bring this disease under control. Intralesional triamcinolone injections, grenz ray, and application of Unna boots may also be helpful. As with any other eczematous condition, moisturizing the skin with a creamy or greasy emollient is fundamentally essential, particularly after a bath or shower, to enhance penetration of the emollient.

Prognosis and Complications

Nummular eczema is a chronic skin condition that can be challenging to control and can be exacerbated. Infections can develop secondary to chronic scratching and may require treatment. Chronic plaques can result in permanent scarring and hyperpigmentation.

Patient Education and Follow-up

Patient should be taught good skin care measures for the prevention and treatment of nummular eczema. Understanding the appropriate use of TCS, including risks and benefits of long-term use, is very important. Patients should see the PCP if there are any signs or symptoms of infection.

CONTACT DERMATITIS

Contact dermatitis is an eczematous dermatitis resulting from contact with or exposure to external irritants or allergens in the environment. There are two types of contact dermatitis: *irritant contact dermatitis* (ICD), a nonimmunologic disease resulting from physical contact with the skin barrier; and *allergic contact dermatitis* (ACD), an immunologic response with a genetic predisposition. ICD is responsible for the majority (approximately 80%) of contact dermatitis seen in outpatient care and virtually anyone in the general population is at risk for developing ICD.

Irritant Contact Dermatitis

The majority of contact dermatitis seen in the clinical setting is ICD. It is the most common cause for occupational skin disease and is estimated to be responsible for 70% to 80% of all occupational skin dermatoses. Occupations with a higher risk for exposure to irritants are as follows: those working in food catering, furniture industry workers, health care providers, housekeeping workers, food service workers, hair stylists, industrial workers exposed to chemical irritants, dry cleaners, metal workers, florist shop employees and designers, and warehouse employees. Factors that can influence and predispose a patient to developing ICD are age, gender, race, preexisting skin disease (such as AD), areas of exposure, and sebaceous activity. Both infants and the elderly can readily be affected by ICD because of a thin and more vulnerable epidermal barrier, and when affected experience a more severe dermatitis. It is speculated that individuals with darker skin pigmentation may have more resistance to irritant reactions, whereas fair-skinned individuals are more vulnerable. ICD is observed more commonly on the upper extremities of women compared to men. Other preexisting skin diseases or eczematous disorders may play a role in the development of ICD.

Pathophysiology

ICD is not due to an immunologic response as in ACD, but rather due to exposure or repeated exposures to an irritating and/or drying substance. The offending agent in ICD may be a caustic chemical or solvent, plant or flower, or abrasive product causing microtrauma. The most common of all irritants is water, sometimes called the *universal solvent*. When water comes in contact with the skin and then allowed to evaporate without sealing the moisture, there is potential to develop an eczematous reaction to the wet–dry cycle, setting the scene for repeated episodes of irritant dermatitis each time the skin is exposed to water. Strong alkaline soaps or solvents may elicit a similar or more robust irritant response. When the skin barrier is compromised, nearly any substance has the potential to produce an inflammatory response, producing a cytotoxic effect, and resulting contact dermatitis.

There are several cellular components that play a role in ICD. It is presumed that cytokines which we know to stimulate an inflammatory response in the skin are primary mediators in T-cell inflammation. There are differences in cell and skin barrier disruption in acute ICD when compared to chronic ICD. The pathogenic route in acute ICD starts with penetration through the stratum corneum and a release of inflammatory mediators, which then activate T cells. When activation has begun, this action continues independently from the offending antigen. In chronic ICD, the stratum corneum has already been altered, and lipids in the stratum corneum, which normally provide barrier protection, are weakened, leading to scaling of the epidermis and transepidermal water loss (TEWL). As the skin works to retain hydration and repair the protective barrier, it is unable to accomplish this due to chronic exposure. The epidermal barrier demonstrates a chronic eczematoid irritant reaction.

Clinical presentation

The intensity of clinical signs and symptoms of ICD depends upon the properties of the irritating substance and the degree of skin barrier impairment at the time of exposure. Environmental factors can also play a role in the severity of ICD and include, but are not limited to, temperature, mechanical pressure on the skin, humidity, concentration of the irritating substance, pH, and time duration of contact with the skin. ICD has a rapid-onset reaction and improves with avoidance of the offending agent.

Acute ICD develops when the skin is exposed to irritating substances. The skin's reaction is immediate and peaks within minutes to hours after the exposure, with the patient reporting burning, stinging, or tenderness. Sharply demarcated erythematous patches with edema and sometimes bullae are evident on skin in the areas of exposure to the irritant substance. Acids and alkaline solutions capable of producing chemical burns are the most common potent irritants resulting in acute ICD.

Chronic ICD results from multiple subthreshold contacts when the skin does not have ample time between exposures to completely recover and restore normal skin barrier function. Lesions of chronic ICD contrast with those of acute ICD, in that erythema is present, but are not as distinctively demarcated and less inflammatory appearing. Other signs present in chronic ICD are scaling, vesicles, lichenification, and hyperkeratosis (Figure 3-8).

DIFFERENTIAL DIAGNOSIS Irritant contact dermatitis
• Allergic contact dermatitis
• Atopic dermatitis
• Scabies
• Psoriasis
• Tinea

Diagnostics

ICD is usually a clinical diagnosis but may require patch testing if ACD is suspected. Bacterial and fungal cultures can help identify infections. A KOH prep is a rapid, in-office test that can identify fungus, and a mineral prep can be for scabies. Biopsy is helpful only in differentiating ICD from other dermatoses like psoriasis.

Prognosis and complications

ICD can be chronic and relapsing, especially if the individual has difficulty avoiding contact with the offending agent. This can be seen when the patient's occupation results in unavoidable exposure to irritants, forcing them to make a choice between finding another occupation and dealing with chronic ICD. The most common complications include secondary infections, scarring, pigmentary changes, and lichen simplex chronicus (LSC). Severe or chronic dermatitis ICD can have a significant impact on the patient's quality of life, which should be addressed by the clinician.

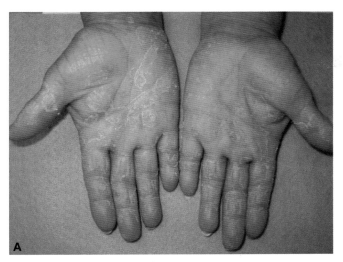 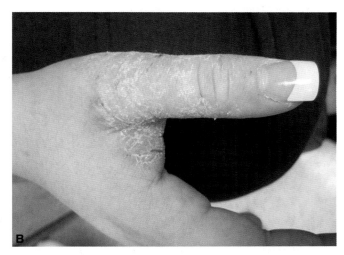

FIG. 3-8. **A:** Irritant contact dermatitis on the hands of a health care worker. **B:** Chronic ICD, becoming fissured and lichenified on a woman who worked as a coffee barista and came in contact with a bleach cloth regularly.

Patient education and follow-up

Patients with ICD should be educated about the appropriate use of TCS, side effects (long and short term), and signs and symptoms of secondary infection. Prevention education is important as patients are their best advocate in identifying and avoiding contact irritants.

Allergic Contact Dermatitis

ACD accounts for roughly 20% of contact dermatitis. Patients may have a very specific dermatitis that develops from wearing jewelry containing nickel or when coming in contact with poison ivy. Identifying the allergen allows the patient to practice avoidance and allowing their dermatitis to improve or resolve. It becomes a more complicated clinical picture when ACD is chronic and when it affects hands, face, or eyelids without known cause of the specific allergen. Allergens and exposure to allergens vary from region to region, and preservatives added to skin care products that have potential to cause contact dermatitis are variable depending on government regulations and what types of preservatives are allowed to be used in any given location (Box 3-2).

ACD affects patients of all ages, gender, and ethnicity. Occupation and hobbies play a significant role in exposures. ACD accounts for the majority of occupational skin diseases affecting the hands. Many patients with these diagnoses will find it necessary to change jobs or will have extended absences from work because of their dermatitis; some even find it necessary to leave the workforce altogether in order to avoid repeated exposures to offending agents.

BOX 3-2	Common Allergens

Bacitracin
Balsam of Peru
Cobalt chloride
Formaldehyde
Fragrance mix
Neomycin sulfate
Nickel sulfate
Propylene glycol
Quaternium-15
Sodium gold thiosulfate
Thimerosal
Thiuram mix

Pathophysiology

ACD is an allergen-specific reaction caused by a type IV delayed hypersensitivity when a patient comes in contact with a specific allergen. When antigen-presenting Langerhans cells find and digest the antigen on the cell surface, the Langerhans cell then moves toward the closest lymph node, presenting the antigen to the T-memory cell. At this point, the now activated T lymphocytes converge back to the skin where the cascade of inflammatory events is triggered (pruritus, erythema, blistering). Initial sensitization must have occurred when the patient is first exposed to the allergen, and the allergen is allowed to come in contact with and penetrate through the skin. Reexposure at a later date, even in a low or minimal concentration, will lead to a release of cytokines and chemotactic factors resulting in an inflammatory, pruritic, weepy dermatitis. This cascade of events occurs rapidly once sensitization is established, within 12 to 48 hours of exposure, and if vesicular, can last for days or weeks before resolution.

Clinical presentation

ACD presents as a well-demarcated, pruritic eczematous eruption, often acute, with edema and vesicles that open and become moist and weepy (Figure 3-9). If ACD continues and becomes chronic, scaly plaques and lichenification may be evident (Figure 3-10). The areas of involvement are typically localized to areas of exposure; however, the dermatitis can become diffuse depending on the vehicle of the causative agent (Figures 3-11 and 3-12). For example, shampoos or cleansing washes which may rinse over larger areas of the body and thus affect other areas as well as the primary point of contact (Figure 3-13).

DIFFERENTIAL DIAGNOSIS Allergic contact dermatitis

- Tinea
- Perioral dermatitis
- Seborrheic dermatitis
- Drug eruptions
- Asteatotic eczema
- Drug-induced photosensitivity

Diagnostics

Patch Testing. The gold standard for diagnosis of ACD is patch testing, which is often needed to identify causative agents for ACD. The Thin-layer Rapid Use Epicutaneous Test (TRUE test), a U.S.

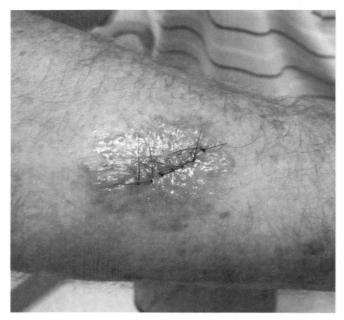

FIG. 3-9. Allergic contact dermatitis from the application of Neosporin on a surgical site.

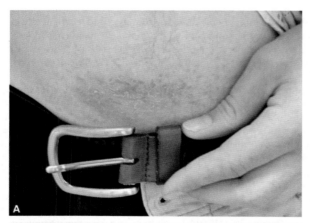

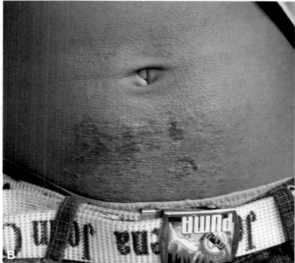

FIG. 3-10. A: Allergic reaction to contact with belt buckle containing nickel. **B:** Chronic allergic contact dermatitis from a belt buckle. The area has become hyperpigmented and lichenified.

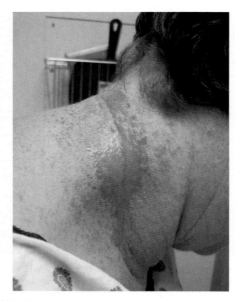

FIG. 3-11. Allergic contact dermatitis from a necklace containing nickel.

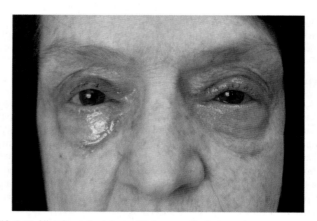

FIG. 3-12. Allergic contact dermatitis from medicated eye drops.

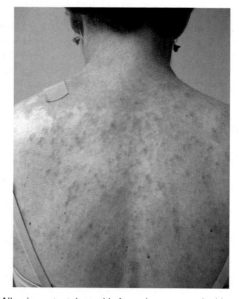

FIG. 3-13. Allergic contact dermatitis from shampoo resulted in eczematous papules and plaques in a washed-out pattern from the scalp.

FDA-approved testing tool, is the most common standard series used for patch testing and consists of a three-panel system of pre-impregnated allergens and screens. Currently, the TRUE test includes 36 allergens, allergen mixes, and controls used to diagnose 90% of the most common allergens seen in ACD. Patients with persistent, unresolved ACD can suffer for months or even years, impacting their ability to live a full and productive life. Through patch testing, causative agents can be identified and eliminated, thereby improving the patient's quality of life. The process of patch testing is complex and requires that experienced clinicians in dermatology or allergy/immunology to both apply and interpret the results of the tests.

Understanding how and when to patch test patients requires training and experience. Patch tests are generally placed on the upper back of the individual and require that the area of skin is clear of dermatitis. This is important and prevents interference from the existing dermatitis. TCS may be necessary to clear dermatitis on the patient's back, but must be discontinued 1 week prior to application of the patch tests. Ideally, systemic corticosteroids should be discontinued 1 month prior to patch application. Patients should be warned that they will not be allowed to take a shower, exercise, bend, or twist their back during the testing time, which lasts for 5 to 7 days.

After the initial application of the patches, patients are asked to return to the office in 48 hours for removal of the patches and the first reading. Sites of application are marked in order to identify the location of specific allergens. A second reading is taken in 72 hours to 7 days after the patches were initially placed. As mentioned, the interpretation of patch test results should be done by knowledgeable and skilled clinicians. There is no consensus on interpretation, but the International Contact Dermatitis Research Group has developed a standardized scoring system often used in the evaluation of skin reactions to allergens. The noted reaction may range from a weak positive to a bullous skin reaction. These results must be interpreted in the context of the patient's clinical presentation and symptoms to determine the clinical relevance of the allergic reaction. All positive results may not be significant. A true test of clinical relevance is resolution of the dermatitis when the offending agent is removed.

Management
Once positive allergens are identified, avoidance is the key treatment for ACD. If dermatitis is present after testing is completed, use of a topical or systemic corticosteroid is appropriate to clear any residual dermatitis. Forewarn patients that it can take up to 6 weeks for dermatitis to completely clear once the offending agent has been removed.

Prognosis and complications
The complications and prognosis of ACD are similar to those associated with ICD.

Referral and consultation
When ACD is chronic or affecting critical areas such as hands and/or face, referral to dermatology or allergy/immunology for patch testing is crucial for diagnosis and treatment. Referral to a specialty clinic or clinicians experienced in patch testing is appropriate and important for patient well-being and quality of life.

Patient education and follow-up
Patients should be provided detailed written information about the causative allergens identified from testing. The chemical name, as well as possible synonymous or brand names, should be provided along with instructions as to how to prevent future exposure. It is important that patients learn how to read product labels and compare them to their chemical list in order to avoid contact.

ASTEATOTIC ECZEMA
Nearly everyone after their sixth decade of life experiences some type of skin dryness (xerosis). For some, it may only be a patch or two of dryness in the winter months, but more often it involves extensive areas or the entire body. Asteatotic eczema (also called *eczema craquelé* or *desiccation dermatitis*) is severely dry skin that is inflamed and fissured. It is linked to outside influences, including drier climates, cold winter weather, and individuals who bathe, swim, or shower often without caring for their skin immediately after out of the water. Asteatotic eczema can be seen in most any part of the world and to a slight degree affects men more than women.

Pathophysiology
Dry skin (xerosis) in an aging individual is not related to a deficiency of oil or sebum production, but rather from functional problems with the stratum corneum. Low levels of intercellular lipids lead to an inability to bind and retain water. The dehydrated cells shrink and become rigid, forming deep fissures in the epidermis and sometimes extending into the dermis. Factors that contribute to or aggravate dryness include low humidity, low ambient temperatures, chronic ultraviolet light, excessive use of soaps, habitual scrubbing, and excessive water exposure. Perfumed soaps and other skin cleansers may provoke the cutaneous nerve fibers, leading to a release of proinflammatory cytokines which then begins the cycle of inflammation.

Clinical Presentation
Asteatotic eczema often presents itself or worsens in winter weather and is referred to as "winter itch." In mild disease, there may be no symptoms, but in moderately or severely affected skin, patients are likely to complain of pruritus, burning, or stinging. Dry or xerotic skin appears dull, dry, and scaly. The scaling associated with general xerosis and with asteatotic eczema is described as fine, bran-like scales. The skin can actually demonstrate a crisscross show of superficial cracks as well as fissures in the horny layer, sometimes referred to as "crazy-paving" or "dried river bed" cracks (Figure 3-14). The affected areas can appear pink or mildly erythematous. In chronic, advanced asteatotic eczema, a background of dull erythema with oozing, crusting, and excoriations can be seen. Vesicles and pustules are generally not seen with asteatotic eczema. There are many factors which can influence and aggravate xerotic skin, including drier climates, detergents with higher alkalinity, showering or bathing excessively, malnutrition, renal insufficiency, hereditary skin conditions (ichthyosis vulgaris), and those with a history of atopy. Eczema craquelé develops when dry skin is perturbed by contact with irritating substances in topical skin preparations.

DIFFERENTIAL DIAGNOSIS   Asteatotic eczema
• Atopic dermatitis
• Allergic contact dermatitis
• Cellulitis
• Stasis dermatitis

Diagnostics
Laboratory studies are not indicated for the diagnosis of asteatotic eczema. Bacterial cultures may be indicated if there is clinical suspicion for infection.

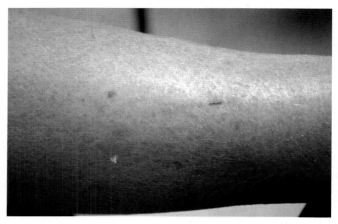

FIG. 3-14. Asteatotic skin typical with dried curled edges and erythema.

Management

Use of a mid-potency TCS ointment for 5 to 7 days is usually sufficient to clear the inflammation from asteatotic eczema and bring it under control. Maintenance can generally be achieved with regular use of a creamy or greasy emollient. Use of urea or lactic acid preparations can also be beneficial for some patients. Patients should be educated to continue moisturization and avoidance of known aggravating factors.

Prognosis and Complications

Asteatotic eczema can be an acute problem that can be resolved. Yet, recurrence is not uncommon in individuals with chronic environments exposure or poor skin care. Secondary infections and inflammation are common complications. Furthermore, scratching behavior may result in ulceration.

Referral and Consultation

A referral to a specialist is generally not indicated unless chronic wounds develop and require wound care.

Patient Education and Follow-up

Although the elderly cannot change the physiologic changes in the skin from aging, they can reduce the environmental triggers and actively prevent dermatitis with good skin care. Patients should be educated about the signs and symptoms of infection and contact their PCP if they present.

DYSHIDROTIC ECZEMA

An intensely pruritic form of eczema, dyshidrotic eczema is characterized by the appearance of vesicles on the hands and feet. It occurs twice as often in females as males. And it can present at any age but most often in the second to fourth decade. Risk factors for dyshidrotic eczema include a history of atopic or ACD, industrial exposure to certain metals (cobalt, nickel, and chromium), and anxiety or stress.

Pathophysiology

The etiology of dyshidrotic eczema is unknown. Unlike hyperhidrosis (excessive sweating of the palms, soles, and axillae), dyshidrotic eczema (also called *pompholyx*) is not related to sweat gland activity. It is thought to be associated with psychogenic factors (stress related), fungal infection, id reaction (literally an eczematous reaction to a fungal infection somewhere else on the body), drug reaction, and in many cases idiopathic.

Clinical Presentation

The clinical picture of dyshidrotic eczema is a vesicular eruption, appearing as clear or white small deep vesicles (described as tapioca pearls) on the palms, fingers, and soles (Figure 3-15). Patients often complain of severe pruritus and sometimes burning pain. It distinctly spares the dorsum of the hands or feet, but may extend to the lateral aspects of the fingers and soles. Once the vesicles dry, scale is usually the most notable symptom.

DIFFERENTIAL DIAGNOSIS   Dyshidrotic eczema
• Palmarplantar pustular psoriasis
• Tinea
• Contact dermatitis
• Bullous impetigo

Diagnostics

Punch biopsy is not necessary but can help to differentiate from psoriasis or tinea if a PAS is performed. Direct immunofluorescence can rule of autoimmune blistering disease. Bacterial culture and sensitivity can identify bacterial pathogens.

Management

Treating the suspected cause (infections, drugs, stress) of dyshidrotic eczema can be curative. Stress and anxiety management may help reduce recurrence. Underlying infection, either bacterial or fungal, should be treated with the appropriate antibiotics, and antihistamines may be helpful. Treatment with high-potency TCS twice daily is the first-line therapy. Once controlled, tapering the TCS to milder-potency TCS or a calcineurin inhibitor can be effective, and

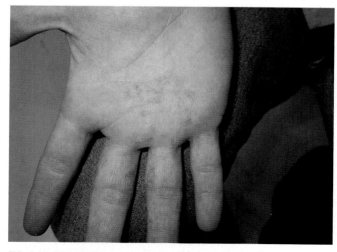

FIG. 3-15. Dyshidrotic eczema with vesicles and erythema on the palms involving the lateral aspects of the finger.

antihistamines may be helpful. If the dyshidrotic eczema is severe, a short-term course of systemic corticosteroids may be indicated. Dermatologists treating recalcitrant disease often use immunosuppressants including methotrexate, cyclosporine, azathioprine, and PUVA (psoralen followed by UV light therapy).

Referral and Consultation

Referral to a dermatologic specialist may be warranted if first-line therapies are not effective or the dyshidrotic eczema is severe or recurrent. In some cases, referral to a psychotherapist may be beneficial and appropriate in controlling stress.

Prognosis and Complications

Dyshidrotic eczema can have a significant impact on an individual's daily living and essential function. It can interfere with interpersonal relationships, employment, and home life, all of which impact the general quality of life.

Patient Education and Follow-up

Instructions should be given to avoid contact with irritants and hand care for prevention and control. Reducing stress and avoiding excessive water exposure may prevent flares. Dietary modifications may be helpful if allergy and patch testing identifies allergens.

SEBORRHEIC DERMATITIS

Seborrheic dermatitis is discussed in chapter 5, Papulosquamous Disorders.

ID REACTION

An id reaction is an inflammatory dermatitis which is the body's response to an infection, inflammatory condition, or substance. It is also referred to as *autosensitization, disseminated eczema,* or *dermatophytids*. It is estimated that at least two-thirds of patients with contact dermatitis develop disseminated eczema, whereas one-third of the patients with a history of stasis dermatitis have developed autosensitization.

Pathophysiology

The pathogenesis of IDs is not clearly understood but thought to be an immune-mediated response of the body to an infection, trauma, or antigens from an inflammatory process. Fungus is the most common pathogen seen that triggers an immunologic response. However, bacteria, mycobacteria, and viruses, such as the pox virus in molluscum, can trigger autosensitization dermatitis. Epidermal antigens from inflammatory skin conditions like contact dermatitis can lead to hypersensitization, resulting in an id reaction

Clinical Presentation

Symptoms of id reaction can vary on the stimuli causing the immune response. Id can be characterized by poorly demarcated eczematous patches, papules, petechiae, or vesicles may present on the extremities, face, and, occasionally, the trunk. The reaction may occur near the sites of infection (i.e., surrounding the molluscum papules) or remotely on distant sites not affected by the primary pathogen or inflammatory process. Thus, an annular plaque of tinea on a patient's face could result in an id reaction located on their hands and fingers (Figure 3-16). Likewise, a patient with stasis dermatitis

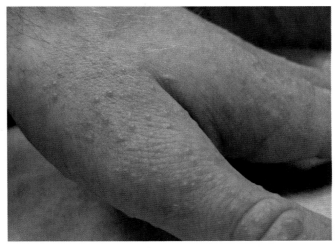

FIG. 3-16. Id reaction with vesicles located on the hands and fingers in a young man with tinea on his leg.

may appear to have a diffuse, papulovesicular eruption spreading to other extremities and even overlying the original stasis dermatitis of the shins.

Autosensitization is not immediate and develops days to weeks after the onset of the initial infection or inflammatory condition. The dermatitis will continue to spread until the underlying condition is treated.

DIFFERENTIAL DIAGNOSIS Id reaction

- Contact dermatitis
- Nummular eczema
- Granuloma annulare
- Autoimmune blistering diseases
- Dyshidrotic eczema
- Viral exanthem
- Scabies
- Drug eruption

Diagnostics

Laboratory studies should include culture and sensitivity or scraping to identify hyphae, scabies mites, or scybala. Punch biopsy has limited diagnostic value and will only exclude eczematous dermatoses. Patch testing will help identify allergens.

Management

The most important therapeutic intervention for id reaction is the treatment of the underlying infection with the appropriate antimicrobial or therapeutic treatment. Use of TCS can provide some relief from the pruritus but is somewhat controversial as some clinicians believe that corticosteroids can suppress the cutaneous immune system and allow further spread of the infection. For weeping patches and plaques, wet dressings or Burow's compresses (aluminum acetate or available as Domboro) can be effective.

Prognosis and Complications

Id reaction is self-limiting and will resolve spontaneously once the associated infection or inflammatory process is treated.

Patient Education and Follow-up

Patients should be instructed to follow up for signs and symptoms of infections.

LICHEN SIMPLEX CHRONICUS

A chronic disorder resulting from excessive scratching and rubbing of the skin, LSC or neurodermatitis is a very frustrating skin disease. It is more commonly seen in adults in the sixth decade of life or older. LSC in children is usually during adolescents. Patients with a history of AD or anxiety have a higher incidence of LSC.

Pathophysiology

The etiology of LSC is thought to be associated with sensitization. LSC can develop from rubbing or scratching in response to pruritus from a primary process like contact dermatitis, insect bites, psoriasis, stress, etc. Perpetuation of the itch–scratch cycle may be further aggravated by psychological stress or anxiety disorders. Environmental factors like heat, irritants, or sweat can contribute to the pruritus.

Clinical Presentation

LSC lesions are identified as hyperpigmented, thick, lichenified plaques with a leathery that evolve over time. Patients may or may not be aware of their habitual scratching and rubbing, and it may occur when the patient is asleep. Secondary erosions may be noted. LSC is located in easy to reach areas like the back of the neck and occipital scalp, extensor aspects of the arms and legs, vulva/scrotum, and perianal area (Figure 3-17).

DIFFERENTIAL DIAGNOSIS Lichen simplex chronicus
• Hypertrophic lichen planus
• Psoriasis
• Nummular eczema
• Lichen sclerosis
• Human papillomavirus
• Tinea

Diagnostics

LSC is usually a clinical diagnosis. Punch biopsy may help identify a primary disease or condition cause pruritus fundamental to the itch–scratch cycle. Cultures for secondary infections may be indicated.

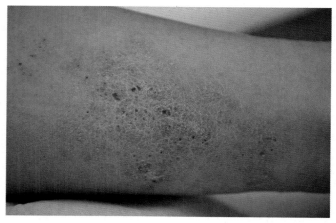

FIG. 3-17. Lichen simplex chronicus from chronic scratching on the lower leg.

Management

Breaking the itch–scratch cycle is most important and can be quite challenging, often requiring a multidisciplinary approach. Antipruritics and emollients can provide immediate relief of pruritus. High-potency TCS with or without occlusion can ease the pruritus and, equally important, provide a barrier to prevent more scratching or rubbing to affected areas. Intralesionally, corticosteroids are effective in controlling pruritus and reducing the size of involved lesions. Treatment goals should also include risk reduction for secondary infections.

Referral and Consultation

Counseling may be necessary and helpful to identify stressors which may cause or exacerbate rubbing and scratching behaviors. LSC has been associated with obsessive compulsive and anxiety disorders where patients treated with selective serotonin reuptake inhibitors (SSRIs) or oral doxepin have shown some improvement.

Prognosis and Complications

Secondary infection, hyperpigmentation, and scarring are the most common complications of LSC. Complete resolution can occur if the patient is successful in halting the scratching behaviors. Patients with LSC easily triggered by stress or cannot break the itch–scratch cycle are likely to experience recurrence.

Patient Education and Follow-up

Prevention and awareness of rubbing or scratching behaviors is important. Patients should be educated that resolution of the symptoms will require more than pharmacologic intervention and be dependent on behavioral modification. If the patient is using TCS, follow-up with the clinician should include routine examination of the site.

CLINICAL PEARLS

- If cost is an issue with regard to emollients, plain white Crisco, found at any grocery store, can be used as an emollient for AD patients.
- For children with extensive flaring of their AD, getting into a bathtub can be an issue; wearing clothing into the bath may help until the skin starts to heal and getting into the water is more comfortable.
- An alternative for bathing when the skin is flared with painful open areas is to use wet pajamas with dry sweats over the top for an hour or longer. It will hydrate the skin and improve the effectiveness of emollients and medication applied immediately after removing them. After a few days, the skin should be healed enough so the child can get into a bathtub without pain.
- The swimming pool is an acceptable alternative to bathing, as children are happier to get into a pool than into a tub of water.

BILLING CODES ICD 10

Allergic contact dermatitis, unspecified	L23-9
Atopic dermatitis, unspecified	L20.9
Autoeczematization	L30.2
Dyshidrotic eczema (pompholyx)	L30.1
Irritant contact dermatitis, unspecified	L24.9
Lichen simplex chronicus	L28.0
Nummular eczema	L30.0
Xerotic eczema (dermatitis)	L30.9

READINGS

Aoyama, H., Tanaka, M., Hara, M., Tabata, N., & Tagami, H. (1999). Nummular eczema: An addition of senile xerosis and unique cutaneous reactivities to environmental aeroallergens. *Dermatology, 199*(2), 135.

Berardesca, E., & Distante, F. (1995). Mechanisms of skin irritations. *Current Problems in Dermatology, 23*, 1–8.

Chamlin, S. L., Mattson, C. L., Frieden, I. J., Williams, M. L., Mancini, A. J., Cella, D., & Chren, M. M. (2005). The price of pruritus. *Archives of Pediatrics & Adolescent Medicine, 159*, 745–749.

Diepgen, T. L. (2001). Atopic dermatitis: The role of environmental and social factors, the European experience. *Journal of the American Academy of Dermatology, 45*, S44–S48.

Ellis, C. N., Drake, L. A., Prendergast, M. M., Abramovits, W., Boguniewicz, M., Daniel, C. R., …Tong, K. B. (2002). Cost of atopic dermatitis and eczema in the United States. *Journal of the American Academy of Dermatology, 46*, 361–370.

Hanifin, J., Gupta, A. K, & Rajagopalan, R. (2002). Intermittent dosing of fluticasone propionate cream for reducing the risk of relapse in atopic dermatitis patients. *British Journal of Dermatology, 147*, 528–537.

Lapidus, C. S., Schwarz, D. F., & Honig, P. J. (1993). Atopic dermatitis in children; who cares? Who pays? *Journal of the American Academy of Dermatology, 28*, 699–703.

Larsen, F. S., Hold, N. V., & Henningsen, K. (1986). Atopic dermatitis. A genetic-epidemiologic study in a population-based twin sample. *Journal of the American Academy of Dermatology, 15*, 487–494.

Lewis-Jones, M. S., & Finlay, A. Y. (1995). The Children's Dermatology Life Quality Index (CDLQI): Initial validation and practical use. *British Journal of Dermatology, 132*, 942–949.

Molin, S., Diepgen, T. L., Ruzicka, T., & Prinz, J. C. (2011). Diagnosing chronic hand eczema by an algorithm: A tool for classification in clinical practice. *Clinical and Experimental Dermatology, 36*(6), 595–601.

Moore, E., Williams, A., Manias, E., & Varigos, G. (2006). Nurse-led clinics reduce severity of childhood atopic eczema: A review of the literature. *British Journal of Dermatology, 155*, 1242–1248.

Palmer, D. N., Irvine, A. D., Terron-Kwiatkowski, A., Zhao, Y., Liao, H., Lee, S. P., … McLean, W. H. (2006). Common loss-of-function variants of the epidermal barrier protein filaggrin are a major predisposing factor for atopic dermatitis. *Nature Genetics, 38*(4), 441–446.

Silverberg, J. I., & Hanifin, J. M. (2013). Adult eczema prevalence and associations with asthma and other health and demographic factors: A US population-based study. *The Journal of Allergy and Clinical Immunology, 132*(5), 1132–1138.

Simpson, E. L., & Hanifin, J. M. (2005). Atopic dermatitis. *Journal of the American Academy of Dermatology, 53*(1), 115–128.

Simpson, E. L., & Hanifin, J. M. (2006). Atopic dermatitis. *The Medical Clinics of North America, 90*(1), 149–167.

Stevens, S. R., & Cooper, K. D. (1996). Allergic skin diseases. In: *Clinical immunology–principles and practice.* St Louis, MO: Mosby.

Su, J. C., Kemp, A. S., Varigos, G. A., & Nolan, T. (1997). Atopic eczema: Its impact on the family and financial cost. *Archives of Disease in Childhood, 76*(2), 159–162.

CHAPTER 4

Acne and Related Disorders

Dorothy Sullivan

Every spring, clinicians receive a deluge of phone calls heralding the seasonal rites of passage: prom, graduation, and weddings, to name a few. The desire to look one's best particularly during life's milestones is human nature. It is estimated that primary care clinicians see up to 22% of patient visits that include dermatologic conditions. Therefore, it is incumbent upon the general practitioner to be well versed on the etiology and management of some of the most prevalent skin disorders, especially those which can be socially debilitating, such as acne vulgaris, rosacea, and hidradenitis suppurativa (HS). In this chapter, we will explore the etiology of these common dermatoses, their potential impact on patients' lives, and current strategies to best manage these often chronic conditions.

ACNE VULGARIS

Acne vulgaris impacts 40 to 50 million people in the United States every year at an estimated annual cost of 2.5 billion dollars. Acne is responsible for 10% of *all* patient encounters and is estimated to account for 4 to 8 million visits to a health care provider each year (Villasenor & Kroshinsky, 2011). Acne is often ascribed to the teenage population yet has been reported throughout the lifespan to include neonates and older adults. The onset of acne frequently correlates with puberty and may occur as early as 8 to 12 years of age among females during adrenarche. Males tend to develop acne somewhat later in adolescence, but develop disease of greater severity. Females tend to have a less severe, but a more chronic course. Episodes of adult-onset acne de novo seem to affect women more than men.

Because of the visible nature of the condition and the potential for permanent scarring, acne is frequently associated with psychological distress, depression, and decrease in self-esteem. The Dermatology Quality of Life Index surveys have shown that patients rank acne as comparable to the morbidity of asthma or epilepsy. Too often acne is dismissed by clinicians as a benign disease and a normal part of maturation. It can, however, have a profound psychosocial impact that has been linked with suicide in rare instances. It is important for the clinician to remain cognizant of the subtle manifestations indicating a deeper, significant psychological turmoil.

Individuals at increased risk for acne include patients with endocrine disorders such as polycystic ovarian syndrome (PCOS), hyperandrogenism, Cushing syndrome, and precocious puberty. There is also a predisposition for acne among patients with at least one parent with a history of severe acne. Acne can be exacerbated by stress, hormonal fluctuations, endocrine disorders, certain medications, and diets with a high glycemic index. Medications that may trigger or worsen acne include topical and systemic corticosteroids, progesterone, testosterone, antidepressants, antiseizure medications, isoniazid, and anticancer drugs, specifically the epidermal growth factor receptor (EGFR) drugs.

Pathophysiology

The pathophysiology of acne is a complex interplay of factors that involves the pilosebaceous unit (Figure 4-1). Previously, the dermatology community believed that acne was initiated by the development of the microcomedo. It is now believed that subclinical inflammation is the initiating event and that the inflammation continues throughout the entire process. Contributing factors include androgens, increased sebum production, altered follicular differentiation, enlargement of pores, and *Propionibacterium acnes* colonization of the follicle. This combination of factors results in the development of the microcomedo, which blocks the pore and eventually results in rupture of the follicular wall, leading to the formation of papules, pustules, and sometimes cysts. *P. acne* continues to trigger inflammatory mediators throughout the active state, and as the process is resolving. Experts disagree as to whether this sequence in the development of *P. acnes* is a primary or secondary event. Research is focused on gaining a better understanding of the pathogenesis of acne, in hopes of developing new and improved targeted therapies.

Acne classification

There are several subtypes of acne. Some of them occur because of physiologic changes associated with normal development.

Neonatal acne and *infantile acne* are discussed in chapter 6.

Mid-childhood acne is observed in children aged 18 months to 7 years and is the most concerning age group. Acne in this age range is rare and implies more significant systemic problems such as Cushing syndrome, premature adrenarche, congenital adrenal hyperplasia, gonadal/adrenal tumors, or true precocious puberty. It is often misidentified as keratosis pilaris, rosacea, perioral dermatitis, or *Demodex*. Patients in this age group who present with chronic, severe, or virilizing acne require further evaluation for systemic disease. An appropriate evaluation would include use of growth charts, bone scans, total/free testosterone, dehydroepiandrosterone (DHEAS), prolactin, LH/FSH, 17-OH progesterone levels, and androstenedione. Both topical and oral therapies are advised, with the exception of prescribed tetracycline products, which are not recommended to children age 8 years and younger.

Preadolescent acne is the fourth type of acne within the childhood spectrum and encompasses ages 8 to 12 years. Typically, comedones are evident on the face and neck, but are less common on the torso. This may be an indicator of emerging puberty as it corresponds to additional sebum production and increase in the size of sebaceous follicles. There is some evidence to suggest that the severity and prevalence of acne in the preteen years is predictive of advanced prepubertal maturity. Treatment with traditional topical therapies is advised until the individual's level of severity and potential for scarring can be assessed.

Adolescent acne is a common occurrence, and about 70% of the time occurs at puberty and lasts, in general, approximately 5 years.

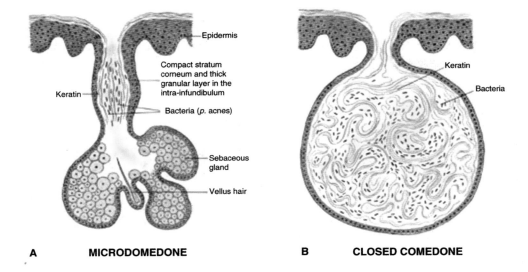

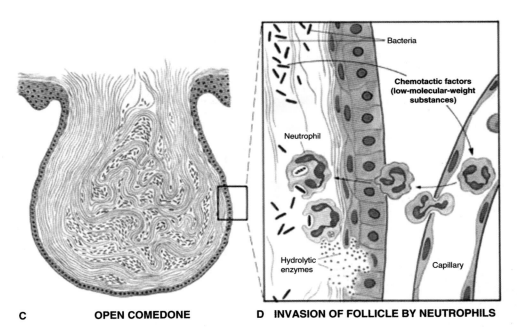

FIG. 4-1. Pathogenesis of acne vulgaris.

It can present simply as comedones and a few papules, or it can progress to multiple inflammatory papules, pustules, and cysts. Individuals will vary with regard to lesion type, extent, location, and development of scarring. It can be present in two severe forms as well.

Acne conglobata is the most severe form of acne and typically arises in adolescent males, although it does not exclude females. It distinguishes itself with nodules, abscess formation, and scars. Comedones may have more than one opening, and cystic lesions often drain. Sinus tracking is not uncommon. Keloid scars, depressed, hypertrophic, boxcar, or ice pick scars may be evident.

Acne fulminans occurs uncommonly but with an explosive onset in the teenage male population. It is accompanied by bone pain at the clavicle and sternum. Patients may experience fever and leukocytosis as well as joint pain, anemia, and liver enlargement. Other acne variants develop as a result of secondary changes imposed by external factors (Table 4-1).

TABLE 4-1	Acne Variants
Acne excoriée	Habitual picking, usually by young women, in a vain attempt to eradicate them
Acne mechanica	Caused by friction or chafing from chin straps, sports padding, or equipment
Chloracne	Due to occupational exposure to toxins like chlorinated or halogenated chemicals Large comedones and pustules face, trunk, genitals, and extremities
Acne cosmetica	Adolescent females who wear a lot of makeup. Comedones, papules, pustules
Acne associated with endocrine abnormalities	Often accompanied by hirsutism, menstrual irregularities, and virilizing characteristics. Pustules and cysts

Clinical Presentation

The clinical presentation of acne is varied and may assume different forms, but the initial lesion is usually an open comedo (blackhead) or a closed comedo and is clinically considered a noninflammatory lesion. The presence of comedones is required for the clinical diagnosis of acne vulgaris.

Inflammatory lesions can be observed as papules, pustules, nodules, or cysts. They are typically found on the face, chest, and back, which are often the sites of greatest concentration of pilosebaceous follicles and sebaceous activity. In addition to being described as noninflammatory or inflammatory, acne may also be classified as mild, moderate, or severe depending upon the type and number of lesions, location, and the presence or absence of scarring. Scarring is the result of prolonged inflammation and is more common with nodulocystic lesions. Additional collagen is laid down in an attempt to heal the deep tissue injury. Figure 4-2 shows an example of atrophic scarring. Early intervention is essential to diminish the formation of scars.

A thorough history is critical when assessing the acne patient and determining a treatment regimen that will promote adherence and optimize outcomes. The many variables that must be considered are listed in Table 4-2.

DIFFERENTIAL DIAGNOSIS Acne

- Milia
- Sebaceous hyperplasia
- Perioral dermatitis
- Rosacea
- Folliculitis (gram positive and gram negative; Pityrosporum)
- Pseudofolliculitis barbae
- Acne keloidalis
- Angiofibromas
- Keratosis pilaris

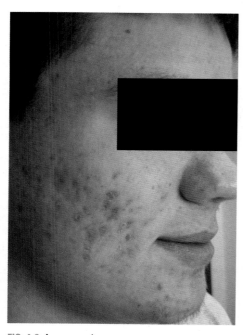

FIG. 4-2. Acne scarring.

TABLE 4-2 Essential History Taking for Acne Vulgaris

QUESTIONS	FOR ASSESSMENT
Location	Face/neck/jawline/chest/back
Onset	Age at initial breakout
Duration/frequency	Waxes & wanes? Cyclical with menses? Chronic?
Current treatment	All OTC and prescription products. Vehicle? Dose? Frequency? What worked? What didn't?
Previous treatments	OTC and prescription products Topical vs. systemic Dose? Frequency? Vehicle? What worked? What didn't?
Prescribed medications	Hormonal (OCP, Spironolactone). Lithium? Allergies to medications?
Pregnancy status	Pregnant? Planning? Breastfeeding? Method of contraception?
Women's health	Premenstrual flares & menstrual history? Increase of androgen-dependent hair? Thinning of scalp hair? Hormones/testing?
General health	Endocrinopathies? PCOS? Stein–Leventhal? Cushing? Behavioral health issues? Crohn's/colitis?
Dermatologic conditions	History of atopy or eczema? Contact dermatitis? Hidradenitis suppurativa?
Family history	Acne or other skin disorders? Hidradenitis suppurativa? Behavioral health?
Nutrition	Dairy products? High glycemic index?
Grooming products	Hair-styling gels? Moisturizers? Cleansing regimen & products used? Makeup?
QUESTIONS	**FOR MANAGEMENT**
Daily schedule	Time constraints? Work/school schedule?
Psychosocial	Self-perception? Social withdrawal? Impact on relationships?
Triggers or exacerbating factors	Seasonal variation? Emotional stress? Foods? Topical products?
Other external factors	Sports activities: use of chin straps/padding/sports bras, etc.? Work environment: hot/humid; Chemicals; Protective clothing/masks?
Cost factors	Insurance limitations? Generic vs. brand?

Adapted from Habif 2010.

Diagnostics

Most often, acne is diagnosed clinically without the need for laboratory assistance. On occasion, the onset of acne may be an indicator of a systemic process or endocrine abnormality necessitating additional diagnostics. DHEAS and free testosterone are good initial screening laboratory studies in evaluating hormonal influences. DHEAS is the best index of adrenal androgen activity. If there is a suspicion of precocious puberty, PCOS, or hyperandrogenism, referral to endocrinology is appropriate,

Management

When selecting a treatment approach for the patient, one must consider morphology, distribution, pathogenesis, severity, history, and patient preference. The goals of treatment are normalizing follicular keratinization, reducing sebaceous gland activity, reducing the follicular bacterial colonization, and minimizing inflammation. Treatment should be started early to prevent permanent sequelae. Ongoing maintenance therapy, particularly with a topical retinoid, is the best strategy to combat the likelihood of relapse.

The updated Global Alliance to Improve Outcomes in Acne Group (2009) recommends the first-line treatment for most patients with acne vulgaris should be topical therapy—specifically a topical retinoid plus an antimicrobial agent. This combination targets multiple pathogenic features and treats acne more effectively. As explained in chapter 2, the vehicle chosen for topical treatment will impact the overall effect. It is important to remember that topically applied products are absorbed percutaneously through the body,

therefore may be contraindicated in pregnancy—particularly retinoids (Tables 4-3 to 4-5).

Systemic therapy

Oral antibiotics suppress the growth of cutaneous flora such as *P. acne* and also have an anti-inflammatory effect. They are generally indicated when there is widespread involvement of face, chest, and back or if there is cystic involvement of the face. Long-term use is not recommended; however, at least a 3-month trial must be given before improvement will be seen (Table 4-6).

Hormones

Hormonal therapy may be necessary when the pathogenesis of a patient's acne is heavily influenced by sebum production. Consideration for hormonal therapy must be made on an individual patient bases. And since many of these patients are young adult females, education and counseling for the patients and their parents are very important.

Oral contraceptive pills (OCPs) are used in acne to suppress testosterone production. This can be especially effective in conditions such as PCOS and can reduce the occurrence of acne and excess facial hair. OCPs approved by the Food and Drug Administration (FDA) for the treatment of acne include Ortho Tri-Cyclen (estrogen and norgestimate), Estrostep (estrogen and norethindrone), and Yaz (estrogen and drospirenone).

| **TABLE 4-3** | Acne Vulgaris: Treatment Matrix | | | |

LEVEL OF SEVERITY	FIRST LINE*	ALTERNATIVES*	NO OR LITTLE RESPONSE	EXAMPLE
Mild Open and closed comedones Facial involvement	*Treatment & Maintenance:* topical retinoids			
	Topical retinoids Mild cleanser	Change topical retinoid or d/c and start azelaic acid Consider topical antimicrobial, and/or salicylic acid	Check for adherence Increase to moderate-level therapy Refer to dermatologist for acne surgery, PDT, chemical peels	
Moderate Comedones plus inflammatory papules and pustules Involving face, chest and/or back Scarring on face, chest, or back escalates level of treatment	*Treatment & Maintenance:* topical retinoids and BPO			
	Topical retinoids, BPO *and* topical antibiotics (single agent or combination), *and/or* oral antibiotics	Consider alternative oral antibiotic In females, hormonal assessment, oral contraceptives, spironolactone	Assess in 8–12 wk Check for adherenceIf persistent inflammation, or evidence of scarring, refer to dermatologist for intralesional steroids, microdermabrasion, PDT, chemical peels, and oral isotretinoin	
Severe Comedones, inflammatory papules, pustules, nodules, cysts, and/or scarring	PCP should initiate treatment including topical retinoids, BPO, oral antibiotics, ± oral contraceptives *and* refer to a dermatologist.			

*Refer to Table 4-4 for a list of topical agents.

BPO, benzoyl peroxide; PDT, photodynamic therapy.

Modified from Gollnick, H., Cunliffe, W., Berson, D., Dreno, B., Finlay, A., Leyden, J. J., . . . Global Alliance to Improve Outcomes in Acne. (2003). Management of acne: A report from Global Alliance to Improve Outcomes in Acne. *Journal of the American Academy of Dermatology, 49*(Suppl. 1), S1–S37.

TABLE 4-4	Topical Agents for Management of Acne		
AGENT	**GENERIC/BRAND**	**PREGNANCY CATEGORY**	**COMMENTS**
Cleansers Keratolytic, anti-inflammatory, antimicrobial	Mild cleansers (nonabrasive)		Twice daily For dry/sensitive skin or irritation from treatment Antibacterials are drying
	BPO wash, creamy wash	C	Bleaches fabrics Keratolytic, anti-inflammatory, antimicrobial
	Salicylic acid 2%	C	Keratolytic
Antimicrobials Decreases bacterial count, prevents bacterial resistance, keratolytic, decreases free fatty acids Antimicrobial	BPO 2.5%–10% (OTC and Rx)	C	Daily wash or leave on gel Irritating Possible allergic contact dermatitis Bleaches fabric
	Sodium sulfacetamide (Plexion, Rosaderm)	C	Twice daily wash
	Azaleic acid 15% gel (Finacea) 20% Cream (Azelex) Once daily	B	Good for skin of color Also comedolytic Decreases hyperpigmentation
Antibiotics Anti-inflammatory Antimicrobial Attacks neutrophils to decrease inflammation	*Clindamycin 1% sol, lotion, gel, (Cleocin T, Clindagel, Evoclin)	B	Daily or twice daily Rare pseudomembranous colitis Bacterial resistance
	*Erythromycin 2% (Akne-Mycin Oint, Ery pads, and solution)	B	Daily or twice daily Good for sensitive or dry skin
	Dapsone (Aczone Gel)	C	Twice daily but not at same time as using BPO (orange skin) Decrease inflammation
Retinoids Keratolytic Comedolytic Anti-inflammatory	Tretinoin, c, g, (Retin A, Retin A Micro, Atralin gel 0.05%	C	Irritating, use on dry face Apply small amount at nighttime Start 2–3/wk and slowly increase Use as maintenance
	Adapalene (Differin 0.1%, L,G 0.3% Cream	C	
	Tazarotene (Tazorac 0.1% cream, gel)	X	

*Always use with BPO.
BPO, benzoyl peroxide; OTC, over the counter.

Patients considering oral contraceptive therapy should be cautioned that the FDA has concluded that birth control pills containing drospirenone may have increased risk for blood clots compared to pills containing other progestins. Patients should be assessed for

TABLE 4-5	Topical combination products for acne*	
COMBINATION PRODUCT	**AGENTS**	
Epiduo gel	Adapalene 0.1% and BPO 2.5% gel	
Benzamycin gel†	Erythromycin 3% and BPO 5%	
Duac gel	Clindamycin 1% and BPO 5%	
Ziana	Clindamycin 1.2% and tretinoin 0.025%	
Veltin gel	Clindamycin 1.2% and tretinoin 0.025%	
Acanya	Clindamycin 1.2% and BPO 2.5%	

BPO, benzoyl peroxide.
*All listed agents are pregnancy category C.
†Available as generic

contraindications and risk factors prior to starting therapy. Other forms of contraception, such as Depo Provera injection or the intrauterine device (IUD) known as Mirena, have been shown to worsen acne, although they are excellent mechanisms for pregnancy prevention.

Spironolactone is a potassium-sparing diuretic and selective aldosterone blocker. It is used off label in dermatology to treat acne and hirsutism in adult women. Spironolactone alters androgen receptors and diminishes sebum production, which results in acne improvement.

The best candidates for successful use of spironolactone are women 25 years of age and older whose acne tends to be distributed on the lower face and mandible, and who complain of increased oiliness and facial hair. Spironolactone may be used concomitantly with oral contraceptives, but not with oral contraceptives containing drospirenone. When these agents are taken together, the body does not process potassium correctly and may lead to increased potassium levels. This can cause breathing difficulties, chest pain, slow or irregular heartbeat, confusion, or muscle weakness.

Spironolactone dosing should begin at 25 to 50 mg per day for 1 to 2 months and then follow-up. Serum potassium and blood

TABLE 4-6	Systemic Therapy for Management of Acne		
AGENT	**GENERIC/BRAND**	**PREGNANCY CATEGORY**	**COMMENTS**
Antibiotics (target *P. acnes*); anti-inflammatory, first-line therapy	Tetracycline 250–500 mg Doxycycline 50–100 mg Minocycline 50–100 mg Erythromycin 250–500 mg Sustained release Doxycycline (Oracea) 40 mg	X—not for use in pregnancy	Use with BPO to reduce drug resistance Do not take with calcium GI upset, photosensitivity Birth control failure risk Vaginal candidiasis Daily or twice daily
Antibiotic alternatives (not recommended for routine use)	Bactrim 200 mg	C	Daily or twice daily Use cautiously for severe refractory cases
	Amoxicillin 250–500 mg	C	Daily or twice daily GI symptoms, vaginal candida, hypersensitivity
	Cephalexin 500 mg	C	Twice daily GI upset, vaginal candida, hypersensitivity
Hormones	OCPs Combined estrogen/progesterone most effective	D	Drospirenone-containing OCP very effective for hormonal acne Drospirenone 3 mg = spironolactone 25 mg
	Spironolactone	C	Start 50 mg/day, increase to twice daily, maximum of 200 mg/day Consult if family history includes breast cancer Avoid use with K⁺ sparing diuretics, ACE inhibitors, K⁺ supplements, lithium Caution with use of OCP containing drospirenone, monitor for hyperkalemia
Retinoids	Isotretinoin; refer to dermatologist	X	

BPO, benzoyl peroxide; OCP, oral contraceptive pill.

pressure should be checked in 1 month. The dose may be increased to a maximum of 100 mg b.i.d. and should be maintained for at least 3 to 6 months. If improved, the dose may be tapered to the lowest possible dose that maintains control. Common side effects include breakthrough bleeding or spotting, menstrual irregularities, headaches, diuresis, dizziness, fatigue, potential hyperkalemia, and breast tenderness. Contraindicated in pregnancy, it should only be considered for nonpregnant women in whom androgen-related acne is suspected or for those who have failed other treatment approaches.

Spironolactone has a black-box warning as mandated by FDA because it can cause feminization of the male fetus.

Retinoids
Isotretinoin is an oral retinoid approved for the treatment of severe nodulocystic acne or acne that has been refractory to treatment. The mechanism of action is not completely understood; however, it is known that it results in inhibition of sebaceous gland activity for months to years. Although very efficacious, it is not without consequence. Use of oral isotretinoin is highly teratogenic and a category X medication. Patients should be referred to a dermatologist or an approved IPledge provider.

Adjunct treatments
Light therapy has been gaining acceptance in recent years for treatment of inflammatory acne and has two primary therapeutic goals: decrease in *P. acnes* and alteration of sebaceous gland function. There is still much research to be conducted regarding the best light source, dose, and frequency of use. Among the treatments being offered are intense pulsed light (IPL), pulsed dye laser (PDL), photodynamic therapy (PDT) with or without photosensitizing agents, specific narrowband light, or visible light. Initial research indicates that these options are *best* used in partnership with other traditional medical therapies—or for those who cannot withstand a typical regimen.

Intralesional injections with corticosteroids (ILC) for large stubborn painful cystic lesions can give great relief to the patient and often will achieve resolution of the lesion within 48 hours of injection. Small amounts of triamcinolone (Kenalog 10 mg/mL) diluted 1:1with lidocaine or normal saline is the treatment of choice. It is recommended that this therapy be used by clinicians skilled in intralesional injections. The risks of atrophy and depigmentation should be discussed in detail prior to the procedure.

Prognosis and Complications

Acne is often chronic in nature, and the treatment course is difficult to predict. Most acne regimens require at least 3 months of faithful use to see evidence of improvement. Although acne can be a self-limiting disease of adolescence, it is often a disease of chronicity and can last throughout late adulthood with unpredictable flares, exacerbations, and scarring. Relapse is not uncommon. Associated scarring and postinflammatory hyperpigmentation may be an enduring legacy which can result in psychological distress and comorbidity. The majority of teenage boys can expect clearing of lesions between 20 and 25 years of age. Adult acne occurs more often in women and can last up to and beyond the fourth decade (Burch & Aeling, 2011, p. 169).

Patient Education and Follow-up

The updated Global Alliance to Improve Outcomes in Acne Group (2009) reports that patients with acne exhibit poor adherence to treatment regimens and follow-up appointments, which contributes to treatment failure. The following recommendations are made:

- Focus on counseling and education by the provider or office staff at each follow-up visit.
- Demonstrate how much medication should be used and how it should be applied.
- Inquire regarding failure to use their medications as directed.
- Assess quality of life as it is known to contribute to adherence.
- Assess for possibility of psychiatric comorbidity.
- Consider medication reminders: texts, cell phone alarm.

Complete Blood Count (CBC) and Liver Function Tests (LFTs) may be indicated if the patient has been on an oral antibiotic for a year or more. Providers should inquire about any joint discomfort or lupus-like symptoms especially if they have been on minocycline. Long-term use of minocycline can also result in blue/gray hyperpigmentation that may be mistaken for bruising by the patient.

Referral and Consultation

If a patient has failed to respond after 3 to 6 months of therapy and/or has evidence of scarring, refer to a dermatologist for other treatment considerations.

CLINICAL PEARLS

- Abrupt-onset acne that is monomorphic in nature, uncommonly severe, or unresponsive to treatment should prompt further investigation, as this may indicate an endocrine disorder, drug-related onset, or another problem of a systemic nature. Referral to a dermatologist can be helpful.
- Topical dapsone gel should not be used concurrently with a topical benzoyl peroxide (BPO) as the combination produces an orange tint to the skin.
- At times, it can be difficult to differentiate rosacea from acne. The presence of comedones would favor acne.
- BPO should always be used when a topical or oral antibiotic is prescribed to minimize bacterial resistance.

ROSACEA

According to the National Rosacea Society, it is estimated that over 16 million people are affected by this condition. Erythema, flushing, blushing, and breakouts often lead to decreased self-esteem and self-confidence, which can impact social and professional relationships.

The onset of rosacea is most common in the middle-aged population between the ages of 30 and 50, but has been reported in children and the elderly. Women are reported to be affected at an earlier age, but rosacea is more severe in men, and the rhinophymatous subtype is almost exclusive to men. It is typically found in patients with Celtic ancestry and with an inherited predisposition. It occurs very infrequently in skin of color.

Pathophysiology

The etiology of rosacea is unknown. Some authors suspect that contributing factors include repeated vasodilation, changes in the pilosebaceous structure, and colonization of microbial agents. Some authors suggest that chronic sun exposure can prompt edema, impair lymphatic drainage, and produce the characteristic telangiectasia and skin thickening. Recent research suggests that a complicated interplay of neuroimmune mechanisms, innate immunity, and frequent inflammation arises and can promote fibrosis (Leyden, 2013).

Clinical Presentation

In general, rosacea has a polymorphic presentation which may include facial erythema, flushing and blushing, the appearance of papules and pustules, mild edema, telangiectasias, and occasionally a disseminated violaceous hue. Ocular symptoms such as burning and stinging may occur and are often ignored. Sebaceous hyperplasia may be observed, and skin thickening, particularly of the nose (rhinophyma), can occur. Rosacea often affects the convex surfaces of the face, including the nose, centrofacial area, and forehead. Although less common, it may also be evident on the chin or brow.

Rosacea has been classified into four subtypes. Each subtype has clinical features that predominate and are unique to its category, although some features may overlap. Subtypes include erythematotelangiectatic type (Figure 4-3), papulopustular (Figure 4-4), phymatous (Figure 4-5), and ocular.

DIFFERENTIAL DIAGNOSIS Rosacea

- Acne vulgaris
- Perioral dermatitis
- Keratosis pilaris rubra
- Chronic solar damage
- Seborrheic dermatitis
- Demodex folliculitis

Diagnostics

Diagnostic workup is not typically required for rosacea unless the condition fails to respond to treatment or is progressively worsening despite good adherence to treatment and trigger avoidance.

If symptoms of light-headedness, sweating, or palpitations accompany the typical flushing and blushing of rosacea, then other

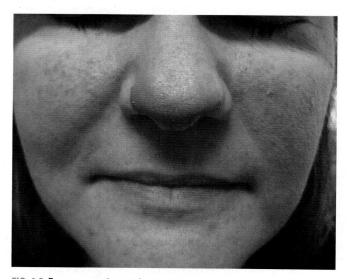

FIG. 4-3. Rosacea, erythematelangectatic type.

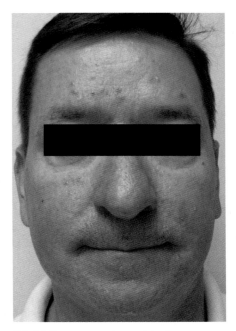

FIG. 4-4. Rosacea, papular-pustular type.

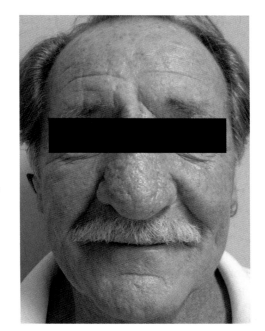

FIG. 4-5. Rosacea rhinophyma.

causes should be suspected such as polycythemia vera, connective tissue disorders (lupus, dermatomyositis), carcinoid syndrome, mastocytosis, and appropriate workup should be performed.

Patients with a suspected diagnosis of rosacea should be questioned as to the presence of eye symptoms such as burning, grittiness, stinging, or itching. Ocular rosacea may exist without significant cutaneous manifestations, and a referral to ophthalmology may be warranted.

Management

Management of rosacea is driven by the subtype and level of severity (Table 4-7). There is global agreement on the need for the following:

- *Photoprotection* for all subtypes: a broad-spectrum UVA/UVB sunscreen should be applied daily at appropriate intervals, depending on outdoor exposure and activities.

TABLE 4-7 Treatment of Rosacea by Subtype

ROSACEA SUBTYPE			
ERYTHROTELANGIECTATIC	**PAPULAR/PUSTULAR**	**PHYMATOUS**	**OCULAR**
Presents as red facial skin/telangiectasias flushing and blushing	Papules and pustules scattered on a background of central facial erythema	Papular fibrotic cobblestone appearing	Red-rimmed eyes; gritty; burning; itchy
Camouflage green-based makeup Topical alpha-2 agonist brimonidine (Mirvaso) daily Laser treatment Avoid vasodilatory medications. β-blockers may be utilized to avoid flushing.	Topical metronidazole cream/lotion/gel (MetroGel or Noritate) 1–2 × daily Topical azelaic acid (Finacea 15% or Azelex 20%) 1 to 2 × daily Topical sulfacetimide/sulfur (Ovace) Doxycycline 20–50 mg b.i.d.; Doxycycline, minocycline 100 mg b.i.d. Tetracycline 500 mg b.i.d. Erythromycin 500 mg b.i.d. if others contraindicated. OCPs may be helpful in those who report cyclical flares. Oral isotretinoin for severe disease. Referral to dermatologist if no improvement with 3 months of topical and oral antibiotic therapy.	If early in disease, oral isotretinoin may be helpful CO$_2$, pulse dye or ablative laser Loop cautery Referral to dermatology for all of the above	Eyelid hygiene essential Eyewash Oral antibiotics Doxycycline Tetracycline Referral to ophthalmologist if not improving

NOTE: Universal recommendations: Daily sunscreen SPF 30–50; mild nonirritating cleaners & moisturizers; trigger avoidance

- *Trigger avoidance*: The list of potential triggers is extensive, but also unique to the individual. The most common triggers provided by the National Rosacea Society include food, alcoholic beverages, skin care products (astringents, exfoliants), emotional influences, health conditions, types of physical exertion, and temperature- or weather-related factors. Topical products reported to be sources of irritation are alcohol, witch hazel, fragrance, menthol, peppermint, and eucalyptus oil.
- *Demodex eradication*: It has been achieved with use of permethrin cream, lindane, BPO, or sulfur-based lotions, and is a promising area of clinical trials.

Referral and Consultation

If a systemic cause such as lupus is suspected, further referral to a rheumatologist is suggested. An ophthalmology consult is warranted if the patient is symptomatic.

Special Considerations

Pediatrics. Rosacea has been observed in the pediatric population. Tetracycline products should not be prescribed to children 8 years of age and under. Erythromycin would be an alternative solution, and topical treatment should be attempted first.

Mature patients. The diagnosis should not be ruled out because of age. It is important to remember that when treating an older patient, tetracycline products can alter coumadin levels and the patient's primary care physician should be notified should this be a concern.

Prognosis and Complications

It is important to emphasize to the patient the benign nature of the condition and also set realistic expectations. There is no cure for rosacea. It is a disease of chronicity that tends to have periods of remission and relapse.

CLINICAL PEARLS

- It is of critical importance not to overlook the possibility of HIV or AIDS, which may present as a papulopustular eruption of the face in early adulthood. Rosacea is seen more frequently in the latter decades of life.
- The characteristic feature, or negative finding, in all forms of rosacea is the absence of comedones, a hallmark sign of acne vulgaris. Although acne and rosacea can coexist, the absence of comedones is more suggestive of rosacea.

PERIORAL DERMATITIS

Perioral dermatitis (more accurately named as periorificial dermatitis) is a common problem most often affecting young women between the ages of 15 and 35. Initially, it was thought to be related to the use of topical corticosteroids on the facial skin. However in recent years, the use of occlusive moisturizers and foundation makeup has been implicated as the etiology, especially in those individuals with no history of topical corticosteroid use. It is not exclusive to the female population and has been identified in children between the ages of 7 months and 13 years with no gender favored. Other suspected causes include candida, *Demodex* mites, topical or inhaled fluorinated corticosteroids, toothpaste, and lip licking. Some authorities argue that it may be a subtype of rosacea or seborrheic dermatitis. Those who suffer from perioral dermatitis are also known

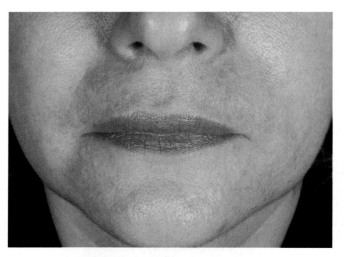

FIG. 4-6. Perioral dermatitis.

to have an increased incidence of atopy (Schalock, 2007). Often patients suffering from this problem complain of skin sensitivity, a burning sensation, and intolerance to heat, water, or cosmetics at affected sites. Pruritus is not an associated symptom.

Clinical Presentation

The appearance of this entity is usually distinctive. Lesions are described as tiny pink discrete and coalescing papules accompanied by scale and clustered around the mouth, nose, or eyes (Figure 4-6). It is usually symmetric in distribution, but can be unilateral. Some authors have described the appearance of perioral dermatitis as looking like acne superimposed on eczema. There is often an area of sparing between the vermillion border and involved skin. Comedones are not present. Typically, the onset is abrupt, and lesions are at the same stage of development. This is in contrast to rosacea, which occurs on the convex surfaces of the face and has lesions which are less homogenous in their stage of development.

DIFFERENTIAL DIAGNOSIS Perioral dermatitis

- Acne
- Rosacea
- Seborrheic dermatitis
- Irritant or allergic contact dermatitis (cinnamon products)
- Gram-negative folliculitis
- Angular cheilitis
- Liplicking dermatitis

Management

Treatment involves discontinuation of any topical corticosteroids or occlusive moisturizers and foundation makeup. Rebound flare can occur upon withdrawal of topical corticosteroids, and patients should be forewarned of this possibility. First-line therapies include a course of oral antibiotics such as Tetracycline or Doxycycline 100 b.i.d. for 4 to 6 weeks and then tapered in the last 2 to 4 weeks of therapy. A topical agent such as metronidazole 0.75% cream or azelaic acid 15% gel twice daily can also be used alone or in combination with the oral agents. Pediatric patients can use topical erythromycin 2%.

Prognosis

The prognosis is favorable, and clearance should be achieved within weeks of treatment with full resolution expected within months. Some individuals have a propensity for recurrences often on an annual basis; most patients experience the problem just once.

HIDRADENITIS SUPPURATIVA (HS)

HS, also known as *acne inversa*, is a persistent disease which most often has its onset after puberty, with the mean age of 38 years. Onset after menopause is rare. Approximately 1% of the population is reported to have HS, but the majority of those individuals will have a form that is less severe. Women are afflicted at least three times more than men; however, men are prone to have a more severe form such as perianal HS. Although there is no evidence to confirm this, there appears to be a higher incidence in African Americans. There is no definitive cause for HS, but there has been a strong association noted between family history, obesity, cigarette smoking, as well as mechanical stress (friction, pressure), and certain drugs (lithium). Common comorbidities or associated diseases include acne vulgaris, acne conglobata, anemia, dissecting cellulitis of the scalp, Crohn disease, and pilonidal cysts.

Pathophysiology

Originally, in 1854, Verneuil believed that HS was a result of apocrine gland dysfunction, but current research has identified blockage of the follicular structure with ensuing rupture of the follicle as the origin of the disorder. Once the follicle bursts, the products of the follicle, including keratin and bacteria, are released into nearby dermis. This process initiates an inflammatory, chemotactic response and results in the development of abscesses and the formation of sinus tracts and scarring.

There is a subtype of HS that is familial in nature and has an autosomal dominant transmission. Among such patients, there have been reports that 34% of those individuals had a first-degree relative with HS. Both males and females appeared to be equally affected. There has been speculation as to whether HS in women is prompted by hyperandrogenism; however, conflicting data have rendered the theory inconclusive.

Clinical Presentation

The most frequent anatomical site for HS is the axillae, but lesions can also occur in the perineum, inframammary area, inguinal folds, medial thighs, nape of the neck, and retroauricular and anogenital areas. In obese patients, lesions often arise in skin folds of the trunk and extremities. New or acute HS is tender (if not painful), red, indurated, and round nodules, as opposed to furuncles, which can have a pointed top and are not symmetrically placed. One of the hallmark signs are the double comedones which communicate under the skin and are distributed in a cord-like or linear manner in the flexural regions.

HS can present as a range of symptoms as well as acute and chronic disease states. One of the most practical approaches to assessment is the use of the Hurley staging system, which can also guide the management of the disease. Depending on the stage and severity, there can be a large range of HS symptoms. Atrophic skin, scar formation, deep sinus tracts, and unwieldy abscesses may all be present. Purulent drainage, active weeping, signs of secondary bacterial infection, and odor may be evident. If there are lesions near the anus, disorders such as Crohn's and fistulas should be suspected.

DIFFERENTIAL DIAGNOSIS Hidradenitis suppurativa

- Abscesses
- Furuncles/carbuncles
- Ruptured epidermal inclusion cyst
- Infected Bartholin cyst
- Cat scratch disease
- Lymphogranuloma venereum
- Lymphadenitis
- Crohn disease

Diagnostics

HS is a clinical diagnosis and cannot be confirmed by biopsy. Although HS lesions are usually sterile, a culture (ideally from wound aspirate) should be performed if a secondary infection is suspected. Occasionally, tissue cultures are obtained for bacterial, fungal, and mycobacterial infections. Patients with a history of Crohn disease or gastrointestinal symptoms should have a biopsy and have further GI evaluation.

A diagnosis of HS is made in the presence of key characteristic findings. *Typical lesions* that are red, painful papules, nodules, and abscesses; cord-like scarring; and double open comedones. A *characteristic distribution* common in the axillae, groin, medial thighs, and anogenital region, less commonly in the breasts, perianal and perineal areas *plus* a *recurrent pattern* of disease since the age of 10 years, including the presence of one active lesion in the axillae or groin, and a history of at least three draining lesions of those areas. If the disease is not active (no active lesions), the patient should have a history of five or more painful and draining lesions from the axillae or groin.

Management

The initial approach for any patient with HS should be to minimize contributing factors, especially smoking cessation and weight loss. Management of disease should be guided by the severity or Hurley stage system (Figure 4-7A–D). Primary care clinicians can usually manage treatment of Hurley stage I HS with oral tetracyclines. Their effectiveness is attributed mostly to the anti-inflammatory action. Since tetracycline is not available, doxycycline 100 mg b.i.d. or minocycline 100 mg bi.d. should be prescribed and continued for 3 to 6 months. Topical clindamycin 1% b.i.d. can also be used as monotherapy or in combination with systemic therapy.

In addition to antimicrobials, cleansers such as chlorhexidine can be used to prevent secondary infection (Table 4-8). Topical tretinoin 0.05% cream has been used to keep the follicles clear but may cause irritation. Most nodules will resolve spontaneously, but occasionally large, fluctuant cysts, or abscesses may require incision and drainage followed by topical compresses with Domeboro solution. Silver-impregnated dressings are used for drainage, while charcoal-impregnated dressings help to control odor. Smaller cysts can be treated with intralesional injections of triamcinolone (Kenalog) 10 mg per mL diluted 1:1 with lidocaine or normal saline.

HS lesions that do not respond after 3 months of therapy or patients who have more advanced disease with scarring (Hurley stage II or III) should be referred to a dermatology for more aggressive management. Pharmacologic management options by experienced dermatology clinicians include metformin, dapsone, isotretinoin or acitretin, and finasteride. Immunosuppressive agents used include prednisone or cyclosporine for short-term therapy of flare or mycophenolate mofetil for longer term suppression.

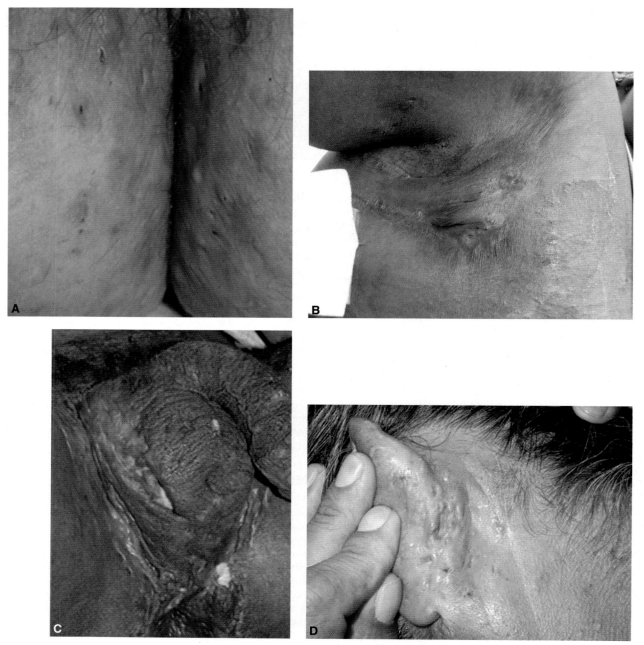

FIG. 4-7. A: Hidradenitis suppurativa, Hurley stage I. Hidradenitis suppurativa can be distinguished from furunculosis by the presence of comedones that may be subtle or marked, as well as poor response to antibiotics, and nondiagnostic cultures. **B:** Hidradenitis suppurativa, Hurley stage II, showing recurrent abscesses with sinus tracts and scarring: single or multiple widely separated lesions. **C:** Hidradenitis suppurativa, Hurley stage III, occurring in the anogenital area can be extremely difficult to manage and a poorer prognosis. It produces mutilating scarring, and the ongoing inflammation should be monitored for malignant transformation. **D:** Hidradenitis suppurativa can occur in the postauricular area.

There are some reports that TNF-α inhibitors—infliximab and etanercept—have been effective, but studies regarding the long-term risk of these drugs for use in HS patients has not been established. Treatment with neurotoxins, radiotherapy, cryotherapy, PDT, and nonablative radiofrequency have reported some effectiveness in a limited number of cases and warrant further evaluation.

Lastly, HS patients with intractable or extensive disease may require wide excision. Despite the risk of recurrence and operative complications, most people report a significant improvement in their quality of life after surgery. Surgical excision with split-thickness grafts for closure has the lowest recurrence rates, probably attributed to extensive tissue excisions. The success of surgical excision is also dependent on the location and severity of the HS. Patients should be warned regarding possible slow healing by secondary intention or delayed healing.

Prognosis and Complications

HS is a chronic skin disease that can result in significant morbidity depending on the level of severity and can progressively

| TABLE 4-8 | Therapeutic Treatment Options for Hidradenitis Suppurativa Based on Hurley Stages |

HURLEY STAGE	EXTENT OF DISEASE IN TISSUE	TREATMENT OPTIONS*	THERAPEUTICS & PATIENT EDUCATION
I	Abscess formation (single or multiple) without sinus tracts and scarring	Oral or topical antibiotics for 3–6 mo Injectable corticosteroids (limited number of lesions) Hormonal therapy Topical retinoids Zinc Cryotherapy Local incision and draining	Stop smoking Avoid friction or tight-fitting clothes Local hygiene Weight loss Avoid mechanical or chemical irritation (i.e., shaving) Avoid follicular occlusion—deodorants or antiperspirants Warm compresses incl. Burow's solution
II	One or more widely separated recurrent abscesses with tract formation and scars	**Above plus:** Referral to dermatology Immunosuppressive therapy Nonnarcotic analgesic Limited excisions CO_2 laser ablation	
III	Multiple interconnected tracts, scar and abscesses throughout an entire area	**Above plus:** Radiation therapy Wide excision	

*Regardless of the stage, some therapies require an experienced dermatology provider for adequate and safe treatment.

worsen over time. The disease can be painfully debilitating. There is no cure for HS, although surgical excision offers the greatest resolution for problematic lesions. Due to constant and repeated scarring, there is a four to five times greater risk of developing cutaneous squamous cell carcinoma and a 50-fold risk in general for increased malignancy. In particular, buccal cancer and primary liver cancer are found to be more common in HS patients. This may be due to the high prevalence of smoking and alcohol abuse among this population so the data may be skewed. Additionally, contractures, strictures, and infection are not uncommon for HS patients. Anal fistulas are seen with perianal HS because of recurrent abscesses.

Clinicians should be keenly aware of the psychosocial impact of HS. Odor and drainage may prevent patients from establishing intimate relationships. The quality of life for an HS patient is comparable to that of patients with moderate to severe psoriasis. The economic impact may be significant because of missed days of work, medical bills, or depression from the disease. Patients with moderate or severe HS should be screened for depression.

Referral and Consultation

The importance of early referral of severe HS patients to a dermatologist cannot be overemphasized. Aggressive treatment with multiple modalities, instituted before extensive scarring occurs, offers the patient reduced risk of morbidity. Consultation with radiation therapy and plastic surgery may be necessary.

Patient Education and Follow-up

It is extremely important to dispel the notion that HS is the result of poor hygiene. The malodorous drainage may lead to this misinterpretation and further humiliation. Education regarding lifestyle modifications is essential to reduce flares or progression of the disease. Patient support groups may be helpful.

ACNE KELOIDALIS NUCHAE

Acne keloidalis nuchae (AKN) is a misleading term originally used by Bazin in 1872 for an entity now known to be unrelated to the pathogenesis of acne vulgaris. Although the etiology remains elusive, it is a disorder that most often presents on the occiput, posterior hairline, and neck with discrete papules which may coalesce into thick hypertrophic plaques. The term *nuchae* is not accurate as it can occur on other parts of the scalp, including the vertex. The patient population most affected is African American males and occasionally African American females. In fact, AKN is reported to comprise 0.5% of all cutaneous diagnoses in Blacks. There has been evidence in the literature of AKN arising in Asian and Hispanic individuals. It is rare in Caucasians, and the male to female incidence is 20:1. It generally begins in adolescence or early adulthood and rarely begins after age 50.

Pathophysiology

Initially, AKN was postulated to be an inflammatory, follicle-based process akin to folliculitis or pseudofolliculitis barbae (PFB). However, this theory has been disproven, and experts now classify AKN as a primary form of cicatricial alopecia.

Some experts believe that frequent aggravation from rough curly hairs in the skin prompts an inflammatory process and subsequent development of lesions. It is known that chronic rubbing from shirt collars, football helmets and close shaving all make acne keloidalis worse. This may be consistent with the hypothesis that chronic irritation may initiate the inflammatory process and possibly explains the emergence of small papules; however, it does not account for the development of a scarring alopecia that worsens over time with some patients. In addition to chronic irritation, other inciting factors have been proposed and include an innocuous chronic bacterial infection, frequent haircuts, curvature of the hair follicles, altered immune process, or increased mast cells in localized areas of the scalp.

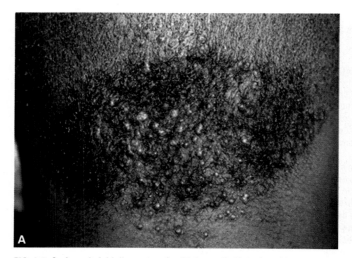
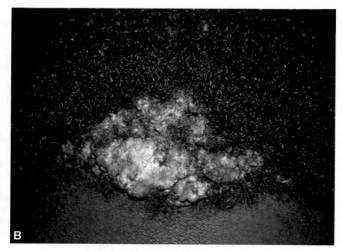

FIG. 4-8. A: Acne keloidalis nuchae (multiple small skin colored hypertrophic papules on the lower scalp and neck). **B:** As acne keloidalis progresses, papules coalesce into plaques with potential to keloid.

Clinical Presentation

AKN can be asymptomatic or pruritic and irritating. Some patients will describe a burning sensation. Its appearance depends on the progression of disease. Early findings may include discrete and coalescing follicular papules and some pustules (Figure 4-8A). Eventually, these may transform into fibrotic, hypertrophic papules and keloidal plaques in advanced disease (Figure 4-8B). Secondary erosions from picking or crust from secondary infection would not be a surprising finding. Comedones are typically not a feature consistent with AKN.

DIFFERENTIAL DIAGNOSIS Acne kelodalis nuchae

- Folliculitis decalvans
- Acne necrotica
- Dissecting folliculitis
- Bacterial, fungal, or viral folliculitis

Diagnostics

AKN is a diagnosis that is made clinically; however, if there is a suspicion of scarring alopecia, biopsy would be recommended. On histologic examination, an inflammatory process, fibroplasia, and vanishing of the sebaceous glands have been observed.

If lesions are weeping or crusted, samples should be taken for culture and sensitivities to rule out a rare occurrence of bacterial or fungal etiology. Other diagnoses should be considered if lesions arise in an unexpected age range or in women.

Management

There is universal agreement that early treatment has the greatest likelihood of ameliorating the problem and disrupting the progression of disease. The goals for treatment include avoidance of exacerbating factors and triggers, arresting disease progression by treating any possible infection, and relieving symptoms (Table 4-9).

Special Considerations

An association of AKN with metabolic syndrome and truncal obesity has been observed in some patients. Thus far, this has not been proven to be a causative factor, and more research is required.

TABLE 4-9	Treatment Options for Acne Keloidalis Nuchae
TREATMENT OPTION	**SUMMARY OF TREATMENT APPROACHES**
Trigger avoidance	Refrain from close shaves, or haircuts, use of tight-fitting or chafing collars, baseball caps, helmets, or sports garments which could cause mechanical irritation to neck or scalp
Topical products	OTC povidone iodine shampoo Topical clindamycin solution 1% b.i.d. Topical mupirocin 2% b.i.d., Clobetasol 0.05% solution b.i.d. for 8 wk, followed by betamethasone valerate 0.02% for 4 wk Tretinoin 0.1% gel at bedtime Tazarotene gel 0.05% or 0.1% at bedtime
Oral products	Doxycycline 100 mg b.i.d. × 2–3 mo Minocycline 50–100 mg b.i.d. × 2–3 mo, then reevaluate
Intralesional injections	Triamcinolone acetonide (Kenalog) 10–40 mg/mL dilute with lidocaine or normal saline Repeat in 6 weeks if needed
Surgical intervention	Deep excision for advanced disease CO_2 laser ablation with primary intention Refer to dermatology surgery
Other modalities	Punch excision, elliptical excision; Liquid nitrogen can cause hypopigmentation and discomfort
Preventive measures	Laser hair removal of unaffected sites with Nd: YAG laser for prevention Refer to dermatologist

Prognosis and Complications

Prognosis for AKN is good if treated early. Treatment is far more difficult and less responsive once scarring occurs. Consequences of progressively worsening disease may include keloid formation, scarring alopecia, chronic discharge, and vulnerability to repeated episodes of secondary infection.

Referral and Consultation

Referral to a dermatology provider should be initiated if there is evidence of scarring, progressive worsening of the condition, or infection.

PSEUDOFOLLICULITIS BARBAE

Despite the similar clinical appearance, PFB is unrelated to the pathogenesis of acne vulgaris. Essentially the outbreaks are a result of a foreign body reaction and a resulting inflammatory process. It is a disorder most associated with the unique features of hair follicle curvature inherited in certain ethnicities. There is a prevalence of 40% to 80% reported in African American males. Hirsute women of color and women who have attempted facial hair removal have also been reported. This condition is typically only found in 3% to 5% of white males who shave. A common contributing factor is frequent shaving and improper shaving technique. Use of depilatories may also aggravate the situation. This is a significant problem in men whose occupation requires them to have a clean-shaven facial appearance, such as in the military.

Pathophysiology

During shaving, tightly curled hair is transected in a somewhat diagonal fashion, which results in a pointed tip at the distal end. This hair then curls back, piercing and reentering the skin a few millimeters from the original follicular opening, causing subsequent inflammation. Certain ethnicities are genetically predisposed because of the unique cellular composition of the hair follicle (Figure 4-9).

Clinical Presentation

Patients typically report painful lesions localized to the beard and neck. This condition presents as skin-colored or erythematous, folliculocentric papules or pustules on the lower face, jaw, chin, and neck. Abscesses or larger clusters of pustules may arise in secondarily infected skin (Figure 4-10).

DIFFERENTIAL DIAGNOSIS Pseudofolliculitis barbae
• Acne vulgaris
• Folliculitis
• Tinea barbae
• Sarcoidosis

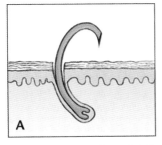 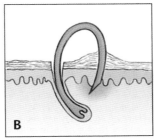 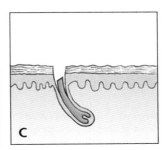 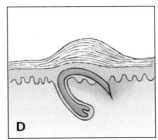

FIG. 4-9. Pathophysiology of pseudofolliculitis barbae. **A:** Curly hair grows from a sharply curved hair root. When shaved, the hair is left with a sharp point. As this hair grows, the sharp tip curves back and pierces the skin. **B:** The sharpened hair penetrates the skin. **C and D:** When hairs are cut too closely, they can penetrate the side of the hair root. Both types of follicular reentry cause a foreign body–like reaction (papule).

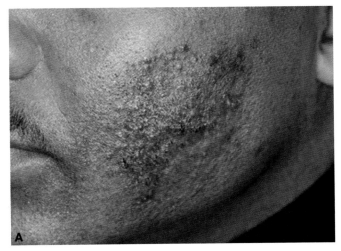 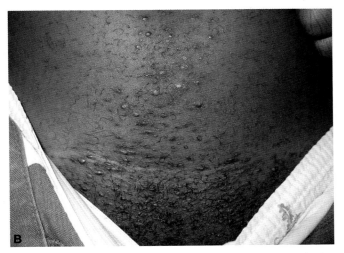

FIG. 4-10. **A:** Pseudofolliculitis barbae occurring locally on the face and beard. **B:** Pseudofolliculitis barbae can occur in other hair-bearing areas, including the abdominal and pubic regions as shown.

Diagnostics

Any clinical findings suggestive of secondary bacterial infection should be swabbed for culture and sensitivity. Likewise, if a fungal etiology is among diagnostic considerations, KOH test can be performed on contents of a pustule. Hairs may also be plucked and plated for fungal culture.

A skin biopsy may reveal fungal elements as well. Any suspicion of sarcoidosis should be confirmed by biopsy.

Management

PFB is a chronic condition whose symptoms can be remedied by permitting the hair to grow out at the affected site. However, this is an impractical solution for many patients. Topical corticosteroids are efficacious in reducing inflammation, but cannot be used for long periods on the face. Topical and oral antibiotics may reduce the inflammatory process as well as combat any suggestion of secondary infection. Topical retinoids, such as tretinoin cream 0.05%, have demonstrated benefit in some early cases. An alternative approach is complete destruction of the hair follicle with laser therapy or electrolysis. Research has shown promising outcomes by pretreating the area with topical eflornithine hydrochloride before standard laser hair removal. Unfortunately, permanent hair removal is not always affordable.

Special Considerations

There is a variant of PFB called pseudofolliculitis pubis, which may occur when the pubic area is shaved. This subset affects both men and women. While PFB is infrequently found in Caucasians, it is reported to be common in Caucasian renal transplant recipients.

Prognosis and Complication

Patients must utilize management strategies to reduce discomfort, inflammation, and potential infection. Postinflammatory hyperpigmentation, scarring, and keloid formation may arise in those who have chronic outbreaks or in patients not appropriately treated.

Referral and Consultation

Referral should be initiated if there is any evidence of early scarring, postinflammatory hyperpigmentation, secondary infection, or keloid formation.

Patient Education and Follow-up

In addition to allowing the hair to grow out, patients should be educated about shaving techniques and facial skin care (Box 4-1). Electric shavers or razors limited to one or two blades may reduce the severity.

BILLING CODES ICD-10

Acne	L70.0
Acne, keloid	L73.0
Herpes simplex	L73.2
Perioral dermatitis	L71.0
Pseudofolliculitis barbae	L73.1
Rosacea, unspecified	L71.9
Rosacea/perioral dermatitis	L71.0

BOX 4-1 **Patient Education: Pseudofolliculitis Barbae**

General principles

Refrain from pulling the skin tightly.
Shave *with* the direction of the hair, not against it.
Use fresh, sharp razors.
Shave with short brief strokes and *do not* shave the same area repeatedly.
A routine with daily shaving has been shown to diminish the severity of pseudofolliculitis barbae.
Completely abandoning shaving can resolve the problem, but is not optional for many people.

Technique

1. Eliminate observable hairs with electric clippers. Leave 1- to 2- mm residual stubble.
2. Cleanse affected site with a gentle acne soap and textured face cloth. If ingrown hairs are observed, use a toothbrush in a circular motion to dislodge the embedded hairs.
3. Remove soap, then use face cloth and warm water to apply a compress for several minutes before shaving.
4. Lather involved skin with favorite shaving cream and massage into affected site.
5. Before the cream dries, begin shaving *with* the grain, *not* against it. Refrain from applying tension.
6. Rinse the area thoroughly with water. Apply an aftershave preparation or lotion which is comforting. Use topical corticosteroids only as directed by your provider's instructions.

READINGS

Alikhan, A., Lynch, P., & Eisen, D. (2009, April). Hidradenitis suppurativa: A comprehensive review. *Journal of the American Academy of Dermatology, 60,* 539–561.

Batra, R. S. (2007). Acne. In K. Arndt, & J. Hsu (Eds.), *Manual of dermatologic therapies* (7th ed., pp. 3–18). Philadelphia, PA: Lippincott Williams & Wilkins.

Blair, G. S., & Allie, N. D. (2011). Spironolactone use for women with acne or hirsutism. *Journal of the Dermatology Nurses' Association, 3,* 374–376.

Burch, J. M., & Aeling, J. L. (2011). Acne and acneiform eruptions. In J. E. Fitzpatrick, & J. G. Morelli (Eds.), *Dermatology secrets plus* (4th ed., pp. 148–155). Philadelphia, PA: Elsevier Mosby.

Cosmatos, I., Matcho, A., Weinstein, R., Montgomery, M., & Stang, P. (2013, March). Analysis of patient claims data to determine the prevalence of hidradenitis suppurativa in the United States. *Journal of the American Academy of Dermatology, 68,* 412–419.

Fu, L. W., & Vender, R. B. (2011). Newer approaches in topical combination therapy for acne. *Skin Therapy Letter, 16*(9), 3–6.

Habif, T. F. (2010). Hair diseases. In *Clinical dermatology* (5th ed., p. 355, 942). China: Elsevier.

Habif, T. P. (2004). *Clinical dermatology: A color guide to diagnosis and therapy* (4th ed.). Philadelphia, PA: Mosby.

Habif, T. P., Campbell, J. L., Chapman, M. S., Dinulos, J. G., & Zug, K. A. (2011). *Skin disease: Diagnosis & treatment* (3rd ed.). China: Elsevier Saunders.

James, W. D., Berger, T. G., & Elston, D. M. (2011). Acne. In *Andrew's diseases of the skin: Clinical dermatology* (11th ed., pp. 228–246). China: Elsevier Saunders.

Letada, P. R. (2012). *Acne keloidalis nuchae.* Retrieved from http://emedicine. medscape.com/article/1072149-overview

Leyden, J. (2013). The evolving view of rosacea. *Journal of the American Academy of Dermatology, 69,* S1.

McMichael, A., Curtis, A. R., Guzman-Sanchez, D., & Kelly, A. P. (2012). Folliculitis and other follicular disorders. In J. L. Bolognia, J. L. Jorizzo, & J. V. Schaffer (Eds.), *Dermatology* (3rd ed., pp. 571–585). China: Elsevier.

Piggott, C. D., & Eichenfeld, L. F. (2010). Overcoming the challenges of pediatric acne. Retrieved from http://bmctoday.net/practical dermatology

Schalock, P. C. (2007). Rosacea and perioral (periorificial) dermatitis. In K. A. Arndt, & J. T. Hsu (Eds.), *Manual of dermatologic therapeutics* (7th ed., pp. 174–179). Phildelphia, PA: Lippincott, Williams & Wilkins.

Sperling, L. C., Sinclair, R. D., & Shabrawl Cohen, L. E. (2012). Cicatricial alopecias. In J. L. Bolognia, J. L. Jorizzo, & J. V. Schaeffer (Eds.), *Dermatology* (3rd ed., pp. 1104). China: Elsevier.

Stein Gold, L. F. (2013, June). What's new in acne and inflammation? *Journal of Drugs in Dermatology, 12,* S67–S69

Sterling, J. B., Sina, B., Gaspare, A., & Deng, A. (2007, April). Acne keloidalis: A novel presentation for tinea capitis. *Journal of the American Academy of Dermatology, 56,* 699–701.

Stern, R. S. (1996). Managed care and the treatment of skin diseases: Dermatologists do it less often. *Archives of Dermatology, 132,* 1039–1142.

Thiboutot, D., Gollnick, H., Bettoli, V., Dreno, B., Kang, S., Leyden, J.,… Global Alliance to Improve Outcomes in Acne. (2009, May). New insights into the management of acne: An update from the Global Alliance to Improve Outcomes in Acne Group. *Journal of the American Academy of Dermatology, 60*(Suppl. 5), S1–50.

Thomas, D. R. (2004). Psychsocial effects of acne. *Journal of Cutaneous Medical Surgery, 8,* 3–5.

Verma, S., & Wollina, V. (2010, December). Acne keloidalis nuchae: Another cutaneous symptom of metabolic syndrome, truncal obesity and impending/overt diabetes mellitus? *American Journal of Clinical Dermatology, 11*(6), 433–436.

Villasenor, J., & Kroshinsky, D. (2011). Acne and Related Disorders. In P. C. Schalock, J. T. Hsu, & K. A. Arndt (Eds.), *Lippincott's Primary Care Dermatology* (pp. 50–67). China: Lippincott Williams & Wilkins.

Xin, Y., Cho, S., Howard, R., & Maggio, K. (2012, October). Topical eflornithine hydrochloride improves the effectiveness of standard laser hair removal for treating pseudo folliculitis barbae: A randomized, double blinded, placebo controlled trial. *Journal of the American Academy of Dermatology, 67,* 694–699.

Zaenglein, A. L., Graber, E. M., & Thiboutot, D. M. (2012). Acne vulgaris and acneiform eruptions. In L. A. Goldsmith, S. I. Katz, B. A. Gilchrest, A. S. Paller, D. J. Leffell, & K. Wolff (Eds.), *Fitzpatrick's dermatology in primary care* (8th ed., pp. 897–917). Philadelphia, PA: Elsevier.

Zaenglein, A. L., & Thiboutot, D. M. (2012). Adnexal Diseases: Acne Vulgaris. In J. L. Bolognia, J. L. Jorizzo, & J. V. Schaeffer (Eds.), *Dermatology* (3rd ed., pp. 545–559). China: Elsevier Saunders.

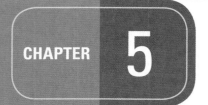
Papulosquamous Disorders

Lakshi M. Aldredge and Jane Tallent

PSORIASIS

Psoriasis is an autoimmune skin condition that affects 2% to 5% of the world population. There is no race that is spared from this disease, although there is a lower incidence in African Americans for unknown reasons. It is equally present among males and females, and onset can occur at any age; however, it is most likely to appear between the ages of 15 and 30 years. Approximately one third of patients with psoriasis have a first-degree relative affected with the disease, and most experts agree that there is strong evidence to demonstrate a genetic family link.

Medications such as β-blockers, lithium, and antimalarials have been associated with inducing psoriasis. Emotional stress, streptococcal and other bacterial infections, and viral infections, such as HIV, can initiate psoriasis as well as inducing flares of the disease. Interestingly, psoriasis has also been triggered by surgery or trauma, with the resulting initial plaque occurring directly over the injury or incision (Koebner phenomenon).

Pathophysiology

The exact cause of psoriasis and psoriatic disease is unknown. It is an immune-mediated disease that can be triggered by medical, emotional, and environmental factors, although in many cases, the sudden onset of disease has no precipitating factors. Being a T-cell-mediated condition, the immune system is thrust into "hyper drive" and a cascade of cytokine-driven sequences occur, which signal increased skin cell production and angiogenesis. In the past two decades, immunological research has demonstrated that specific cytokines, such as TNF-α and interleukins (IL) 12 and 23, as well as numerous other immune mediators, are key players in the development and progression of psoriatic disease.

Clinical Presentation

Cutaneous symptoms of psoriasis can occur in several forms and is subsequently named based upon clinical presentation.

Plaque psoriasis

The thick, red plaques of classic *plaque psoriasis* affect approximately 80% to 90% of patients. Plaques can range from a violaceous red to pinkish red which may be covered with a thin or thick adherent silvery scale. Lesions have well-demarcated borders and occur anywhere on the body, but typically favor the scalp and extensor surfaces of the knees and elbows (Figure 5-1). This is compared to eczema, which favors flexural surfaces and is typically not well-demarcated. Removal of scale from a psoriasis plaque will reveal punctate blood vessels that bleed (*Auspitz* sign) and aid in the clinical diagnosis of psoriasis. The severity of disease can range from limited scalp involvement (mild disease) to widespread or severe disease involving greater than 5% of the body surface area (Figure 5-2).

Scalp psoriasis

Scalp psoriasis, which often appears as a "cap" of thick, silvery, adherent scale on an erythematous (even violaceous) base, can be a very challenging form of psoriasis and is often mistaken for seborrhea or seborrheic dermatitis (SD) (Figure 5-3). Scalp psoriasis can be a particularly distressing manifestation for patients due to the visibility of the plaques, the significant pruritus, and the extensive scaling that sheds on clothing.

Palmoplantar psoriasis

Psoriasis can be localized on the palms and/or soles in a condition known as *palmoplantar psoriasis*. Lesions can present as erythematous papules, patches, deep-seated vesicles, and pustules. Fissures can form on the palms and fingers, along with dystrophic nail changes. Because of the pustular nature of this type of psoriasis, many providers may conclude that it is a bacterial or viral infection; however, culture of these sterile papules does not reveal any microorganisms.

Guttate psoriasis

Guttate psoriasis occurs in 2% of patients with psoriasis who are usually younger than 30 years, and is characterized by round 1- to 10-mm, salmon-pink papules ("dew-drops") with a fine white scale (Figure 5-4). In many cases, it is preceded by a streptococcal throat (strep throat) or sinus infection; however, the pathophysiologic association between the infection and disease is not clearly understood.

Inverse psoriasis

Psoriasis that occurs in the intertriginous areas of the skin is called *inverse psoriasis* and is often mistaken for a fungal or candidal infection. These conditions can present as thin, erythematous, shiny patches with little to no scale. The folds of the axillae, groin, and intergluteal, and inframammary areas are the most common locations. It is not unusual for patients to be treated with topical antifungals for months before making the diagnosis of inverse psoriasis.

Erythrodermic psoriasis

A more severe form of psoriasis which presents with full-body (>90% BSA) erythema and scaling is referred to as *erythroderma* (Figure 5-5). This condition may be triggered by environmental factors or as a response to medication. Interestingly, patients with plaque psoriasis who may be treated with systemic corticosteroids may show an initial remission, and then experience a severe "rebound," resulting in erythrodermic psoriasis. Most dermatology providers do not treat any form of psoriasis with systemic corticosteroids for this very reason. Patients with erythroderma often require hospitalization and are quite ill.

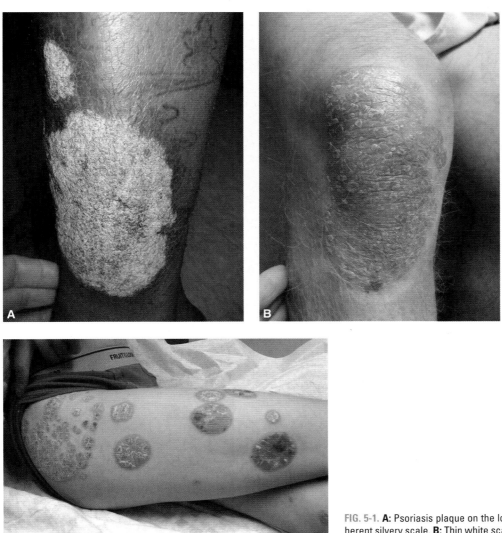

FIG. 5-1. **A:** Psoriasis plaque on the lower leg with thick adherent silvery scale. **B:** Thin white scale on psoriasis plaque on knees. **C:** Psoriasis plaques on a 9-year-old boy.

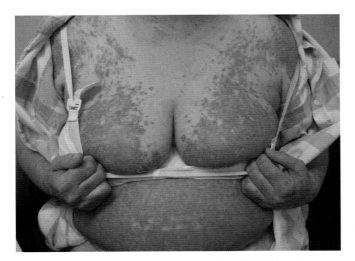

FIG. 5-2. Severe plaque psoriasis covering more than 10% of body surface area.

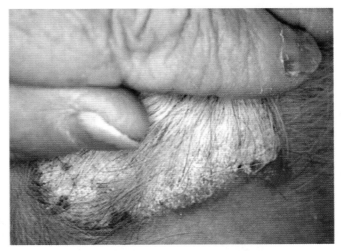

FIG. 5-3. Scalp psoriasis with thick, silvery adherent scale on erythematous base. The patient's nails are also affected.

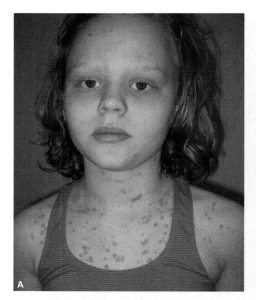
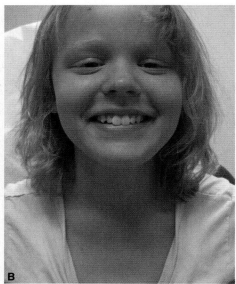

FIG. 5-4. **A:** Guttate psoriasis on a 10-year-old child. **B:** Clearance after treatment with methotrexate and home light box therapy.

Psoriatic nails

Most patients with psoriatic disease have finger and toenail involvement. Thickened, dystrophic, and yellow nails, which may separate from the nail bed, are often mistaken for fungal disease. In more subtle involvement, pinpoint "pitting" may be observed and is classically associated with psoriatic arthritis (PsA) (Figure 5-6). "Oil spots" are a nail finding in some patients with psoriasis and present as pink or tan round areas within the nail. Nail involvement can be incredibly disfiguring as well as painful for patients, and presents a challenge for providers to manage (Figure 5-7). Severe dystrophy of the nails may require removal of the entire nail and nail matrix in order to alleviate painful symptoms.

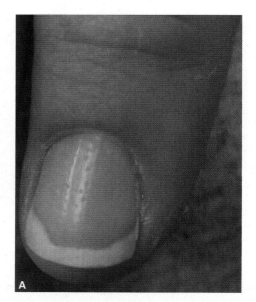

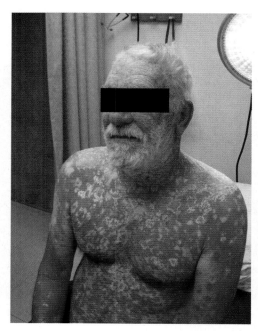

FIG. 5-5. Erythroderma.

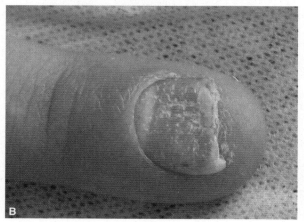

FIG. 5-6. **A:** Nail pitting can be a subtle clue for psoriatic disease. **B:** Nail dystrophy in psoriasis is commonly misdiagnosed as fungal nail infection (onychomycosis).

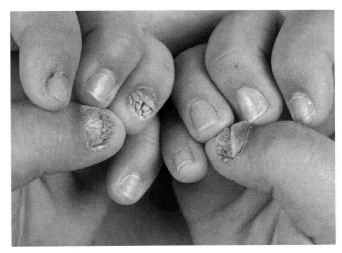

FIG. 5-7. Psoriasis with subungual hyperkeratosis and destruction of nail plates.

DIFFERENTIAL DIAGNOSIS Psoriasis

- Atopic dermatitis
- Contact dermatitis
- Squamous cell carcinoma
- Seborrheic dermatitis
- Xerosis
- Dermatophytic infections
- Cutaneous T-cell lymphoma
- Nummular eczema
- Tinea corporis and capitis
- Onychomycosis

Comorbidities

Psoriasis was initially believed to be limited to the skin. However, because it is an immune-mediated disease, it is now clear that the inflammation that occurs in the skin can also be found in other systems, including the joints, heart, brain, and other organs. Patients with more severe psoriasis have shown an increased incidence of joint disease (psoriatic arthritis), cardiovascular disease, hypertension, obesity, diabetes, and other immune-mediated conditions such as Crohn disease. Additionally, there are numerous psychological disorders that can be associated with psoriasis, including depression, increased risk of suicide, alcoholism, and social isolation.

Understanding the concept that psoriasis is associated with other inflammatory diseases is critical for two reasons. First, it heightens the clinical suspicion of practitioners to screen patients with psoriasis for associated comorbidities as soon as psoriasis is diagnosed (Table 5-1). Second, the education and prevention of these diseases can start earlier in life.

Cardiovascular disease

Patients with severe plaque psoriasis may be self-conscious of their appearance and therefore avoid participating in exercise or social activities. The lack of physical activities can result in increased weight gain, hypertension, diabetes, and chronic pain syndromes. Conversely, the chronic inflammatory nature of psoriasis itself may lead to other inflammatory conditions such as cardiovascular disease and myocardial infarction.

TABLE 5-1	Monitoring of Comorbidities in Patients with Psoriasis*
COMORBIDITY	**MONITORING PARAMETERS**
Cardiovascular disease	Blood pressure, lipids, BMI, tobacco use, physical exercise, pedal edema, dyspnea, tobacco, and alcohol
Diabetes mellitus	HgbA1c, glucose monitoring, diet, physical exercise
Metabolic syndrome	Lipids, glucose and insulin levels, HgbA1c, CVD, BMI
Depression	Suicidal or homicidal ideations or attempts, emotional lability, relationship stability, work patterns, alcohol and drug use, family history of depression
Malignancy	Family history of cancer, age-appropriate cancer screenings, positive review of symptoms or new symptom onset, lymphadenopathy or hepatosplenomegaly, chest imaging (smokers)
Psoriatic arthritis	Early morning stiffness in hands/knees/feet, joint deformity or sausage digits, nail pitting, oil spots, difficulty performing activities of daily living due to joint pain (buttoning shirt, opening food cans), changes in radiographic imaging of hands/feet

*Many of the parameters overlap conditions and are not exclusive.

Metabolic syndrome

Studies have demonstrated that there is an increased risk of metabolic syndrome in patients with psoriasis. Clinicians should assess psoriatic patients for the coexistence of disorders, which include obesity, hyperlipidemia, hypertension, insulin resistance, and prothrombic and proinflammatory state. Metabolic syndrome raises an individual's risk for heart disease, stroke, and diabetes.

Depression

One quarter of patients with psoriasis suffer from depression. Social isolation may contribute to increased risk of depression and anxiety, smoking, alcoholism, job instability, and financial problems. In addition to depression, patients with psoriatic disease often contend with low self-esteem and chronic pain issues. Patients report difficulties maintaining relationships due to fears of being ostracized because of their skin disease. Young patients often fear participating in sports or social events as they are concerned their peers may think that their condition is "contagious."

Malignancy

The increased risk of cancer in patients with psoriatic diseases is controversial. Because psoriasis is an immune-mediated disease, some psoriasis experts hypothesize that this may be associated with an increased risk of lymphoma and solid tumor cancers. Although phototherapy with narrow-band ultraviolet radiation is a common treatment for skin psoriasis, it has a low but nonetheless significant risk for the development of squamous and basal cell carcinomas. Lastly, the overall increased risk of smoking and alcohol use in patients with psoriasis makes it difficult to determine whether these factors also contribute to cancer risk rather than the psoriatic disease itself.

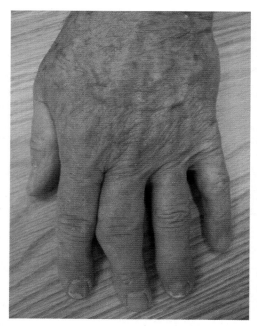

FIG. 5-8. Psoriatic arthritis with dactylitis ("sausage joint") and deformity.

Psoriatic arthritis

Psoriasis is typically identified as a skin disease, yet approximately 10% to 30% of these patients develop associated joint disease referred to as PsA. The inflammatory mechanisms that form thickened skin plaques also result in bony destruction and overgrowth in joints. Patients with PsA suffer from significant joint pain and dystrophy. In addition to examining the skin, it is imperative that the clinician obtain a thorough history of joint pain and family history of rheumatologic diseases, as well as conduct a physical examination of hand and foot joints. Patients may have dactylitis (sausage digits), asymmetrical oligoarticular (few joints) arthritis, distal interphalangeal arthropathy, and joint deformity (Figure 5-8). Patients with psoriasis should be assessed yearly and if PsA is suspected, should be referred to rheumatology. Early diagnosis and aggressive treatment with systemic therapies can prevent permanent joint destruction and significantly improve the quality of life (QOL) for psoriatic patients.

Diagnostics

Psoriasis is usually a clinical diagnosis after conducting a detailed patient history, physical examination, and documentation of their medication (prescribed and over-the-counter). In more complex or atypical presentations, a punch biopsy of the affected skin can aid in the diagnosis. Laboratory studies are usually not helpful in diagnosing psoriasis but are critical in identifying comorbidities. Radiology studies are indicated if the patient is suspected of PsA.

Equally important in the assessment and diagnosis of a patient with psoriasis is the perceived impact on their QOL from psoriatic disease. QOL can be measured with a 10-point questionnaire, **Der**matology **L**ife **Q**uality **I**ndex (www.dermatology.org.uk). A clinician may diagnose the patient with mild cutaneous disease; however, it may be incredibly distressing for the patient. Of course, screening tools for depression, anxiety, and substance abuse should be utilized when there is clinical concern.

Management

Unfortunately, there is no cure for psoriasis, and control of the disease is the goal of management. Once diagnosed, treatment of the psoriasis patient is focused on symptom management, disease control, reducing the risk for comorbidities, and optimizing QOL. Developing a plan of care for a psoriasis patient should consider the type of psoriasis, location, severity and extent of disease, age, symptoms and comorbidities, response to previous treatments, pregnancy (or intent) and lactation, access to treatment facilities, economic factors related to insurance coverage and cost of care, and QOL. The severity of the disease can be a starting point for the clinician in selecting appropriate treatment options. Here are some guidelines.

Mild-to-moderate psoriasis

Most primary care providers who have a basic understanding of psoriasis should feel comfortable treating mild-to-moderate skin disease. Good skin care including emollients should be employed even before prescribing therapy. Topical corticosteroids (TCS) are the **first-line treatment** for mild disease; however, patients should be warned about the side effects with prolonged use (see chapter 2). Use of TCS should be avoided or limited on the face, axillae, and genitals. Topical immunomodulators (TIMS) are often selected for treatment in these areas. **Reevaluate** adult patients in 4 weeks and children in 2 weeks, to assess their response to therapy. If there is an inadequate response, evaluate the patient's understanding and use of TCS, consider changing the class of TCS, or add another topical agent (TCS chart on inside of back cover).

CLINICAL PEARLS

TCS for treatment of mild-to-moderate psoriasis:

- Evaluate response in 4 weeks (2 weeks for children).
- Once disease is controlled, taper to twice a week or lower potency.
- If the skin does not improve, assess the patient to determine whether medication is being used properly before switching the class of TCS or adding another topical agent.
- Ointments are preferable for thicker plaques with adherent scale.
- Solutions, gels, foams, and lotions are preferable for hair-bearing areas.
- Avoid use of potent or very potent TCS for more than 2 weeks or use on the face, genitals, intertriginous or flexural areas due to risk of skin atrophy.
- Provide drug holidays from TCS by rotating other topicals such as vitamin D analogs or keratolytics.
- If skin symptoms worsen after use of TCS, consider superinfection with dermatophyte.
- For thicker scales, consider application of keratolytic or topical tazarotene prior to application of TCS for better absorption.

Vitamin D derivatives can be used as adjuvant topical therapy and are safe to use in steroid-sparing regions; however, they may cause some skin irritation initially. Coal tar has been used for centuries to treat psoriasis but is less common now; it decreases the rapid proliferation of skin and reduces inflammation. It can be very effective for controlling the itch associated with psoriasis. Keratolytics help thin the plaques of psoriasis and improve the penetration of TCS (Table 5-2).

Management of scalp psoriasis can be frustrating for both the patient and the clinician (Figure 5-9). The first-line treatment for scalp psoriasis is the initiation of topical therapies at the first sign of erythema, scaling, or scalp pruritus. Tar preparations, salicylic acid, and oils are recommended for mild disease and are now available in easier-to-use shampoos, solutions, gels, and foams. Some are used as overnight applications for a greater effect. Mild-to-moderate scalp

TABLE 5-2 Topical Therapies for Psoriasis

CLASSIFICATION	AGENT/FORMULATION	DOSING	ADVERSE EVENTS	KEY CONSIDERATIONS
Topical corticosteroids (TCS) (see chapter 2 and TCS chart inside back cover)	Mild/moderate psoriasis or sensitive areas (face, eyelids, axillae, genitals): mild-to moderate-potency TCS Moderate/severe disease or thick skin areas: potent to very potent TCS	Apply thin film directly to lesions daily or b.i.d. for 2–4 wk	SE: acne, irritation, telangiectasias, xerosis, skin atrophy, striae, hypopigmentation, and rebound when discontinued. Increased risk of cataract and glaucoma Adrenal suppression if long term	Slows proliferation of keratinocytes and reduces inflammation Assess children after 2 wk and adults after 4 wk. Taper to 1–2 times a week if controlled. LIMIT the quantity and number of refills in to ensure patient follow-up Caution if using occlusion which increases potency and side effects
Topical immunomodulators (see chapter 3)	Calcineurin inhibitors: tacrolimus (Protopic)* ointment FDA approved: 0.1% for >16 yr and older; 0.03% for 2–15 yr of age	Apply thin film to lesions b.i.d.	May cause burning and irritation but usually subsides in first 2 wk	Anti-inflammatory Patient education regarding SE increases adherence. Can be used on face, eyelids, and flexural areas without risk of skin atrophy or telangiectasis
Vitamin D₃ analogs	Calcitriol (Vectical) Calcipotriene (Dovonex) Combination of calcipotriene and betamethasone propionate (Taclonex)	Apply thin layer q.d.-b.i.d. to affected areas for up to 8 wk Combination applied once daily	May cause irritation Can lower vitamin D levels (especially in children) Possible elevation of serum calcium level	Blocks hyperproliferation of keratinocytes and anti-inflammatory properties Safe for use on face and intertriginous areas Combination therapy (with TCS) is more effective and more expensive Mix with petrolatum to reduce irritation
Vitamin A analogs (retinoids)	0.05% and 0.1% tazarotene gel (Tazorac)	Apply at night, followed by mid- to high-potency TCS in a.m. Start with 0.05% can increase to 0.1%	May cause scaling and irritation Pregnancy category X (not be used by women considering pregnancy, who are pregnant or nursing)	Apply zinc oxide or moisturizer to healthy skin around the plaque to prevent irritation Optimal efficacy when used as combination rather than monotherapy
Tar preparations (OTC)	Many brands	Massage into scalp and leave on for 5–10 min, then rinse.	Can stain clothing, bathtubs, or skin Irritation and photosensitivity for up to 24 hr after application	Often used as adjunctive therapy Helpful for pruritus, especially the scalp
Keratolytic agents	Shampoos, lotions, creams, and gels containing salicylic acid, lactic acid, urea	Shampoos: apply to scalp, wait 5–10 min, then rinse Apply creams/lotions daily to plaques	Can cause nausea and tinnitus if used over large areas of the body Can cause atrophy of healthy skin	Softens thick plaques and removes scale Enhances penetration of other topicals EXCEPT salicylic acid inactivates vitamin D₃ analogs, so should not be used together.

*Black-box warning.

involvement may require the addition of TCS, vitamin D analogs, or both. Patients should be advised not to pick or scratch the scale of their scalp, which puts them at increased risk for infection. Scalp psoriasis that is severe should be referred to a dermatologist.

Moderate-to-severe psoriasis

Moderate-to-severe psoriatic disease warrants a referral to a dermatology practitioner experienced in psoriasis care. The definition of "moderate to severe" has varied definition and complicated metrics that are used in clinical trials, but are not very practical in primary care. For the purposes of this text, the parameters of moderate-to-severe psoriasis and indications for referral are outlined in Table 5-3.

Phototherapy can be a very effective modality for moderate or severe psoriasis. However, if phototherapy is not available or effective, systemic therapies must be considered. These traditional agents have been utilized in the management of psoriasis for decades; however, they do pose significant health risks, not limited to, but including liver, kidney, cardiovascular, and blood dyscrasias. *Biologics* are the newest therapeutic agents for the management of moderate-to-severe psoriasis and with some also indicated for the treatment of PsA. These systemic agents directly target specific chemical mediators within the immune systemic that are associated with psoriatic disease. Table 5-3 provides an overview of treatment options in the management of moderate-to-severe psoriasis. These agents should be prescribed and managed by a dermatology provider.

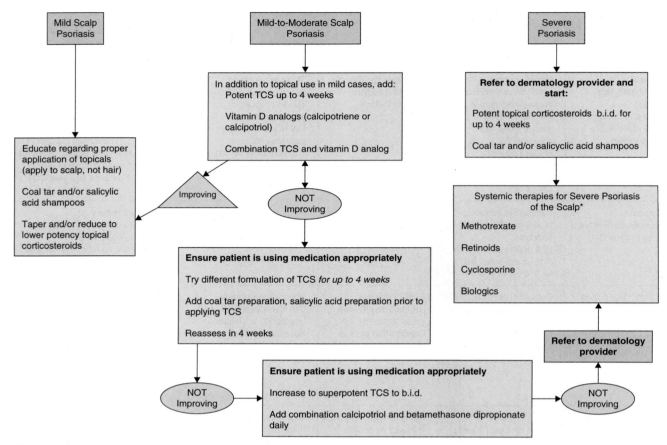

FIG. 5-9. Algorithm for treatment of scalp psoriasis. TCS, topical corticosteroids. *To be managed by a dermatology provider.

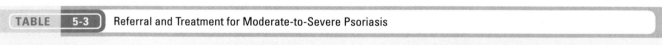

TABLE 5-3	Referral and Treatment for Moderate-to-Severe Psoriasis

WHEN TO REFER

Disease is not responding or adverse response to topical therapy
Patients with severe or extensive disease (>5% BSA)*
Diagnostic uncertainty
Disease involving the face/head, genitals, or palmar-plantar area
Nail disease
Guttate psoriasis that may require phototherapy
Any disease which has a major impact on patient's quality of life or psychosocial well-being
Immediate attention for erythroderma
Children and pregnant women

TREATMENT MODALITY	OPTIONS
Phototherapy	Narrow-band UVB, excimer laser, chemophototherapy (PUVA), home light box therapy
Systemic, biologic agents	TNF-α inhibitors adalimumab, etanercept, infliximab, interleukin-12 and -23 agonists (ustekinumab)
Systemic, oral agents (nonbiologic)	Methotrexate, retinoids (acitretin), immunosuppressants

*1% BSA is approximately the area of one outstretched hand.

Special Considerations

Psoriasis can be unpredictable during pregnancy, with remission or severe flare. Pregnant females or those trying to conceive who have mild disease can be managed with emollients, TCS, or vitamin D_3 analogs. If phototherapy is considered or second-line therapies are required for moderate-to-severe psoriasis, pregnant females should be managed by a dermatologist.

Mild psoriasis in children may be managed with TCS as a first-line therapy. Children with moderate-to-severe disease should be referred immediately to a dermatologist, where phototherapy (depending on their age), methotrexate, biologics, or a combination may be used.

Referral and Consultation

Psoriasis that does not present with a classic presentation or respond to common treatment modalities should be referred to a dermatology provider to ensure the correct diagnosis. Furthermore, it cannot be overemphasized that patients with moderate and severe psoriasis should be referred early and managed by a dermatologist to reduce morbidity. Patients with signs or symptoms of joint stiffness and pain should be referred to a rheumatologist for evaluation of PsA. In severe cases of depression or suicidal ideation, a mental health provider should be involved in the management of care as these patients have a significantly increased risk of suicide.

Patient Education and Follow-up

Patients with psoriasis require ongoing education and support for their chronic disease management, which can greatly impact their QOL. Patients with psoriasis should be reevaluated yearly. With an additional focus on comorbidities and PsA related to psoriasis, both dermatologist and primary care clinicians have the opportunity to reduce mortality and morbidity through routine screening, management, and recommendations to reduce risk factors. Skin care and skin cancer prevention should not be forgotten especially for patients receiving phototherapy or immunosuppression. Fortunately, there are numerous tools and resources available that support psoriasis education and counseling for both patients and providers.

CLINICAL PEARLS

Clinicians should assess and discuss the following:

- Patient expectations of disease course (triggers, waxing/waning nature of disease)
- Importance of compliance with treatment regimens
- Prevention of cardiovascular disease and type II diabetes
- Smoking cessation aids
- Avoidance of alcohol and other illicit drugs
- Weight management and fitness promotion
- QOL and depression
- Age-appropriate cancer screenings
- Vaccination protocols (especially with biologic treatment regimens)

SEBORRHEIC DERMATITIS

SD is a recurring, papulosquamous skin disorder that causes erythema and waxy, yellowish scale. It occurs in approximately 50% of the population and has no racial predilection. The well-known problem of *dandruff* is the mildest form of SD, making it far more common and probably underdiagnosed. Males are affected slightly more than females, and there is a 1% to 5% worldwide distribution.

There is an increased prevalence in individuals with Down syndrome, Parkinson disease, and neurologic disorders (including head injury, stroke, mood disorders), and in those who are immunocompromised. SD tends to be chronic, with remissions and exacerbations often improving in the summer and worsening in the winter. Certain medications have been associated with the development or exacerbation of SD and include lithium, psoralens, and interferon.

Pathophysiology

Although the pathogenesis is not fully understood, SD is associated with the lipophilic yeast *Malassezia*, a normal inhabitant of the skin. Many believe there is an abnormal inflammatory response against the yeast *Malassezia furfur* (pityrosporum), combined with increased sebum levels, and individual susceptibility. Persons prone to this dermatitis also tend to have a skin barrier dysfunction.

Clinical Presentation

SD has a distinctive pattern in different age groups; pediatric and adult forms exist. This section will cover SD in adults (see chapter 6 for pediatric SD). This condition commonly involves the scalp, forehead, eyebrows, glabella, nasolabial folds, ears, and postauricular skin. Less often, the axillae, inguinal folds, and trunk are involved, and distribution is often symmetric. In men, it can erupt in the sternal area with a fine papular erythematous, scaly rash, sometimes in an annular pattern and may be evident over the upper back. SD presents as areas of erythema covered by dry or moist greasy white scale in the sebum rich areas of the skin (Figure 5-10A). Hypopigmentation is seen in skin of color, but there is little to moderate discomfort. In the scalp, it ranges from mild patchy scaling to widespread, thick, adherent crusts with pruritus (Figure 5-10B). Skin sensitivity is common, and it can be exacerbated by heat, sunlight, fever, and irritating topical therapy. A common practice among African Americans is the daily application of oils to the scalp, a practice which may lead to further buildup of scale and worsen the dermatitis.

DIFFERENTIAL DIAGNOSIS Seborrheic dermatitis

- Rosacea
- Psoriasis
- Lupus erythematosus
- Periorbital dermatitis
- Tinea versicolor
- Contact dermatitis (irritant or allergic)
- Atopic dermatitis
- Pityriasis rosea
- Candidiasis
- Tinea faciale
- Tinea corporis

Diagnostics

A clinical diagnosis of SD is usually made based on a history of waxing and waning severity, and the typical presentation and distribution of involvement. An erythematous eruption on the central face is characteristic of several different disorders and can be challenging to distinguish. In SD, the erythema and scale extend directly from the cheeks to the nose involving the folds (Figure 5-11A). SD is often confused with the facial rash of systemic lupus erythematosus (SLE). In the "butterfly" distribution of SLE, there is sparing of the area beside the nose, nasolabial and mesolabial

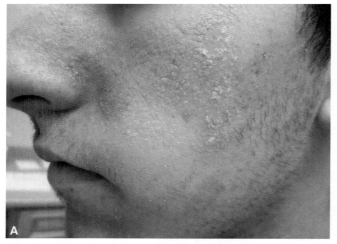

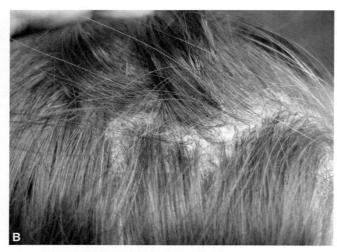

FIG. 5-10. **A:** Waxy scale of seborrheic dermatitis. **B:** Scalp-adherent crust.

folds (Figure 5-11B). The color is often brighter red, and there may be photosensitivity. In rosacea, there may be redness, dilated vessels, and often papules and pustules in the central face, but there is minimal scale (Figure 5-11C). SD may also be seen in the eyebrows, behind the ears, and scalp and will confirm the diagnosis. It can be very difficult to differentiate SD from psoriasis and there may, in fact, be an overlapping condition referred to as "sebopsoriasis." The scale associated with SD is typically not adherent compared to psoriasis, where the plaque is difficult to remove and may cause bleeding. A skin biopsy is rarely needed but can support the diagnosis.

Management

The mainstay of therapy is the use of topical azole antifungals because of their effect on the *Malassezia*. SD tends to be chronic and

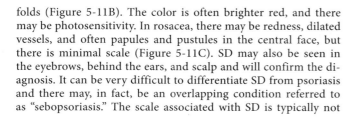

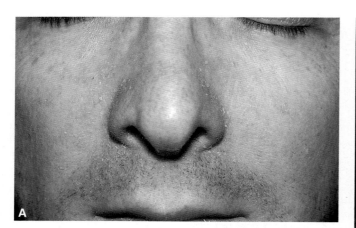

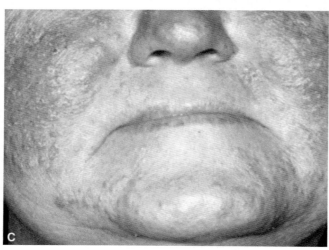

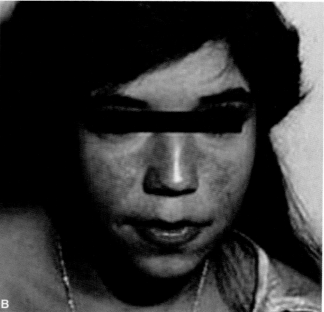

FIG. 5-11. **A:** Classic seborrheic dermatitis involving the nasolabial folds. **B:** Classic "butterfly" rash of systemic lupus erythematosus sparing the nasolabial folds. **C:** Acne rosacea. Note the erythema, papules, and pustules appear across cheeks and nose.

recurrent primarily because once the patient sees improvement, treatment is often discontinued. The *Malassezia* organism then continues to grow slowly, and in a few weeks the symptoms recur.

It may be beneficial, especially in adult patients prone to frequent recurrences of facial SD, to combine a TCS or TIMS with the antifungal for a short period of time. The response to therapy may be slower with TIMS alone. Clinicians using TCS should taper the frequency of application as opposed to abrupt withdrawal.

Daily shampooing or lathering for a longer time with shampoos may help reduce recurrences as well. Sensitive skin care measures to improve the barrier function of skin include nonsoap cleansers,

and mild, fragrance-free moisturizers are of utmost importance as well as choosing medications with nonirritating vehicles. Medicated shampoos can be used for washing the face and ears, with caution to avoid the orbits of the eye. Table 5-4 provides an overview of treatment options in the management of SD.

CLINICAL PEARL

- Sudden onset of severe disease or SD that is resistant to treatment may be a cutaneous sign of HIV.

TABLE 5-4 Treatment for Seborrheic Dermatitis[†]

SEVERITY*	SELF-CARE	SHAMPOOS	TOPICAL AGENTS	COMMENTS
Mild	Shampoo daily (once weekly for African Americans) Antifungal or dandruff shampoo, OTC, or Rx products (apply to wet scalp, lather, wait 5 min, rinse) Facial cleansing to remove oil and scale (can use antifungal shampoo as wash) Apply a moisturizing or barrier cream	Ketoconazole 1%[†] or 2% (Nizoral) Ciclopirox 1% (Loprox) Selenium sulfide 2.5% (Selsun) Zinc pyrithione 1% and 2%[†] (Head & Shoulders)	Ketoconazole 2% C, G, F Ciclopirox 1% C, L Butenafine C, G Terbinafine C, G	If facial rash persists, consider adding a topical antifungal to the face b.i.d.
Moderate	Follow measures for mild disease P&S solution (leave on overnight, wash out in the morning)	*Keratolytic shampoos:* Salicylic acid 2% shampoo, tar shampoo, P&S shampoo[†]	*Corticosteroids—scalp:* Clobex‡ Sh, Capex‡ Sh Fluocinolone acetate 0.01% in peanut oil (Derma-Smoothe F/S) Fluocinolone solution 0 Fluocinonide 0.05% Betamethasone diproprionate 0.05% Clobetasol 0.05%, spray *Face and body topicals:* Metronidazole cream 0.75% b.i.d. Metronidazole gel 1.0% q.d. Azelaic acid 15% b.i.d. Sodium sulfacetamide lotion, gel wash, shampoo (Klaron, Ovace, Mexar) Promiseb b.i.d.—t.i.d. Hyaluronic acid 0.2% (Bionect) C, G, Sp *Corticosteroids—face and body:* Hydrocortisone 1 & 2.5%[†], Desonide 0.05%[†] cream and lotion *Immunomodulators:* Tacrolimus ointment (Protopic)[†] # 0.03 and 0.1% Pimecrolimus cream (Elidel) [†]#	If there is thick, adherent scale on the scalp, use a keratolytic agent Low- to mid-potency topical corticosteroids may be applied to the scalp daily or b.i.d., 2–4 wk for scalp and 1–2 wk for face, then taper A combination of therapies may be most effective
Severe	Overnight Derma-Smoothe F/S scalp oil‡ at night with cap Apply antifungal in a.m. and another in p.m.	Follow measures for mild disease	If scalp scale persists despite frequent shampooing, increase the topical corticosteroid to mid to high potency (i.e., clobetasol b.i.d.) Consider other topical agents for facial eruption If necessary, use a mild anti-inflammatory lotion to the face such as Desonide 0.05%[†] b.i.d. to improve the redness, but only for short period	Reconsider diagnosis, conditions like rosacea and seborrhea often coexist In severe or recalcitrant cases, refer to dermatologist

*There is no accepted standard for assessing the severity of SD.

[†]Available over the counter

‡Scalp only.

#Black-box warning.

C, cream; F, foam; G, gel; Sp, spray.

Prognosis and Complications

Adult SD has a chronic relapsing course with remissions and exacerbations. Patients feel well, and systemic signs are absent. Although complications are rare, erythrodermic forms can occur and may be associated with underlying HIV.

Patient Education and Follow-up

The treatment of SD, as discussed above, generally involves shampooing several times a week if not daily. African American hair generally is not shampooed as often, so understanding individual cultural practices is important to the success of the treatment. Daily oiling may also contribute to worsening, so patients are encouraged to use the ketoconazole cream or gel in place of their oil at least several times per week. Shampoo should be encouraged at least twice as often as usual.

Follow up in 6 to 8 weeks to review treatment and management if the condition is not improved. Patients need to be educated about the chronicity of this condition and should realistically hope to "control, not cure."

PITYRIASIS ROSEA

Pityriasis rosea (PR) is a common, self-limiting, papulosquamous dermatosis that usually affects young healthy individuals. The majority of cases are seen in patients between the ages of 10 and 35, and females are affected more often than males. There is no racial predilection, and is more common in the spring and fall.

Pathophysiology

Observational studies support a viral etiology, although that has been difficult to confirm. Documentation of clustered cases among household members, seasonal variation, intolerance to ampicillin, and response to acyclovir at the onset of disease supports this theory. Current research has greatly focused on the causal association between the human herpes virus 6 and 7 (HHV-6 and HHV-7) and this condition, but it remains controversial.

Clinical Presentation

Classic PR presents with a solitary 2- to 4-cm patch or plaque on the trunk, which can precede the typical rash by 1 to 2 weeks and is known as the "herald patch" (Figure 5-12A). Lesions are often pink to salmon-colored with a fine, scaly center and advancing border. The herald patch may be as small as 1.0 cm or as large as 10 cm but only occurs about 10% of the time. This is followed by a generalized eruption within days to weeks of the original lesion. The rash of PR consists of multiple pink, round-to-ovoid, papules, and plaques with a fine "collarette scale" on the border (Figure 5-12B). Minute pustules can also be seen in this early eruptive phase.

PR has a symmetrical distribution following the long axis of skin tension lines often resembling a Christmas or fir tree pattern on the trunk. The face is often spared, although the neck is a common occurrence. Palms and soles are usually spared. Approximately 25% of patients complain about pruritus, and a few report prodromal low-grade fever, chills, headache, fatigue, myalgias, and lymphadenopathy. The rash usually lasts for 6 to 8 weeks and then spontaneously resolves. Some cases last up to 5 months or more.

DIFFERENTIAL DIAGNOSIS Pityriasis rosea
• Secondary syphilis
• Tinea versicolor
• Drug eruption
• Nummular eczema
• Guttate psoriasis
• Pityriasis lichenoides

Diagnostics

The diagnosis of PR is made on the basis of the characteristic clinical presentation. A biopsy will not be diagnostic as the histology is nonspecific, but it can assist in ruling out other differential diagnoses. A KOH prep can identify fungal or yeast infections. Distribution and nail involvement are key if the clinician favors a diagnosis of psoriasis. An RPR or VDRL should be obtained if there is a suspicion or

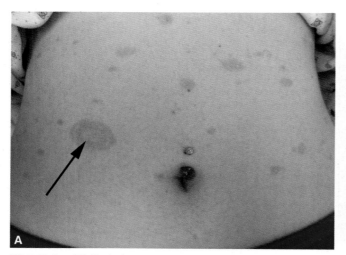
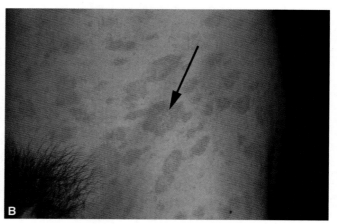

FIG. 5-12. **A** and **B**: Pityriasis rosea. Note the "herald patch" (*arrow*).

history of high-risk sexual contact, a previous genital ulcer, or significant involvement of the palms and soles to rule out secondary syphilis.

Management

PR does not typically require any treatment other than symptomatic care. Pruritus may be severe, and therapy with oral antihistamines such as cetirizine or loratadine during the day may be helpful. Hydroxyzine 25 to 50 mg or diphenhydramine 12.5 to 25 mg have sedating effects and are recommended to be taken at bedtime. A mild TCS lotion such as desonide 0.05% can be applied twice daily for relief of itch.

Extensive PR with severe pruritus is uncommon but may respond to ultraviolet (UVB) light or natural sunlight. The use of antivirals has been debated as some clinicians believe that it is useful in patients with severe disease associated with flu-like symptoms. Acyclovir 400–800 mg five times daily for a week are the suggested dosages. Oral erythromycin has been found to eliminate and/or reduce the severity of PR.

Special Considerations

Pregnancy. PR is associated with HHV-6 and HHV-7 infection. Premature delivery and fetal demise have been observed in pregnant patients with PR, especially if it occurs within the first 15 weeks of gestation. Referral to obstetrics is important for pregnant women with PR for a discussion about the risks of potential fetal complications and possible benefits of acyclovir (Category B). Women may contact the Acyclovir in Pregnancy Registry, established in 1984 by the manufacturer and the Centers for Disease Control and Prevention.

CLINICAL PEARL

- Lymphadenopathy is a rare finding in PR. If present, it is important to rule out syphilis and obtain RPR/VDRL.

Prognosis and Complications

PR is self-limiting and has an excellent prognosis. The eruption may be cosmetically unpleasing for some patients. Some patients have reported recurrences.

Referral and Consultation

If symptoms are prolonged or not relieved by systemic or topical medications, reevaluate the patient and reconsider the diagnosis. Differential diagnoses such as pityriasis lichenoides, a more chronic disorder, should be considered, and referral to a dermatologist is recommended.

Patient Education and Follow-up

Follow-up is recommended for any patients who cannot manage their symptoms or in whom the rash does not clear in several months. Patients often need reassurance about the benign nature of PR. If the patient is seen in the early phase, they should be advised that the rash may worsen and spread and that is the expected progression.

LICHEN PLANUS

Lichen planus (LP) is an inflammatory, mucocutaneous condition estimated to occur in 1% of the population. It most commonly affects middle-aged adults, with a slightly higher prevalence in females. Studies report a high incidence of hepatitis C virus (HCV), chronic hepatitis, and primary biliary cirrhosis in patients with LP. It has also been associated with other immune-mediated conditions involving the skin such as vitiligo, alopecia areata, lichen sclerosis, and dermatomyositis.

Pathophysiology

LP is thought to be related to T-cell-mediated damage to the basal keratinocytes of the skin, mucous membranes, hair follicles, or nails. The etiology is unclear, but observations suggest a relationship between exposure to an antigen and the development of LP. Viruses, in particular, HCV, medications, and contact allergens have been implicated.

Clinical Presentation

The cutaneous lesions of LP are often described as having five "P" qualities: pruritic, purple, planar (flat topped), polygonal (or polyangular), papules. These lesions are present most commonly on the flexural surfaces of wrists and forearms, the dorsal hands, and anterior aspect of the lower legs (Figure 5-13A). Initially, lesions are small violaceous, slightly shiny papules. Overtime, they may coalesce into larger plaques. Characteristic fine white lines called *"Wickhams striae"* or grey-white puncta may evolve as lesions age. In addition to the classic characteristics described above, other morphologies can be seen, which include hypertrophic, atrophic, erosive, follicular, annular, linear, guttate, actinic, bullous, and ulcerative lesions.

Oral LP has many forms, and may occur separately or concurrently. The reticular form is most common and appears as white plaques with a lace-like pattern affecting the buccal mucosa or lateral tongue (Figure 5-13B). Mucous membrane involvement may be severe and erosive. Lesions may be found on the conjunctiva, vulva, glans penis, anus, tonsils, larynx, and throughout the GI tract. LP in the genital area is discussed in chapter 21.

Lichen planopilaris refers to involvement of the scalp hair and presents as erythematous, perifollicular scale, which may lead to a permanent scarring alopecia if not treated promptly. This may occur alone or in conjunction with other cutaneous involvement. Nail changes which represent scarring are seen in approximately 10% of patients with LP. Look for lateral thinning, longitudinal ridging, thickening, and pterygium (overgrowth of the cuticle) on the proximal nail fold. See chapter 14 for discussion of hair and nail changes in LP. Linear eruptions may develop in areas of trauma/scratching (Koebner phenomenon; Figure 5-13C).

Always consider drugs as an underlying cause of LP. Drug-induced LP usually occurs within months of starting the offending agent. It is important to consider that the eruption may range from 10 days to several years after starting, and multiple drugs may be considered.

Diagnostics

LP is a clinical diagnosis most often based on the distinctive appearance and distribution of lesions. Particular attention to the oral mucosa, nail units, and scalp may support the diagnosis. A lichenoid drug

DIFFERENTIAL DIAGNOSIS Lichen planus

- Cutaneous Lichen Planus
  - Lichenoid drug eruption
  - Subacute lupus erythematosis
  - Psoriasis
  - Granuloma annulare
  - Warts
  - Pityriasis rosea
  - Tinea corporis
  - Mycosis fungoides
  - Lichen simplex chronicus
  - Secondary syphilis
  - Chronic graft-vs.-host disease
  - Squamous cell carcinoma
- Nail Lichen Planus
  - Alopecia areata
  - Onychomycosis
  - Psoriasis
- Hair Lichen Planus
  - Alopecia areata
  - Discoid lupus erythematosis
  - Other scarring alopecias
- Mucous Membrane Lichen Planus
  - Squamous cell carcinoma
  - Pemphigus vulgaris
  - Bullous pemphigoid
  - Benign mucus membrane
  - Pemphigus
  - Lichen sclerosis
  - Herpes simplex virus
  - Drug eruption

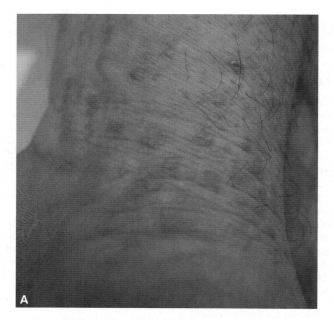

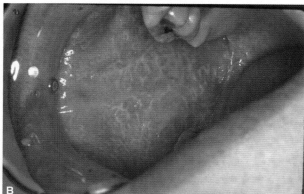

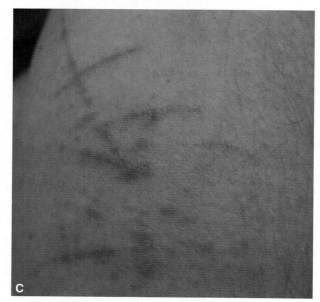

reaction may differ from classic LP by its generalized distribution, older mean age, photo distribution, and lack of mucosal involvement.

A skin punch biopsy will confirm the diagnosis of LP. Classic pathology shows a lichenoid interface dermatitis without parakeratosis or eosinophils. Direct immunofluorescence (DIF) reveals globular deposits of IgG, IgM, IgA, and complement and linear basement membrane deposits of fibrin and fibrinogen. Serologic tests for hepatitis C should be considered especially in geographic regions where LP is more commonly associated with hepatitis. High-risk regions include the Mediterranean basin and the United States.

Management

Although LP often resolves spontaneously, treatment is often requested because of severe pruritus. Oral antihistamines and topical antipruritic agents are used to manage itching. In localized disease TCS and topical immune modulators are used to both control pruritus and promote resolution of lesions. For genital and oral LP, TCS are the first-line treatment. Steroid-sparing agents may be used for maintenance. Widespread disease may necessitate systemic therapy with corticosteroids or other agents. Topical anesthetics may be used for pain management and water-based lubricants for sexual activity. Drug-induced LP must be ruled out before starting any therapy as withdrawal of the potential offending agent will result in resolution of lesions. Table 5-5 provides an overview of treatment options for management of LP.

FIG. 5-13. A: Lichen planus on the wrists showing the five "P" qualities. **B:** Oral lichen planus. **C:** Koebnerized lichen planus. Note the linear presentation from scratching.

TABLE 5-5	Treatment for Lichen Planus	
	PRIMARY CARE	**DERMATOLOGY**
Cutaneous	Topicals antipruritics Oral antihistamines Topical corticosteroids: mid to high potency (class 1 or 2); apply b.i.d. for 2–3 wk only to lesions Calcineurin inhibitors (steroid sparing)*	Intralesional triamcinolone (localized) Phototherapy or chemophototherapy Oral corticosteroids Dapsone Hydroxychloroquine Immunosuppressants
Genital	*Vaginal* Tacrolimus vaginal suppositories (compounded) Tacrolimus 0.1% (compounded) cream with Replens-like base *Vulvar* Superpotent topical corticosteroids	Systemic corticosteroids Systemic retinoids Hydroxychloroquine Azathioprine Mycophenolate mofetil Dapsone
Oral	Topical corticosteroids†(mix with adhesive dental paste or triamcinolone 0.1% using a custom tray); tacrolimus 0.1% Topical retinoids Lidocaine Consider antimycotic	Systemic retinoids Cyclosporine mouthwash Cyclosporine oral Hydroxychloroquine Azathioprine Mycophenolate mofetil Photodynamic therapy

*Topical calcineurin inhibitors can burn, especially on inflamed skin, and long-term safety is unknown. Avoid long-term/continuous use.

†Consider concurrent treatment for oral candidiasis, as increased risk is associated with corticosteroid use.

Prognosis and Complications

The duration is dependent on the LP variant. LP may spontaneously resolve, typically after a year or may follow a chronic, remitting course. Hypertrophic, oral, and nail LP tend to be more persistent. Ulcerative LP tends to be lifelong.

Referral and Consultation

Refer all patients with erosive LP to a specialist (ophthalmologist, oral surgeon, gynecologist, or dermatologist) for appropriate treatment. Refer all patients with severe cutaneous LP for consideration of systemic therapy to a dermatologist.

Patient Education and Follow-up

All patients given TCS and/or oral corticosteroids should be warned that prolonged use may lead to cutaneous and systemic side effects. See chapter 2 for side effects of corticosteroid. The "black-box warnings" associated with the use of calcineurin inhibitors should be carefully explained. Advise patients with genital mucosal involvement that topical treatments are available to help alleviate pain and improve sexual function.

Oral LP requires good oral hygiene. Regular brushing and use of dental floss may prevent tooth decay and gingival damage.

Management of pruritus and pain may be particularly challenging, and close follow-up is recommended. Ideally, patients should be seen 2 to 4 weeks after the initiation of treatment. Follow-up is recommended for any patient whose symptoms interfere with activities of daily living, which include eating, sleeping, the ability to engage in sexual activity, and coping with a potentially chronic skin disease.

ERYTHRODERMA

Erythroderma is defined as a generalized redness and scaling of the skin associated with extensive exfoliation. It is not a specific disease entity, but a manifestation of other diseases, including preexisting dermatoses such as atopic dermatitis, psoriasis, and drug reactions. The cause remains unknown (idiopathic) in approximately 30% of cases. Erythroderma that is not due to eczema usually develops in patients older than 40 years. It is slightly more common in males than in females.

Pathophysiology

The generalized redness is due to increased skin blood perfusion causing temperature dysregulation which results in heat loss and hypothermia. The basal metabolic rate then rises to compensate for this heat loss, and high cardiac output failure may occur. There is also an extensive exfoliation which contributes to hypoalbuminemia. Edema may be observed because of a fluid shift into the extracellular spaces. Immune reactions may include increased γ-globulins, serum IgE, and CD4 T-cell lymphocytopenia.

Clinical Presentation

Signs and symptoms of erythroderma include generalized redness (erythema) and edema of 90% or more of the skin surface; scaling (fine flakes or large sheets), typically 2 to 6 days after the onset of redness, starting on flexural skin (Figure 5-5); serous drainage, resulting in an unpleasant odor as clothes and dressings stick to skin; pruritus, severe in some cases (may be associated with excoriations); keratoderma—thickening of palmer surface of hands and plantar surface of feet; thick scale on the scalp associated with alopecia as symptoms persist. Nails may become thickened and shed overtime. Eyelid swelling/edema may result in ectropion. Lymphadenopathy may be present.

Long-standing erythroderma may result in pigmentary changes, resembling vitiligo, especially in individuals with skin of color. Pustules and crusting with secondary infection can develop. Systemic symptoms may include fever, chills, hypothermia, electrolyte imbalances and dehydration secondary to fluid loss, low serum albumin due to protein loss, and increased metabolic rate. Heart failure associated with untreated tachycardia is common in the elderly.

DIFFERENTIAL DIAGNOSIS erythroderma

- Atopic dermatitis
- Contact dermatitis
- Cutaneous T-cell lymphoma
- Stevens–Johnson syndrome
- Staphylococcal scalded skin syndrome
- Graft-versus-host disease
- Lichen planus
- Pemphigus foliaceus
- Pityriasis rubra pilaris
- Psoriasis
- Seborrheic dermatitis

Diagnostics

Initially, a thorough history is needed to identify an underlying disease. Recent drug history may identify a possible drug etiology. In pemphigus foliaceous, there will likely be the presence of superficial blisters which may be hard to distinguish from overall crust. Pityriasis rubra pilaris will have characteristic "islands of sparing." Examine the patient for other signs of psoriasis looking at the scalp, fingernails, and gluteal cleft as well as scaly plaques on the elbows and knees. The patient may exhibit the oral manifestations of LP or nail changes of the same.

Skin biopsy can support clinical findings and confirm diagnosis in 40% of cases. More often erythroderma will mask the underlying disease's distinctive features. The most common histopathologic findings will reveal a subacute or chronic dermatitis. Repeat biopsies and hematologic studies may be necessary to detect specific conditions such as T-cell lymphoma. Laboratory studies may reveal an increased erythrocyte sedimentation rate, anemia, hypoalbuminemia, and hyperglobulinemia. IgE will be elevated when erythroderma is associated with atopic dermatitis. Peripheral blood smears and bone marrow evaluation may assist in a leukemia work-up.

Immunophenotyping, flow cytometry, and B- and T-cell rearrangement can confirm the diagnosis of lymphoma. Cultures may show secondary bacterial overgrowth or detect herpes virus. Skin scrapings may reveal hyphae of fungal infection or scabies.

Management

In drug-induced erythroderma, the offending medication must be withdrawn, and it may be prudent to discontinue all unnecessary medications initially. These patients are at risk for cardiac failure and acute respiratory distress syndrome and require hospitalization. Management includes nutritional support, body temperature regulation, and fluid and electrolyte replacement. Application of a mid-strength TCS such as triamcinolone 0.1% cream or ointment b.i.d. under occlusion (wet dressings or sauna suit, see chapter 2) after soaking is standard care. Once improved, gentle skin care should be started with the application of bland emollients.

Antihistamines such as hydroxyzine 25 to 50 mg q6h (2 mg/kg/day) or cetirizine 10 mg b.i.d. may help alleviate pruritus and provide much needed sedation. Systemic antibiotics for signs and symptoms of secondary infection may be warranted. Systemic corticosteroids may be given and need to be tapered over a 2- to 3-week period; however, this should be avoided if possible in patients with psoriasis and staphylococcal scalded skin syndrome. Immunosuppressive systemic agents such as acitretin, cyclosporine, methotrexate, and azathioprine may be needed for psoriatic or idiopathic erythroderma.

Special Considerations

Elderly patients may require nutritional intervention as preexisting malnutrition is not uncommon.

Prognosis and Complications

The prognosis is dependent on the underlying etiology.

Referral and Consultation

Refer all patients with erythroderma to a dermatologist at an inpatient hospital setting.

Patient Education and Follow-up

Educate patients on the specifics of the underlying cause of their erythroderma and the importance of diligent management of underlying disease, if any.

Follow discharged patients on a regular outpatient basis for management of their underlying disease. For patients with idiopathic erythroderma, serial biopsies may be necessary to rule out an underlying lymphoma.

PITYRIASIS LICHENOIDES

Pityriasis lichenoides or Mucha–Habermann disease is a rare skin disorder of unknown origin. It has both acute and chronic variations known as pityriasis lichenoides et varioliformis acuta (PLEVA) and pityriasis lichenoides chronica (PLC), respectively. PLEVA and PLC are two ends of a disease spectrum. There is also a rare, ulceronecrotic febrile form of PLEVA associated with high fever and constitutional symptoms.

The incidence of this disease has not been established in the United States. Internationally, approximately 44,000 patients were seen in three catchment areas of Great Britain and 17 cases were reported. In the pediatric population, there is a male predominance. The age of onset ranges from 3 to 15 years, with a mean age of 9.3 years. Most cases appear before age 30, and there is no racial predilection.

Pathophysiology

Pityriasis lichenoides is a T-cell lymphoproliferative disorder. A cell-mediated mechanism has been suggested based on a T-cell lymphocytic infiltrate which is composed of monoclonal CD8+ T lymphocytes. The presence of CD30+ cells is occasionally seen in pityriasis lichenoides, which leads some authors to view this as a self-healing lymphoproliferative disease. An infective etiology has been suggested, but no pathogen has been identified. An association with toxoplasmosis has been identified.

Clinical Presentation

PLEVA presents with a sudden onset of asymptomatic crops of small erythematous papules, typically affecting children and young adults (Figure 5-14). The lesions appear spontaneously, resolve within weeks, and reappear at a later date. The lesions typically come and go

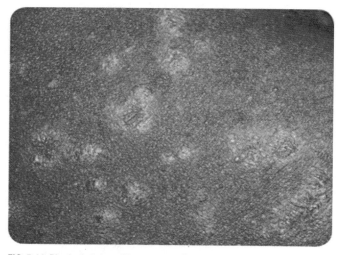

FIG. 5-14. Pityriasis lichenoides chronica (PLC).

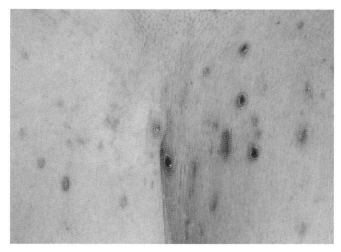

FIG. 5-15. Papular, purpuric, and ulcerative lesions of pityriasis lichenoides et varioliformis acuta (PLEVA).

in crops so variations of individual lesions may appear concurrently as papules rapidly progress to vesicles or pustules with crusting, necrosis, ulceration, and varicella-like scarring. They vary in number from a few lesions to hundreds. They favor the trunk, buttocks, and proximal extremities. Lesions of the scalp, face, palms, and soles are seen infrequently. In general, PLEVA is considered a benign disorder with spontaneous resolution of symptoms in 1 to 3 years. In very rare instances, progression to cutaneous T-cell lymphoma (CTCL) has been reported.

PLC is a chronic variation of PLEVA. Typical lesions are scaly erythematous papules which are slow to develop and take months to resolve. PLC lesions favor the lateral trunk (Figure 5-15) and proximal extremities. Patients may have 10 to 100s of lesions, but typically, less than 50. PLC tends to last for many years, occasionally leaving hypopigmented areas which are also slow to resolve. PLC is also considered a benign disease. There are rare instances of patients who progress to T-cell lymphoma and therefore it is important to follow these patients long term.

DIFFERENTIAL DIAGNOSIS Pityriasis lichenoides
• Lymphomatoid papulosis (LyP)
• Varicella
• Pityriasis rosea
• Lichen planus
• Guttate psoriasis
• Gianotti–Crosti syndrome
• Small-vessel vasculitis

Diagnostics

LyP is typically seen in older patients, lesions are more nodular, and predominately have CD30+ cells on skin biopsy. Varicella is usually accompanied by a prodrome of mild fever, malaise, and myalgia. The presence of a "Herald Patch" may help make a diagnosis of PR. LP lesions are pruritic and may exhibit the five Ps. Guttate psoriasis lesions are pruritic and monomorphous and rarely crusted. Papular acrodermatitis of childhood typically spares the trunk, may have pruritus, and follows a viral illness. Patient history and biopsy will help confirm a diagnosis of arthropod reaction.

Consider biopsy of lesions that become indurated, atrophied, ulcerated, or eroded, or have persistent erythema or poikiloderma (this term refers to the presence of cutaneous atrophy, telangiectasia, and hyper- and hypopigmentation).

Skin biopsy will typically confirm the diagnosis exhibiting a perivascular interface dermatitis. Variations include a denser, wedge-shaped infiltrate in the acute phases of the disease. Lymphocytes predominate in the infiltrate, occasionally mixed with neutrophils. Parakeratosis associated with edema to extensive necrosis is dependent on lesion development. Erythrocyte extravasation is commonly seen. These findings appear milder in chronic lesions with features that include parakeratosis, a more subtle interface lymphocytic infiltrate accompanied by focal keratinocyte necrosis and mild erythrocyte extravasation.

Management

Therapeutic trials often group PLEVA and PLC together so management strategies are similar. The lesions are typically not symptomatic and resolve spontaneously without treatment. First-line treatment for adults is phototherapy, and both narrow-band UVB (NBUVB) and psoralen plus UVA (PUVA) can be used. In children, however, erythromycin, at a dose of 40 mg per kg in a younger child and 250 mg q.i.d. in adolescents, is recommended for 6 weeks.

For more severe cases, referral to a dermatologist may be needed for consideration of systemic antibiotics, as well as topical and systemic corticosteroids, systemic retinoids, and immunosuppressants such as cyclosporine and methotrexate. If children do not respond to erythromycin, phototherapy is tried as second-line therapy.

Prognosis and Complications

There is evidence to predict the outcome based on the distribution of lesions. For example, the average clinical course with lesions limited to the extremities is 33 months, and patients with wide distribution average a shorter clinical course of 11 months. Although generally considered a benign condition, PL merits awareness as there is a less than 2% chance of cases progressing to cutaneous lymphoma. The ulceronecrotic variation may progress to cutaneous lymphoma and has a mortality rate of 25%

Referral and Consultation

Refer all patients with PL to a dermatologist for biopsy confirmation and/or administration of phototherapy and systemic agents.

Patient Education and Follow-up

Patients with long-term disease or disease that is refractory to treatment should be followed periodically by a dermatologist. If patients are receiving phototherapy, they should be followed every 6 to 8 weeks.

PARAPSORIASIS

Parapsoriasis refers to a group of skin disorders in the papulosquamous category. The present term refers to two specific cutaneous disorders that are characterized by T-cell-predominant infiltrates of the skin and are referred to as small plaque parapsoriasis (SPP) and large plaque parapsoriasis (LPP). Both conditions are asymptomatic chronic dermatoses. Parapsoriasis is most often seen in the middle-aged to elderly individual with a peak incidence in the fifth decade of life. It affects all races and geographic regions. There is a male predominance, greater in small plaque disease. There are no accurate statistics on incidence and frequency.

Pathophysiology

The etiology of SPP and LPP is unknown. There is a superficial dermal infiltrate composed primarily of CD4+ T cells. Dominant T-cell clonality is evident in many cases of LPP and only a few cases of SPP. It is thought that these diseases most likely signify different stages in a continuum of lymphoproliferative disorders from chronic dermatitis to a malignant state of CTCL. Both SPP and LPP can be regarded as forms of clonal dermatitis, with only LPP having any significant risk of transformation to overt CTCL.

Clinical Presentation

In general, parapsoriasis appears as red scaly, sometimes salmon-colored patches or slightly elevated plaques that resemble psoriasis clinically.

DIFFERENTIAL DIAGNOSIS parapsoriasis
Small Plaque/Large Plaque
• Pityriasis rosea/mycosis fungoides
• Drug eruption
• Pityriasis lichenoides chronica/psoriasis
• Psoriasis/poikiloderma
• Nummular dermatitis/connective tissue disease
• Secondary syphilis
• Cutaneous T-cell lymphoma

Small plaque parapsoriasis

This often presents as oval to round pink, well-demarcated, minimally scaly plaques of up to 5 cm in diameter with a "cigarette paper" -like scale. Plaques may be seen over the entire body, but favor sun-protected skin such as the trunk, buttocks, and lower extremities. Lesions with a yellow hue are called xanthoerythrodermia

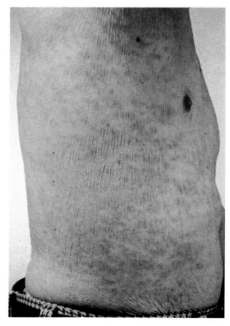

FIG. 5-16. Small plaque parapsoriasis, digitate pattern.

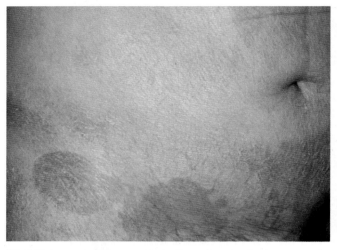

FIG. 5-17. Large plaque parapsoriasis. These large, scaly plaques may be evolving into cutaneous T-cell lymphoma.

perstans. Finger-like patches distributed symmetrically on the flank are described as digitate dermatoses (Figure 5-16). These lesions break the 5 cm rule of SPP and may elongate to 10 cm.

Large plaque parapsoriasis

This presents with larger (>6 cm) round or irregularly shaped, faint erythematous plaques on the trunk, buttocks, and proximal extremities. LPP frequently has a "bathing suit" distribution. The surface has minimal scale, with an atrophic "cigarette paper" quality (Figure 5-17).

Management

Patients with SPP should be reassured that progression to CTCL is very rare. Treatment can be as desired to control symptoms. In contrast, patients with LPs should be treated despite the absence of symptoms because of the potential for progression to CTCL. Initial treatment may include the use of antihistamines and TCS for both types. Dry and sensitive skin care and emollients should be incorporated to reduce scaling. SPP can be treated with NBUVB if topicals fail.

LPP should be treated with phototherapy preferably PUVA. Other topical agents for LPP can be tried, but patients should be referred to a dermatologist.

Prognosis and Complications

SPP is a benign condition that lasts several months to years and often spontaneously resolves without treatment over time. LPP can remain stable for many years; however, there is potential for the disease to progress to CTCL. The 5-year survival rate remains high and is greater than 90%.

Referral and Consultation

All patients with LPP should be referred to a dermatologist. Long-term follow-up is imperative, and periodic biopsies should be performed especially if there is any change in cutaneous presentation.

Patient Education and Follow-up

Patients with SPP can be reassured that this is considered a benign, chronic condition and does not progress to more significant disease.

Close follow-up every 1 to 3 months is needed for patients undergoing treatment for LPP and then at least annually. Biopsy should be considered for any patient with an increased number of lesions, increase in lesion size >5 cm, or development of induration, atrophy, or lymphadenopathy.

BILLING CODES ICD-10

Lichen planus (subacute)	L43.3
Bullous lichen planus	L43.1
Follicular lichen planus	L66.1
Hypertrophic lichen planus	L43.0
Lichenoid drug eruption	L43.2
Pityriasis lichenoides acute	L41.0
Pityriasis lichenoides chronic	L41.1
Pityriasis rosea	L42
Psoriasis	L40.0
Large plaque parapsoriasis	L41.4
Small plaque parapsoriasis	L41.3
Seborrheic dermatitis	L21.9
Unspecified erythematous condition	L53.9

READINGS

Avanlowo, O., Akinkuabe, A., & Olumide, Y. (2010, Jan–Mar). The pityriasis rosea calendar: A 7 year review of seasonal variation, age and sex distribution. *Nigerian Quarterly Journal of Hospital Medicine, 20*(1), 29–31.

Bhutani, T., Hong, J., & Koo, J. (2011). *Contemporary diagnosis and management of psoriasis* (5th ed.). Newton, PA: Handbooks in Health Care Co.

Broccolo, F., Drago, F., Careddu, A. M., Foglieni, C., Turbino, L., Cocuzza, C. E., . Malnati, M. S. (2005, Jun). Additional evidence that pityriasis rosea is associated with reactivation of human herpesvirus-6 and -7. *Journal of Investigative Dermatology, 124*(6), 1234–1240.

Drago, F., Brocollo, F., Zaccaria, E., Malnati, M., Cocuzza, C., Lusso, P., & Rebora, A. (2008, May). Pregnancy outcome in patients with pityriasis rosea. *Journal of American Academy of Dermatology, 58*(5 Suppl. 1), S78–S83.

Esposito, M., Saraceno, R., Giunta, A., Maccarone, M., & Chimenti, S. (2006). An Italian study on psoriasis and depression. *Dermatology. 212*(2), 123–127.

Gelfand, J. M., Shin, D. B., Neimann, A. L., Wang, X., Margolis, D.J., & Troxel, A. B. (2006). The risk of lymphoma in patients with psoriasis. *Journal of Investigative Dermatology, 126*(10), 2194–2201.

Gudjonsson, J. E., & Elder, J. T. (2007). Psoriasis: Epidemiology. *Clinics in Dermatology, 25*, 535–546.

Horn, E. J., Fox, K. M., Patel, V., Chiou, C-F, Dann, F., & Lebwohl, M. Are patients with psoriasis undertreated? Results of National Psoriasis Foundation survey. *Journal of the American Academy of Dermatology, 57*(6), 957–962.

Hsu, S., Papp, K. A., Lebwohl, M. G., Bagel, J., Blauvelt, A., Duffin, K. C., & Crowley, J., . National Psoriasis Foundation Medical Board. (2012). Consensus guidelines for the management of plaque psoriasis. *Archives of Dermatology, 148*(1), 95–102.

Kimball, A. B., Gladman, D., Gelfand, J. M., Gordon, K., Horn, E. J., & Korman, N.J., . National Psoriasis Foundation. (2008). National Psoriasis Foundation clinical concensus on psoriasis co morbidities and recommendations for screening. *Journal of the American Academy of Dermatology, 58*(6), 1031–1042.

Lebwohl, M., Heyman, W., Berth-Jones, J., & Coulson, I. (2010). Pityrisis lichenoides chronica. In *Treatment of skin disease* (3rd ed., pp. 565–570). Philadelphia, PA: Saunders Elsevier.

Lebwohl, M, Heyman, W., Berth-Jones, J., & Coulson, I (2010). Lichen planus. In *Treatment of skin disease* (3rd ed., pp. 383–386). Philadelphia, PA: Saunders Elsevier.

Menter, A., Korman, N.J., Elmets, C.A, Feldman, S. R., Gelfand, J.M., & Gordon, K.B., . Bhushan, R. (2011). Guidelines of care for the management of psoriasis and psoriatic arthritis. *Journal of the American Academy of Dermatology, 65*(1), 137–174.

Ramsay, B., & O'Reagan, M. (1988). A survey of the social and psychological effects of psoriasis. *British Journal of Dermatology, 118,* 195–201.

Van de Kerkhof, P. C. M., & Schalkwijk, J. (2008). Psoriasis. In J. L. Bolognia, J. L. Jorizzo, & R. P. Rapini (Eds.), *Dermatology* (2nd ed., pp. 115–135). Philadelphia, PA: Mosby Elsevier.

Wood, G. S., & Reizner, G. Other Papulosquamous Disorders. In J. L. Bolognia, J. L. Jorizzo, & R.P. Rapini (Eds.), *Dermatology* (2nd ed., pp. 144–146). Philadelphia, PA: Mosby Elsevier.

Victoria Garcia-Albea

CUTANEOUS DISORDERS OF THE NEWBORN

Newborn skin is different from adult skin in several ways: It is thinner, less hairy, and the attachment between the epidermis and dermis is weaker. Infants have a body surface area to weight ratio that is up to five times higher than adults. For these reasons, infant skin is at a higher risk for injury, percutaneous absorption, and skin infection. Additionally, infants have a higher rate of transepidermal water loss, which can lead to dehydration, electrolyte imbalance, and temperature instability.

NEWBORN SKIN CARE

At birth, the skin is covered with vernix caseosa, a grayish-white thick greasy material. Newborns lack the normal skin flora that protects against infection. There may be one or two surgical wounds present after birth—the umbilical stump and the circumcision site. To prevent infection, skin care should involve gentle cleansing with nontoxic, nonabrasive material. Wipe the vernix caseosa from the face, but allow the vernix on the rest of the body to come off by itself.

Newborns do not need to be bathed daily. Washing the buttocks and perianal area with warm soapy water at diaper changes will suffice. Once weekly bathing should be quick, to prevent thermoregulatory problems, followed by application of topical emollients to prevent transepidermal water loss and improve barrier function. Safe ingredients for neonates include white petrolatum ointment and lanolin. Parents should look for products that are fragrance- and dye-free.

There is no single standard of care for the umbilical stump. Avoid the use of povidone-iodine, as absorption of iodine can cause transient hypothyroxinemia or hypothyroidism. The cord site can be left dry, without bandages until the crust falls off on its own, usually about 10 days after birth. The site can become irritated, red, and sometimes painful, usually from diapers or clothing rubbing or pulling on the scab.

Infection of the umbilical stump is not common but can occur and may present as periumbilical erythema and induration (*omphalitis*). *Staphylococcus aureus*, introduced through the cut umbilical stump, is the most common pathogen and requires treatment to prevent sepsis. Systemic antibiotics are first line, but preventing infection is the primary focus. Daily washing with regular soap and water is usually enough to prevent infection.

Care of the circumcision site is similar to that of the umbilical stump. Keep the area clean by washing the area gently with soap and water at least once a day. Apply petrolatum ointment to the tip of the penis at each diaper change to prevent the penis from sticking to the diaper. The penis may initially be red, swollen, and bruised, and can have an yellow crust. Infection is rare; perform a culture if there is pus or drainage. The wound will heal in about 7 to 10 days.

SUBCUTANEOUS FAT NECROSIS

Subcutaneous fat necrosis (SCFN) is a benign panniculitis that affects healthy full-term newborns. It usually begins during the first few days to weeks of life.

Pathophysiology

The cause is unknown. It may be related to perinatal trauma, asphyxia, hypothermia, and hypercalcemia.

Clinical Presentation

SCFN is usually painless, but occasionally can be tender or uncomfortable, making infants cry when handled. There may be one or several erythematous or bruise-like, well-defined, firm nodules or large plaques, but they are not warm to touch. SCFN occurs most often on the cheeks, back, buttocks, arms, and thighs (Figure 6-1).

DIFFERENTIAL DIAGNOSIS Subcutaneous fat necrosis
• Cellulitis
• Erysipelas
• Sclerema neonatorum
• Nevus comedonicus
• Child abuse

Diagnostics

A punch biopsy of affected skin will confirm the diagnosis. This diagnosis can sometimes be made clinically. Serum calcium should be evaluated.

Management

Hypercalcemia is rare, but can be treated with low calcium and vitamin D intake or systemic corticosteroid therapy.

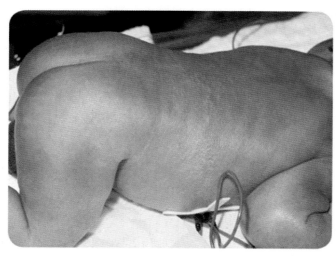

FIG. 6-1. Superficial red nodules of varying size due to subcutaneous fat necrosis.

Prognosis and Complications

SCFN is self-limited. Most lesions heal spontaneously, though lesions can become fluctuant with necrotic fat, ulcerate, and scar. Some heal with temporary skin depression, which resolves over time without treatment.

Referral and Consultation

Dermatology should be consulted. In severe or ulcerated cases, a surgical consultation may be required for debridement.

Patient Education and Follow-up

Parents should be reassured that most cases of SCFN spontaneously resolve without significant sequelae. If hypercalcemia is present, serum calcium levels should be monitored regularly and patients placed on a low calcium and vitamin D diet.

MILIARIA

Miliaria crystallina and *miliaria rubra* (prickly heat) commonly occur in infancy. The onset of miliaria crystallina peaks at one week of life. Miliaria rubra can present in infants and adults, and usually follows a move to a tropical climate.

Pathophysiology

Miliaria is caused by an occlusion of the sweat glands, resulting in retention and rupture. Crystallina occurs higher in the epidermis, at the stratum corneum, compared to rubra, which occurs deeper in the epidermis.

Clinical Presentation

Clear, superficial pinpoint vesicles without inflammation are the classic presentation of miliaria crystallina. Lesions rupture in 1 or 2 days, leaving behind a fine scale. In infants, it occurs on the head, neck, and upper trunk. In older children, it favors the sun-exposed areas. *Miliaria rubra* is characterized by slightly larger 2- to 4-mm erythematous papules or vesicles, and occurs after excessive sweating. These lesions tend to favor flexural areas, including the neck, antecubital fossa, popliteal fossae, axillae, and groin, or in localized areas that have been occluded. Rubra also tends to be quite itchy or may sting, and may last for weeks. Secondary bacterial infections can occur, changing the morphology to pustules or honey-crusted lesions.

DIFFERENTIAL DIAGNOSIS   Miliaria
• Cutaneous candidiasis
• Varicella
• Erythema toxicum neonatorum
• Folliculitis
• Herpes simplex virus
• Pityrosporum folliculitis
• Pseudomonas folliculitis

Diagnostics

Miliaria is a clinical diagnosis. If the diagnosis is uncertain, a biopsy could be helpful. A Tzanck examination negative for multinucleated giant cells will rule out HSV and a negative KOH test eliminates a yeast or fungal etiology.

Management

Miliaria crystallina does not require treatment because it is asymptomatic and benign. Treatment of miliaria rubra includes avoiding excessive heat and humidity to minimize sweating, dressing in lightweight cotton clothing, limiting activity, taking cool baths, and using air conditioning. For infants, a mild-potency topical corticosteroid (TCS) may be used but should be limited to no more than 2 weeks. If a secondary bacterial infection has been identified by culture and sensitivity, mupirocin 2% ointment three times daily for 10 days is safe and usually effective for infants.

Referral and Consultation

If the diagnosis is unclear or the symptoms are severe, a referral to a pediatric dermatologist is warranted.

Prognosis and Complications

Miliaria crystallina is self-limited, and resolves without complications in a few days. Miliaria rubra spontaneously resolves when patients are moved to cooler environments, but will recur when sweating is stimulated.

Patient Education and Follow-up

For infants, the emphasis should be on the avoidance of over dressing. Patient education should also include avoiding high heat and humidity (above).

ACNE NEONATORUM

Acne neonatorum refers to neonatal acne and infantile acne. Neonatal acne usually begins within the first few weeks of life and resolves by 6 months of age. Infantile acne occurs in males to females 5:1, and starts at 6 to 12 months old.

Pathophysiology

The etiology of most neonatal acne is unknown, but may be related to hormonal stimulation of sebaceous glands by maternal androgens. Infantile acne, which starts later, tends to be more severe and persistent than neonatal acne, and may occasionally be associated with an underlying systemic disease or hormonal abnormality.

Clinical Presentation

Neonatal acne and infantile acne resemble acne vulgaris, with involvement usually on the face only. Open and closed comedones are most common; inflammatory papules and pustules are seen occasionally. Rarely, deep papules, nodules, and cysts can present with infantile acne. When neonatal acne is associated with *Malassezia* yeast overgrowth, lesions appear more pustular.

DIFFERENTIAL DIAGNOSIS   Acne neonatorum
• Miliaria
• Rosacea
• Contact dermatitis
• Seborrheic dermatitis
• Folliculitis

Diagnostics

Direct examination of pustule contents with KOH test shows yeast. A bacterial culture and sensitivity may be indicated if there is suspicion of infection. If acne is especially severe or persistent, diagnostic tests for abnormal androgen production should be considered.

Management

Treatment is not usually needed, as most cases are mild. Neonatal acne tends to resolve spontaneously in 1 to 2 weeks. Cleansing with gentle soap and water daily can clear many cases. Mild inflammatory acne can be treated safely in patients of all ages. Topical antibiotics, such as erythromycin or clindamycin, are not recommended as monotherapy because they take a long time to start working and are associated with high rates of bacterial resistance. Instead, Eichenfield et al. (2013) recommends using benzoyl peroxide 2.5%, 5%, or 10% and clindamycin 1% in conjunction (Duac, Benzaclin, Acanya). In moderate to severe acne cases, dermatology specialists may use topical retinoids. Most are used off-label for children under 12 years old, except for combination adapalene plus benzoyl peroxide gel 0.1%/2.5% (Epiduo) which is approved for those 9 years and older. Patients with *Malassezia* can be treated with topical antifungal creams or shampoos, like ketoconazole 2% or selenium sulfide 2.5%.

Prognosis and Complications

Nearly all cases of acne neonatorum resolve spontaneously. Treatment may hasten resolution.

Referral and Consultation

If severe, patients should be referred to a dermatologist. Refer to endocrinologist if there are any signs of virilization or growth abnormalities.

ERYTHEMA TOXICUM NEONATORUM

Erythema toxicum neonatorum (ETN) is a benign, self-limiting eruption seen in full-term neonates. It most often begins in the first 2 to 4 days of life.

Pathophysiology

ETN is idiopathic.

Clinical Presentation

Erythematous macules and papules occur anywhere on the body, usually sparing the palms and soles. Lesions may be blotchy and irregular, and can vary in size from 1- to 3-mm papules and pustules to larger pink plaques that are several centimeters in diameter (Figure 6-2).

DIFFERENTIAL DIAGNOSIS Erythema toxicum neonatorum

* Transient neonatal pustular melanosis
* Milia
* Miliaria
* Candidiasis
* Herpes simplex virus
* Folliculitis

Diagnostics

ETN is a clinical diagnosis, and skin biopsy is rarely indicated.

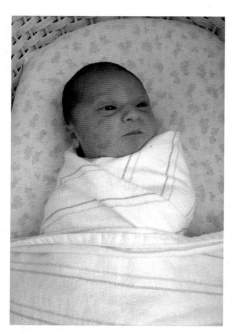

FIG. 6-2. Erythema toxicum neonatorum.

Management

No treatment is necessary.

Prognosis and Complications

ETN is self-limiting, and patients rarely have complications.

Patient Education and Follow-up

ETN may be concerning to parents, so reassurance and parent education are important. No follow-up is necessary unless the characteristics of the eruption change.

Seborrheic Dermatitis

In children, seborrheic dermatitis is a benign, erythematous scaly or crusting dermatosis common in infants and adolescents. Parents may call it "cradle cap."

Pathophysiology

The exact cause of seborrheic dermatitis is unknown. It occurs in "seborrheic areas" (see chapter 5) which contain the highest concentration of sebaceous glands, suggesting an association with sebum and sebaceous glands. The yeast, *Malassezia furfur*, has also been implicated.

Clinical Presentation

In infants, scalp involvement has variable erythema with thin, white-yellow scale (Figure 6-3). In the diaper area, lesions are redder and may have scale with accentuation in the skin folds (Figure 6-4). In older children and adolescents, central facial and nasolabial folds can have red to salmon-colored with greasy scale and sharply defined borders. Pinpoint red papules may present near the nasal ala. They may complain of dandruff. Pruritus is usually minimal.

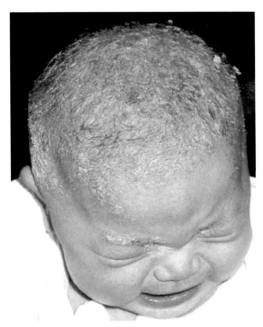

FIG. 6-3. Seborrheic dermatitis. Note the thick yellow scale, background erythema, and typical seborrheic distribution.

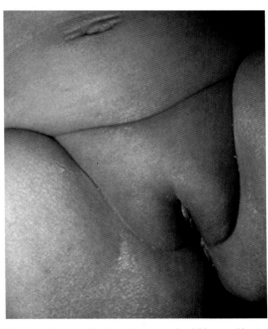

FIG. 6-4. Seborrheic dermatitis is most common in children and is manifested by skin fold redness and scale.

DIFFERENTIAL DIAGNOSIS Seborrheic dermatitis

- Atopic dermatitis
- Acneiform dermatoses
- Contact dermatitis
- Psoriasis
- Langerhans cell histiocytosis
- "Leiner's phenotype" of immunodeficiency

Diagnostics

Seborrheic dermatitis is usually diagnosed clinically. However, the diagnosis can be difficult and must be differentiated from other papulosquamous, eczematous, and infectious dermatoses. If seborrheic dermatitis occurs in a child with failure to thrive and diarrhea, evaluate for immunodeficiency. Figure 6-5 shows an algorithm for use in diagnosing scaly scalp.

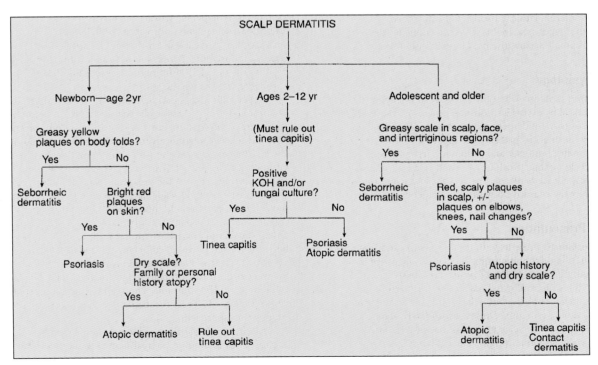

FIG. 6-5. Algorithm for diagnosis of a scaly scalp.

Management

Infantile seborrheic dermatitis can resolve in as little as 3 to 4 weeks, even without treatment. Therefore, because it is benign, watchful waiting and reassurance are acceptable. If treatment is desired for infants and children, application of mineral or baby oil can be left on the scalp overnight. A shampoo in the morning will allow for gentle removal of the scale with a soft brush or toothbrush. Over-the-counter keratolytic or antiseborrheic shampoos containing zinc, salicylic acid, or tar may be used safely. Antifungal shampoos, such as ketoconazole and ciclopirox, are used if *M. furfur* is suspected. Low-potency TCS (used twice daily for up to 2 weeks) and calcineurin inhibitors can reduce inflammation and help control pruritus. Tea tree oil is a naturopathic alternative used by many, but lacks supporting studies. See chapter 5 for more information about seborrheic dermatitis in adults.

Secondary bacterial infection is most common in the diaper or intertriginous areas. If oozing occurs, a culture should be obtained and antimicrobials prescribed as needed. Children who scratch or pick off waxy plaques from their scalp are also at increased risk for bacterial infection.

Prognosis and Complications

It usually spontaneously resolves by 8 to 12 months of age. In adolescents and adults, the condition may wax and wane.

Patient Education and Follow-up

Seborrheic dermatitis has no cure. Reassure parents that infantile cradle cap will self-resolve. In older children and adolescents, seborrheic dermatitis has a more chronic course. Daily use of medicated shampoos and antipruritic agents can control symptoms.

DIAPER DERMATITIS

Diaper dermatitis, also called *napkin dermatitis* or *diaper rash*, is one of the most common skin conditions of childhood, affecting about 25% of children under 2 years old. "Diaper dermatitis" describes a number of different clinical disorders characterized by acute inflammation in the diaper area. In this section, chafing dermatitis (the most common), irritant dermatitis, and diaper candidiasis are discussed.

Pathophysiology

Inflammation develops when the integrity of the epidermal barrier is compromised by excessive moisture, heat, or irritation. The warm, moist environment of diapers can exacerbate skin irritation.

Chafing dermatitis presents in areas with the most friction (thighs, genitalia, buttocks, and abdomen). Irritant dermatitis results from direct skin contact with urine, stool, or chemicals (soap, detergent, creams). *Candida albicans* lives in the lower intestine of infants and is usually the causative organism in diaper candidiasis.

Clinical Presentation

Chafing dermatitis presents with mild erythema and fine scale and is due to friction or rubbing from the diaper. Leg openings or waist are commonly affected. *Irritant contact dermatitis* causes bright red erythema, fine scale, and skin breakdown or superficial erosions on the convex surfaces of the buttocks, vulva, lower abdomen, proximal thighs, and perineum. *Diaper candidiasis* appears as bright red plaques with white scale at the border located on the buttocks, lower abdomen, and inner thighs. The hallmark features are satellite bright pink-red papules and pustules. Also, examine the oral mucosa to screen for oral thrush.

DIFFERENTIAL DIAGNOSIS Diaper dermatitis

- Seborrheic dermatitis
- Psoriasis
- Intertrigo
- Folliculitis
- Impetigo
- Scabies
- Nutritional deficiency (e.g., acrodermatitis enteropathica)
- Contact dermatitis
- Atopic dermatitis
- Granuloma gluteale infantum
- Langerhans cell histiocytosis
- Epidermolysis bullosa
- Tinea cruris
- Streptococcal perianal cellulitis

Diagnostics

First, differentiate between the types of diaper dermatitis above, then rule out yeast and bacterial infections. If *C. albicans* is present, microscopic KOH examination will show budding yeasts with pseudohyphae. See Skills Section for how to do a KOH test. Bacterial culture and sensitivity may be helpful. Fungal infection is rare in infants.

Management

Treatment depends on the underlying cause. For chafing dermatitis, reduce the friction by loosening the securing tabs, buying a larger-size diaper, or using barrier creams (reduce frictions). Primary management for irritant dermatitis is to keep the area as clean and dry as possible. Skin will improve with frequent diaper changes; nonirritating, fragrance-free wipes; chemical-free disposable diapers or cloth diapers; exposure to air whenever possible; and liberal use of barrier creams (petrolatum, zinc). In the absence of candidiasis, conservative use of low-potency (nonfluorinated) TCS can be used cautiously for up to 2 weeks, sooner if the dermatitis resolves. Hydrocortisone 2.5% ointment and desonide 0.05% ointment are safe and effective choices.

Diaper candidiasis can be treated with topical antiyeast/fungal creams (nystatin, clotrimazole, ketoconazole). It should be noted, there are combination antifungal/corticosteroid products available, which are commonly used. Using a combination product means that even after the acute inflammation has been calmed, additional treatment with the TCS is necessary if the parent is going to continue to treat the yeast infection. Nystatin/triamcinolone (mid-potency TCS) is available as Mycolog II and is FDA approved for children >2 years old, but should not be used under occlusion (diapers or plastic pants). Clotrimazole/betamethasone dipropionate, available as Lotrisone, contains a high-potency TCS and has been prescribed by some clinicians for diaper dermatitis. It should be noted that it is FDA approved for children 17 years and older for treatment of tinea for no longer than 2 weeks. It should NOT to be used under occlusion. The manufacturer reports that use in children under 17 years for diaper dermatitis has reported adrenal suppression approaching 30%.

The authors suggest use of separate agents to allow the clinician and caregiver to modify the treatment without requiring the administration of both drugs (mild TCS and antifungal) for diaper dermatitis. Oral fluconazole is used for severe cases.

Prognosis and Complications

Once the cause of diaper dermatitis is determined, treatment and management can be administered, and clearance should be completed within days to weeks. Any diaper dermatitis present for more than 3 days is at high risk for developing a secondary candidiasis. Chafing dermatitis and diaper candidiasis are both prone to recurrences. Provide anticipatory guidance about prevention (see Management section).

Patient Education and Follow-up

Prevention is the focus of patient education for all diaper dermatoses. Close follow-up is not needed, as parents should notice improvement a few days after starting treatment. If improvement is not rapid, and in severe or complicated cases, more frequent monitoring may be indicated with phone calls or in-office check-ups, especially if oral medications are required. If treated with TCS, the clinician must educate that caregiver about the administration, risk, benefits, and side effects of therapy.

THRUSH

Infants contract thrush (oral candidiasis) during delivery, nursing from contaminated nipples, contact with contaminated hands, or from improper sterilization of bottles and nipples. Oral thrush in children and adolescents can occur secondary to corticosteroid inhalers used for asthma.

Pathophysiology

Pathogenesis of thrush due to *C. albicans* is the same as for diaper candidiasis.

Clinical Presentation

Thrush appears as white or gray pseudomembranous or velvety patches and plaques on red mucosa that bleeds easily. It affects the tongue, hard and soft palates, buccal mucosa, and gingivae. It can be painful or asymptomatic.

DIFFERENTIAL DIAGNOSIS Thrush

- Aphthous stomatitis
- Candidiasis
- Herpes simplex virus
- Cytomegalovirus
- Blastomycosis
- Esophagitis
- Pharyngitis
- Enteroviral infection
- Human immunodeficiency virus infection
- Histiocytosis

Diagnostics

Diagnosis is often based on clinical findings. To confirm the presence of yeast, gently rub a cotton applicator or tongue depressor on the area to remove some of the plaques and perform a KOH test.

Management

The most common treatment for infants is 2 mL of nystatin 100,000 units per mL, deposited on the inside of each cheek with a dropper, four times a day for 1 to 2 weeks. For infants, the parents should massage the suspension on the mucosa. Mothers who are breastfeeding should also apply the solution to their nipples four times a day. Administer medication between meals to allow for longer contact time. Medicated troches or suppositories used in the tip/slit of a pacifier or bottle are not recommended as it has not been evaluated in controlled studies, and there is a risk for aspiration.

Oral antifungal medications such as fluconazole (Diflucan) should be used if there is a risk for widespread disease. Older children can use nystatin or clotrimazole oral tablets or troches. If corticosteroid inhalers are used for asthma, ensure that the child has good technique with administration, good oral hygiene, and rinse with water after using inhaler.

Special Considerations

Recurrence. Examine for maternal vaginal candidiasis or contaminated nipples or pacifiers. Most treatment failures are due to improper medication application, not resistance, but *Candida* species are becoming resistant to itraconazole.

Immunosupression. Thrush in immunocompromised children can be severe and may require oral treatment. Candidal esophagitis is a common complication, which can cause dysphagia, respiratory distress, and anorexia.

Prognosis and Complications

Most cases are uncomplicated and clear in 1 to 2 weeks.

Patient Education and Follow-up

Follow-up should be at least 2 weeks after treatment is initiated, to evaluate response to therapy and ensure complete resolution.

APLASIA CUTIS CONGENITA

Aplasia cutis congenita (ACC) refers to the absence of epidermis, dermis, and sometimes, subcutaneous tissue, and is present at birth. Most cases are sporadic, but familial cases have been reported. ACC can occur in association with epidermal nevi, premature rupture of membranes, limb abnormalities, epidermolysis bullosa, malformation syndromes, and infections.

Pathophysiology

ACC represents an interruption in intrauterine skin development, but the etiology is not known. Genetic factors, trauma, vascular compromise, intrauterine infections, and teratogens have been suggested, most notably the thyroid medication methimazole (MMI). Parents often assume it is due to the use of forceps during delivery—scratching the scalp and leaving a scar. However, the defect occurs during gestation, as an absence of the skin, and sometimes, subcutaneous tissue.

Clinical Presentation

At birth, ACC can present as an ulcer, superficial erosion, atrophic plaque, or a well-formed scar (Figure 6-6). Lesions that occur early in gestation have time to heal into a scar that will be present at birth. Lesions that occur later in gestation appear as ulceration at birth. Most are 1 to 2 cm in diameter; larger lesions are more likely to extend to deeper structures.

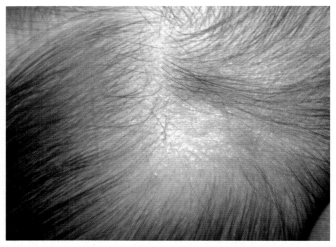

FIG. 6-6. Aplasia cutis congenita. Note that these lesions can be quite subtle.

If a membrane is present, it is called *membranous aplasia cutis*. Seventy percent of cases occur as a single lesion on the scalp, but it can occur anywhere on the body. Scalp lesions are usually located near the hair whorl at the vertex. The *hair collar sign* is when ACC is surrounded by a ring of long, dark hair. This is a marker for ACC and can indicate deeper involvement.

DIFFERENTIAL DIAGNOSIS Aplasia cutis congenita

- Birth trauma (e.g., from forceps)
- Nevus sebaceous

Diagnostics

ACC is diagnosed clinically.

Management

Most lesions do not require treatment, but depends on the size, location, and depth of the lesion. Small ACC lesions are managed like any other localized wound. The area should be kept clean and moist with petrolatum, Aquaphor, or silver sulfadiazine ointments that promote healing and prevent further tissue damage. Antibiotics should be used only for culture-confirmed secondary bacterial infections. Infants with full-thickness lesions may require imaging and surgical management.

Prognosis and Complications

Most small lesions heal into a smooth, subtle scar with alopecia within a few weeks or months. Lesions over 4 cm in diameter have the potential for hemmorhage, venous thrombosis, and meningitis. These patients should have CT scan or MRI imaging.

Referral and Consultation

For large and obvious lesions, consult plastic surgery for reconstruction and to prevent complications.

Patient Education and Follow-up

While lesions are healing, follow-up should be regular to monitor progress and screen for secondary infection. Once healing is complete, follow-up is as needed.

NEONATAL LUPUS ERYTHEMATOSUS

Neonatal lupus erythematosus (NLE) is an autoimmune disease that occurs in infants whose mothers have systemic lupus erythematosus (SLE); or a tendency for SLE, rheumatoid arthritis, Sjögren syndrome, or mixed connective tissue disease. This occurs in less than 2% of births to women with autoimmune diseases.

Pathophysiology

NLE occurs when autoimmune antibodies are passively transferred to the neonate. Only about half of these mothers have a previously diagnosed connective tissue disease. When cardiac manifestations like heart block occurs, it usually develops in utero.

Clinical Presentation

Almost one quarter of infants with NLE have systemic symptoms at birth. Congenital heart block is most common. NLE can also affect the liver, spleen, and lymphatic and hematologic systems.

About half of patients display cutaneous symptoms at some point, including discoid lesions, scaly atrophic plaques, and telangiectasias. Facial erythema is common, especially around the periorbital areas (raccoon eyes). Cutaneous signs may be present at birth, and typically resolve without sequelae within weeks to months (Figures 6-7 and 6-8).

Diagnostics

Diagnosis is based on cutaneous findings, systemic symptoms, and laboratory studies. Further workup includes thorough history and physical examination, CBC with platelets, liver function tests, antinuclear antibody (ANA), urinalysis, and serum complements C_3 and C_4. If bradycardia or a heart murmur is detected, electrocardiography and echocardiography should be performed. A skin biopsy should be performed, which will show histological features of lupus erythematosus.

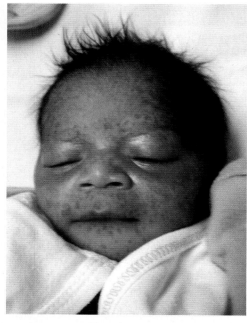

FIG. 6-7. Neonatal lupus erythematosus. Note the marked facial and periorbital erythema "raccoon eyes."

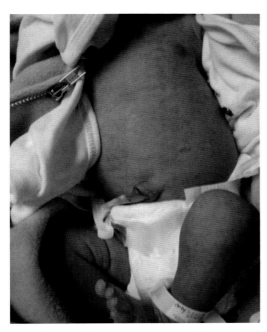

FIG. 6-8. Neonatal lupus erythematosus, trunk.

Management

Treatment with low- to mid-potency TCS or topical calcineurin inhibitors can improve erythema, but will not reduce permanent skin changes. Treatment should address any associated systemic disease and complications.

Prognosis and Complications

Skin lesions usually fade by age 6 to 12 months of age, as maternal antibodies wane, but can last longer. One quarter of patients have permanent telangiectasia, hyper- or hypopigmentation, atrophic scars, and/or alopecia.

Special Considerations

Pregnancy. Mothers with one child with NLE have a 22% risk of having another child with NLE.

Referral and Consultation

If neonatal lupus is suspected, consult a dermatologist and a cardiologist.

Patient Education and Follow-up

Reassure parents that patients do not have a higher risk of developing SLE or other autoimmune disorders. These patients should have regular well-child visits with a pediatrician and any other specialties needed to manage other complications.

VASCULAR DISORDERS OF INFANCY

Vascular lesions can be classified into two categories: tumors and malformations. Although both can be present at birth, their pathogenesis, clinical presentation, and evolution during the first few months of life are different. Understanding the progression of various vascular lesions can aid in an accurate diagnosis. Vascular lesions may be associated with or be an indication of systemic disease or genetic syndromes. In this chapter, specific vascular tumors and malformations will be discussed, but tumor and malformation syndromes will not be extensively covered.

VASCULAR TUMORS

Vascular tumors are benign vascular growths that include infantile hemangiomas and pyogenic granulomas. They also include tufted angioma and kaposiform hemangioendothelioma, which will not be discussed in this chapter.

INFANTILE HEMANGIOMA

Infantile hemangiomas (IHs) or *hemangiomas of infancy* are the most common benign soft tissue tumor of childhood. They occur in 4 to 10% of full-term infants. IHs are more common in girls than in boys (3 to 5:1) and premature infants. Most are not present at birth, but develop in the first 4 weeks of life, and are often first noticed by the parents.

Pathophysiology

IHs can be categorized as superficial, deep, or mixed, and are described by phases. The *proliferation phase* occurs within the first 8 weeks of life, much earlier than previously thought, and is characterized by rapid growth. The *plateau phase* follows for up to 6 months and usually has no growth of the lesion. Then the *involutional phase* follows where there is dramatic color change from bright red to dull red, purple, or gray. The center of the hemangioma begins to involute or flatten. Lesions become smaller, softer, and less warm. Involution is completed by age 10 years in 90% of cases.

Clinical Presentation

Superficial hemangiomas present as bright red, flat or raised papules, plaques, or nodules. *Deep* hemangiomas appear as subcutaneous nodules with an overlying blue discoloration and may have telangiectasias or a prominent venous network. *Mixed* hemangiomas, the most common type, have both a superficial and deep component causing them to appear bright red with a nodular blue component. All types tend to be compressible, slightly more solid than a lipoma, but not as firm as a lymph node or cyst. They are most common on the head and neck, but can appear anywhere on the body, including internally (Figure 6-9).

> **DIFFERENTIAL DIAGNOSIS** Infantile hemangioma
> - Vascular malformation
> - Trauma

Diagnostics

IHs are usually diagnosed clinically with the help of the history of the lesion as provided by parents, photos, or in-office monitoring. Hemangiomas can be differentiated from vascular malformations, as the latter are more likely to be present at birth and do not proliferate or involute. If the distinction cannot be made based on history and physical examination, it is highly recommended that an experienced dermatology provider or surgical specialist evaluate the patient. If the IH has any high-risk features, specialists will need additional imaging, biopsy, and other studies to carefully diagnose the extent and severity of the vascular tumor (Table 6-1).

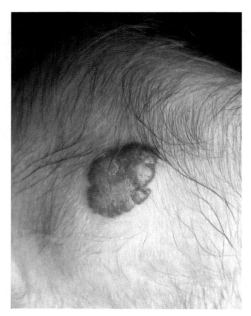

FIG. 6-9. Infantile hemangioma. This is a superficial infantile hemangioma commonly found on the scalp with characteristic bright red color.

Management

Most IHs can be monitored and do not require treatment. The management goals are to prevent life-threatening complications, minimize disfigurement, prevent or reverse functional impairment, and reduce psychosocial stress.

Until a few years ago, oral corticosteroids were the gold standard of treatment for large, life-threatening or function-threatening hemangiomas. These are still used to hasten involution in some cases. Current therapies include the oral β-blocker propranolol, which has been shown to rapidly stop proliferation and induce involution. The topical β-blocker, timolol, is also effective. However, children must be monitored closely for the side effects of these medications, which include hypoglycemia, hypotension, and bronchospasm. Multidisciplinary teams providing care have protocols for initiation and monitoring of treatment.

Prognosis and Complications

Approximately 10% to 15% of IHs ulcerate, usually during the proliferation phase, and is most common in the diaper area. When the skin breaks down, the IH bleeds, causes pain, and increases risk for secondary infection and possible scarring. Care of ulcerated IHs includes warm compresses, topical antibiotics, and petrolatum-based nonstick gauze dressings. A culture and sensitivity of deeply ulcerated lesions that have drainage or exudate should prompt appropriate use of oral antibiotics. Pulsed dye laser (PDL) can be used to treat and reduce pain of ulcerated hemangiomas.

Once the IH has involuted, there are usually residual telangiectasias, atrophy, scarring, or a fibro-fatty mass (like a lipoma).

Referral and Consultation

High-risk IHs that are life-threatening and function-threatening require prompt referral to a specialists, ideally a multidisciplinary team dedicated to children with vascular anomalies (usually academic centers), for evaluation and treatment.

TABLE 6-1	Features of High-Risk Infantile Hemangiomas
LOCATION	**ASSOCIATED RISKS**
Periorbital hemangiomas	Impaired development of normal binocular vision, amblyopia, astigmatism, strabismus, proptosis, and optic atrophy
Nasal tip hemangiomas	Distortion of nasal anatomy and disfigurement
Lip hemangiomas	Increased risk of ulceration, bleeding, scarring Feeding problems
Ear hemangiomas	Possible obstruction of the auditory canal and conductive hearing loss Cosmetically problematic
"Beard area" hemangiomas (neck, lower lip, chin, preauricular, mandibular area)	Increased risk for airway obstruction, feeding difficulties, respiratory stridor, and hoarseness Patients may require immediate laryngoscopy
Genital and perineal hemangiomas	Frequent ulceration and bleeding Increased risk for infection, pain, and scarring
Lumbosacral hemangiomas	Possible occult spinal dysraphism or spinal cord defect (tethered cord most common) Anorectal, urogenital, and renal abnormalities
Segmental hemangiomas	Higher incidence of urogenital anomalies
PHACES syndrome	Genetic disorder with constellation of features: P—posterior fossa abnormality (brain and especially cerebellum) H—hemangiomas (head, face, and/or neck) A—arterial anomalies (brain) C—cardiac anomalies or aortic coarctation E—eye abnormalities S—sternal clefting, supraumbilical abdominal raphe, or thyroid abnormalities
Five or more lesions anywhere on the body	At risk for visceral involvement, further workup is recommended

PYOGENIC GRANULOMA

A pyogenic granuloma (PG) is a common benign lobular capillary hemangioma. The incidence is higher in children and pregnant women.

Pathogenesis

The etiology is unknown, but they often develop following minor trauma; PGs are exophytic papules comprised of blood vessels.

Clinical Presentation

Presenting as a well-circumscribed, small (<1 cm) red papule, PGs grow rapidly, can ulcerate and bleed easily (Figure 6-10). The most common site is on the face and acral areas.

DIFFERENTIAL DIAGNOSIS Pyogenic granuloma
• Melanocytic nevus
• Glomus tumor
• Hemangioma
• Irritated nevus
• Verruca vulgaris
• Spitz nevus

Diagnostics

Diagnosis is confirmed with a skin biopsy.

Management

PGs are benign, but if not removed, they can persist. Shave removal or excision followed by electrocautery is sufficient to remove most lesions. Recurrence is common.

Referral and Consultation

Refer to a dermatologist, plastic surgeon, or general surgeon for excision and biopsy.

Patient Education and Follow-up

Reassure the patient and family that these are benign. No follow-up is needed.

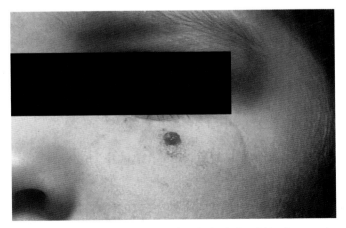

FIG. 6-10. A child suddenly developed a single dark red bleeding papule, which is common with a pyogenic granuloma.

VASCULAR MALFORMATIONS

A vascular malformation is an abnormal development of blood vessels that occurs without any endothelial cell growth or proliferation. Vascular malformations are present at birth, and do not undergo rapid progression, or involute. Thus, vascular malformations are permanent. They are categorized by the predominant vessel involved, including capillary, venous, and arteriovenous malformation (AVM).

SALMON PATCH

A salmon patch, also known as *nevus simple,* is a common capillary malformation that occurs in 30% to 40% of all newborns.

Clinical Presentation

Most present as a light pink patch on the posterior neck and are commonly referred to as a *stork bite.* They can be on the occipital scalp, eyelids, forehead or eyelids (*angel kiss*), glabella, nose or naso-labial area. Lesions become more pronounced when infants cry, hold their breath, strain during defecation, or physically exert themselves.

Management

Salmon patches are benign and have no associated developmental risks, and therefore do not require treatment.

Prognosis and Complications

Ninety-five percent of facial lesions fade by age 2 years. Some neck lesions fade over time, while others may remain visible for a lifetime. They are usually covered by hair and are therefore minimally cosmetically bothersome.

Patient Education and Follow-up

Reassure and educate parents that lesions become more pronounced during crying, straining to defecate, etc.

PORT WINE STAIN

A port wine stain (PWS) or *nevus flammeus* is the most common type of vascular malformation, especially in Caucasian newborns. These can be associated with Sturge–Weber syndrome, Parkes–Weber syndrome, Klippel–Trenaunay syndrome, Hyperkeratotic cutaneous capillary-venous malformation, and Proteus syndrome.

Clinical Presentation

Initially appearing as pink patches, PWS get their name from the dark red color that develops with age (Figure 6-11). They can occur anywhere on the body but are most common on the face, and are almost always unilateral. PWS can become raised or develop nodules and blebs, and can affect the growth of underlying tissue. Unlike infantile he mangiomas, PWS are static and do not undergo a proliferation phase.

DIFFERENTIAL DIAGNOSIS Port wine stain
• Birth trauma
• Infantile hemangiomas
• Salmon patch
• Cellulitis
• Morphea

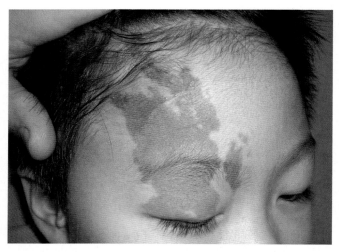

FIG. 6-11. Port wine stain.

Diagnostics

PWS are a clinical diagnosis, but can be indistinguishable from IHs at birth. Monitoring for proliferation or involution can help make the diagnosis, and a skin biopsy would confirm it.

Management

The size of the lesion, location, and possible associated syndromes will influence the clinician's plan of care. Most PWS are small and benign and require no treatment. If cosmesis is a concern, the patch can usually be covered up with makeup such as Dermablend. PDL can effectively treat PWS. Evidence suggests that the earlier the PWS are treated with laser, the better they respond.

Referral and Consultation

Laser treatment for PWS requires referral to a cardiovascular or dermatology specialist experienced in treatment of PWS in children. If there is any suspicion for an associated syndrome like Sturge–Weber, a prompt referral to a dermatologist, neurologist, and ophthalmologist is essential. If the PWS is in the trigeminal area, patients must be followed up by an ophthalmologist, as there is a high risk of glaucoma.

Prognosis and Complications

Most PWS are uncomplicated and may fade slightly over time. Lesions covering an extremity should be carefully evaluated for risk of venous stasis, varicosities, lymphedema, ulcerations, and Klippel–Trenaunay syndrome. Patients with facial PWS may have Sturge–Weber syndrome, glaucoma, or complications of the central nervous system. Even when not associated with a genetic syndrome, these lesions are almost always of cosmetic importance because of their size and location.

VENOUS MALFORMATIONS

Venous malformations (VMs) are the most common of all vascular anomalies. Although they are congenital, they may not be clinically obvious until infancy, childhood, or adulthood. The exact etiology is not well understood, but most appear to be sporadic. There are familial cases caused by autosomal dominant inheritance (i.e., Klippel–Trenaunay syndrome).

Pathophysiology

A VM is a slow-flow vascular malformation resulting from the abnormal development of venules or veins. Some VMs may also present with a lymphatic malformation (LM) and arterial malformation (AM). The exact etiology is not well understood, but most appear to be sporadic. There are familial cases caused by autosomal dominant inheritance.

Clinical Presentation

At birth, a VM may appear as blue or purple nodules, but may not be detectable for a few years. Initially, they are asymptomatic, soft, and compressible. When the limb is in a dependent position, the lesion can become engorged with blood. As lesions enlarge, they can become nodular with swelling and pain. Blood clots can form following trauma or venous stasis.

DIFFERENTIAL DIAGNOSIS Venous malformation
• Infantile hemangioma
• Trauma
• Blood clot

Diagnostics

VMs can be diagnosed with CT scan, MRI, or doppler ultrasonography.

Management

VMs are difficult to treat and are typically managed by a pediatric vascular anomaly team. Compression stockings reduce pain, swelling, and risk of coagulopathy. Surgery, physical therapy, and sclerotherapy are also effective. Low-dose aspirin can help prevent thrombotic events. Some authors advocate for early surgical intervention to prevent symptoms and to reduce long-term complications.

Prognosis and Complications

Complications of VMs include thromboses, pain as lesions enlarge and put pressure on surrounding structures, disfigurement and possible psychosocial distress, limited mobility, and localized intravascular coagulopathy. Klippel–Trenaunay syndrome (VM and LM) often results in abnormal development of the underlying soft tissue and bone growth in the limb. Infections are quite common.

Referral and Consultation

Refer patients to a dermatologist and/or surgeon.

Patient Education and Follow-up

Inform parents that lesions are difficult to treat. Follow-up in a pediatric specialty clinic is advised.

ARTERIOVENOUS MALFORMATION

AVM is a rare vascular malformation involving both arteries and veins. These are the most serious type of vascular anomaly and can cause functional deformity, cardiovascular compromise, and cosmetic concerns. Lesions are present at birth, but if there is minimal skin involvement, they may not be detected until years later.

Pathophysiology

AVMs are high-flow lesions resulting from the shunting between the artery and vein, bypassing the capillaries.

Clinical Presentation

Lesions vary from small red patches to thin vascular plaques or large pulsating masses with an audible bruit. The overlying skin may be thickened. Most start out as a vascular blush that begins to expand and bleed. Lesions grow faster during puberty or other hormonal changes. Often, signs and symptoms of AVMs may not be clinically obvious until the second or third decade of life. They can undergo frequent, dramatic, and rapid growth spurts, which are caused by a number of environmental factors. Some are internal and are only detected when patients become symptomatic.

DIFFERENTIAL DIAGNOSIS Arteriovenous malformation

- Infantile hemangioma
- Port wine stain
- Trauma
- Venous malformation

Diagnostics

Ultrasound, CT, MRI, or angiography is required for diagnosis.

Management

Treatment depends on the age of the patient, comorbidities, and the size, location, and severity of the AVM. Options include monitoring, excision, amputation, or embolization. When localized to the skin, excision and embolization can be curative.

Special Considerations

Although stable in childhood, AVMs may worsen during pregnancy because of increased blood pressure and volume.

Prognosis and Complications

Prognosis depends on the location of the AVM. They can be life-threatening because of the risk of massive bleeding from cutaneous and internal lesions. Scalp or facial lesions can cause seizures and headaches.

Referral and Consultation

Refer patients to a multidisciplinary team experienced in management of vascular anomalies. Dermatology, cardiology, neurology, and other specialists may be involved.

Patient Education and Follow-up

Monitor patients regularly for signs and symptoms of AVM reexpansion or cardiovascular compromise.

EXANTHEM

An exanthem is a local or widespread skin eruption usually in response to a viral infection. It can also be in response to bacterial illnesses, toxins produced by pathogens, or drug ingestion. The term *exanthem* actually refers to lesions found on the skin while *enanthem* refers to those on the mucosa. Some causative infectious agents can be potentially harmful to specific patient populations, such as pregnant women or the immunocompromised patient.

Vaccinations are available to prevent and control many infectious diseases, including several childhood exanthems discussed in this chapter. Each year, the CDC's Advisory Committee on Immunization Practices (ACIP) publishes recommended vaccine schedules that guide clinician practice and public health (http://www.cdc.gov/vaccines/schedules/).

Evaluation should include a thorough history, review of systems, and physical examination. Lesion morphology, distribution pattern, prodrome, concurrent symptoms, known exposures, and local epidemiology are key for an accurate diagnosis. If a vesicular component is present in the exanthem, it can be helpful in generating a differential diagnosis based on morphology (Table 6-2).

VARICELLA

Varicella zoster virus (VZV) is a member of the herpesvirus family and is the causative agent of varicella (*chicken pox*) and herpes zoster (*shingles*), which is more common in adults and is discussed in more detail in chapter 10. Active disease or vaccination usually confers lifetime immunity. Recurrence can occur, but is uncommon.

Pathophysiology

Primary infection with VZV causes the cutaneous eruption known commonly as *chicken pox*, which is highly contagious via respiratory droplet spread. Patients are contagious until at least 5 days after the appearance of the rash, or until all of the lesions are dried and crusted.

TABLE 6-2 Differential Diagnosis of Exanthem on the Basis of Morphology

MORBILLIFORM ERUPTIONS	PAPULAR VESICULAR ERUPTIONS
Rubeola (measles)	Herpes simplex
Roseola erythema	Varicella zoster (chickenpox)
Infectious mononucleosis	Herpes zoster (shingles)
Pityriasis rosea	Coxsackievirus (especially HFM)
Hepatitis	Influenza
Mumps	Echoviruses
Adenoviruses	Variola
Parvoviruses (especially B19)	Vaccina (cowpox)
Echoviruses	
Ebstein–Barr virus (EBV)	
Coxsackieviruses syncytial virus (RSV)	
Cytomegalovirus	
Dengue	
Morbilliform with petechiae	
Rubella	
Ebstein–Barr virus	
RSV	
Echoviruses	
Hepatitis	
Measles (atypical)	
Dengue	
Coxsackievirus A9	

Modified from Weston, L.L., Lane, A.T. & Morelli, J.G. (2007). *Color Textbook of Dermatology*, 4th Ed. St. Louis, Mosby.

Clinical Presentation

There is a prodrome with VZV characterized by malaise, fever, chills, headache, and arthralgia. Within 1 to 2 days, erythematous macules and papules appear, which quickly evolve into vesicles and pustules (Figure 6-12). Lesions develop for several days then become dried and crusted by day 6 or 7.

> **DIFFERENTIAL DIAGNOSIS** Varicella zoster virus
>
> - Disseminated herpes simplex virus
> - Eczema herpeticum
> - Bullous impetigo
> - Arthropod assaults (bites or stings)
> - Drug reaction
> - Measles
> - Urticaria
> - Dermatitis herpetiformis
> - Small pox infection
> - Other viral exanthems

Diagnostics

Diagnosis of primary VZV is based on history and physical findings and, if necessary, can be confirmed with viral culture of a vesicle for PCR. Serum IgG and IgM antibody titers are not recommended for diagnosis because they are less sensitive.

Management

Treatment is symptomatic for otherwise healthy patients. Oral analgesics for pain, and oral antihistamines, cool compresses, and colloidal baths for pruritus can be effective. Use of topical and oral antibiotics should be reserved for cases of secondary infection.

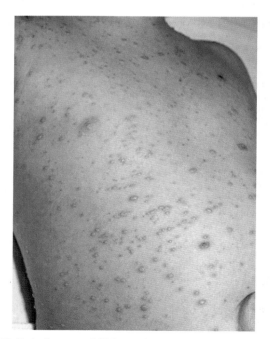

FIG. 6-12. Varicella zoster (chickenpox) with red macules, vesicles, and crusted vesicles on the trunk of a child.

Vaccination

There is a live attenuated vaccine available; refer to http://www.cdc.gov/vaccines/schedules.

Prognosis and Complications

For most immunocompetent patients, VZV infection is a mild and self-limited illness, with adults having a greater risk for complications compared to children. Secondary bacterial infection, usually due to *S. aureus* or group A *strep*, is the most common complication and can result in scarring. Disseminated VZV and pneumonia are less common but potentially lethal complications from VZV, requiring immediate hospitalization and intravenous antiviral therapy.

Special Considerations

Immunosuppression. Complications such as recurrence, disseminated infection, secondary infections, or pneumonia are more common in patients who are immunocompromised.

Pregnancy. VZV infection during pregnancy can cause congenital varicella syndrome, which will not be discussed in this chapter.

Patient Education and Follow-up

The course of disease usually lasts 5 to 10 days. Most children recover without complications. Once lesions are dried and crusted, and the fever resolves, patients may return to daycare or school. Until then, patients are highly contagious, and should not be in public.

MEASLES

Measles, or *rubeola,* is a highly contagious respiratory virus. Since the introduction of the measles vaccine 1963, The incidence in the United States dropped dramatically. Recent outbreaks have been reported and attributed to people who contracted the virus outside the country (such as while on vacation). People who are not vaccinated are at risk of contracting the virus and spreading it to others.

Pathophysiology

The virus is spread via respiratory droplets.

Clinical Presentation

Patients with measles appear very ill, with a high fever, red mucous membranes, and the three "C"s: coryza, cough, and conjunctivitis. *Koplik spots,* gray-white to red papules on the buccal mucosa, are pathognomonic for measles. Skin lesions are red to purple-red macules and papules, which can become confluent. Lesions start on the face or behind the ears and spread cephalocaudally and will fade in the same order that they appeared.

> **DIFFERENTIAL DIAGNOSIS** Measles
>
> - Drug reaction
> - Other viral exanthems
> - Toxic shock syndrome
> - Systemic lupus erythematosus
> - Serum sickness
> - Syphilis

Diagnostics

Diagnosis is based on history and clinical findings and can be confirmed with laboratory studies. The CDC recommends reverse-transcriptase polymerase chain reaction (RT-PCR) and IgM blood testing. Ideally, serum should be collected within 3 days of the onset of the rash. All suspected or laboratory confirmed cases must be reported to the CDC.

Management

Treatment is supportive; no antiviral therapy exists for measles.

Vaccination

A measles vaccine is available as a combination with mumps and rubella.

Prognosis and Complications

Complications include pneumonia, bronchitis, otitis, gastroenteritis, myocarditis, and encephalitis.

Special Considerations

Pregnancy. Measles is not teratogenic, but can cause miscarriage and premature labor.

Patient Education and Follow-up

There is no cure for measles. However, most patients recover without complications in 7 to 10 days. Children with measles should be kept out of daycare and school until 4 to 5 days after the rash initially appeared.

Some parents worry that the vaccine for measles can cause autism. This concern has been proven false by numerous research studies. Parents who do not vaccinate their children can cause outbreaks of measles, mumps, and rubella.

SCARLET FEVER

Scarlet fever, or *scarlatina*, results from a *group A β-hemolytic Streptococcus* (GABHS) infection. It is rare in infants and is most common in 1- to 10-year-olds. Rheumatic fever results when certain strains of GABHS pharyngitis go untreated.

Pathophysiology

Exotoxins from a GABHS infection cause the characteristic rash of scarlet fever. While most cases are associated with GABHS infections of the pharynx and tonsils, it can originate from the skin as well. Patients previously exposed to GABHS have no antibodies to it and therefore develop the exanthem. Patients over 10 years old have usually had exposures and have developed antibodies and therefore do not develop the rash. The difference between "strep throat" and scarlet fever is that in scarlet fever, a rash accompanies the sore throat. GABHS is transmitted via respiratory secretions.

Scarlet fever is contagious from about 4 to 5 days before the onset of the rash, until about 4 to 5 days after it fades, or 24 hours after antibiotics are initiated.

Clinical Presentation

Scarlet fever presents with the abrupt onset of fever, sore throat, headache, and chills. On day 1 or 2, the tongue develops a white coating with red, edematous papillae. The coating peels off by day 4

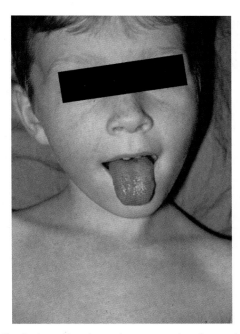

FIG. 6-13. Scarlet fever. Note the erythematous rash on face and chest, and "strawberry" tongue.

or 5, leaving the tongue bright red with prominent papillae, referred to as a "strawberry" tongue (Figure 6-13).

One to five days *after* the onset of fever, a fine, erythematous macular and papular eruption appears on the ears, chest, and axillae (Figure 6-14). The exanthem spreads to the trunk and extremities, accentuated in the flexural areas with petechiae and hyperpigmentation *Pastia's lines.* This morphology is referred to as *scarlatiniform,* which is a term used to describe other rashes with similar characteristics.

The face may be flushed with circumoral pallor. The skin has a classic "sandpaper" or rough texture. In patients with dark skin, the erythema can be difficult to appreciate, but skin will still have the

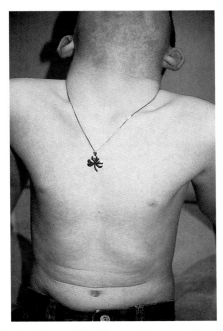

FIG. 6-14. Scarlet fever, with diffuse erythematous, "sandpaper" rash, accentuated on the neck.

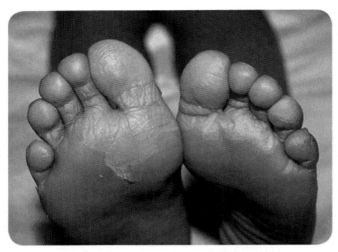

FIG. 6-15. Scarlet fever. Note the desquamation, which is common on the hands and feet.

"sandpaper" texture. The exanthem lasts 4 to 5 days, followed by desquamation (Figure 6-15). There may be painful anterior cervical adenopathy. Rhinorrhea and cough are notably absent in most cases.

> ### DIFFERENTIAL DIAGNOSIS   Scarlet fever
> - Viral infection, including hepatitis
> - Kawasaki disease
> - *Mycoplasma* infection
> - *Chlamydia* infection
> - Hypersensitivity reaction
> - Drug eruption

Diagnostics

Diagnosis is based on clinical findings and laboratory testing. Throat culture will be positive for GABHS. Antistreptococcal (ASO) serologic testing can be useful.

Management

Most patients can be managed in the outpatient setting, with supportive care. The treatment of choice for scarlet fever is penicillin. First-generation cephalosporin (some risk of cross reaction) and macrolides provide alternative treatment for patients with penicillin allergy. Intramuscular penicillin G is used when compliance is a concern. There is no vaccine available.

Prognosis and Complications

Complications include pneumonia, pericarditis, meningitis, hepatitis, post-streptococcal glomerulonephritis, and rheumatic fever. The timeliness of antibiotic therapy is key in the prevention of *acute rheumatic fever*.

Patient Education and Follow-up

If patients appear toxic or are experiencing decreased fluid intake, referral to the emergency department may be necessary. Antipyretics, cool baths, and increased fluid intake help to alleviate symptoms. Parents should be reassured that previously healthy children tend to fully recover in a matter of days. Children can return to school or daycare when they are afebrile and have been on an antibiotic for at least 24 hours.

RUBELLA

Rubella, also known as *German measles* or *three-day measles,* is a viral exanthem caused by an RNA virus in the Togaviridae family.

Pathophysiology

The virus is spread through droplet contact from nasopharyngeal secretions. The disease is self-limiting, but is contagious from onset of symptoms until 7 days after the onset of the rash.

Clinical Presentation

A prodrome, occurring 2 to 5 days before the skin eruption, presents as a low-grade fever (compared to the high fever associated with measles), headache, malaise, eye pain, myalgias, sore throat, rhinorrhea, and cough. Up to 50% of cases are asymptomatic. The exanthem is light pink, "rose-pink," macules and papules that begin on the head, spread to the trunk cephalocaudally, and become confluent.

Lesions begin to fade about 1 to 3 days later, in the same order in which they initially appeared. In severe cases, there may be fine flaky desquamation. The enanthem, *Forchheimer spots,* consists of erythematous and petechial macules on the soft palate.

Patients can develop generalized lymphadenopathy in suboccipital, postauricular, and cervical areas. Arthralgias and arthritis (fingers, wrists, or knees) may be a complaint, especially in adolescent females, and may continue for several months after the infection has resolved.

> ### DIFFERENTIAL DIAGNOSIS   Rubella
> - Hypersensitivity reaction
> - Contact dermatitis
> - Scarlet fever
> - Other viral exanthems

Diagnostics

The vague and often mild symptoms of rubella can make the clinical diagnosis challenging. Serology for rubella-specific IgM antibody identifies recent infection. Rubella titers taken 1 to 2 weeks apart, showing a fourfold or greater increase indicates acute infection. Nasal secretions can be cultured for the virus.

Management

Management is symptomatic. NSAIDs are used for arthralgias.

Vaccination

A vaccine is available as a combination with mumps and measles vaccine.

Special Considerations

Pregnancy. Rubella is teratogenic. *Congenital rubella syndrome* (CRS) results from viral infection during pregnancy and can cause miscarriage, stillbirth, and birth defects, including cataracts, congenital heart disease, hearing impairment, and developmental delay. Mothers who are not immune to rubella are at risk for CRS and therefore should avoid all contact or exposure with individuals suspected of being infected.

Prognosis and Complications

Arthritis may continue for several weeks following the resolution of infection.

Patient Education and Follow-up

Patients should be monitored for adequate fluid intake during illness. Once symptoms improve, no special follow-up is needed, unless complications occur.

ERYTHEMA INFECTIOSUM

Erythema infectiosum (EI), also called *fifth disease* or *human parvovirus,* is caused by parvovirus B19. Patients are contagious for 5 to 7 days after symptoms first appear.

Pathophysiology

EI is spread by respiratory droplets, through blood products, and from mother to fetus. It usually affects preschoolers and school-aged children, with a peak incidence in the spring and winter.

Clinical Presentation

EI consists of three stages, beginning with a prodrome of headache, fever, and chills, with or without rhinorrhea and cough. The rash may be exacerbated with sun exposure, heat, and physical activity

Stage 1: Two to three days after the prodrome begins, the classic "slapped-cheek" rash appears as bright red facial erythema on the cheeks, sparing the nasal bridge and perioral areas.
Stage II: One to four days after the facial rash, the patient develops the characteristic pink, lacy (reticulated) erythematous, macular eruption on the trunk and extremities, sparing the palms and soles (Figure 6-16). This can be pruritic.

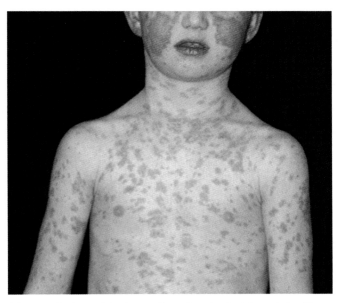

FIG. 6-16. Erythema infectiosum. Note the classic "slapped-cheek" appearance, with erythematous papules and plaques also on the trunk and extremities.

Stage III: It takes about 2 to 3 weeks for the exanthem on the trunk and extremities to fade completely, during which time it may wax and wane. The waxing and waning comprises stage III.

DIFFERENTIAL DIAGNOSIS Erythema infectiosum
- Phototoxic reaction
- Systemic lupus erythematosus
- Other viral exanthems
- Contact dermatitis
- Rosacea
- Drug reaction

Diagnostics

Serology for IgG antibodies to parvovirus can be detected 3 weeks after infection, which is approximately when the rash and arthralgias appear. Thus, the labs are of limited value since the patient is no longer contagious.

Management

Treatment is symptomatic and supportive. Most cases are mild, without complications.

Referral and Consultation

Pregnant women exposed to Parvovirus B19 should be referred to their obstetrician for monitoring and management.

Prognosis and Complications

Parvovirus B19 affects red blood cell (RBC) production, causing transient anemia. Patients with low RBC production, increased RBC destruction or loss, including sickle cell disease, iron deficiency anemia, thalassemia, and glucose-6-phosphate dehydrogenase (G6PD) deficiency, can develop transient aplastic crisis. Arthritis may occur, and is more common in females. It favors the fingers, hands, wrists, ankles, and knees, and resolves spontaneously.

Special Considerations

Pregnancy. Mothers can be infected without showing any symptoms. About 30% to 66% of adult females are immune, so their fetuses are not at risk. In most cases of maternal infection, the fetus is delivered without developmental or neurologic problems. The highest risk for fetal compromise occurs before 20 weeks gestation. Parvovirus B19 is not teratogenic, but *congenital infection* can cause anemia, high-output congestive heart failure, hydrops fetalis, and intrauterine fetal demise. Most fetal losses occur between 9 and 28 weeks gestation. Severely affected surviving fetuses can be treated with *in utero* digitalization and blood transfusions.

Patient Education and Follow-up

EI is self-limiting. Treatment is supportive, as there is no cure. Most cases are mild, and patients tend to make a full recovery. Patients with aplastic crisis may need RBC transfusions. Patients are contagious until the onset of the rash. Once the rash appears, they can return to daycare or school.

ROSEOLA

Roseola, *roseola infantum, exanthema subitum,* or *sixth disease*, is a mild and common exanthem that usually occurs in children under 2 years old.

Pathophysiology

Roseola is caused by human herpes virus types 6 and 7 and is thought to be spread via saliva. Horizontal transmission from mother to child has been well documented.

Clinical Presentation

Typically a mild and short-lived infection, roseola presents with 3 to 5 days of high fever, with or without irritability, diarrhea, bulging fontanelle, cough, cervical lymphadenopathy, and eyelid edema, in an otherwise well-appearing child.

The classic presentation is a cutaneous eruption that presents just as the fever breaks. The lesions are subtle, light pink, erythematous macules and papules on the face, neck and extremities, and sometimes chest. The rash usually resolves in 1 to 3 days.

> **DIFFERENTIAL DIAGNOSIS** Roseola
> - Measles
> - Rubella
> - Other viral illnesses
> - Drug reaction

Diagnostics

Diagnosis is based on history and physical findings, and in rare severe cases, exclusion of other illnesses and diseases. HHV-6 and -7 can be isolated in the saliva and stool of infected patients. Most infants have transplacental antibodies until about 6 months of age. After 6 months of age, most infants are seronegative, and are susceptible to infection.

Management

Treatment of roseola is symptomatic and supportive.

Prognosis and Complications

Most children recover without long-term sequelae.

Patient Education and Follow-up

Follow-up is not necessary unless infection is severe or complicated.

HAND-FOOT-AND-MOUTH DISEASE

Hand-foot-and-mouth disease (HFM) is caused by an enterovirus, and has been linked to multiple coxsackievirus subtypes. It is most common in children 1 to 4 years old.

Pathophysiology

HFM is spread via fecal–oral exposure, with an incubation period of 3 to 5 days.

Clinical Presentation

Patients with HFM experience a prodrome of fever and malaise, followed by the characteristic exanthem of gray-white vesicular lesions on the palms and soles (Figure 6-17). There is also a classic enanthem of discrete vesicles and erosions on the buccal mucosa, palate, tongue, uvula, gingivae, and anterior tonsillar pillars (Figure 6-18). There may be cervical and submandibular lymphadenopathy.

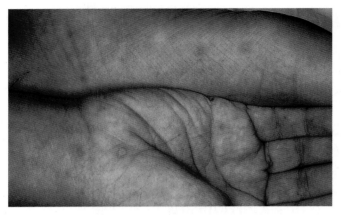

FIG. 6-17. Coxsackie, hand-foot-and-mouth disease. A hand and a foot of this child show isolated vesicles compared with the grouped vesicles seen in the patient with a herpetic infection.

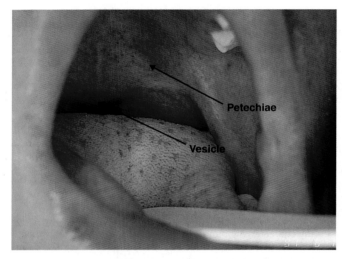

FIG. 6-18. Scattered petechiae appear centrally, and there is a vesicle posteriorly at the junction of the hard and soft palates. Coxsackievirus produces lesions toward the posterior of the oropharynx, whereas herpes simplex virus appears anteriorly.

> **DIFFERENTIAL DIAGNOSIS** Hand-foot-and-mouth disease
> - Erythema multiforme
> - Herpes simplex
> - Other viral exanthems

Diagnostics

Diagnosis of HFM is usually based on clinical findings. Viral culture can be collected from an intact vesicle. An important clue to diagnosis is local epidemiology. Outbreaks are common in summer and fall, but sporadic cases occur throughout the year.

Management

HFM is a mild, short-lived infection with only supportive treatment. Over-the-counter antipyretics and analgesics (acetaminophen and ibuprofen) can be used for fever and pain. Monitor infants and toddlers for dehydration from painful oral erosions.

"Magic mouthwash" is a common off-label pain medication used for HFM in children. There are several versions available. This author

prefers a mixture of diphenhydramine and Maalox (calcium carbonate), with or without viscous lidocaine 2%. The ratio is one to one of each ingredient. Only add lidocaine if the child is able to spit the solution out because if lidocaine is ingested, there is a risk of arrhythmia. Magic mouthwash is administered every 4 to 6 hours as needed for pain associated with oral vesicles and erosions. It should be swished around in the mouth for 30 seconds and then spit out. Of course, this can be a difficult feat in toddlers.

Salt-water mouth rinses using ½ teaspoon of salt in 8 ounces of warm water may be soothing. Encourage increased fluid intake of cold water and milk, especially if the patient has a fever. Acidic juices and sodas can cause burning pain if there are erosions.

Prognosis and Complications

Illness spontaneously resolves after about 7 to 10 days, with a low risk for complications. Lesions are painful, which can cause anorexia and dehydration. Fever can cause febrile seizures.

Patient Education and Follow-up

It is important to counsel parents on pain management, fever control, and prevention of dehydration. Instruct parents to watch for dry mucous membranes, sunken fontanelle, weight loss or decreased urine output. Follow-up is required if the patient becomes lethargic or irritable, or has other signs or symptoms of dehydration.

GIANOTTI–CROSTI SYNDROME

Gianotti–Crosti syndrome or *papular acrodermatitis of childhood* is a common viral exanthem, most common in children between 1 and 6 years of age.

Pathophysiology

The cause of Gianotti–Crosti syndrome is unknown. Several viruses have been implicated, including hepatitis B, Epstein–Barr virus, cytomegalovirus, coxsackievirus, adenovirus, respiratory syncytial virus, parainfluenza virus, parvovirus B19, rotavirus, and HHV-6.

Clinical Presentation

There is a prodrome of upper respiratory symptoms, fever, and lymphadenopathy. A few days later, edematous, erythematous, monomorphous papules and papulovesicles appear. As the name *acrodermatitis* implies, lesions typically occur on the acral surfaces (face, extensor surfaces of extremities; Figure 6-19). The buttocks may be involved, but the trunk is almost always spared. There may be larger coalescing erythematous plaques, localized purpura, and mild pruritus.

DIFFERENTIAL DIAGNOSIS Gianotti–Crosti syndrome

- Other viral illnesses
- Contact dermatitis
- Phototoxic dermatitis

Diagnostics

Diagnosis is based on history and physical findings. Viral cultures from nasal secretions or saliva may be helpful.

Management

Treatment is supportive. If pruritus is severe, use mild TCS like desonide 0.05% ointment twice daily for 1 week on the face and

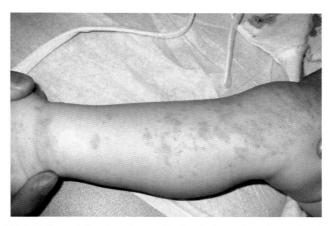

FIG. 6-19. Gianotti–Crosti syndrome affecting the leg and usually sparing the trunk.

mid-potency triamcinolone 0.1% ointment twice daily for up to 2 weeks on the extremities.

Special Considerations

It was once suggested that all patients with Gianotti–Crosti syndrome be tested for hepatitis. Screen patients for any potential risk factors and examine for jaundice, hepatosplenomegaly, and lymphadenopathy. In the absence of risk factors or symptoms, serum studies are not indicated.

Referral and Consultation

If hepatitis is detected, referral to appropriate specialists is recommended.

Patient Education and Follow-up

It can take 8 to 12 weeks for the exanthem to completely resolve, and patients without hepatitis recover fully. If TCS are prescribed, counsel patients on the proper usage, risks, and side effects. Postinflammatory hypopigmentation can last several months, but will fade on its own.

STAPHYLOCOCCAL SCALDED SKIN SYNDROME

Staphylococcal scalded skin syndrome (SSSS) is a bacterial infection that causes a skin eruption giving the burned or scalded appearance. It is quite rare in anyone over 6 years old, unless they have immunosuppression or renal disease. Males are affected more often than females, and it is less common in black children.

Pathophysiology

SSSS occurs in children who are infected with *S. aureus*. However, it is not the organism that causes the cutaneous symptoms. It is the endotoxins produced by the bacteria that cause epidermal separation (blisters) and exfoliation. SSSS occurs mostly in children because they lack protection from antitoxin antibodies and have decreased ability for renal excretion of the toxins (similar to scarlet fever).

Clinical Presentation

SSSS begins with a localized *S. aureus* infection, usually involving the conjunctivae, nares, perioral area, perineum, or umbilicus. Patients

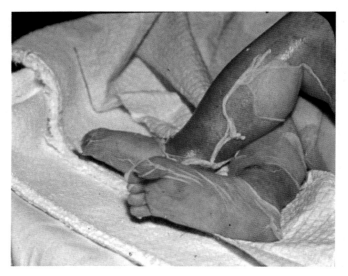

FIG. 6-20. SSSS with erythema and extensive desquamation.

have fever, periorbital and perioral edema, malaise, lethargy, irritability, and poor feeding. The skin becomes diffusely erythematous with large, thin, fragile bullae, which easily rupture, leaving denuded, tender, hemorrhagic skin (Figure 6-20). The eruption is exaggerated in the flexural creases, but may involve the entire skin surface area. The *Nikolsky sign* (gentle pressure next to a blister causes the blister to extend) will be present. The oral mucosa and conjunctiva are usually NOT involved as compared to toxic epidermal necrolysis (TEN), which does have mucosal involvement.

DIFFERENTIAL DIAGNOSIS	Staphylococcal scalded skin syndrome

- Stevens–Johnson syndrome
- Toxic epidermal necrolysis
- Toxic shock syndrome
- Drug reaction
- Thermal or chemical burn
- Child abuse
- Erysipelas
- Erythema multiforme
- Scarlet fever
- Pemphigus

Diagnostics

Diagnosis is based on clinical findings, but is confirmed with bacterial cultures. The best places to collect samples are the conjunctivae, nares, or nasopharynx. Culture of fluid from bullae will be negative. If the diagnosis is unclear, or if TEN is suspected, a skin biopsy is recommended.

Management

Patients may require hospitalization for supportive care to maintain fluid and electrolyte balance, for pain management and fever control, and to prevent secondary infection. Treatment of choice is penicillinase-resistant penicillin, first- or second-generation cephalosporins, clindamycin, or sulfamethoxazole/trimethoprim; antibiotics are often given parenterally. Vancomycin can treat methicillin-resistant *S. aureus* (MRSA).

Referral and Consultation

Numerous specialists may be consulted if complications occur or hospitalization is necessary. If TEN is suspected, consult a dermatologist. If an urgent appointment with a dermatologist is not possible, refer to the emergency department.

Prognosis and Complications

With proper management, patients recover without complications. Patients experiencing extensive desquamation are at risk for thermoregulatory problems, fluid loss, electrolyte imbalance, secondary infection, and sepsis. Pneumonia, septic arthritis, endocarditis, or pyomyositis are also complications that can develop. Although the skin heals without scarring, there may be postinflammatory hypo- or hyperpigmentation.

Patient Education and Follow-up

Once the infection is eradicated, fluid levels have been stabilized, and local wound care has been performed, patients will be discharged from the hospital. Frequent and regular follow-up should be performed until there has been complete resolution.

GENETIC DISORDERS
Neurofibromas and Neurofibromatosis

Neurofibromas are benign tumors that are made up of neuromesenchymal tissue. They commonly occur as a single lesion in healthy people. When accompanied by other clinical criteria, they can be a marker of *neurofibromatosis* (NF), which is an autosomal dominant genetic disorder with an increased propensity to develop tumors of the nerve sheath.

There are two distinct types of NF: NF type 1 (NF1) or von Recklinghausen disease and NF type 2 (NF2) or bilateral acoustic or central neurofibromatosis. Over 90% of NF cases are NF1. This chapter will only discuss NF1. Both sexes and all races are equally affected. If an at-risk patient does not meet diagnostic criteria by age 10 years, he/she is unlikely to be affected.

Pathophysiology
Neurofibromas are an out-pouching of a benign tumor of the nerve sheath.

Clinical presentation
There is great variability in the severity of neurofibromatosis. Most patients have very mild skin disease. More serious involvement or complications from NF typically present in childhood or adolescence.

Cutaneous neurofibromas are soft, skin-colored papules, 2mm to 2cm in diameter (Figure 6-21). Occasionally, they can be red, blue, or brown. As they enlarge, they may become globular, pear-shaped, or pedunculated. Neurofibromas display the "buttonhole" sign, defined as easy invagination into the dermis when direct pressure is applied on top of the lesion.

Subcutaneous neurofibromas are firmer, occur deeper in the dermis, and are less well circumscribed than cutaneous neurofibromas. *Plexiform neurofibromas* are tender, firm nodules or masses in the subcutaneous tissue. They can occur in the skin, fascia, muscle, and internal structures.

The presence of neurofibromas alone is not diagnostic for NF, but it should alert the clinician to look for other clinical signs of the disease, including café au lait macules and axillary or inguinal

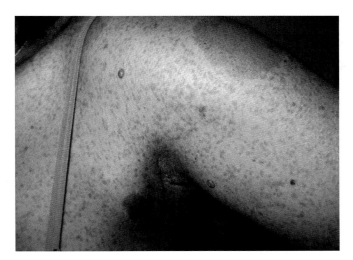

FIG. 6-21. Patient with neurofibromatosis and multiple, large (>1.5 cm) café au lait macules, axillary freckling, and neurofibromas.

freckling (Crowe's sign). The number of cutaneous lesions does not correlate with disease severity. Ocular manifestations of NF1 include plexiform neurofibromas, Lisch nodules, and optic gliomas. Other features include short stature, macrocephaly, hypertension, hearing loss, learning disabilities, cardiovascular complications, and skeletal anomalies.

DIFFERENTIAL DIAGNOSIS Neurofibromatosis

- Café au lait macule
- Nevus spilus
- Partial unilateral lentiginoses
- McCune–Albright syndrome
- Congenital melanocytic nevi

Diagnostics

Table 6-3 lists diagnostic criteria for NF1 and 2. Genetic testing is available for NF1.

TABLE 6-3	Diagnostic Criteria for Neurofibromatosis Types 1 and 2
NEUROFIBROMATOSIS TYPE 1	**NEUROFIBROMATOSIS TYPE 2**
Must have at least two of the following: Six café au lait macules at least 0.5 cm in diameter before puberty or at least 1.5 cm in diameter after puberty Axillary freckling A plexiform neurofibroma Two or more derma neurofibromas Two or more Lisch nodules Optic nerve glioma Pathognomonic skeletal dysplasia An affected first-degree relative	Bilateral vestibular schwannomas seen on MRI or a first-degree relative with NF2 *and* unilateral vestibular schwannoma or two of the following: Meningioma Glioma Schwannoma Juvenile posterior subcapsular cataract

Management

Neurofibromas require no treatment unless they are symptomatic or cosmetically disturbing the patient.

Referral and consultation

If NF1 is suspected, refer patients to a dermatologist, neurologist, or genetic counselor. Once the diagnosis is established, care may be transferred to a multidisciplinary team specializing in NF. Referral should occur as early as possible to optimize patient outcomes.

Prognosis and complications

Patients with NF1 have a 5% lifetime risk of developing malignancy, including malignant peripheral nerve sheath tumors, nonlymphocytic leukemia, carcinoid, and pheochromocytomas. Patients may develop multiple small juvenile xanthogranulomas.

Patient education and follow-up

Counsel patients about the benign nature of neurofibromas or the association with underlying disease. Perform a physical and developmental examination, detailed family history, and examination of family members if indicated. Perform appropriate diagnostic tests if there are positive findings at any time. Patients should have annual ophthalmology examinations and complete blood counts.

Tuberous Sclerosis Complex

Tuberous sclerosis (TS) is an autosomal dominant genetic disorder characterized by excessive development of hamartomas of the skin, brain, eyes, heart, kidneys, lungs, and bones. Harmartomas are abnormal development of cells the skin resulting in benign, tumor-like masses. Our focus is on the cutaneous signs and symptoms of TS, yet systemic disease can occur and should always be considered during the evaluation of these patients. Most patients diagnosed with TS are between 2 and 6 years of age. It affects all races equally, and there is no sex predilection.

Pathophysiology

TS is caused by a mutation in one of two genes: *TSC1*, which encodes hamartin, and *TSC2*, which encodes tuberin. These mutations demonstrate variable expressivity. Patients with *TSC1* mutation tend to have milder disease.

Clinical presentation

There are many cutaneous and systemic features of TS. Cutaneous and dental manifestations are present in nearly all patients with TS. These skin findings can easily be detected on physical examination.

Hypopigmented macules or patches can range from millimeters to centimeters in diameter, and do not evolve over time. They can be anywhere on the body, but are usually on the trunk. They can take the shape of a "thumbprint," "confetti," or "ash leaf."

Facial angiofibromas are hamartomas that contain fibrous and vascular tissue. They are 1- to 4-mm pink-to-red, smooth, dome-shaped soft papules commonly found on the face, especially around the nose. These features can mimic acne in teenagers (Figure 6-22). Histoligically, similar lesions can occur unilaterally on the forehead and are called *fibrous cephalic (forehead) plaques.*

Collagenomas are connective tissue nevi on the forehead, cheeks, scalp, or trunk. On the trunk, they are called *shagreen patches* and are more likely to be present at birth (Figure 6-23). There may be one

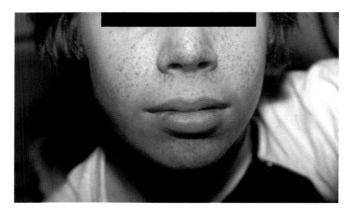

FIG. 6-22. Patient with tuberous sclerosis and facial angiofibromas.

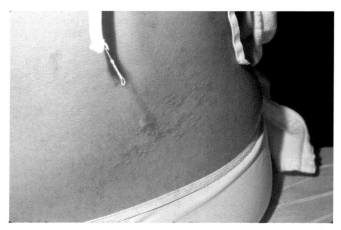

FIG. 6-23. Patient with tuberous sclerosis and a shagreen patch on the lower back.

or many flesh color papules in varied sizes and may have a leathery texture and follicular openings.

Periungual fibromas are benign periungal papules that are more common on the toenails and proximal nail folds. The small tumors can be tender, bleed, and cause longitudinal droves in the nail.

DIFFERENTIAL DIAGNOSIS Tuberous sclerosis

- Acne
- Vitiligo
- Nail trauma
- Nevus depigmentosus
- Nevus anemicus
- Other genetic disorders

Diagnostics

Diagnosis can be a challenge because the manifestations may initially be very subtle and can involve many organ systems. Diagnostic criteria, set forth in the *Recommendations of the 2012 International Tuberous Sclerosis Complex Consensus Conference* (Northrup et al., 2013), identifies the genetic and clinical (major and minor) criteria for a definitive, probable, and possible diagnosis of TS (Table 6-4). Blood tests for TSC1 and TSC2 mutations are available. Although pediatric neurologists are the specialists responsible for the diagnosis and management, primary care and other clinicians are vital in identifying patients with high clinical suspicion. Since dermatologic and dental manifestations are present in almost 100% of patients, a good skin examination could reveal markers for the disease and prompt referral for evaluation and diagnostics.

Management

Treatment is directed at the patient's symptoms. Skin lesions do not require treatment because they are benign. Angiofibromas can be treated with laser or surgical excision if they are a cosmetic concern.

Referral and consultation

If TS is suspected, refer to a dermatologist, neurologist, or genetic counselor. Care is multidisciplinary; referral to a specialty center is recommended once diagnosis is made.

Prognosis and complications

Prognosis depends on disease severity and the extent of neurologic involvement.

Patient education and follow-up

Parents should receive genetic counseling, especially if they are considering having more children. Patient follow-up depends on disease severity and system involvement and involving the appropriate specialists.

TABLE 6-4 Cutaneous Manifestations in the Diagnostic Criteria for Tuberous Sclerosus

CUTANEOUS/DERMATOLOGIC SYMPTOM	CRITERIA	PROPORTION WITH CUTANEOUS MANIFESTATION	ONSET OF SYMPTOMS
Hypomelanotic macules ($\geq$ 3, at least 5 mm diameter)	Major	90%	Birth or infancy
Angiofibromas ($\geq$ 3), or Fibrous cephalic (forehead) plaque	Major Major	75% 25%	2–5 years of age Usually present at birth
Ungual fibromas ($\geq$ 2)	Major	20% in children; 80% adults	Second decade or later
Shagreen patch	Major	50%	First decade of life
"Confetti" skin lesions	Minor	5%–58%	First decade of life

BILLING CODES ICD-10

Aplasia cutis congenita	Q82.8, Q84.8
Arteriovenous malformation	Q28.2
Benign skin neoplasm	D36
Candidial stomatitis	B37.0
Candidiasis, skin and nails	B37.2
Candidiasis, unspecified	B37.9
Chafing and intertrigo	L30.4
Diaper dermatitis	L22
Erythema infectiosum	B08.3
Erythema toxicum neonatorum	P83.1
Gianotti–Crosti syndrome	L44.4
Hand-foot-and-mouth disease	B08.4
Hemangioma	D18.00, D18.01
Herpes zoster (shingles)	B02
Herpes zoster without complications	B02.9
Infantile acne	L70.4
Measles without complications	B05.9
Miliaria crystallina and miliaria rubra	L74.0
Neurofibromatosis	Q85.00
Port wine stain	Q82.5
Pyogenic granuloma	L98.0
Roseola	B08.20
Rubella without complications	B06.9
Rubella with other complications	B06.8
Salmon patch	Q27.9
Scarlet fever	A38.9
Scarlet fever with other complications	A38.8
Seborrheic dermatitis	L21.9
Staphylococcal scalded skin syndrome	L00
Subcutaneous fat necrosis	P15.6
Systemic lupus erythematosus	M32.9
Tuberous sclerosis	Q85.1
Varicella (chicken pox)	B01
Varicella without complications	B01.9
Venous malformation	Q27.9

READINGS

Adegboyega, P. A., & Qui, S. (2005). Hemangioma versus vascular malformation: Presence of nerve bundle is a diagnostic clue for vascular malformation. *Archives of Pathology and Laboratory Medicine, 129*(6), 772–775.

Buckmiller, L. M., Richter, G. T. & Suen, J. Y. (2010). Diagnosis and management of hemangiomas and vascular malformations of the head and neck. *Oral Diseases, 16*(5), 405–418.

Centers for Disease Control and Prevention. (2012). *Measles serology*. Retrieved from: http://www.cdc.gov/measles/lab-tools/serology.html

deGraaf, M., Breur, J. M., Rahael, M. F., Vos, M. Breugem, C. C. & Pasmans, S. G. (2011). Adverse effects of propranolol when used in the treatment of hemangiomas: A case series or 28 infants. *Journal of the American Academy of Dermatology, 65*(2), 320–327.

Eichenfield, L. F., Krakowski, A. C., Piggott, C., Del Rosso, J., Baldwin, H., Friedlander, S. F., . . . Thiboutot, D. M. (2013). Evidence-based recommendations for the diagnosis and treatment of pediatric acne. *Pediatrics, 131*(Suppl. 3), S163–S186.

Liu, A. S., Mulliken, J. B., Zurakowski, D. Fishman, S. J., & Greene, A. K. (2010). Extracranial arteriovenous malformations: Natural progression and recurrence after treatment. *Plastic and Reconstructive Surgery, 125*(4), 1185–1194.

Melancon, J. M., Dohil, M. A., & Eichenfield, L. F. (2012). Facial port wine stain: When to worry? *Pediatric Dermatology, 29*(4), 548.

Northrup, H., Krueger, D. A., & International Tuberous Sclerosis Complex Consensus Group. (2013). Tuberous Sclerosis Complex Diagnostic Criteria Update: Recommendations of the 2012 International Tuberous Sclerosis Complex Consensus Conference. *Pediatric Neurology, 49*(4), 243–254.

O'Connor, N. R., McLaughlin, M. R., & Ham, P. (2008). Newborn skin: Part I. Common rashes. *American Family Physician, 77*(1), 47–52.

Paller, A. S. & Mancini, A. J. (2011). *Hurwitz Clinical Pediatric Dermatology* (4th ed.). Philadelphia, PA: Elsevier Saunders.

Pride, H. B., Tollefson, M., & Silverman, R. (2013). What's new in pediatric dermatology? Part I. Diagnosis and pathogenesis. *Journal of the American Academy of Dermatology, 68*(6), 885–896.

Pride, H. B., Tollefson, M., & Silverman, R. (2013). What's new in pediatric dermatology? Part II. Treatment. *Journal of the American Academy of Dermatology, 68*(6), 899–909.

Schwartz, R. A., Janusz, C. A., & Janniger, C. K. (2006). Seborrheic dermatitis: An overview. *American Family Physician, 74*(1), 125–132.

CHAPTER 7

Pigmented Lesions and Melanoma

Theodore D. Scott

Patients often seek evaluation of their nevi (often referred to as moles by patients) because of a concern for possible malignancy or disconcerting appearance. Primary care clinicians are strategically positioned to assess skin lesions not only when it is the patient's chief complaint but also during office visits for other health concerns. Skin examinations, integrated into patient visits, are opportunities for early recognition and treatment of skin cancer. The simple practice of having patients remove their shirt when listening to lung sounds can provide the clinician with the opportunity to visualize their back, one of the common areas for melanoma.

The examination of a patient with numerous pigmented lesions can be challenging for both novice and experienced clinicians. There are multiple tools and common characteristics that can help health care providers discern benign lesions from those that warrant further investigation. For lesions that do suggest possible pathology, this chapter will address the various sampling techniques and initial interpretation of the pathology report.

PATHOPHYSIOLOGY OF PIGMENTED SKIN LESIONS

Pigmented skin lesions are due to melanocytes that develop from dendritic cells in the neural crest of the embryo and migrate to the epidermis. Melanosomes, contained in the melanocytes, produce *melanin,* which provides the skin with its color. There is about one melanocyte for each ten basal keratinocytes (Figure 7-1). Variation in the color of skin among races is due to the size and distribution of melanosomes, not number of melanocytes. Individuals with dark skin have larger melanocytes that are distributed more linearly along the basement membrane. Likewise, light-skinned people have smaller-sized melanocytes which are clustered together as well as containing less melanin.

Exposure to both natural and artificial ultraviolet radiation (UVR) increases the production of melanin, which results in larger melanocytes, giving lighter skin a tanned appearance. Other physiologic variables that influence the production of melanin include estrogen and progesterone. This can be seen with patient complaints of darkening nevi or melasma during pregnancy, hormone replacement therapy, and use of oral contraceptives.

Melanin also has a protective function as it both absorbs and scatters UVR, which protects the keratinocytes from DNA mutation that can lead to oncogenesis. This small measure of protection (about SPF 4) contributes to the social practice of going to tanning beds to acquire a "base tan" before vacation. This creates a challenge for clinicians in teaching patients about the increased skin cancer risk from UVR for all types of skin.

BENIGN PIGMENTED LESIONS

Patients seek care from both primary care and dermatology providers for the complaint of a changing nevus. Often the patient reports that a nevus has raised, developed hair, changed color, or become speckled. They rely on the clinician's assessment to reassure them that it is benign or proceed with appropriate diagnostics if it is suspicious for malignancy. However, all "brown spots" are not nevi, and understanding the pathophysiology and risk for malignancy of pigmented lesions can improve the clinician's accuracy for risk, diagnosis, and patient satisfaction.

Epidermal Melanocytic Neoplasms

Most pigmented epidermal lesions are benign and have a vast variation in clinical presentation. The characteristics of lesions are based upon the number, size, amount of melanin, and distribution of the melanocytes at the dermoepidermal junction (DEJ).

Lentigos

Lentigines (the plural of lentigo and pronounced len-tij´ĭ-nēz) present as pigmented macules that have an increased number of melanocytes or increased amount of melanin. Despite their benign pathology, patients may request treatment to minimize their appearance. They occur in a number of different clinical forms.

Ephelides, commonly known as freckles, are characterized by hyperpigmented brown macules found on sun-exposed areas during childhood. The number of ephelides usually increases with sun exposure in the summer and may almost completely fade during the winter. They are due to an increase in size of the melanocytes, not number of the melanocytes, and are evidence of UVR damage (Figure 7-2).

Lentigo simplex is larger and darker than an ephelides and can also appear during childhood. They are not affected by sun exposure and therefore do not fade in the winter months. A lentigo simplex can occur anywhere on the body as solitary, hyperpigmented brown 0.5- to 1.5-cm macule. They are characterized by an increased number of melanocytes at the dermal–epidermal junction. These benign lesions require no treatment (Figure 7-3).

Solar lentigines are a common response to sun exposure in fair-skinned, blue-eyed, and blonde or red-haired individuals. Like ephelides, their onset is during childhood and they are distributed in large numbers (sometimes coalescing) in sun-exposed areas of the face, neck, shoulders, arms, and dorsal hands (Figure 7-4). Unlike ephelides, these do not fade when the patient stays out of the sun. Pigmentation is the result of increased melanin production due to prolonged UV exposure. Treatment is not necessary unless the patient is seeking cosmetic improvement, which can be difficult if they are extensive. A clinical skin examination should be performed to identify abnormal lesions or "ugly duckling" amid the solar lentigines.

Labial, penile, and vulvar lentigines are a proliferation of melanocytes, with an increase in the number of dendrite melanocytes, which are different from the melanocytes found in typical keratinocytes. These lentigines occur on the labia, vulva, mucosa of the lips and glans penis. Solitary lesions are usually not concerning and require no treatment (Figure 7-5). However, numerous hyperpigmented

Superficial

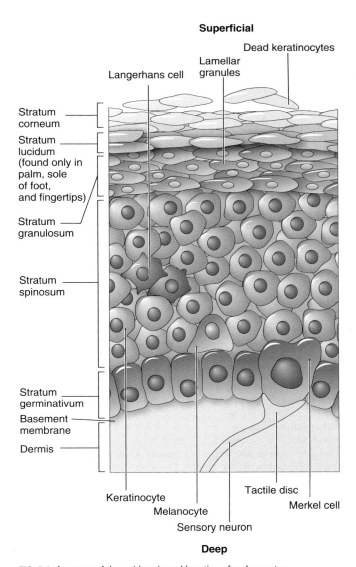

FIG. 7-1. Anatomy of the epidermis and location of melanocytes.

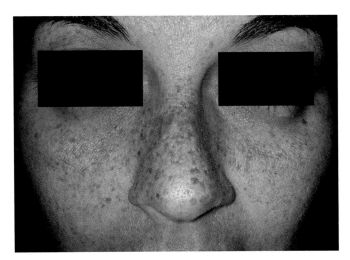

FIG. 7-2. Ephelides or common freckles are the result of UVR exposure and usually fade in the winter.

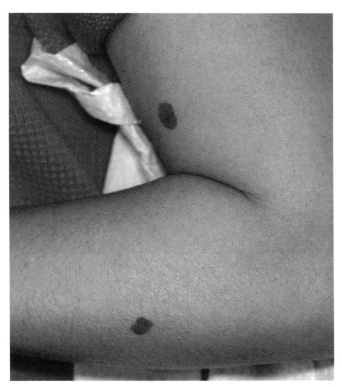

FIG. 7-3. Lentigo simplex.

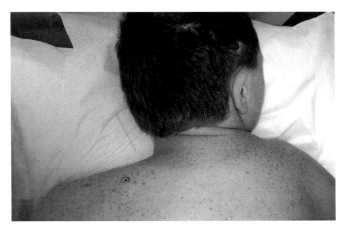

FIG. 7-4. Solar lentigines from sun exposure do not fade in the winter. Noted "ugly duckling" lesion upon examination.

brown macules noted on the lips, mucosal surfaces, and genitalia, should alert the clinician for potential Peutz–Jeghers syndrome (Figure 7-6). Patients diagnosed with this syndrome during childhood are at higher risk for gastrointestinal adenocarcinomas and breast and ovarian cancers.

Café au lait macule

These uniformly pigmented, light brown macules and patches are known as café au lait lesions and typically appear at birth or during infancy. They are usually flat, ovoid in shape, and lighter brown than congenital nevi (Figure 7-7). Twenty percent of the population has one café au lait macule, which is considered normal. Multiple café au lait macules, however, can be associated with the autosomal dominant genodermatoses, neurofibromatosis type 1 and type 2 (NF1 and NF2,

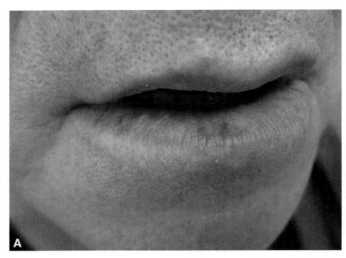
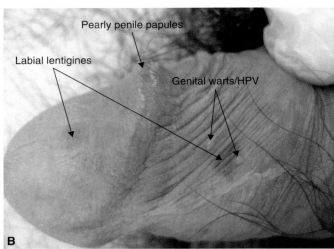

FIG. 7-5. **A:** Labial lentigines more common on the lower lip. **B:** Penile lentigines in addition to pearly penile papules and HPV.

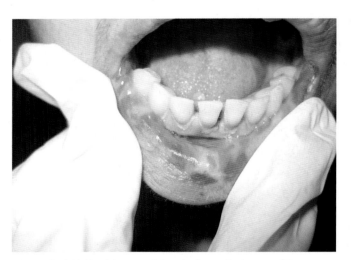

FIG. 7-6. Orolabial lentigines suspicious for Peutz–Jeghers syndrome.

respectively). A full skin examination should be performed to assess for the number and size of café au lait macules/patches, presence of neurofibromas and axillary freckling. Patients with clinical presentation suspicious for NF1 or NF2 should be referred for neurologic and developmental evaluation (see chapter 6). In adults, a full skin examination should be performed for skin cancer screening.

Nevus spilus

Nevus spilus is a congenital epidermal nevus with an appearance similar to a café au lait. It typically presents in infancy as a light brown patch with darker hyperpigmented brown macules or speckles (also called speckled lentiginous nevus) within the lesion. Most are located on the trunk or lower extremities and are benign (Figure 7-8).

Becker's nevus

A Becker's nevus (Becker's melanosis) is typically a very large, light brown to tan patch with or without an increased amount of darker hair growth. The most common location is on the shoulders, upper chest, or back, becoming more evident during adolescence, with a higher incidence in males. Becker's nevi are epidermal nevi involving

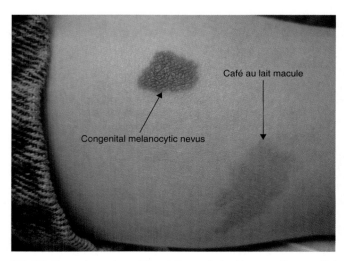

FIG. 7-7. Comparison of a café au lait macule beside a small congenital melanocytic nevus.

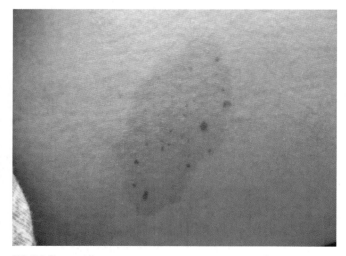

FIG. 7-8. Nevus spilus.

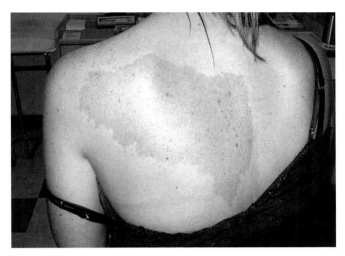

FIG. 7-9. Becker's nevus classic presentation on the shoulder or upper chest.

keratinocytes, hair follicles and melanoctyes. They are usually unilateral and may be associated with ipsilateral hypoplasia of breast and skeletal anomalies, including scoliosis, spina bifida occulta, or ipsilateral hypoplasia of a limb (Figure 7-9).

Dermal Melanocytic Neoplasms

Mongolian spots

Commonly located over the sacrum of infants, Mongolian spots are dark blue-brown patches that occur in infants usually with dark skin tones. The hyperpigmented blue color is from elongated melanocytes, giving the patch the appearance of a bruise. Given the location of the lesion and bruise-like appearance on an infant or child, many providers have mistaken this for a sign of child abuse (Figure 7-10). They are benign and usually fade significantly by adulthood. It is uncommon, but possible for adults to develop this type of dermal melanocytosis (Figure 7-11).

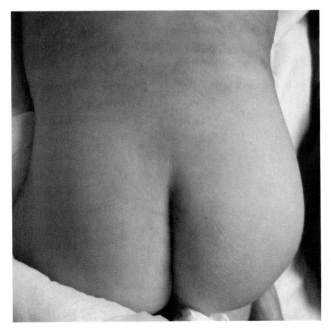

FIG. 7-10. Dermal melanocytosis or common Mongolian spot commonly located over the sacrum.

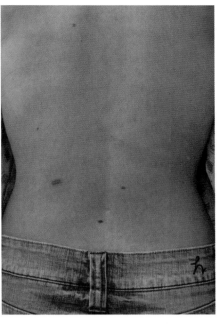

FIG. 7-11. Less common dermal melanocytosis in a Caucasian adult.

Nevus of Ota and Ito

Nevus of Ota is oculodermal melanocytosis. It is thought to be due to the failure of the melanocytes to migrate from the dermis up to the epidermis during embryonic development. Patients present with a dark blue hyperpigmented patch, usually with a unilateral distribution along the trigeminal nerve (V1 and V2 branches). The underlying mucosa, conjunctiva, and tympanic membranes may be also be pigmented and may darken with age. There is an increased prevalence in women and Asian, African American, and Indian races (Figure 7-12). The less common nevus of Ito is similar, but involves the lateral supraclavicular or lateral brachial nerve distribution.

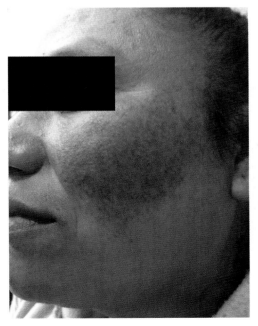

FIG. 7-12. Nevus of Ota.

Like any pigmented lesion, these should be monitored for signs and symptoms of melanoma. Glaucoma has been associated with nevus of Ota. Although usually benign, these lesions can have a psychological impact on the patient's body image. Camouflage makeup is often used, but topicals have no effect. Q-switched laser, requiring repeated treatments, provides the most promising cosmetic results.

Melanonychia striata

Brown longitudinal stria (plural is striae) that occurs in the nail is called melanonychia striata. This can be a normal variant that is common in patients with darker skin and is typically consistent pattern present in several nails. The streak of pigmentation is thin, uniform, and does not involve the nail folds. Clinicians should carefully assess all nails for atypical features that may indicate a developing periungual melanoma and prompting a referral to a dermatologist for evaluation (Box 7-1).

Melanocytic Nevi

Pigmented nevi are composed of nevus cells (nevocytes) that are derived from melanocytes located in nests near the DEJ. Nevocytes are similar to melanocytes, but are nondendritic cells and larger in size. Some nevus cells remain at the DEJ while others eventually migrate down into the dermis, accounting for some of the normal physiologic changes that can occur throughout the life span. And since most common nevi have a very low risk for malignancy, understanding the normal characteristics and evolution of nevi can reduce the number of unnecessary biopsies on benign nevi, which can be costly, scarring, and stressful for patients. It can also help assist the clinician to recognize atypical features or suspicious symptoms indicating risk for melanoma and necessitate a biopsy.

The subtypes of nevi can be classified in several ways, including *onset* of the lesion, *location* of the nested cells, and *type* of cells (Box 7-2). There can be an overlap in the classification of the same lesion. For example, an *intradermal* nevus is an *acquired* nevus located in the dermis. Nonetheless, these categories can help you understand the pathophysiology and clinical presentation.

Congenital nevi

Nevomelanocytes clustered in the deeper dermis and subcutaneous that appear at birth, or within the first 6 months of infancy, are called congenital melanocytic nevi (CMN; Figure 7-13). CMN occur in approximately 2% to 6% of newborns and have been historically categorized according to the predicted adult size (PAS). This has guided clinicians in anticipating the risk for malignancy and management options (Table 7-1).

Although all CMN have the risk of developing melanoma, small- and medium-sized lesions carry the lowest risk (<1%), which would most likely occur after puberty. In contrast, large (also called giant or garment) nevi have an estimated lifetime risk of up to 5%, with half of these melanomas occurring before the age of 5 years. Yet many experts argue that lesion characteristics, in addition to size, should be considered in the classification criteria and ultimately risk stratification. Krengel et al. (2013) proposed new criteria in hopes of providing a better prognostic tool to measure risk and guide care.

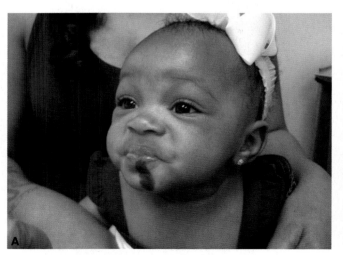

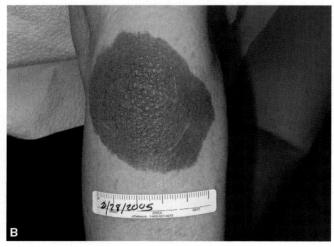

FIG. 7-13. A: Child with medium-sized CMN on the lip and chin of infant with significant cosmetic impact. **B:** Medium CMN.

TABLE 7-1	Risk Stratification Based on Size of Congenital Melanocytic Nevi	
	SIZE OF LESION	**MANAGEMENT**
Small	<1.5 cm diameter	Greatest risk for malignancy occurs *after* puberty If no atypical features: Routine prophylaxis excision is controversial Regular self skin checks—ABCDEs Annual clinical examinations or with any changes Documented baseline photo of lesion UVR avoidance and protection Elective excisions can be delayed until puberty If any concern: PCPs may monitor small lesions if they are confident in their skin assessment skills Refer to a dermatologist for regular monitoring or biopsy of medium lesions, atypical symptoms, or if PCP is unsure.
Medium	≥1.5 to 10 cm diameter	
Large/Giant	>20 cm or ≥10% BSA	Greatest risk for malignancy occurs *before* puberty Refer immediately to dermatologist: If located over head or spine due to increased risk for neurocutaneous melanocytosis Coordination of care with a neurologist, plastic surgeon, and other specialists Counseling patient and parents Lifelong monitoring and UVR avoidance

PCP, primary care provider; UVR, ultraviolet radiation

Modified from Kopf, A.W., Bart, R.S. & Hennessey, P. (1979). Congenital Nevocytic nevi and malignant melanoma. *Journal of the American Academy of Dermatology, 1*(2), 123–130.

Lesions characteristics were added to the classification system as variables influencing risk for malignancy (Box 7-3). The stratification of CMN sizes was also expanded to include a separate "giant size" category. Large CMN overlying the spinal column and skull have been associated with neurocutaneous melanocytosis (NCM) with symptoms of increased cranial pressure, vascular birthmarks, spinal cord compression, tethered spinal cord, or leptomeningeal melanoma.

Clinical Presentation

The initial presentation of small or medium CMNs can be varied from pink to dark brown and with some color variation including speckled appearance. They are usually well circumscribed and may have hypertrichosis. As the child ages, CMNs commonly rise into a plaque. Large CMNs may develop a cobblestone surface with color variation. Garment or bathing suit nevi may involve any area of the body and have a dermatomal distribution. A segmental or circumferential distribution can be associated with underlying musculoskeletal abnormalities.

All CMNs, like any pigmented lesion, should be assessed for clinical characteristics of melanoma using the classic *ABCDE* checklist (Box 7-4). The common variation of color and irregular borders of large and giant CMN can make this risk assessment very complex. Additionally, particular attention should be given to the development of satellite lesions, nodularity, and ulceration.

BOX 7-3 Proposed Characteristics of Congenital Melanocytic Nevi That Increase Risk for Malignancy

Size
Number of medium CMN
Location
Number of satellite nevi by 1 year of age
Heterogeneity of color
Rugosity
Hypertrichosis
Extensive nodules

Adapted from Krengel, S., Scope, A., Dusza, S.W., Vonthein, R., & Marghoob, A. A. (2013). New recommendations for the categorization of cutaneous features of congenital melanocytic nevi. *Journal of the American Academy of Dermatology, 68*(3), 441–451.

BOX 7-4 **ABCDE Checklist for Lesion Characteristics of Melanoma**

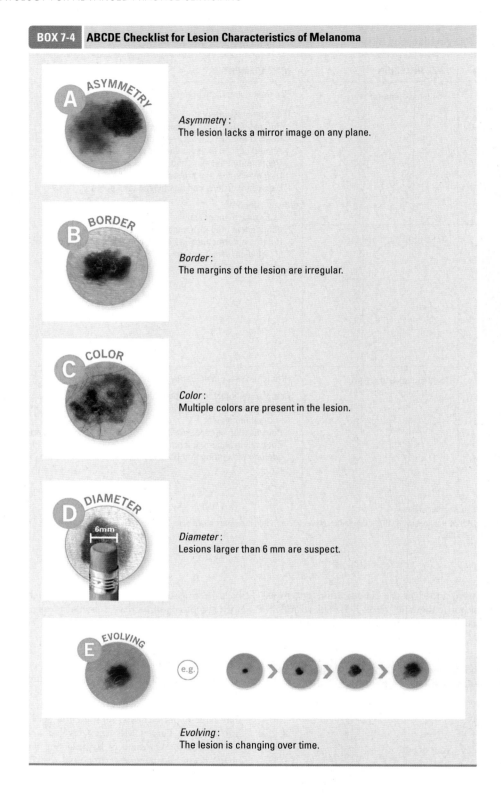

Asymmetry:
The lesion lacks a mirror image on any plane.

Border:
The margins of the lesion are irregular.

Color:
Multiple colors are present in the lesion.

Diameter:
Lesions larger than 6 mm are suspect.

Evolving:
The lesion is changing over time.

Diagnostics

Primary care clinicians should document the specific characteristics of any congenital nevus during the physical exam of a newborn or child. The size, number and location of each lesion should be noted. The PAS should be estimated since the lesion grows proportionally with the patient into adulthood and stratifies the patient risk for melanoma. To calculate the PAS, multiply the diameter of the lesion (in millimeters) by 2 if it is located on the head, or 3 if it is on the trunk. This determines the size for classification.

Changes in a CMN or suspicious features indicate the need for a biopsy. However, this can be difficult since most CMN are large in size, making excisional biopsy (preferred method for any lesion suspicious for melanoma) by nonsurgical clinician impossible. A punch biopsy offers little value for determining an accurate assessment of risk and management since the sample would only be from a small portion of the lesion. A normal histology report may give a false sense of safety because the punch specimen does not represent the melanocytic features of the entire lesion. Therefore, there is a risk of misdiagnosing a possible melanoma with a punch biopsy. It is recommended that clinicians refer the patient to a dermatologist or plastic surgeon when a biopsy is indicated.

Management

Every CMN should be evaluated on a case by case basis given the size, location, suspicious features, symptoms (if any), parents' concern for malignancy and potential disfigurement, or loss of function from surgery. It should be noted, however, that treatment of CMN continues to be controversial as dermatologists, dermatopathologists, and surgical specialists worldwide vary in their management approach.

Primary care providers (PCPs) who elect to monitor small CMN should be confident in their ability to accurately assess potential malignant changes. Patients with a medium-sized and large CMN should be referred to a dermatologist for evaluation, management, and monitoring. Referral to a dermatologist should occur early in childhood. Surgical excision of these large lesions during early childhood may have better outcomes because infants and children have greater laxity in their skin. Further, many large and giant CMNs can require serial surgeries to achieve the best cosmetic outcomes (Figure 7-14). Atypical features such as ulcerations, erosions, or nodules have become increasingly important in weighing the decision for surgical management of CMN.

Infants born with a large CMN that are notably at risk for NCM should be referred immediately for coordinated evaluation and care with a dermatologist, neurologist, ophthalmologist, and other specialists as appropriate. Imaging of the brain and spine is usually performed within the first few months of life, as well as neurological and developmental assessment. Patients with evidence of CNS involvement often require neurosurgical intervention.

One of the most important aspects of care for patients with large or giant CMNs is appropriate psychological assessment and counseling. Whether or not the lesion is excised, CMN can be severely disfiguring or may result in a permanent loss of function. Parents should be carefully counseled about all of the risks, benefits, and complications so that they can make an informed decision for treatment.

Patient Education and Follow-up

PCPs should emphasize the importance of lifelong clinical skin examinations and routine self-examinations for all patients with CMN, regardless of the size. Additionally, patients with a history of NCM should be diligent maintaining routine physical examinations (including lymph nodes), age appropriate screening, and neurological evaluations for metastasis or new primary melanoma. The nevus or scars from excision should always be examined closely for recurrence or any atypia.

The foundation for education of patients with CMN is to avoid excessive UVR and to monitor for any changes in the nevus. Employing the ABCDE skin cancer guidelines are helpful for all patients. Furthermore, CMN patients must be acutely sensitive to other symptoms that may suggest transition into malignancy, including new satellite lesions, ulcerations, tenderness, and changes in surface growths like nodules.

Acquired melanocytic nevi

Most people have benign, acquired melanocytic nevi (AMN) or "nevi" that typically appear during childhood and can occur anywhere on the body. Patients at higher risk for developing AMN are those with a family history of multiple nevi, repeated UVR exposure (including tanning beds), male gender, and occupational exposure like truck drivers and construction workers.

Clinical Presentation

Common nevi are usually classified based upon the location of the nevus cells in the skin (Box 7-2). Nevi can occur anywhere on the body, but are increased on areas of sun exposure. Depending on their location, nevi can have a wide variation of appearance such as on the palms, soles, and scalp (Figure 7-15). Common nevi begin in childhood as *junctional nevi*, appearing as round or oval, flat brown macules usually less than 6 mm in diameter. Normal changes characteristically occur during adolescence and adulthood where some (not all) of the nevus cells migrate downward into the dermis. The resulting *compound nevi* become slightly elevated and sometimes darker or with a halo effect. During adulthood, these nevi may continue to migrate so that all of the nevus cells relocated in the dermis. These *intradermal nevi* are more raised and have dome or nodular appearance (Table 7-2).

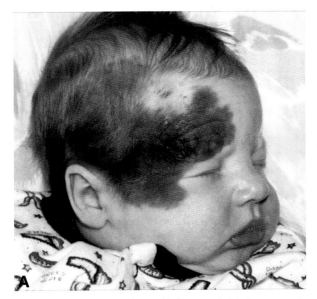
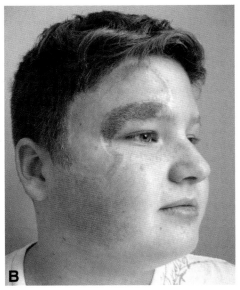

FIG. 7-14. **A:** Giant CMN on newborn with increased risk for neurocutaneous melanocytosis due to location on head. **B:** Excision of congenital nevus and appearance 10 years later.

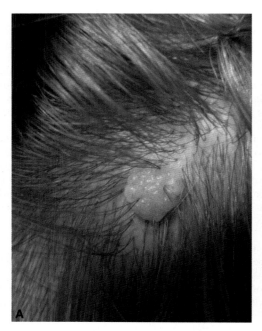
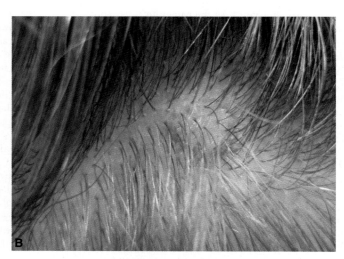

FIG. 7-15. **A:** Polypoid dermal nevus on scalp. **B:** Halo-type appearance of a nevus on the scalp.

The clinical appearance of benign nevi changes with aging and involute or fade around the sixth or seventh decade. You may have noticed that geriatric patients have very few nevi (but may have a lot of seborrheic keratoses). Growing or symptomatic changes in a nevus on an elderly patient should elicit concern for transformation into a malignancy. Therefore, understanding the normal characteristics and age-associated changes are essential to identifying suspicious or atypical nevi.

Spitz Nevus

A *Spitz nevus* is derived from spindle-shaped melanocytes and clinically presents as a single pink to brown papule on the extremities or face (Figure 7-16). Although they are usually solitary, multiple lesions have been reported. Most Spitz nevi appear during the first two decades of life, with 50% occurring in children under 10 years of age. These lesions may appear very innocuous and are commonly mistaken for a pyogenic granuloma or wart. Clinicians must include benign juvenile melanoma as an important differential diagnosis as it can be very aggressive and impact management.

There is some controversy in the management of Spitz nevus as to whether they should be completely excised or simply observed. PCPs would be prudent to biopsy lesions suspicious for Spitz nevi and send for histopathological analysis. Consultation with a pediatric dermatologist and dermatopathologist is highly recommended for diagnosed Spitz nevi, especially when there is family history of melanoma or equivocal biopsy report. Clinical and histopathologic correlation is paramount for the correct diagnosis and plan of care. Diagnosed Spitzoid melanomas may prompt a sentinel lymph node biopsy.

Halo Nevus

Also known as a Sutton's nevus, halo nevus is the development of a hypopigmented halo surrounding an AMN (Figure 7-17A). They usually appear on the trunk during adolescence and may be associated with a concomitant vitiligo. The patient may have several AMN lesions developing a halo phenomenon and in different stages of transformation. Although the etiology is uncertain, many opine that it is an autoimmune response to the normal melanocytes and nevus cells that causes pigment regression. Oftentimes, the AMN involutes completely, leaving a hypopigmented macule or normal skin color (Figure 7-17B). Most are benign but warrant a full skin examination. The AMN inside the halo is the lesion that should be evaluated for atypical features using the ABCDE checklist.

Blue Nevus

A blue nevus is an acquired or congenital melanocytic lesion resulting from Tyndall effect secondary to the depth of the pigmented cells. Presenting as dark blue to black (<0.5 cm) well-circumscribed papules, they can easily be mistaken for melanoma (Figure 7-18). It can be difficult for a primary care clinician to visually differentiate between a blue nevus and melanoma without histopathology. Clinical signs that help differentiate a common blue nevus from a melanoma are the presence of normal skin markings, homogenous color and surface, symmetry, and well-defined border—usually not seen in melanoma.

The common blue nevus is benign and does not require biopsy if does not have features suspicious for melanoma. However, a variant type, cellular blue nevus, does have an increased risk for malignancy. Cellular blue nevi are larger (>1 cm), nodular, and found on the scalp or sacral region. Some blue nevi may have a combination of both types. In the presence of multiple blue nevi, patients should be referred to a dermatologist to rule out Carney complex (NAME/LAMB syndrome) with associated atrial myxomas.

DYSPLASTIC NEVI

Dysplastic nevi (DN), also called *atypical nevi*, *Clark's nevi*, and *atypical melanocytic nevi*, are found in about 5% of the adult Caucasian population. There is an equal prevalence in men and women. The onset of DN can begin during adolescence and extend into the fifth and sixth decades of life. Individuals who report a frequent history of sun exposure, especially sunburns, before the age of 20 years have a higher incidence of DN. Yet there is no evidence to establish a causal relationship between UVR and DN.

TABLE 7-2 Characteristics of Acquired Melanocytic Nevi (Common Moles)

TYPE OF MOLE	FEATURES	EXAMPLES	LOCATION OF NEVUS CELLS
Junctional nevus	Childhood Flat or slightly elevated Uniform, flesh, brown Well defined < 6 mm diameter Scalp-brown halo		Dermal-epidermal junction.
Compound nevus	Adolescents & adults Macule withpapule/nodule Large variation Fried-egg or halo look Brown or flesh Course hair sometimes Increasing elevation with age		Dermal-epidermal junction with some nevus cells in dermis.
Dermal nevus	Adulthood Dome, verrucal, polypoid, or stalk base Flesh to brown shades Can be translucent Anywhere but frequent on head and neck Larger up to 1 cm		Nevus cells migrated into dermis.

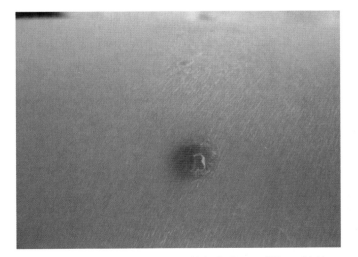

FIG. 7-16. Suspected Spitz nevus on the thigh of a 7-year-old boy with histopathology significant for spitzoid melanoma.

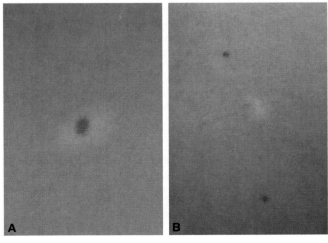

FIG. 7-17. **A:** Hypopigmented halo around AMN without suspicious features. **B:** Complete pigment regression of halo nevus.

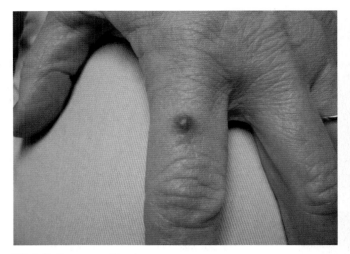

FIG. 7-18. Blue nevus of hand.

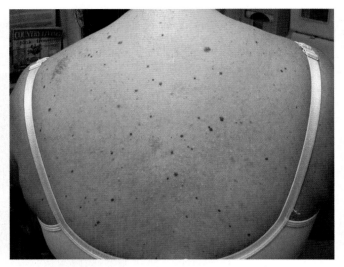

FIG. 7-19. Large number of nevi on patient with DNS.

DN are an independent risk factor for melanoma and considered by most as a *potential* precursor lesion. Although DN should alert clinicians to an increased risk for melanoma, it should be carefully noted that only 10% of melanomas arise in DN compared to 90% arising de novo on normal skin. Consequently, clinicians should be cautioned not to equate risk of one or two DN with that of patients with dysplastic nevus syndrome (DNS). DN have histopathologic and clinical characteristics that differ from common benign nevi as described in the previous section and are therefore important to identify.

Pathophysiology

The pathogenesis of DN is unknown. Research is focused on genetic factors such as germline mutations and environmental factors (i.e., UVR exposure). The result is an alteration in the nevus cells in both their appearance (cellular atypic) and arrangement (architectural atypia). These changes equate to an increased risk for malignant transformation into melanoma.

DNS, also called *atypical* or *B-K mole syndrome*, is a familial association of multiple DN and inherited melanoma attributed to a mutation of CDKN2A tumor-suppressing gene. CDKN2A mutations have been associated with increased risk for pancreatic cancers and is concerning for patients with DNS. These patients have a 500-fold increased risk for developing melanoma, typically at an earlier age onset. DNS patients often present with more than 100 pigmented nevi on their body (Figure 7-19).

Clinical Presentation

The initial presentation of a DN is most likely during adolescence or adulthood, and not during childhood like common benign nevi. The timing of lesion can be a helpful diagnostic clue. Other characteristics of a DN that should trigger clinical suspicion include large size, asymmetry, flat, and varied color or pigmentation (Figure 7-20). Discriminating between benign nevi and DN can be difficult for any clinician. Keeping in mind the characteristics of common nevi, a comparison between benign and atypical features can be helpful (Table 7-3). And of course, clinicians should always be mindful of the classic *ABCDE* guidelines used by both patients and clinicians for early recognition of melanoma.

Diagnostics

Skin examination

The foundation of any skin cancer screening is a full body skin examination especially in patients with more than 50 nevi. Patients at high risk for DN, or with a personal or family history of DN, should have full skin examination each year by an experienced clinician. A "peek-a-boo" examination can be incomplete and risks a missed diagnosis of DN or malignancy. A skin examination incorporated into a well physical can begin with global look for any "ugly duckling" lesions that stand out. For clinicians who are not confident in their ability to recognize precursor or cancerous lesions, a referral to dermatology is highly recommended. Furthermore, any changes in nevi reported by the patient should be investigated and biopsied as necessary.

Biopsy

The diagnosis of a DN cannot be made clinically and can only be made histologically. Pigmented lesions with suspicious features should be biopsied with a 2-mm clearance from the lesion margin. Punch biopsy is preferred for pigmented lesions; however, saucerization with adequate depth into the reticular dermis is acceptable.

Dermatoscopy

Dermoscopy (epiluminescent microscopy) can be valuable in the assessment of pigmented lesions. The value of dermoscopy as an assessment tool is dependent on the user's knowledge, training, and experience in evaluating the suspicious characteristics of malignancy. Some dermatoscopes use nonpolarized light, while most consist of a polarized light source and 10 × magnification that allows the clinician to identify lesion characteristics that are suspicious for melanoma. The polarized light reduces the reflection of light off the surface of the epidermis and allows for observation of deep structures, pigment, and vascular patterns that are not visible to the naked eye. Dermoscopy utilized by an experienced clinician may reduce the number of unnecessary biopsies and increase diagnostic accuracy of melanoma.

Histopathology

All clinicians would be prudent to send any mole or lesion removed from a patient for histologic examination. The histology

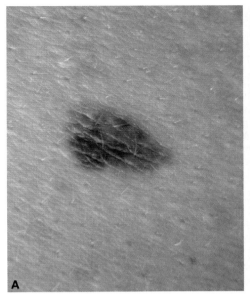
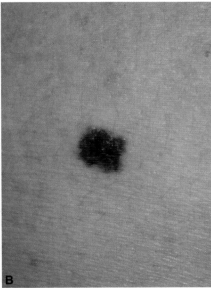
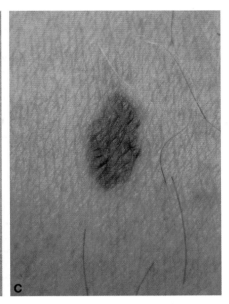

FIG. 7-20. **A–C:** Dysplastic nevi.

TABLE 7-3	Comparison of Benign Acquired Melanocytic Nevi and Dysplastic Nevi

NORMAL NEVI	DYSPLASTIC NEVI
Onset childhood	Onset adolescence to adulthood
Usually <5 mm	Usually >6 mm
Symmetrical	Asymmetry
Well-defined border	Poorly defined border
Consistent color	Variegated color
Uniform surface	Irregular surface
Unchanging	Changing appearance

of pigmented lesions should be evaluated by a pathologist, but more favorably by a dermatopathologist who specializes in pathology of the skin. The atypia of a DN is usually reported as mild, moderate, or severe. Or it may be standardized into categories (I, II, or III) for coding purposes. Clinicians who biopsy a lesion should be capable of interpreting the significance of the pathology report which determines the patient's plan of care. If there is any question or doubt about the pathology, the clinician should collaborate with the dermatopathologist or clinician experienced in dermatology.

The degree of atypia and management may be categorized as:

- *Mild Atypia* (category I) has melanocytes with nuclei that are ovoid or ellipsoid-shaped, hyperchromatic, and smaller (or nonexistent) than nuclei of basal keratinocytes.
- *Moderate Atypia* (category II) includes melanocytes with large nuclei (1–2 times the size of basal keratinocyte nuclei), hyperchromatic, ellipsoid- or rhomboid-shaped, with a small nucleolus visible in the center of the nucleus.
- *Severe Atypia* (category III) is characterized as spindle- or epithelioid-shaped, hyperchromatic nuclei larger than basal

keratinocytes (2 or more times or greater than nuclei of basal keratinocytes), but with distinct nucleoli.

There is variability in the grading of atypia among dermatopathologists, which emphasizes the difficulty in differentiating severe atypia from melanoma. A severely atypical DN is considered, by many dermatology specialists, to be analogous to a melanoma in situ.

DIFFERENTIAL DIAGNOSIS Dysplastic nevi

- Blue nevus
- Dermatofibroma
- Lentigo
- Melanoma
- Melanocytic nevi
- Seborrheic keratosis
- Spitz nevus

Management

The management of all DN is predicated on the degree of atypia identified in the histopathology report and mindfulness of the patient's medical history and risk factors for melanoma. Additionally, the clinician should note the presence or absence (clearance) of atypia on the margins of the biopsy specimen sent for analysis. This may impact the plan of care, as well as anticipate the recurrence of a pigmented lesion at the site of biopsy.

DN with mild cytologic atypia usually does not require reexcision even when atypical cells are present on the biopsy margins. Unfortunately, the management of a DN with moderate atypia (category II) and clear margins is not as straight forward and currently debated. Many dermatologists, dermatology surgeons, and dermatopathologists prefer to have moderate atypical DN reexcised with conservative margins. Their belief is that it is beneficial to excise surrounding tissues to ensure there are no more atypical cells are present for potential mutation. The decision for reexcision may be further influenced by the patient's or family's history of DN and melanoma. Conversely, other dermatology specialists do not reexcise moderately atypical DN with clear margins in all areas, believing the specimen was fully excised based on the histopathology. Specimens collected by shave biopsy may transect the base of the lesion, leaving cells on the margin and typically require reexcision.

There is no uncertainty about the need for reexcision of all severely atypical DN (category III). A reexcision of 5-mm margins is usually considered adequate, but should be confirmed with histopathology. Nonsurgical clinicians receiving a pathology report with a severe DN should refer the patient to a dermatologist or surgeon.

Patient Education and Follow-up

Patients with a history of DN should be taught to perform regular self skin checks and follow-up with annual clinical examinations. Many dermatology practitioners follow patients with a history of severe DNs at even more frequent intervals. Patient education about DN is the same as for a patient with melanoma. With an emphasis on sun avoidance and protection, patients should understand the risk of UVR. Patients with known family CDKN2A mutations should have clinical skin examinations starting at the age of 10 years and yearly monitoring.

CLINICAL PEARLS

- DN are considered possible precursor lesions to melanoma.
- Patients with a personal or family history of DN or melanoma are at higher risk for melanoma.
- Patients with DN should perform self-examinations, with particular attention to the *ABCDE* guidelines, and regular clinical skin examinations for early detection and treatment.
- Reducing UVR exposure is the single most important aspect of prevention. Hats, sunglasses, photo-protective clothing, and sun screen of SPF 30 or higher are recommended.

MELANOMA

The American Cancer Society estimates that 9,480 people will die of melanoma in 2013, with a lifetime risk of 1 out of 60 for a person living in North America. Melanoma, the deadliest of all the skin cancers, is responsible for 75% of the deaths associated with skin cancer (ACS, 2013). Even more shocking is that melanoma is the most common cancer in 25- to 29-year-olds and the leading cause of *cancer deaths* in females aged 25 to 30. And in an even younger population (15- to 29-year-olds), melanoma is the second leading cancer. This morbidity and mortality is startling when placed in the context—this disease has its greatest impact on young adults contemplating college, career development, and establishing their families. In short, it strikes young adults in the prime of their lives.

Melanoma can occur anywhere on the body, including the not-so-common areas. Genitals, soles, postauricular, and oral mucosa are not typically examined by clinicians but may be affected. The highest incidence of cutaneous melanoma is on the back, chest, and arms in white males, while the most common locations for white females are their backs, arms, and legs. In patients with dark skin tones, palmar, plantar, mucosal, and subungual areas are the most common locations.

BOX 7-5 Risk Factors for Melanoma

Unprotected UVR exposure, especially chronic, severe intermittent, or blistering sunburns
Fair complexion, blue or green eyes, blond or red hair with the tendency to freckle or burn
The presence of large number of nevi or history of DN and DNS
Large or garment CMN
Family and/or personal history of melanoma
CDKN2K, BRAF, NRAS, MC1R and *BRCA2* mutations
Xeroderma pigmentosum
Immunosuppressed patients

All patients should be assessed for risk factors for melanoma. Intermittent sun exposure (weekends and vacations) with painful sunburns during childhood and adolescence is the major predisposing risk factor for melanoma. However, other genetic and environmental risk factors can increase an individual's risk (Box 7-5). Individuals are at increased risk for melanoma if they have a family history of melanoma or DNS. If a first-degree relative (parent, sibling, or offspring) has a history of diagnosed melanoma, then the risk of developing melanoma doubles for an individual and is significantly higher if there are three or more family members with a history.

Pathophysiology

Melanoma is a cancer originating from the melanocytes, which are the pigment-producing cells in the epidermis. The term *malignant melanoma* is becoming obsolete because the word "malignant" is redundant as there are no benign melanomas. *BRAF* is a protein kinase within the RAS-RAF signaling pathway. The RAS-RAF pathway, a type of mitogen-activated protein kinase (MAPK) pathway, regulates the expression of genes. These genes encode proteins that control many essential cellular functions, such as cell proliferation and cell survival. Mutations in the *BRAF* gene result in constitutive activation of the *BRAF* protein (Figure 7-21). Approximately 50% of melanomas harbor oncogenic *BRAF* mutations at position V600. Recent research shows that patients with mutation of the BRAF gene have a higher incidence of melanoma as well as familial pancreatic and melanoma syndromes in mutations of the CDKN2A germline. The genomics of cutaneous melanoma are vastly expanding in search of risks and mutations that predispose individuals to cutaneous melanoma.

Clinical Presentation

A skin examination for the early detection of melanoma is a low-cost, straightforward screening tool (only requires a visual examination) that can have a significant impact on patient outcomes. A complete skin examination should include the "not so common" areas, including the scalp, postauricular, axillae, interdigital spaces, genitals, gluteal cleft, palms, and soles. Inspection of the oral mucosa and eyes should be considered if the patient has not had a screening by their dentist and ophthalmologist.

Although the *ABCDE* checklist for melanoma is helpful, caution should be used in discounting lesions that do not fit into these classic criteria (Box 7-4). Melanoma can look like anything, especially in individuals with red or blonde hair who may develop melanoma that is only lightly pigmented or amelanotic. Lesions can be macular, papular, or nodular. The surface may be smooth or rough and vary

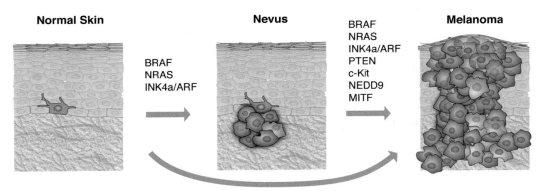

FIG. 7-21. Gene mutations in the development of melanoma.

in pigmentation from pink to brown to gray, blue or black. Some patients may report a sudden onset of burning, pruritus, ulceration, or tenderness of a lesion which could signify potential malignancy. Likewise, melanoma can arise in a previously benign lesion, like a dermal nevus or freckle, that the patient has had for years. This emphasizes the importance of listening to patients with worrisome complaints about a specific changing lesion.

There are four clinical subtypes of melanoma with associated characteristics or distribution. The most common type of melanoma is superficial spreading subtype (70%), followed by nodular melanomas (10%–15%), lentigo maligna melanomas (LMM) (5%–10%), and acral lentiginous (7%).

Superficial spreading melanoma

Superficial spreading melanoma (SSM) is characterized by a flat or slightly raised (papular) appearance. The pigment is usually variegated with brown, black, blue, or pink colors. Most are symmetrical, but are greater than 6 mm in diameter and have irregular borders. SSM is commonly found on the trunk in both genders, with an onset in the fourth or fifth decade of life. Of the subtypes, SSM is most associated with a pre-existing nevus and grows very slowly. These lesions are beginning the vertical growth phase and becoming invasive, as will be discussed later in this section (Figure 7-22).

Invasive melanoma is most commonly noted on the trunk and sun-exposed areas of the head and neck in both sexes. These melanomas have progressed in the vertical growth phase and are invading the dermis. Invasive melanoma can be any color and are rarely amelanotic (without pigment). They can easily be mistaken for basal cell carcinoma or squamous cell carcinoma (Figure 7-23).

Nodular melanomas

Nodular melanomas usually occur on the extremities or back. Typically reported as a rapidly growing dark brown to black papule or dome-shaped nodule, the surface is friable and prone to ulceration. This is the most aggressive type of melanoma and more often develops de novo instead of from a preexisting nevi. Nodular melanoma has usually advanced at the time of initial diagnosis (Figure 7-24).

Lentigo maligna and lentigo maligna melanoma

Lentigo maligna (LM) is synonymous with melanoma in situ (MIS), while *LMM* is considered a progression toward invasive melanoma. These melanomas develop on the sun-exposed regions, with cheeks, nose, and temples being the most common sites, usually during the sixth and seventh decades of life. LM and LMM appear as irregular, mottled brown macules with variegated pigment and

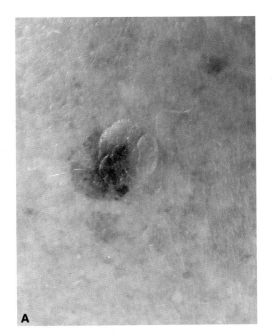

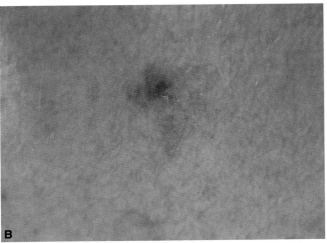

FIG. 7-22. **A:** SSM arising in a dermal nevus. **B:** SSM.

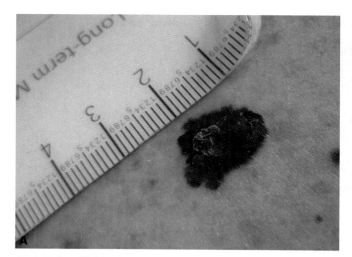

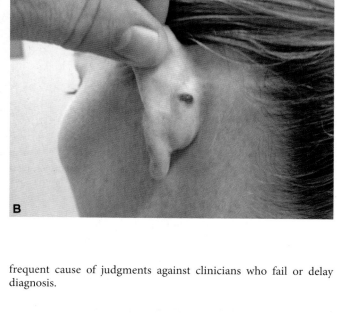

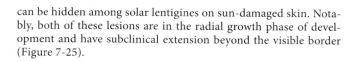

FIG. 7-23. **A** and **B:** Invasive melanoma.

can be hidden among solar lentigines on sun-damaged skin. Notably, both of these lesions are in the radial growth phase of development and have subclinical extension beyond the visible border (Figure 7-25).

Acral melanomas

Acral lentiginous melanoma (ALM) is a less common type of melanoma, yet it accounts for 20% of diagnosed melanomas in darker pigmented individuals (Fitzpatrick type IV to VI) compared to 2% in Caucasians. Unlike other melanomas types, ALM has a lower association with BRAF mutations. Pigmented macules develop on the palms, soles, and subungual (beneath the nail plate) areas. The highest incidence is on the plantar aspect of the foot and is easily mistaken for a hematoma (Figure 7-26). ALM is frequently misdiagnosed or delayed, resulting in a poor 5-year survival rate of 25% to 51% (Miranda, 2012) (Figure 7-27).

Subungual lesions present with diffuse nail discoloration or longitudinal pigmentation that may extend to the proximal nail fold, commonly referred to as the *Hutchinson sign* (Figure 7-28). Nail findings noted on exam may be a red flag and indicate the need for biopsy (Box 7-1). Subungual melanomas are the most commonly missed lesion on clinical examinations and account for the most

frequent cause of judgments against clinicians who fail or delay diagnosis.

DIFFERENTIAL DIAGNOSIS Melanoma
• Cherry angioma
• Junctional or compound nevi
• Kaposi sarcoma
• Pigmented basal cell carcinoma
• Pyogenic granuloma
• Seborrheic keratosis

Diagnostics

Biopsy

Biopsy is essential for the diagnosis of melanoma. Excisional biopsy (excising the complete lesion with 1 to 2 mm beyond the edge and full depth of the dermis) is the recommended method of sampling. Punch biopsies are appropriate for small lesions if you can remove the entire lesion with one punch. A deep shave (sometimes referred to as

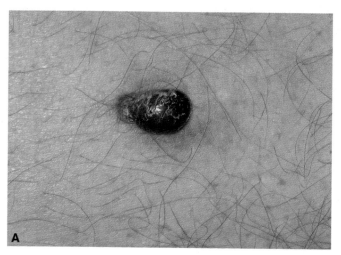

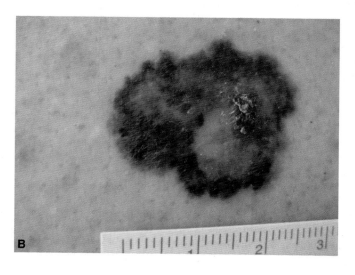

FIG. 7-24. **A** and **B:** Nodular melanoma.

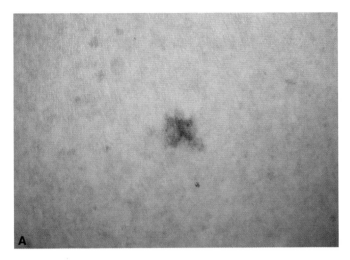

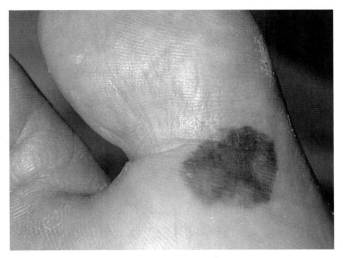

FIG. 7-26. Acral lentiginous melanoma.

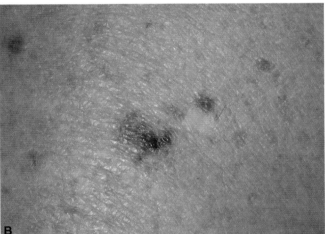

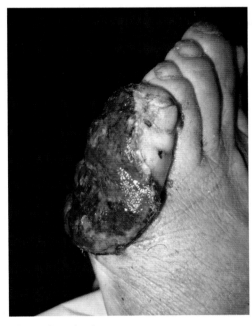

FIG. 7-27. Advanced acral melanoma.

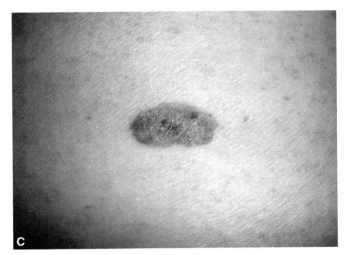

FIG. 7-25. **A:** Lentigo maligna. **B** and **C:** Melanoma in situ.

It cannot be overemphasized that when a clinician is not skilled in biopsy or excision, they should collaborate with a qualified clinician who can perform the biopsy right away. The patient should not be left to wait weeks for an appointment. A phone call from provider to provider may be necessary to facilitate patient access for a prompt appointment. Developing a relationship with a local dermatologist or surgical provider who will accommodate urgent requests can be invaluable. In this scenario, we would recommend that the patient's appointment be scheduled before they leave your office and a follow-up confirmation with the patient to ensure that they have completed the biopsy and received the appropriate management from the specialist if indicated.

Histopathology

The histopathologic characteristics of a biopsied lesion are critical to determining the diagnosis as well as the type melanoma. Many

a scoop) biopsy to the reticular dermis for small lesions is acceptable, but requires much practice to perfect. An incisional biopsy may be performed for lesions that are too large to excise for biopsy. Furthermore, if the lesion is on the face or cosmetically sensitive areas, consider a referral to a Mohs or plastic surgeon but without delay.

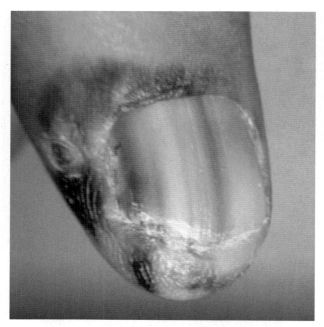

FIG. 7-28. Subungual melanoma. Note the pigment on the surrounding cuticle: a positive Hutchinson's sign.

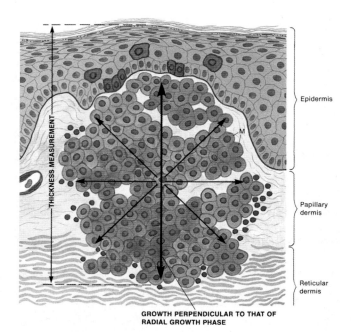

FIG. 7-29. Breslow's depth measurement of invasion by melanoma.

histologic characteristics reported about the melanoma are key variables used to stage or classify the tumor, predict morbidity, and guide treatment. Therefore, the clinician can impact the diagnostic value of the biopsy by providing a quality specimen (discussed above) and key clinical information on the pathology request form, including the following: a photograph (if available), pertinent medical history, and complete description of the lesion. Details such as "0.8 cm blue and black variegated papule with irregular border and central ulceration located on left upper chest at the MCL" can be helpful, while "a bump on chest" will be of little value to the dermatopathologist.

The *depth* of the lesion will be reported in the histopathology report and is the most predictive factor in staging melanoma. Two methods are used for reporting lesion depth. *Breslow's depth* measurement (in millimeters) is the accepted standard currently used in AJCC Melanoma Tumor Classification and measures the invasion of the lesion from the top of the epidermis to the deepest point of melanocyte proliferation (Figure 7-29). You may also see some histopathology that report the *Clarks level,* but this is becoming less frequently reported.

The histopathology report will note tumor characteristics like the presence of microscopic ulceration which upgrades a tumor's seriousness and can move it into a later stage. Mitotic rate (cancer cell division) has been introduced into the staging system based on recent evidence that it is also an independent factor predicting prognosis. Perineural or perivascular invasion will be noted if present. The presence of any or all of these features suggests a more aggressive disease and will impact the staging of the lesion.

Sentinel lymph node biopsy

The depth of a melanoma usually guides the surgeon's decision to perform a *sentinel lymph node biopsy* (SLNB). Lesions with a thickness of 1 mm or greater are more likely to metastasize to the lymph vessels and then regional lymph nodes. Accordingly, SLNB is usually recommended for lesions 1 to 4 mm in thickness or if the lesion is less than 1 mm and has noted ulceration. An SLNB to assess for lymph node involvement is often performed at the same time as the surgical

excision of the primary melanoma. A radionucleotide (Technetium Tc 99m) and methylene blue dye are injected at the site of the primary melanoma. The regional lymph node basin is scanned for the presence of the isotope or "hot" node. Any lymph nodes found with uptake of the blue dye is then excised and sent for pathology. A positive SLNB indicates metastasis to lymph nodes and the possible need for further lymph node dissection of the regional basin. It may also indicate the need for further diagnostics such as serologies and positron emission tomography (PET scan) to assess for distant metastases. Negative SLNB does not rule out metastasis, but has a better prognosis over time.

Management

Staging of melanoma (or any cancer) helps clinicians classify the severity of the primary tumor and possible metastasis of the cancer patient. It is invaluable in calculating the patient's prognosis and guidelines for treatment. Other factors such as patient's health and comorbidities may influence treatment choices and plan of care.

Modalities

Surgical excision with histologically proven clear surgical margins, is the gold standard of treatment for all biopsy-proven primary melanoma. While most primary care clinicians refer these patients to dermatologists or dermatology surgeons, some elect to perform the surgical excision. Providers should have competent surgical skills and current knowledge regarding the recommendations by the National Cancer Institute, which guides most dermatologists, Mohs and oncology surgeons (NCI, 2013). The recommended surgical margins are as follows:

- MIS: 0.5 cm-margin
- Melanomas <1 mm depth: 1.0 cm-margin
- Melanomas 1 to 4 mm in depth: 2.0 cm-margin
- Melanomas >4 mm in depth: ≥ 2.0 cm-margin

Oncologists and surgeons may consider alternative treatment with radiation, cryotherapy, and topical immunomodulators for a large MIS and LMM that would disfigure a patient or in a patient who is a poor surgical candidate. For these patients, referral to a dermatologist is essential. Mohs surgery can be beneficial in areas where full surgical margins are not possible or where cosmetic concerns are significant. This technique remains somewhat controversial as some experts believe that it is difficult to visualize melanoma cells in a fresh frozen specimen. The introduction of immunohistological stains should make this a more utilized technique in the future.

Chemotherapy

In spite of the advances in new drug therapies, these drugs do not cure metastatic melanoma. They offer only the hope of slowing the progression and extending life during advanced stages of the disease.

Interferon alfa-2b is the only Food and Drug Administration (FDA)-approved adjunctive therapy for stage IIIB–IIIC melanoma with an improved survival rate and disease-free period. Yet the toxicities and side effects of the drugs, especially the high-dose regimen with the longest survival rate, can be difficult for the patients to tolerate and advance beyond the 3-month induction phase of therapy.

Vaccines currently being studied in clinical trial offer an antigen-directed approach by stimulating an immune response to melanoma-associated tumor cells. They have reported lower toxicities but some hypersensitivity reactions. At this time, vaccine trials have not offered any significant improvement in survival rates and are not FDA approved.

Once distant metastasis occurs, the 5-year prognosis for survival plummets, with limited therapies available by experienced oncologists. Ongoing clinical trials continue to evaluate potential treatments based on the newly described oncogenic BRAF signaling pathway. In the past 2 years, new options have been approved by the FDA for the treatment of patients with late-stage (metastatic) melanoma. *Ipilimumab* (YERVOY) is a monoclonal antibody that enhances the patient's natural antitumor response and blocking the cytotoxic T-lymphocyte antigen 4 (CTLA-4). And *Vemurafenib* (ZELBORAF) is a targeted therapy for metastatic melanoma patients with a known BRAF mutation. It is a kinase inhibitor that boosts T-cell activation to kill the melanoma tumor cells. While these are the first drugs approved to treat melanoma, their chemotherapy side effects can cause severe disability, organ failure, and death during or after infusion.

Prognosis and Complications

The 5- and 10-year survival rates for melanoma are published by the ACS and based on the AJCC 2008 Staging Database (ACS, 2011). The diagnosis and surgical treatment of early melanoma (stage I) has a 97% 5-year survival rate, which means it is eminently curable. And, with continued follow-up, a patient should have a normal life span. Moreover, the ACS emphasizes the drastic decrease in survival for patients with metastatic melanoma or advanced stages (III and IV) where the 5-year survival rate plummets to 78% and 15%, respectively. Additional factors that increase the risk for morbidity include diagnosis in elderly, African Americans, acral melanomas, and immunosuppressed patients.

Patient Education and Follow-up

Prevention education is the clinician's greatest tool in reducing the incidence of melanoma in their patients. The following teaching points are aimed at prevention and early recognition:

- Monthly patient self-examinations are highly recommended (reinforced at each visit).
- Frequent clinical skin examinations by a dermatology provider for patients with a history of melanoma. Examination every 4 to 6 months after diagnosis is needed for the first few years.

- The *most* important factor is avoidance of UVR exposure, including tanning bed use.
- Protect yourself from the sun (see chapter 2).
- Melanoma is curable with early detection and treatment.
- Let your dentist, ophthalmologist, and gynecologist know about your history of melanoma.
- Counsel your family (parents, siblings, and children) about their increased risk for melanoma.
- Recommend reliable sources for patient information like the Skin Cancer Foundation.

Clinicians should emphasize the importance of clinical follow-up after diagnoses of melanoma to reduce the risk of mortality and morbidity. While there are many varied beliefs and opinions regarding the monitoring of patients diagnosed with primary cutaneous melanoma without metastasis, the American Academy of Dermatology provides an evidence-based algorithmic approach to the diagnoses, treatment, and management. During the initial 2 years following diagnosis, patients should have a total skin examination every 4 to 6 months, then 1 to 2 years thereafter. For patients with metastatic disease, the oncologist should recommend and guide follow-up management and monitoring in collaboration with dermatologist.

CLINICAL PEARLS

Early recognition and diagnosis of melanoma

- Stand back for a "five-foot view" of the patient's skin and look for the "ugly duckling."
- Not all melanomas are brown or pigmented.
- LISTEN to patients with a heightened concern about a *specific* lesion and consider biopsy even if the lesion has benign characteristics.
- Make sure to look in all the cracks and crevices and palms and soles.
- Ask about sun-protective behaviors at each office visit and teach prevention.
- Biopsy the entire suspicious lesion. A small biopsy of a large lesion can lead to a false negative result and fatal outcome.
- Refer early and often if you have any doubts or if you are unable to biopsy.

BILLING CODES ICD-10

Dysplastic nevus	D48.5
Melanocytic nevi	D22
lip	D22.0
eyelid	D22.1
ear	D22.2
other unspecified areas face	D22.3
scalp and neck	D22.4
trunk	D22.5
upper limb incl. shoulder	D22.6
lower limb incl hip	D22.7
unspecified	D22.9
Blue nevus	D22.M8780
Congenital melanocytic nevus	D22.
Halo nevomelanocytic nevus	D22.M8723/0
Mongolian spot	
Nevus of Ota	D22.
Nevus spilus	D22.
Spitz nevus	D22. M8772

READINGS

Ali, A. (2010). Dermatology: A pictorial review. New York, NY: McGraw-Hill Medical.

American Cancer Society. (2011, June). *Melanoma skin cancer overview.* http://www.cancer.org/acs/groups/cid/documents/webcontent/003063-pdf.pdf

American Cancer Society (ACS). (2013). *American Cancer Society Facts and Figures.* Retrieved on November 15, 2013, from http://www.cancer.org/research/cancerfactsstatistics/cancerfactsfigures2013/index

Chen, L., James, N., Barker, C., Busam, K., & Marghoob, A. (2013). Desmoplastic melanoma: A review. *Journal of the American Academy of Dermatology, 68*(5), 825–833. doi: 10.1016/j.jaad.2012.10.041

Edge, S. B. (2010). *AJCC Cancer Staging Manual* (7th ed.). New York, NY: Springer.

Fox, M., Lao, C., Schwartz, J., Frohm, M., Bichakjian, C., & Johnson, T. (2013). Management options for metastatic melanoma in the era of novel therapies: A primer for the practicing dermatologist: Part I: Management of stage III disease. *Journal of the American Academy of Dermatology, 68*(1), e1–1.e9. doi: 10.1016/j.jaad.2012.09.040

Fox, M., Lao, C., Schwartz, J., Frohm, M., Bichakjian, C., & Johnson, T. (2013). Management options for metastatic melanoma in the era of novel therapies: A primer for the practicing dermatologist: Part II: Management of stage IV disease. *Journal of the American Academy of Dermatology, 68*(1), e1–e13. doi: 10.1016/j.jaad.2012.09.041

Goodson, A. G., & Grossman, D. (2009). Strategies for early melanoma detection: Approaches to the patient with nevi. *Journal of the American Academy of Dermatology, 60*(5), 719–735. doi: 10.1016/j.jaad.2008.10.065

Gershenwald, J. E., & Ross, M. I. (2011). Sentinel-lymph-node biopsy for cutaneous melanoma. *New England Journal of Medicine, 364*(18), 1738–1745. doi: 10.1056/NEJMct1002967

Kopf, A.W., Bart, R. S. & Hennessey, P. (1979). Congenital nevocytic nevi and malignant melanoma. *Journal of American Academy of Dermatology, 1*(2), 123–130.

Krengel, S., Scope, A., Dusza, S. W., Vonthein, R., & Marghoob, A. A. (2013). New recommendations for the categorization of cutaneous features of congenital melanocytic nevi. *Journal of the American Academy of Dermatology, 68*(3), 441–451.

Marghoob, A. A. (2012). *Nevogenesis mechanisms and clinical implications of nevus development.* Berlin: Springer-Verlag. doi: 10.1007/978-3-642-28397-0

Marghoob, A. A., Borrego, J. P., & Halpern, A. C. (2003). Congenital melanocytic nevi: Treatment modalities and management options. *Seminars in Cutaneous Medicine and Surgery, 2*(1), 21–32.

Miranda, B. H., Haughton, D. N., & Fahmy, F. S. (2012). Subungual melanoma: An important tip. *Journal of Plastic, Reconstructive & Aesthetic Surgery, 65*(10), 1422–1424. doi: 10.1016/j.bjps.2012.03.001

Naeyaert, J. M., & Brochez, L. (2003). Dysplastic nevi. *New England Journal of Medicine, 349*(23), 2233–2240. doi: 10.1056/NEJMcp023017

National Cancer Institute (NCI). (2013). *Melanoma Home Page.* Retrieved from http://www.cancer.gov/cancertopics/types/melanoma

Price, H. N., & Schaffer, J. V. (2010). Congenital melanocytic nevi-when to worry and how to treat: Facts and controversies. *Clinics in Dermatology, 28*(3), 293–302.

Rapini, R. P. (2012). *Practical dermatopathology* (2nd ed.). Philadelphia, PA: Elsevier/Saunders.

Russak, J. E., & Rigel, D. S. (2012). *Melanoma and pigmented lesions.* Philadelphia, PA: Saunders.

Sober, A. J., Chuang, T-Y., Duvic, M., Farmer, E. R., Grichnik, J. M., Halpern, A. C., . . . the Guidelines/Outcomes Committee. (2001). Guidelines of care for primary cutaneous melanoma. *Journal of the American Academy of Dermatology, 45*(4), 579–586.

Wong, S. J., Balch, C. M., Hurley, P., Agarwala, S. S., Akhurst, T. J., Cochran, A., & Lyman, G. H. (2012). Sentinel lymph node biopsy for melanoma: American Society of Clinical Oncology and Society of Surgical Oncology Joint Clinical Practice Guideline. *Journal of Clinical Oncology, 30*(23), 2912–2918. doi: 10.1200/JCO.2011.40.3519.

CHAPTER 8

Precancerous and Nonmelanoma Skin Cancers

Victoria Lazareth

Each year, 2 million Americans develop nonmelanoma skin cancers (NMSC), costing health care nearly $500 million. Untreated or incompletely treated tumors lead to disfigurement, nerve damage, functional impairment, and even death. Advanced practice clinicians (APCs) can provide early diagnosis and treatment of NMSC, reducing patient morbidity and mortality. Additionally, APCs can provide valuable preventative education regarding sun safety and early detection of skin cancer through clinical and self-examinations.

PRECANCEROUS LESIONS

Actinic keratoses (AKs) are extremely common lesions which develop in increasing number with cumulative sun exposure and advancing age. Approximately one in five Americans will develop AKs in their lifetime. Patients who develop AKs tend to have fair skin and a history of chronic or intense, intermittent sun exposure, and often have clinical signs of photoaging, including freckles, lentigines, and pigmentary dyschromia. AKs may present years after the sun exposure. These precancerous lesions constitute one of the most common reasons for patients to present to a clinician.

While it is estimated that up to 20% of AKs may develop into squamous cell carcinoma (SCC), there is no way to discern clinically if a given lesion will progress. Lesions which become large, thickened, tender, or ulcerated are worrisome for SCC. AKs may resolve spontaneously with sun-protective measures, but persistent lesions are usually treated both for symptomatic relief and to prevent their progression into skin cancer.

Pathophysiology

The epidermal layer of the skin is composed of keratinocytes, which slowly migrate from the base to the surface of the epidermis (Figure 8-1). Ultraviolet radiation (UVR) damage to the keratinocytes can result in premalignant transformation. AKs are altered keratinocytes within the epidermis and are thought to represent an intermediary step along the continuum of development to SCC. These atypical keratinocytes show an increased mitotic rate, which have the potential to develop into SCC. If the atypical keratinocytes extend across the full extent of the epidermis, they are designated as localized or in situ SCC.

Clinical Presentation

AKs initially present as a skin color to pink to red, rough areas with a texture likened to that of sandpaper (Figure 8-2). Lesions may develop thick scale, which may evolve into sharp papules or plaques, which may in turn become crusted or bleed when removed. AKs are better detected by feel than by sight; so a tactile examination with the fingertips over sun-exposed areas (i.e., nasal dorsum, helical rims of the ears, and dorsal hands) should be performed.

Discerning an advancing AK from SCC in situ (SCCIS) requires histologic diagnosis made by the dermatopathologist or pathologist.

Therefore, AKs with suspicious features, including sensitivity to touch or sun exposure, spontaneous bleeding, size larger than 1 cm, or location adjacent to a previously diagnosed NMSC, warrant a biopsy.

Several variants of AK exist:

Pigmented actinic keratoses (PAKs) are identical to AKs with a brown, blue, or black hue which results from melanocytes within the lesion. PAKs are more often seen in individuals with darker skin tones.

Hypertrophic AKs are lesions which have become very thick, scaly, or crusty plaques. They are often large, yellow, and crusty (Figure 8-3). A biopsy is often needed to exclude SCC.

A *cutaneous horn* is a hyperkeratotic papule which becomes protruberant (Figure 8-4). Similar lesions may develop from benign seborrheic keratoses or warts; so a biopsy is necessary to identify SCCIS.

Actinic cheilitis is the designation for AKs of the lower lip (Figure 8-5). These lesions are rough, scaly, fissures, or plaques which may be white or hyperpigmented. It is not uncommon for them to become tender, bleed, or ulcerate. Actinic cheilitis persists longer than an HSV lesion and doesn't resolve with emollients typically helpful for chapped or dry lips.

DIFFERENTIAL DIAGNOSIS Actinic keratoses

- Squamous cell carcinoma
- Lichenoid keratosis
- Basal cell carcinoma
- Psoriasis
- Eczema
- Seborrheic keratosis
- Chondrodermatitis nodularis helicis
- Solar lentigo
- Melanoma
- Wart
- Herpes simplex virus

Diagnostics

Lesions which are presumed to be AKs but have not resolved with initial therapy, as well as a cutaneous horn, should also be biopsied. AKs which are becoming larger, thicker, tender, or ulcerated are worrisome for SCC and require histologic evaluation. The shave biopsy is an efficient, well-tolerated procedure that can provide a sufficient tissue sample for histology (described in chapter 24). Yet, if the sample is too shallow and does not include a portion of the dermis, an invasive SCC could be misdiagnosed as an in situ lesion, risking incomplete treatment and recurrence.

Management

There are many treatment options for AKs, including watchful waiting with careful sun-safety measures. Consideration must be given to patient selection, efficacy, risks, side effects, psychosocial

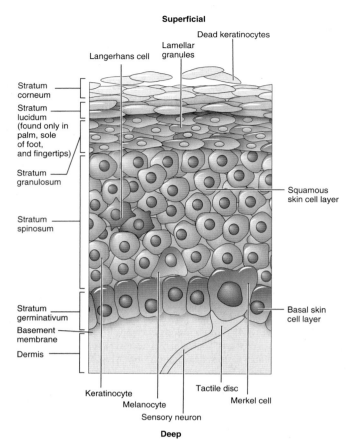

FIG. 8-1. Anatomy of the epidermis.

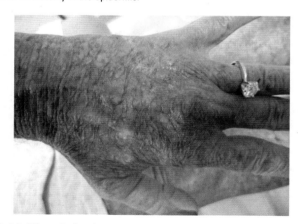

FIG. 8-2. AKs on the hand.

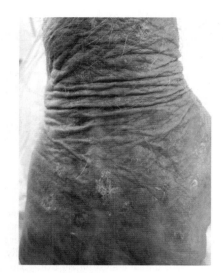

FIG. 8-3. Hypertrophic AKs on the hand.

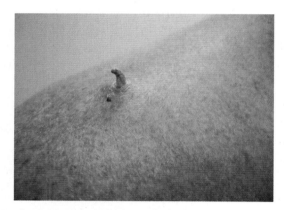

FIG. 8-4. Cutaneous horn on the shoulder.

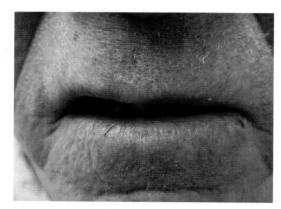

FIG. 8-5. Actinic cheilitis on the lower lip.

variables, cosmesis, compliance, cost, and duration of therapy in selecting the best treatment option for a given patient. Competent primary care providers often provide effective treatment for patients with a few, well-defined AKs using FDA-approved immunotherapy and cryosurgery (Table 8-1). However, off-label treatment with immunotherapy and more advanced procedures should be referred to experienced dermatology specialists to avoid the risk of misdiagnosis, inadequate treatment, and complications.

Local therapy

When there are a few clearly identified AKs, localized therapy can provide prompt and effective treatment. The knowledge and experience of the clinician providing treatment will impact the patient's experience and treatment outcomes.

Cryotherapy is the most widely used modality to treat AKs. It is a quick, effective, and generally well-tolerated in-office procedure. The lesions are destroyed by freezing with liquid nitrogen (−196.5°C), which crystallizes the tumor cells, producing necrosis and tissue destruction. Blisters often form and dry into crusts, usually healing within 1 to 2 weeks. Potential adverse effects include pain, hypopigmentation, or scarring, which may be of concern in cosmetically sensitive areas. The advantage is that it requires one visit for treatment, and

TABLE 8-1	Treatment Modalities for Actinic Keratoses	
TREATMENT MODALITY (BRAND NAME)	**REDUCTION OF LESIONS**
Cryotherapy	88%
Imiquimod (*Aldara, Zyclara*)	87%
5-fluorouracil (*Efudex, Carac, Fluoroplex*)	86%
Ingenol mebutate (*Picato*)	85%
Diclofenac (*Solaraze*)	64%
Photodynamic therapy	78%
Chemical peels: *glycolic acid, salicylic acid, trichloroacetic acid*	High
Dermabrasion, laser resurfacing	High

has been traditionally covered by insurers compared to prescription immunotherapies which can be more costly.

Curettage can be used to debulk hypertrophic AKs immediately following a shave biopsy, which is sent for histology to exclude invasive SCC. The provider uses a curette to scrape off the friable, damaged keratinocytes until normal, firm dermal tissue is reached. Electrocautery is used to control any bleeding. The procedure should only be performed by clinicians trained and experienced with this technique. Disadvantages of curettage include risk of hypopigmented, atrophic and/or hypertrophic scarring.

Field therapy

Patients can present with clinically well-defined AKs, as well as subclinical lesions in moderately and severely photodamaged skin. There are medical and procedural options that can provide *field treatment* to larger areas, treating both types of lesions.

Immunotherapy may be considered for both local and field therapy. There are several FDA-approved topical agents outlined in Table 8-2 with varied mechanism of action, dosages, contraindications, side effects, and duration of therapy. In general, patients receiving topical therapy are advised to avoid application to the

TABLE 8-2	Topical Actinic Keratoses Immunotherapy			
DRUG AND MECHANISM OF ACTION	**GENERIC AND BRANDDOSING**	**SIDE EFFECTS**	**CLINICAL GUIDANCE**
Imiquimod* Immunomodulator	*Imiquimod* 5% cream; *Aldara* 5% cream: apply twice per week at bedtime for 16 wk *Zyclara* 2.5% cream: Nightly for 2 wk; off for 2 wk; then repeat for 2 more wk (Zyclara 3.75% indicated for HPV)	Redness, edema, scale, pruritus, erosions, crusts, burning, URI, flu-like symptoms, headache, photosensitivity	Should not use topical corticosteroids Treatment should be stopped when erosions or ulcerations develop
5-Fluorouracil* Antineoplastic and antimetabolite	*5-Fluorouracil* 2% and 5% cream, 2% solution; *Efudex* 5% cream; *Fluoroplex* 1% cream or solution. Apply b.i.d. for 2–6 wk *Carac* 0.5% microsphere: apply once daily for up to 4 wk	Redness, edema, scale, pruritus, maculopapular rash, erosions or ulcers, N/V, diarrhea, stomatitis headache, photosensitivity	Can use topical corticosteroid to calm SE after therapy Treatment should be stopped when erosions or ulcerations develop
Ingenol mebutate Cytotoxic	*Picato* 0.015% or 0.05% gel Face and scalp: 0.015% gel once daily for 3 consecutive days. Trunk and extremities: 0.05% gel once daily for 2 consecutive days	Redness, edema, scale, burning, pruritus, erosions or ulcers, potential application site pain, infection, periorbital edema, nasopharyngitis, headache	Only 2–3 days application Side effects last longer than actual treatment duration
Diclofenac sodium 3% gel Nonsteroidal anti-inflammatory	*Solaraze* 3% gel Apply b.i.d. for 60–90 days Often used in combination with *hyaluronic acid* for increase percutaneous absorption	Redness, edema, scale, pruritus, erosions or ulcers **Hematologic:** Blood coagulation disorder, burning sensation in eyes, keratitis, lacrimal drainage, increased intraocular pressure **Contraindicated:** hypersensitivity to diclofenac or NSAIDS	Avoid concomitant use of NSAIDs Well tolerated in sensitive individuals sensitive to other treatments

*Only imiquimod 5% and 5-fluorouracil 5% are FDA approved for the treatment of superficial basal cell carcinoma using different dosage recommendations.

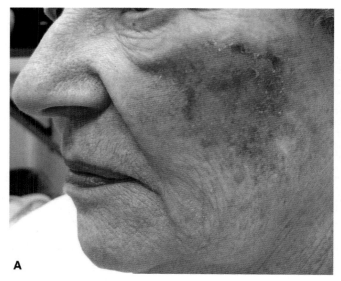
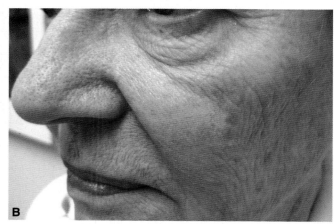

FIG. 8-6. **A:** AKs treated with topical 5-fluorouracil. **B:** One month after completed treatment.

mucous membranes and UVR exposure during and immediately after therapy. Use of shade, full-brimmed hat, and sun screen are suggested if patients will be outdoors. Common side effects for almost all topical therapies include allergic contact dermatitis, burning, crusting, dryness, edema, erosion, erythema, hyperpigmentation, irritation, pain, soreness, and ulceration (Figure 8-6A). Patients may struggle with the red, crusted appearance during treatment, but are usually pleased with the final cosmetic results. On the other hand, the advantages of topical immunotherapy are treatment of subclinical lesions and cosmetic outcomes (Figure 8-6B).

Photodynamic therapy (PDT) is a form of phototherapy which utilizes a photosensitizing agent which is activated by a timed exposure to a light source. This process selectively causes destruction of the damaged cells. Many patients compare the experience to that of a severe sunburn. PDT has a better cosmetic result than cryotherapy and 5-FU; however, the treatment causes significant discomfort and burning. Patients must avoid all sun exposure for at least 3 days posttreatment. PDT is performed in dermatology offices.

Dermabrasion is an in-office procedure used occasionally for treatment of AKs. It physically removes the surface of the epidermis using a surgical sanding tool or laser therapy. The skin is red and abraded initially, but then heals with healthy keratinocytes.

Chemical peels (medium depth), using trichloroacetic acid or glycolic acid, exfoliate the stratum corneum and can be effective. The skin can become very red and irritated initially, but then skin heals with a soft, smooth texture. Deep chemical peels are rarely used due to risk of systemic and cutaneous complications.

Laser resurfacing with carbon dioxide or erbium: YAG lasers are used for the treatment of extensive actinic damage and epithelial dysplasia implicated in the development of aggressive skin cancer. Sustained efficacy with laser resurfacing has not been established.

Special Consideration

Regular preventive strategies and early treatment of precancerous AKs and SCCIS are very important in the immunosuppressed patient. These lesions can rapidly develop into aggressive, invasive skin cancers.

Prognosis and Complications

There are few, if any, complications associated with treatment of AKs by experienced providers. Complications like scarring and systemic

side effects vary with each modality. Patients may report resolution after treatment only to experience recurrence after new sun exposure. Up to 20% of AKs may progress to invasive SCC.

Referral and Consultation

Patients with an extensive number of AKs, poorly defined lesions, and those resistant to treatment should be referred to dermatology. Primary care APC's would be prudent to maintain a low threshold for referral to dermatology or plastic surgery.

Patient Education and Follow-up

AKs are preventable with consistent, careful sun-protective and sun-safety measures. Regular application of sunscreen has been shown to actually decrease the number of AKs and thereby significantly decrease SCC development by almost 40%. Patients treated for AKs must be counseled about the effectiveness, risk for recurrence, and progression. Recommended follow-up after completed treatment is 6 to 12 months.

SQUAMOUS CELL CARCINOMA

While the incidence of many cancers has been on the decline, SCC has *doubled* over the past 40 years. This development is likely due, at least in part, to an increasing exposure of the population to UVR—especially UVB radiation. Patients who develop SCCs tend to be fair with a history of chronic or intense, intermittent sun exposure and have clinical signs of solar elastosis, including freckles, lentigines, and pigmentary dyschromia.

SCC occurs more often in men and in older patients. While basal cell carcinoma (BCC) is the most common skin cancer in patients of Caucasian, Hispanic, Chinese, and Japanese descent, SCC is the most common type of skin cancer that occurs in African Americans and Asian Indians. Melanin provides a sun-protection factor (SPF) of approximately 13.4 in African American skin, compared to 3.4 in Caucasian skin, which unfortunately creates the misconception that dark skin is not vulnerable to skin cancer. SCC lesions in people with dark skin tones are often diagnosed at later stages and may be more advanced and potentially fatal. SCCs occurring in these patients are often secondary to scarring or chronic inflammation. The metastatic rate of SCC caused by chronic UVR in Caucasians is <10%, whereas SCC caused by chronic scarring in blacks is nearly 30%.

Other subsets of patients are also at increased risk for developing SCC. A history of lymphoproliferative disease is an independent risk factor for SCC, which does not revert back to normal with control of the disease. HIV patients are more susceptible to human papilloma virus (HPV) infections and therefore three times more likely to develop SCC than the general population. The health of 30,000 Americans who are organ transplant recipients (OTRs) rely on immunosuppression to prevent rejection of the new organ. Unfortunately, this increases their risk of skin infections and skin cancers. By 20 years post transplantation, 40% of OTRs in the United States will eventually develop skin cancers, especially SCCs which behave far more aggressively than those in the immunocompetent patient.

Pathophysiology

SCC is a malignant epithelial tumor arising from a proliferation of keratinocytes (squamous cells) from the epidermis. Damage to the keratinocytes results in a mutation of cellular DNA. Irregular nests of the damaged cells form a tumor which invades into the dermis.

Clinical Presentation

Invasive SCC presents as papules, plaques, or nodules which develop in sun-exposed areas, including areas of thinning hair at the scalp and at the anterior lower extremities (Figure 8-7). Tumors may have a smooth or hyperkeratotic surface or they may develop a cutaneous horn. The SCC grows slowly, becoming increasingly indurated over time, and may eventually ulcerate. Invasive SCC may bleed, become tender or painful.

"High-risk" SCCs are tumors which present a high risk for recurrence or metastasis. Lesion characteristics and patient history are vital for an accurate assessment of risk in SCC (Table 8-3).

Location. Seventy percent of SCCs develop at the head and neck and 15% at the upper extremities (Figure 8-8A). SCCs which develop at the ears, lips, tongue, genitalia, and distal extremities have a much higher rate of recurrence than those that develop at other locations. Additionally, the scalp is increasingly being considered a high-risk location as SCC can penetrate the bony outer table of the skull (Figure 8-8B).

Size. SCCs which are greater than 2 cm have up to three times the metastatic rate of smaller tumors.

Etiology. SCCs which develop in scars, sinus tracts, chronic ulcers, and areas of previous radiation also present higher rates of recurrence (Figure 8-9).

Cellular Behavior. Certain SCC cellular subtypes may also present aggressive behavior. Those which are poorly differentiated invade nerves or blood vessels, or those which develop in isolation as single cells present a particularly high risk for recurrence.

Subtypes of SCC

SCCIS is an AK which has progressed through the full thickness of the epidermis and extended into the hair follicles (*follicular* or *adnexal extension*). Clinically, SCCIS is thicker than an AK and has an erythematous base (Figure 8-10). They enlarge and become increasingly tender, bleed easily, or ulcerate.

Bowen disease is an SCCIS which develops in hair-bearing epithelium, often in areas with limited sun exposure such as the trunk or extremities (Figure 8-11).

Bowenoid papulomatosis (BP) is Bowen disease thought to be induced by HPV. Lesions are solitary, sharply defined, red papules or plaques which ooze or crust. BP is usually located on the genitals, and can affect both males and females. Up to 5% of BP may become invasive carcinoma.

Erythroplasia of Queyrat is an SCCIS that develops in the mucosal epithelium (glans and prepuce of the penis) often in older, uncircumcised males. It presents as a solitary, *sharply* defined, shiny, red plaque which may ulcerate but is generally nontender. Up to 30% of cases may become invasive carcinoma.

Keratoacanthoma (KA) is a low-grade SCC variant which develops in sun-exposed areas (Figure 8-12). Clinically, it presents as a 1- to 2.5-cm dome-shaped, skin color to red, firm nodule which can be tender. KAs have central, hyperkeratotic crusting or horn, often described as a volcano. Tumors grow very quickly and *may* involute within 6 months.

Verrucous carcinoma (VC) is also a low-grade SCC variant developing in the genital or oral regions, but can be found on the sole of the foot and other sites of chronic irritation and inflammation (Figure 8-13). VC is an exophytic, verrucal, or fungating tumor associated with the HPV. It is not an aggressive tumor; however, the location of the lesions can create high morbidity for the patient.

DIFFERENTIAL DIAGNOSIS Squamous cell carcinoma

- Actinic keratoses
- Basal cell carcinoma
- Seborrheic keratosis
- Psoriasis
- Eczema
- Verruca vulgaris
- Melanoma
- Extramammary Paget disease

It is worthwhile to note an important differential diagnosis, *extramammary Paget disease* (EMPD). It is a rare, slow-growing intraepithelial adenocarcinoma derived from keratinocytes in the epidermis which can affect anogenital skin (outside of the mammary gland). It occurs more often in older women. Lesions are large, eczematous, and erythematous plaques which may be asymptomatic or painful. EMPD is characteristically very pruritic (Figure 8-14). The differential for EMPD includes eczematous dermatitis, psoriasis, tinea, seborrheic dermatitis, lichen sclerosis, and lichen planus. Suspicious lesions should be biopsied if they do not resolve after 6 weeks of treatment. There is a 12% rate of recurrence after Mohs micrographic surgery (MMS), and 25% of patients have a nonassociated genitourinary, rectal, or breast carcinoma.

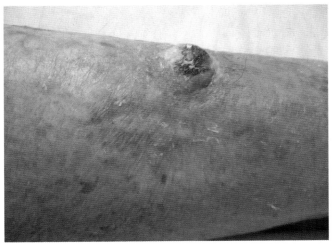

FIG. 8-7. Invasive SCC of the left shin.

TABLE 8-3 Characteristics of Nonmelanoma Skin Cancer.

TYPE OF TUMOR	LOCATION	SIZE/DEPTH	HISTOLOGY	HISTORY
Low-risk BCC	Any location including <6 mm in the H-zone (postauricular scalp, ears, preauricular cheek, temples, periorbital, eyelids, nose, lips, chin, mandible), hands and feet	<10 mm on head, forehead, cheeks, neck <20 mm on all other areas	sBCC or nodular BCC Lacks perineural invasion	Primary tumor, well-defined Immunocompetent patient No history of radiation therapy at site
Low-risk SCC	Trunk and extremities-excluding hands and feet	<20mm Depth: epidermal: SCCIS or Bowen disease	Well-differentiated	Primary tumor, well-defined Immunocompetent patient No history of radiation therapy at site
High-risk BCC	H-zone Hands and feet	>10 mm at the head, forehead, cheeks, neck >20 mm in all other areas	Micronodular Morpheaform Sclerosing Perineural invasion Poorly defined	Recurrent tumor Immunocompromised patient History of radiation therapy at site
High-risk SCC	Scalp, face, ears, mucosa, digits; tumors arsing in scars, chronic ulcers, burns, sinus tracts, gentialia	>20 mm Invasive	Moderately differentiated Poorly differentiated Perineural Single cell	Recurrent tumor, poorly defined Older age Male gender History of radiation/PUVA therapy at site Arsenic ingestion Immunocompromised patient RDEB

H-Zone, high risk zone (Figure 8-27); BCC, basal cell carcinoma; sBCC, superficial BCC; PUVA, psoralen plus ultraviolet A radiation; RDEB, recessive dystrophic epidermolysis bullosa; SCC, squamous cell carcinoma; SCCIS, squamous cell carcinoma in situ. From Lazareth, V. (2013). Management of non-melanoma skin cancer. *Seminars in Oncology Nursing, 29*(3), 182–194.

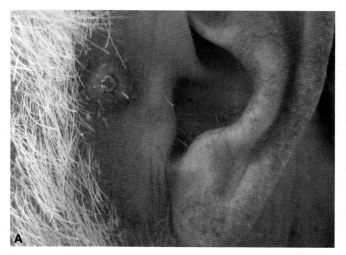
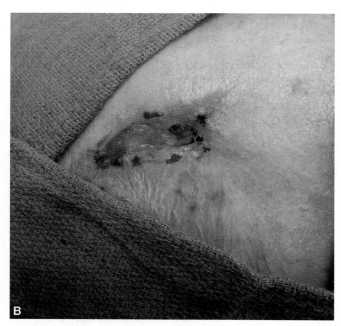

FIG. 8-8. A: SCC on the left preauricular cheek. **B:** Large SCC on the left parietal scalp.

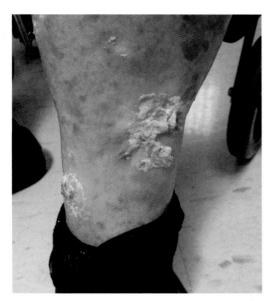

FIG. 8-9. SCC in traumatic scars.

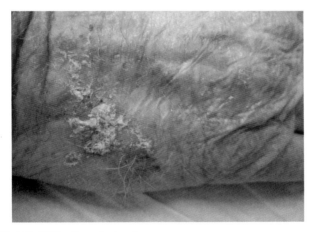

FIG. 8-10. SCC in situ on the hand.

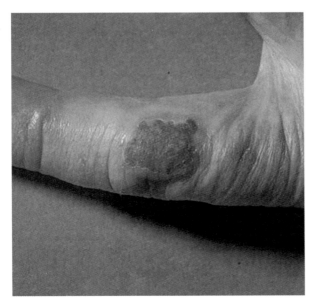

FIG. 8-11. Bowen disease on the finger.

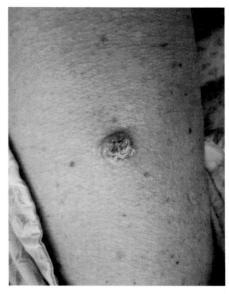

FIG. 8-12. Keratoacanthoma on the upper arm.

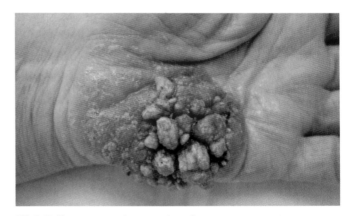

FIG. 8-13. Verrucous carcinoma on the palm.

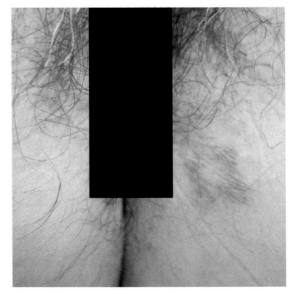

FIG. 8-14. Extramammary Paget disease on the left perineum.

Diagnosis

A shave biopsy should be performed to confirm the diagnosis of SCC. If the sample obtained is too shallow and does not include a portion of the dermal–epidermal junction, an invasive SCC could be misdiagnosed as in situ lesion, risking incomplete treatment with potential for an aggressive recurrence. A repeat biopsy should be performed.

Providers should biopsy suspicious lesions which arise in highly sensitive areas, even though they may bleed profusely or will not heal for weeks. Not doing so will risk recurrence or metastases. Imaging studies may be indicated for clinically palpable nodes or other high-risk tumors without nodes. Sentinel lymph node biopsy is being considered as a new tool in staging head and neck SCC.

Management

Treatment modalities for SCC depend on the subtype and may include immunotherapy, standard surgical excision, MMS, radiation therapy (XRT), or a combination. APCs should refer patients with a biopsy-proven SCC to a dermatologist or Mohs surgeon for management as these tumors can be deceptively aggressive (Figure 8-15).

Immunotherapy

The off-label use of imiquimod or 5-fluorouracil for the treatment of SCCIS should be reserved for use by experienced dermatologists and Mohs surgeons.

Surgical excision

Standard surgical excision is the gold standard for management of many cutaneous neoplasms, including most SCCIS. Using local anesthesia in the outpatient setting, the entire tumor plus several millimeters of healthy tissue for a safety margin, is surgically removed. The resultant wound is closed with sutures, and excised tissue sent for histopathologic analysis (Figure 8-16).

Advantages of excision include relatively low cost, favorable patient tolerability, outpatient care, and cosmetic result. Conversely, costs can increase when skin flaps/grafts are required to repair large

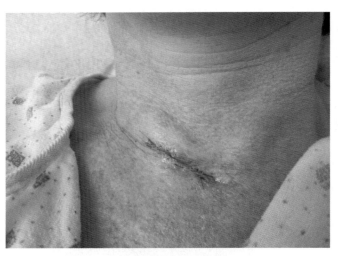

FIG. 8-16. Surgical excision of a cutaneous neoplasm at the anterior neck.

surgical wounds, or if the tumor recurs after initial excision requiring a subsequent procedure. Another disadvantage is the activity restrictions during the immediate postoperative period of a surgical excision.

Surgical excision offers a 5-year cure rate of over 90% for most tumors. Tissue excised during the procedure is evaluated by pathology to assure that tissue margins are free of cancerous cells. However, only about 1% of the tissue block is assessed using the "bread loaf" technique for margin control of the tumor.

Mohs micrographic surgery

MMS is the standard of care for all high-risk skin cancers, high-risk patients, low-risk tumors in cosmetically sensitive areas or those close to vital organs because of its high cure rate and tissue-sparing technique areas. The primary goal of MMS is to completely eradicate a tumor by examining 100% of the margins while maximally preserving normal tissue. MMS has a cure rate of 94% to 97% for primary SCC.

MMS is typically performed in an ambulatory surgical suite. Mohs surgeons are dermatologists who go on to attend an extensive 1-year fellowship training program to establish integrated, but separate and distinct, roles as cancer surgeon, dermatopathologist, and reconstructive surgeon. The Mohs procedure entails the surgical removal of skin cancer layer by layer, then examining the tissue under a microscope while the patients wait until healthy, cancer-free tissue "clear margins" around the tumor is reached. The surgeon precisely identifies and removes the entire tumor while leaving the surrounding healthy tissue intact. Then the wound is surgically repaired (Figure 8-17 A–C).

In addition to the above, advantages of MMS include the highest possible cure rate and outpatient surgical procedure. Disadvantages include the relatively limited access to Mohs surgeons nationwide, increased cost of the frozen sections performed during the procedure compared to conventional histology, and time-consuming nature of the procedure (Table 8-4). Dermatology and nondermatology providers can refer to the *AAD/ACMS/ASDSA/ ASMS 2012 appropriate use criteria for Mohs micrographic surgery: A report of the American Academy of Dermatology, American College of Mohs Surgery, American Society for Dermatologic Surgery Association, and the American Society for Mohs Surgery* regarding the most appropriate circumstances to refer a patient for MMS.

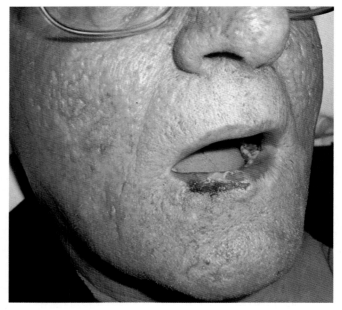

FIG. 8-15. High-risk SCC on the lower lip.

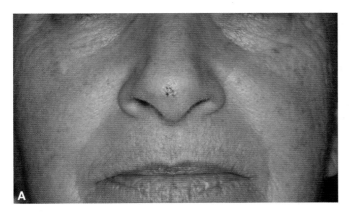

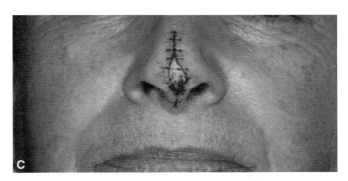

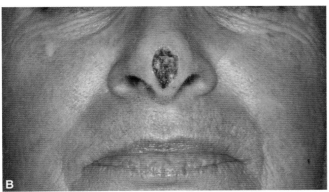

FIG. 8-17. Mohs micrographic surgery. **A:** Preoperative view. **B:** Postoperative view. **C:** Repair.

Radiation therapy

XRT can be successfully employed to treat NMSC and has the benefit of sparing normal, healthy tissue. The cure rate for primary NMSCs treated with XRT is over 90%, with a recurrence rate of approximately 9%.

A typical course of radiation requires multiple treatments over several weeks, with some tumors requiring up to 30 treatments. There are many potential adverse effects such as permanent alopecia, chronic radiation dermatitis, and delayed radiation necrosis, which may present with initial therapy or years later.

TABLE 8-4 Surgical Excision versus Mohs Micrographic Surgery	
SURGICAL EXCISION	**MOHS MICROGRAPHIC SURGERY**
Description Standard for surgical management of most NMSC Removal of the entire tumor plus healthy skin margins BCC needs 3–5-mm margins SCC needs 4–6-mm margins SCC large tumor needs 10-mm margins Cure rate: small, nodular primary BCCs is 95%	***Description*** Gold standard for high-risk tumors, high-risk patients, and low-risk tumors in cosmetically sensitive areas Complete removal of tumor by examining 100% of the margin maximizing the preservation of healthy tissue
Advantages Relatively low cost Favorable patient tolerability and cosmetic result	***Advantages*** High cure rate: primary BCC is 99%; and primary SCC is 97% Lowest rate of tumor recurrence Smaller margins create smaller surgical defects Functional and cosmetic benefit of tissue sparing at ears, eyes, lips, digits, genitals
Disadvantages 1-cm margins for large SCC is equivalent to melanoma Increased cost if flaps or grafts are required Increased costs associated with tumor recurrence	***Disadvantages*** Relatively limited number of Mohs surgeons Increased cost of frozen sections compared to conventional histology Time-consuming procedure Not foolproof as there may be skip areas of tumor

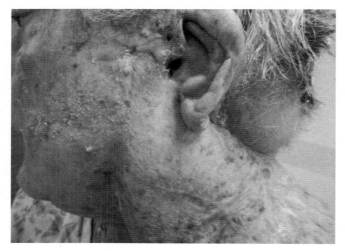

FIG. 8-18. Metastatic SCC at the left parotid.

XRT is very expensive, does not provide margin control, can only be delivered once to a given site, and there is a small risk of developing additional skin cancers in a treated area. There are significant potential adverse reactions to XRT, so radiation treatment of NMSC is usually reserved for patients who are poor surgical candidates, adjuvant therapy for incompletely excised tumors, or tumors which have spread to lymph nodes. XRT can be utilized for metastatic SCC to the parotid gland and adjacent lymph nodes which can be a challenging problem associated with SCCs arising in the head and neck area (Figure 8-18).

Special Consideration

OTRs require special consideration as the development of SCC is considered to be a sentinel event in these patients and warrants referral to a dermatologist. Optimal patient outcomes for OTRs with SCC will require collaborative efforts between the transplant team, dermatology, and primary care.

Prognosis and Complications

SCC is generally responsive to treatment, especially when treated early. If untreated, SCC can invade the subcuticular layer, cartilage, bone and can eventually spread to the lymphatic system leading to metastasis to solid organs, most often the lungs and the liver. Tumors which have the greatest potential for metastasis are those which are large (>2 cm), are located on or near the ears and lips, are poorly differentiated, or are invading nerves.

A patient who has had one skin cancer has an increased risk of developing another skin cancer, including melanoma. A patient who has had a first SCC has up to a 50% risk of a second SCC within 5 years. Additionally, these patients have twice the risk of developing other malignancies, such as lung, colon, and breast cancers.

Referral and Consultation

While most SCCs can be managed without high risk for recurrence, this cancer can be deceptive as certain locations and subtypes can have small but aggressive tumors. Patients diagnosed with SCC should be referred to a dermatologist for further evaluation of the subtype, locations, risk factors, and comorbidities, and review appropriate treatment options with the patient to establish a plan of care. Patients may require plastic surgery, oculoplastics, ENT, or radiation oncology. Nonetheless, patients should maintain follow-up and regular monitoring with a dermatology specialist.

There can be confusion as to the appropriateness of referral to plastic surgeon for patients with skin cancer. As a general rule of thumb, referral to either a procedural dermatologist or a plastic surgeon is appropriate for excision of a SCC at low risk for recurrence. However, a high-risk lesion is best managed by a Mohs surgeon.

Patient Education and Follow-up

SCC patients are advised to follow up at 3- to 6-month intervals for the first year and then at 6- to 12-month intervals thereafter. It is essential to assess the effects of treatment, identify tumor recurrence, and assure early detection of any type of a new skin cancer. Lymph nodes should be carefully assessed for enlargement or tenderness. High-risk SCC patients, like those with recurrent tumors, genetic predisposition, immune suppression, and high-risk subtype, should be monitored by dermatology specialists with regular skin and lymphatic examinations. Patients with invasive SCC with proven regional spread are at high risk for metastatic disease and may require further monitoring by radiation oncology.

The importance of skin cancer education cannot be overemphasized. APCs have an opportunity to educate their SSC patients every time they are seen in the office, regardless of the complaint. In addition to the ABCDEs for early detection, patients should be counseled about sun safety. Written materials can provide helpful hints for the patient to take home (Box 8-1).

BASAL CELL CARCINOMA

BCC is the most common human malignancy. Fair-skinned individuals are particularly susceptible at areas of sun-exposed skin, notably, the head, neck, and upper back (Figure 8-19). A long history of intense, intermittent sun exposure or of incidental blistering sunburns is common. Yet, BCC is rarely seen on the sun-exposed dorsum of the hands or lower extremities. Approximately 20% of BCCs arise in areas which are relatively sun protected, such as behind the ears. BCC can also develop at sites of chemical exposure or chronic trauma.

It is most common in Caucasians, Asians, and light-skinned Hispanics and is rarely seen in people with dark skin color. The incidence of BCC is higher in middle-aged to older adults, with males being more affected than females. Approximately 40% of patients who have had a primary BCC will develop a *new* BCC within 5 years of their first occurrence. The development of BCC in immunosuppressed patients, especially OTRs and those with chronic lymphocytic leukemia, is particularly significant as these tumors tend to be more aggressive. There is a 10-fold increased risk of BCC in OTRs previously diagnosed with a BCC.

Pathophysiology

Basal keratinocytes are present in the epidermis and adnexal structures, which include the hair follicles. Damage to these cells is caused by radiation treatments, unprotected exposure to UVR over many years, and intense exposure to UVR from tanning beds or phototherapy. This exposure compromises the ability of the skin to repair or destroy the damaged cells. It impairs the intrinsic genetic mechanisms within the DNA of epidermal cells, which should protect the cells from malignant transformation.

BOX 8-1 Sun Safety Patient Education

You don't have to avoid sunlight completely, and outdoor activity is important for good health. However, some people think about sun protection only when they spend a day at the beach, lake, or pool. Sun exposure adds up day after day, and exposure to too much sunlight can be harmful. There are some easy steps you can take to limit your exposure to UV rays.

Seek Shade A very important way to limit your exposure to UV light is to avoid being outdoors in direct sunlight for too long especially between the hours of 10 a.m. and 4 p.m., even on cloudy days, when UV light is strongest. Be especially careful on the beach or in areas with sand, water, and snow as they reflect sunlight, increasing the amount of UV radiation you receive. Typical car, home, and office windows block most of the UVB rays but only a smaller portion of UVA rays; so even if you don't feel you're getting burned, your skin may still get some damage.

Wear a Hat A hat with tightly woven fabric, a 2- to 3-inch brim all around and a dark, nonreflective underside to the brim is ideal because it protects the scalp, forehead, ears, eyes, and nose, which are often exposed to intense sun. A shade cap which has about 7 inches of fabric draping down the sides and back will provide more protection for the neck and can be found in sports and outdoor supply stores. (A baseball cap protects the front and top of the head but not the nose, ears, or neck where skin cancers commonly develop).

Wear Sunglasses UV-blocking sunglasses are important for protecting the delicate skin around the eyes, as well as the eyes themselves. Research has shown that long hours in the sun without eye protection increases your chances of developing some eye diseases such as cataracts and melanoma. The ideal sunglasses should block 99% to 100% of UVA and UVB radiation. Labels that say "UV absorption up to 400 nm" or "Meets ANSI UV Requirements" mean the glasses block at least 99% of UV rays. Large-framed and wraparound sunglasses are more likely to protect your eyes from light coming in from different angles. Darker glasses are not necessarily better because UV protection comes from an invisible chemical applied to the lenses, not from the color or darkness of the lenses.

Clothing Wear clothing to protect as much skin as possible when you are out in the sun. Long-sleeved shirts and long pants, or long skirts cover the most skin and are the most protective. Dark colors generally provide more protection than light colors. A tightly woven fabric protects better than loosely woven clothing. Some companies such as Coolibar, L.L.Bean, and Columbia now make clothing that is lightweight, comfortable, and protects against UV exposure even when wet. Some children's swimsuits are now made from sun-protective fabric and are designed to cover the child from the neck to the knees.

Sunscreen Sunscreen products contain one or more active drug ingredients which absorb, scatter, or reflect UV light, and which are regulated as over-the-counter (OTC) drugs by the U.S. FDA. Sunscreen can help to protect your skin against the sun's UV rays, though sunscreen should not be used as a way to prolong your time in the sun.

Sunscreens are available in many forms—lotions, creams, ointments, gels, sprays, wipes, and lip balms. Sunscreens with SPF values of 30 or higher and which have broad-spectrum protection against both UVA and UVB rays are recommended. Sunscreen should be reapplied often for maximal protection. Ideally, about 1 ounce of sunscreen should be reapplied at least every 2 hours and even more often if swimming or sweating.

Sunscreen products labeled "broad spectrum" provide some protection against both UVA and UVB rays, but at this time there is no standard system for measuring protection from UVA rays. Products that contain avobenzone (Parsol 1789), ecamsule, zinc oxide, or titanium dioxide can provide some protection from most UVA rays. The sun-protection factor "SPF" number is the level of protection the sunscreen provides against UVB rays; a higher number means more protection. SPF 15 sunscreens filter out about 93% of UVB rays, while SPF 30 sunscreens filter out about 97%, and SPF 50 sunscreens filter out about 98%.

Choosing a Sunscreen Physical sunscreens (titanium dioxide, zinc oxide) act to reflect and scatter both visible and UV light, yet tend to be thick, stain clothing, and clog pores. Chemical sunscreens (PABA) absorb UV radiation, and typically have a limited spectrum of protection. Combination sunscreens include Johnson and Johnson Minesol Sunscreen, LaRoche-Posay Anthelios SX Daily Moisturizing Cream, Anthelios SX™ 40 Sunscreen, Neutrogena UltraSheer Dry Touch/Age Shield® Sunscreen (with Helioplex), and RoC Tinosorb.

Avoid Tanning Beds and Sunlamps Tanning lamps give out UVA and usually UVB rays as well. This intense exposure to both UVA and UVB rays causes long-term skin damage which contributes to the development of skin cancer. Tanning bed use has been linked with an increased risk of melanom the deadliest form of skin cancer, especially if tanning is started before the age of 30. If you want a tan, consider using a sunless tanning lotion, which can provide a darker look without the danger.

Children Children tend to spend more time outdoors than adults, can burn more easily, and may not be aware of the dangers. Caregivers should protect children from excess sun exposure by using the steps above. If you or your child burns easily, be extra careful to cover up, limit exposure, and apply sunscreens specially formulated for children. Children need smaller versions of real, protective adult sunglasses—not toy sunglasses. Babies younger than 6 months should be kept out of direct sunlight and should be protected from the sun by using umbrellas, hats, and protective clothing.

Vitamin D Vitamin D is an essential nutrient that is vital for strong bones, a healthy immune system, and may help to lower the risk for some cancers. Your skin makes vitamin D naturally when you are in the sun. How much vitamin D you make depends on many things, including how old you are, how dark your skin is, and how strong the sunlight is where you live. Dermatologists recommend that vitamin D should be safely obtained from a healthy diet that includes dairy products and fish, which are naturally rich in vitamin D, milk and cereals which are fortified with vitamin D, and/or vitamin D supplements—not from UV exposure.

Clinical Presentation

Many years may pass before damaged cells amass into a lesion which grows slowly and invades healthy tissue. Patient begin to take notice of the growth as it thickens over time and eventually ulcerates, creating the characteristic rolled borders at the periphery (Figure 8-20). Often the sore waxes and wanes but never fully heals, and may bleed with minimal trauma.

BCC lesions can easily be disregarded by patients as there may be no bleeding or sensitivity initially. BCCs may exhibit periods of rapid growth; however, they rarely metastasize to distant organs.

Basal cell carcinoma subtypes

Nodular BCCs (nBCCs) are the most common subtype and are at low risk for recurrence (Figure 8-21). A lack of melanocytes within

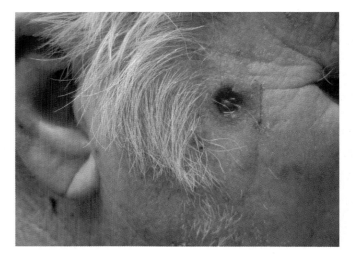

FIG. 8-19. BCC at the malar cheek.

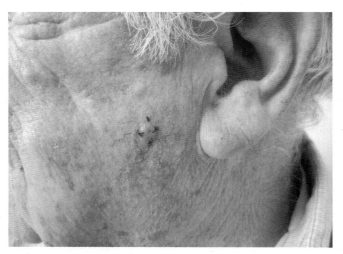

FIG. 8-21. Nodular BCC at the cheek.

the tumor can give it a pearly or translucent appearance. Eventually the center erodes or ulcerates, creating rolled borders. The tumor grows larger and deeper, and small vessels known as telangiectasias can be visible within the border. The tissue is friable, leading to scarring. Occasionally, nBCCs will have flecks of pigment rendering a mottled blue or brown color (Figure 8-22). These tumors are known as pigmented BCC (pBCC) and can resemble seborrheic keratoses or melanoma. The differential diagnosis of nBCC includes angiofibroma (fibrous papule), sebaceous hyperplasia, trichoepithelioma, molluscum contagiosum, and intradermal nevus.

Superficial BCC (sBCC) constitutes 17% of all BCCs (Figure 8-23). As the name implies, these lesions are confined to the surface of the epidermis. They present as well-defined, scaly, rough, pink to red macules, or thin plaques which often develop on the trunk and extremities. sBCCs grow slowly, but may become sensitive or bleed spontaneously. The diagnosis may be delayed because the tumor may resemble eczema, psoriasis, AKs, Bowen disease, and EMPD.

Micronodular BCCs (mnBCCs) appear similar to nBCC clinically, but behave much more aggressively. They often have significant subclinical spread, commonly referred to as "the iceberg phenomenon," and have a high risk for recurrence (Figure 8-24).

Infiltrative BCCs may resemble a KA or SCC (Figure 8-25). These tumors also behave aggressively and extend both peripherally

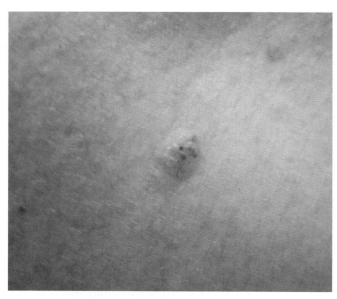

FIG. 8-22. Pigmented BCC on the chest.

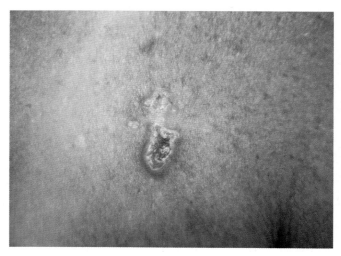

FIG. 8-20. BCC showing rolled border.

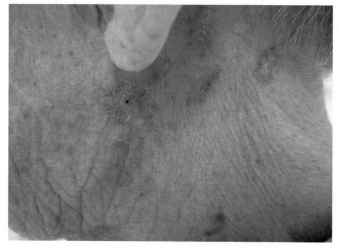

FIG. 8-23. Superficial BCC on the neck and post auricular area.

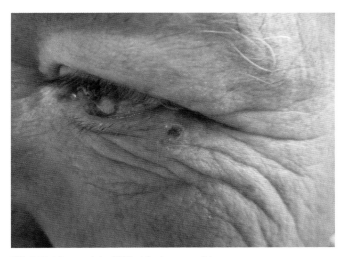

FIG. 8-24. Micronodular BCC at the lower eyelid.

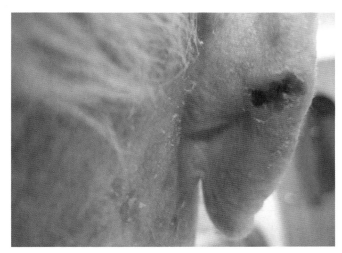

FIG. 8-25. Infiltrative BCC at the posterior ear.

and vertically (depth). As such, it accounts for the high risk for recurrence.

Morpheaform or *sclerosing BCCs* represent only 1% of all BCCs; and are characteristically sclerotic plaques with a waxy, atrophic, white surface (Figure 8-26). They are commonly asymptomatic and easily mistaken for a scar or scleroderma. Morpheaform BCCs extend far beyond the visible surface, resulting in very high rates of recurrence.

Nevoid basal cell syndrome is a rare autosomal dominant disease caused by a mutation of the tumor suppressor *PTCH* gene. Multiple BCCs develop in childhood and are associated with pitted palms and soles, cysts at the jaw, calcification of falx cerebri, skeletal abnormalities, and coarse facial features.

DIFFERENTIAL DIAGNOSIS Basal cell carcinoma

- Angiofibroma
- Fibrous papule
- Sebaceous hyperplasia
- Trichoepithelioma
- Molluscum contagiosum
- Intradermal nevus
- Amelanotic melanoma
- Morphea
- Eczema
- Psoriasis
- Actinic keratoses
- Bowen disease
- Extramammary Paget disease
- Keratoacanthoma
- Squamous cell carcinoma

Diagnostics

Once skin cancer is suspected, a skin biopsy must be obtained both to confirm the diagnosis of BCC and also to identify its subtype. This is extremely important as aggressive subtypes have a higher risk for recurrence and more aggressive behavior upon recurrence. The decision to perform a shave, punch, or curettage biopsy should be determined by the location and size of the lesion in addition to

the differential diagnosis. Shave biopsy is a simple, effective means to diagnose BCC (discussed earlier in SCC). A deep shave (or *scoop*) biopsy or two separate punch biopsies are advised if melanoma (including amelanotic melanoma) is in the differential diagnosis. This would allow for the evaluation of the depth of tumor invasion. A punch biopsy may be preferential in certain locations as the cosmetic result is often superior to that of a shave biopsy (see chapter 24).

Management

Most BCCs are curable when treated promptly; however, some have a high rate of recurrence. Treatment of BCC is indicated to prevent ulceration, gross disfigurement, and invasion into the local subcuticular layer, nerve, muscle, cartilage, and bone. When evaluating treatment options for biopsy-proven BCC, the provider must first determine the tumor subtype and risk for recurrence (Box 8-1). Tumor size, location, and patient history will also impact the clinician's treatment approach. A visual reminder of the "H-zone," representing high-risk locations on the head, can be helpful to clinicians (Figure 8-27).

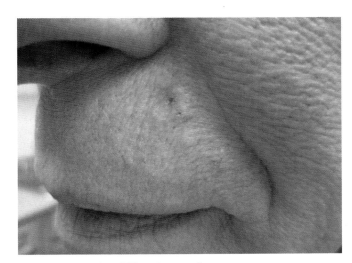

FIG. 8-26. Morpheaform BCC on the upper lip.

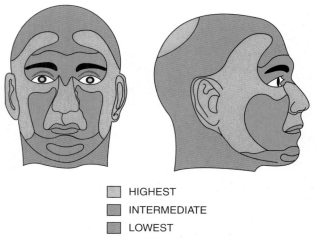

■ HIGHEST
■ INTERMEDIATE
■ LOWEST

FIG. 8-27. "H-zone" showing most common areas of skin cancer recurrence.

Low-risk basal cell carcinoma

Topical immunotherapy may be used alone or in combination with other treatment modalities. Although both agents were discussed earlier in the treatment of AKs, the recommended dosages are different for treatment of BCCs. Topical 5-fluorouricil 5%, an antineoplastic antimetabolite can be used effectively but only for *sBCCs*, not invasive lesions. Cream is applied by the patient to the tumor area twice daily for 6 weeks. Imiquimod 5% stimulates immune responses resulting in antiviral, antitumor, and immune-regulatory properties. Imiquimod is indicated for treatment of *sBCC* with a maximum diameter of 2 cm on the neck, trunk, or extremities (excluding hands or feet). The patient applies it to area daily at bedtime, 5 days per week for 6 to 12 weeks. Common side effects, advantages, and disadvantages are discussed in Table 8-2.

Cryosurgery, freezing with liquid nitrogen at −196.5°C, crystalizes the tumor cells, induces localized frostbite, and produces necrosis and tissue destruction of the tumor. It c an be used for the destruction of low-risk BCC. There is, however, considerable risk for tumor recurrence which can develop undetected in the deep dermis. Cryosurgery should not be confused with *cryotherapy,* which is a common technique used to treat common benign growths such as warts or molluscum. Cryosurgery is an aggressive treatment and should only be performed by dermatology specialists experienced in this procedure. The advantage is that the procedure is quick, in-office, and low cost. However, cryosurgery can be painful, requires lengthy wound care, and may cause hypopigmentation or scarring.

Electrodesiccation and curettage (ED&C) may be used to treat small, low-risk BCCs at low-risk locations (i.e., the neck, trunk, and extremities). After local anesthetics are given, friable tumor cells are easily curetted off until normal, firm dermal tissue is reached. Any remaining tissue is destroyed with electrocautery, which also controls any bleeding. The wound is then left to heal by secondary intention. Clinicians performing ED&C, especially in cosmetically sensitive areas, should be sure to discuss the risks and side effects before the procedure. Disadvantages of ED&C include slow healing, the risk for hypopigmented, atrophic and/or hypertrophic scarring, tissue contraction, and the lack of margin control. Burns, fire, and interference with cardiac defibrillators are rare but may cause serious potential adverse effects. Advantages of ED&C include the speed of the procedure and its relatively low cost. Recurrence rates are low at 3% to 6% for primary BCC < 1 cm.

Simple surgical excision is the treatment of choice for the management of low-risk BCCs. Excision of small, primary nBCCs at the head, neck, trunk, and extremities can be very effective, with a 5-year cure rate of 95%. Not surprisingly, the risk of recurrence increases when using simple surgical excision in the treatment of high-risk BCCs (Table 8-3). The procedure, advantages, and disadvantages are the same as discussed in *Management of SCC.* Of note, the operative time and expense for surgical excision are greater than those required for treatment with ED&C or cryosurgery.

High-risk basal cell carcinoma

Simple surgical excision is not the treatment of choice for high-risk BCCs where MMS has a much higher cure rate, but may be an appropriate treatment modality for some patient circumstances. Examples include lack of proximity to a Mohs surgeon or the inability of an elderly patient to tolerate a lengthy procedure. However, whenever possible, assessment of all margins is optimal for high-risk tumors.

MMS, as detailed in the *Management of SCC,* is considered the gold standard for high-risk nonmelanoma skin cancer (Figure 8-28). MMS is associated with the lowest recurrence rates for primary BCC at only 1% (Table 8-4).

Radiation therapy

XRT can be successfully employed to treat patients with NMSC and may be a favorable option for BCC arising on or near the eyelids, nose, ears, and lips. The procedure, advantages, and disadvantages are also discussed in *Management of SCC.*

Special Consideration

It is not unusual for frail elders or patients who are affected by comorbidities to present with BCCs. These patients and their families may question the appropriateness of treatment for BCC lesions which grow slowly and rarely metastasize. In some situations, it may be reasonable to consider less aggressive therapeutic modalities such as cryosurgery or ED&C rather than attempting multiple XRT sessions or a lengthy MMS. Treatment decisions for BCCs in complex elderly patients with significant comorbidities should begin with a thoughtful discussion between the patient, family, and dermatology provider.

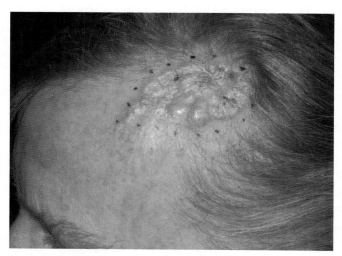

FIG. 8-28. High-risk BCC.

Prognosis and Complications

Patients may misunderstand that biopsy alone is curative. In fact, even after treatment, it is not uncommon for patients to have the misconception that BCCs are not cancerous growths. When left untreated, BCCs can invade local soft tissue, nerves, cartilage, and bone, resulting in deformity and morbidity.

The prognosis for the majority of BCCs is excellent. Even large lesions and those in sensitive locations have very high cure rates with appropriate treatment, but they do have increased risk for invading nerves, vessels, cartilage, and bone if treatment is delayed or inadequate. Although the rate of metastasis for BCC is less than 1%, they can be extremely aggressive and result in high mortality rates. Approximately 40% of patients who have had a primary BCC will develop a *new* BCC within 5 years of the first. And approximately 80% of *recurrent* BCCs will manifest within 5 years of treatment.

Referral and Consultation

While BCC grows slowly, rarely metastasizes, and is generally easily managed in the outpatient setting, it *is* a cancer. Any patient with a histologically confirmed BCC should be referred to a dermatologist for consultation. The dermatology specialist will review appropriate treatment options with the patient and establish a plan of care. If additional specialists (i.e., plastic surgeon or radiation oncologist) are necessary, the dermatologist can coordinate the appropriate treatment and continue to monitor the patient for tumor recurrence and for new lesions.

Patient Education and Follow-up

Patients should follow up with the dermatologist at 6-month intervals for the first year following a BCC, then annually thereafter. It is important to assess the effects of treatment and to identify any tumor recurrence or a new skin cancer as early as possible. Patient education for skin cancer prevention and early detection is the foundation of high-quality patient care (Box 8-1).

As with all skin cancers, patient morbidity from BCC will be minimized by early detection. Providers can help to prevent this common cancer by identifying patients at risk for skin cancer, detecting potentially cancerous lesions, and referring patients to a dermatologist as appropriate. Performing a complete skin cancer screening examination carefully and methodically with optimal tangential light will increase the likelihood of identifying even very small, asymptomatic lesions.

OTHER CUTANEOUS MALIGNANCIES
Merkel Cell Carcinoma

Merkel cell carcinoma (MCC) is an uncommon, aggressive neuroendocrine (sensory cell) carcinoma of the skin with a rapidly increasing rate of occurrence. The development of MCC is strongly associated with ages over 65 years, fair skin or a history of extensive sun exposure, and chronic immune suppression. Susceptible patients include older Caucasians and those with a history of organ transplantation, HIV/AIDS, leukemia, and lymphoma. In fact, MCC is 15 times more likely to develop in OTRs and at a significantly younger age than in their immunocompetent counterparts.

Pathophysiology

Merkel cells are neuroendocrine cells which reside in the epidermal basal layer and are presumably the origin of this tumor. The etiology of MCC suggests a possible infectious component with a growth pattern classified as circumscribed or infiltrative. The tumors are fast growing and aggressive with a propensity for early, in-transit regional, nodal, and distant metastasis.

Clinical presentation

MCCs are firm, smooth, shiny, dome-shaped, skin colored to red, nontender nodules with telangiectasia which develop rapidly and asymptomatically over approximately 6 months. Lesions vary from small 2-mm to large 8-cm-size nodules usually found on sun-exposed areas of the head and neck. Yet, tumors can also occur on the trunk or extremities (Figure 8-29). MCCs have high rates of recurrence, often far from the original tumor, and have high rates of metastatic spread.

DIFFERENTIAL DIAGNOSIS Merkel cell carcinoma

- Basal cell carcinoma
- Squamous cell carcinoma
- B-cell lymphoma
- Sebaceous cyst
- Cutaneous lymphoma
- Melanoma
- Cutaneous metastasis of carcinoma

Diagnostics

Although these lesions are often overlooked during their initial development, a shave or punch biopsy is appropriate for diagnosis.

Management

Once diagnosed, the tumor requires immediate referral for management to surgical oncology and a Mohs surgeon. Patients will undergo wide excision with concomitant sentinel lymph node biopsy.

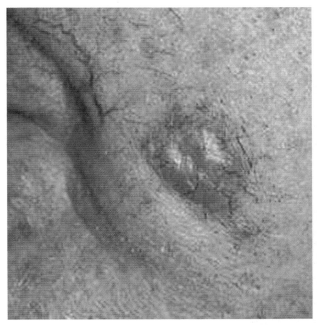

FIG. 8-29. MCC on the cheek.

Prognosis and complications

MCCs are aggressive tumors with a propensity for early, in-transit regional, nodal, and distant metastasis indicating the need for sentinel lymph node biopsy with *all* primary MCCs. Most tumors recur within 8 to 24 months. Despite surgical excision, 45% to 91% of patients develop regional node involvement, and 18% to 52% of patients develop distant metastasis. The 5-year survival rate is 40% to 75% for a primary tumor.

Referral and consultation

Patients with MCC are at high risk for metastasis, requiring rapid consultation and management by an oncologist, Mohs surgeon, and dermatologist.

Patient education and follow-up

Patients with a history of MCC should be followed at 3-month intervals by a dermatologist and an oncologist. Primary care clinicians should be vigilant in ensuring the patient complete age-appropriate health screening examinations in addition to other diagnostics as indication for new complaints.

Atypical Fibroxanthoma

Atypical fibroxanthoma is an intradermal, spindle cell tumor of mesenchymal origin occurring most commonly on the head and neck (Figure 8-30). The lesions most often present as small, firm nodules with eroded or crusted surfaces in patients with fair skin or a history of extensive sun exposure. Atypical fibroxanthoma has a low-to-moderate potential for metastasis. Tumor recurrence is most commonly due to incomplete excision. The recommended treatment is MMS.

Dermatofibrosarcoma Protuberans

Dermatofibrosarcoma protuberans (DFSP) is a relatively unusual primary cutaneous malignancy which is classified as a low-grade sarcoma. DFSP is a dermal tumor which has a propensity for deep invasion and extensive subclinical spread (Figure 8-31). It has a subtle appearance and grows slowly. DFSP presents as one or multiple ill-defined, erythematous, firm nodules or plaques. Most lesions occur on the trunk, particularly at the shoulder or abdomen, though they can also develop at the head and neck. DFSP

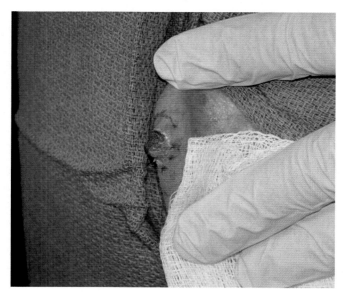

FIG. 8-30. Atypical fibroxanthoma at the left helix.

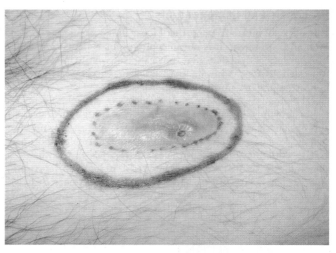

FIG. 8-31. Dermatofibrosarcoma protuberans at the abdomen.

affects young- to middle-aged adults and may be associated with trauma.

Tentacle-like extensions of tumor create a high incidence of local recurrence. The slow-growing, poorly defined nature of the lesions often results in delayed diagnosis, which allows tumors to become quite large. Lesions can invade subcutaneous tissue, muscle, fascia, and bone, but metastasis is rare. Excision of DFSP with 3-cm margins even to fascia has a recurrence rate of 20%. MMS, with a recurrence rate of 1.6%, is therefore the treatment of choice.

Microcystic Adnexal Carcinoma

Microcystic adnexal carcinoma (MAC) usually presents as a deeply invasive, poorly defined plaque which may be red or hemorrhagic. The lesions are frequently located periorally, perinasally, periocularly, or on the scalp. MAC often develops in previously irradiated skin. The tumor often invades nerves and may invade subcutaneous fat, muscle, cartilage, bone, salivary glands, and lymph nodes. MAC is unlikely to metastasize; however, tumor recurrence can occur many years following initial excision.

Sebaceous Carcinoma

Sebaceous carcinoma (SC) is a rare, invasive tumor which most often appears at the upper eyelids. It often presents as a painless, yellow nodule or plaque. It is associated with Muir–Torre syndrome. SC is an aggressive tumor which can invade orbital structures. Approximately one in four patients experience regional lymph node metastasis, with possible distal spread to muscle, liver, spleen, viscera, and brain.

PRIMARY CUTANEOUS LYMPHOMAS

Cutaneous T-Cell Lymphoma

Cutaneous T-cell lymphoma (CTCL) is a class of non-Hodgkin lymphoma that is not a skin cancer, but manifests its symptoms in the skin. The cause of this non-Hodgkin lymphoma is unclear. There is a higher incidence in African Americans than in Caucasians and those over 60 years old. Males are twice more likely to develop CTCL than females. Patients with CTCL have an increased incidence of secondary cancers, especially lymphoma.

The disease presents in the skin, but can also affect lymph nodes, blood, and internal organs. A mutation of the T cells in the immune system can result in the migration of the malignant T cells to the skin. They can cause a variety of lesions to develop and may produce erythema and itching of the skin. The most common subtypes of CTCL are mycosis fungoides (MF) and Sezary syndrome.

Mycosis fungoides

Patient with MF have skin lesions which are persistent and become increasingly progressive. The importance of recognizing potential MF should not be underemphasized as it can easily be misdiagnosed for common dermatoses such as eczema and tinea. The categories of MF include patch, plaque tumor, and erythrodermic stages. It is not uncommon for initial lesions to be ill-defined, scaly plaques which require repeated biopsies before the diagnosis is made. Eventually, the lesions present with mixed morphology and lesions from all stages and/or erythroderma which can be localized or widespread (Figure 8-32). Patches are often large (>5 cm) and vary in size, shape, and color. Plaques are well defined and are dusky to violaceous red color. The tumor stage usually means a more aggressive form of MF. Tumors are red and dusky and may ulcerate. They commonly occur around the head, neck, groin, breasts, and axillary areas. Advanced disease may present with erythroderma, severe scale, bright red patches or plaques covering ≥80% BSA. It is often accompanied by intense pruritus, fever, chills, and malaise.

Diagnosis is often delayed as the lesions are misdiagnosed as dermatoses like eczema or psoriasis. The histopathological criteria can be difficult to identify due to inflammation in the skin. Working with a dermatopathologist can be helpful in determining the diagnosis of MF. Differential diagnosis of MF includes eczema, psoriasis, parapsoriasis, photodermatitis, and drug reaction.

Once suspected, MF should be referred to an experienced dermatology provider who can further evaluate and stage the disease. Staging, based on the primary tumor, regional lymph nodes, metastasis, and serum studies, provides treatment guidelines and prognostic value. Treatment options of limited cutaneous involvement include topical corticosteroids, topical chemotherapy (nitrogen mustard), topical retinoids, local radiation, and narrow-band UVB phototherapy.

Sezary syndrome

Sezary syndrome (SS) is an advanced form of MF. Approximately 10% of patients with MF have atypical lymphocytes (Sezary cells) in their blood and erythroderma of 80% to 90% of their body surface area. The skin may become flaky, and patients may experience feeling hot, sore, or sensitive accompanied by intense pruritus.

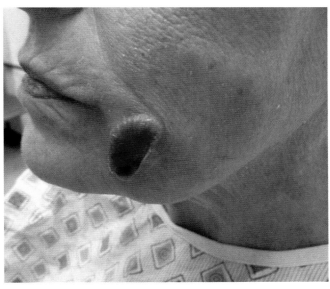

FIG. 8-33. Cutaneous B-cell lymphoma at the lower cheek.

Additional symptoms may include hyperkeratosis at the palms and soles, alopecia, onychodystrophy, and ptosis.

Because SS is chronic and systemic, systemic therapies are required. Treatment options include systemic retinoids, immunotherapies, extracorporeal photophoresis, chemotherapy, and bone marrow or stem cell transplantation. Patients with CTCL should be immediately referred to a dermatology provider experienced in managing the disease.

Cutaneous B-Cell Lymphoma

A mutation of the B cells of the immune system can result in the migration of the malignant B cells to the skin or lymphoproliferation. The disease seems to start as a hyperreactive inflammatory response related to an immunodeficiency disorder, a viral infection, or a bacterial infection.

Lesions present as solitary or multiple red nodules or plaques on the head, trunk, or extremities (Figure 8-33). The differential diagnosis includes B-cell pseudolymphoma, CTCL, or BCC. The prognosis of the most common marginal zone B-cell lymphomas (MZL) is excellent with a 5-year survival rate of greater than 90%. Treatment options include surgical excision for a solitary lesion, antibiotic therapy (doxycycline or cefotaxime), or radiotherapy for multiple lesions.

BILLING CODES ICD-10	
Actinic cheilitis	L57.0
Actinic keratosis	C33. M8090/3
Basal cell carcinoma	C44.91
Biopsy	L85.8
Cutaneous horn	L87.9
Extramammary Paget disease	M8076/2-3
Invasive squamous cell carcinoma	C44.92
Keratoacanthoma	C44. L44
Merkel cell carcinoma	D48-5
Neoplasm of uncertain behavior	L57.9
Photoaging	M8070/2

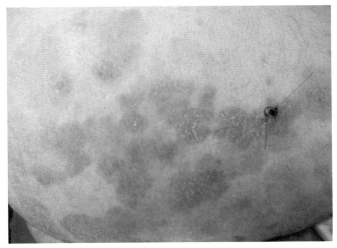

FIG. 8-32. CTCL at the left buttock.

READINGS

Ad Hoc Task Force, Connolly, S. M., Baker, D. R., Coldiron, B. M., Fazio, M. J., Storrs, P. A., ... Wisco, O. J. (2012). AAD/ACMS/ASDSA, ASMS 2012 appropriate use criteria for Mohs micrographic surgery: A report of the American Academy of Dermatology, American College of Mohs Surgery, American Society for Dermatologic Surgery Association and the American Society for Mohs Surgery. *Journal of the American Academy of Dermatology, 67*(4), 531–550.

Agar, N. S., Wedgeworth, E., Crichton, S., Mitchell, T. J., Cox, M., Ferreira, S., ... Whittaker, S. J. (2010). Survival outcomes and prognostic factors in Mycoses fungoides/Sezary syndrome: Validation of the revised International Society for Cutaneous Lymphomas/European Organization for Research and Treatment of Cancer staging proposal. *Journal of Clinical Oncology, 28*(31), 4730.

Alam, M., Ratner, D. (2001). Cutaneous squamous-cell carcinoma. *The New England Journal of Medicine, 344*(13), 975–983.

American Cancer Society. (n.d.). Cancer facts and figures 2013. http://www.cancer.org/acs/groups/content/@epidemiologysurveilance/documents/document/acspc-036845.pdf.

Clayman, G. L., Lee, J. J., Holsinger, F. C., Zhou, X., Duvic, M., El-Naggar, A. K., ... Lipmann, S. M. (2005). Mortality risk from squamous cell skin cancer. *Journal of Clinical Oncology, 23*(4), 759–765.

Farasat, S., Yu, S., Neel, V.A., Nehal, K. S., Lardaro, T., Mihm, M. C., ... Liégeois, N. J. (2011). A new American Joint Committee on Cancer staging system for cutaneous squamous cell carcinoma: Creation and rationale for inclusion of tumor (T) characteristics. *Journal of the American Academy of Dermatology, 64*(6), 1051–1059.

Frankel, D. H., Hanusa, B. H., Zitelli, J. A. (1992). New primary nonmelanoma skin cancer in patients with a history of squamous cell carcinoma of the skin: Implications and recommendations for follow-up. *Journal of the American Academy of Dermatology, 26*(5 pt. 1), 720–726.

Gloster, H. M., Neal, K. (2006). Skin cancer in skin of color. *Journal of the American Academy of Dermatology, 55*, 741–760.

Gogia, R., Binstock, M., Hirose, R., Boscardin, W. J., Chren, M. M., & Arron, S. T. Fitzpatrick skin phototype is an independent predictor of squamous cell carcinoma risk after solid organ transplantation. *Journal of the American Academy of Dermatology, 68*(4), 585–591.

Karagas, M. R., Stukel, T. A., Greenberg, E. R., Baron, J. A., Mott, L. A., Stern, R. S. (1992). Risk of subsequent basal cell carcinoma and squamous cell carcinoma of the skin among patients with prior skin cancer. Skin Cancer Prevention Study Group. *The Journal of the American Medical Association, 267*(24), 3305–3310.

Kuflik, E. G. Cryosurgery for skin cancer: 30-year experience and cure rates. (2004). *Dermatologic Surgery: Official Publication for American Society of Dermatologic Surgery, 30*(2 pt. 2), 297–300.

Lazareth, V. L. (2010). Dermatologic care of the transplant patient: Part I. *Journal of the Dermatology Nurses' Association, 2*(2), 59–63.

Lindelof, B., Sigurgeirsson, B., Gabel, H., & Stern, R. S. Incidence of skin cancer in 5356 patients following organ transplantation. (2000). *The British Journal of Dermatology, 143*(3), 513–519.

Marcil, I., Stern, R. S. (2000). Risk of developing a subsequent nonmelanoma skin cancer in patients with a history of nonmelanoma skin cancer: A critical review of the literature and meta-analysis. *Archives of Dermatology, 136*(12), 1524–1530.

Marghoob, A., Kopf, A. W., Bart, R. S., Sanfilippo, L., Silverman, M. K., Lee, P. ... Abadir, M. (1993). Risk of another basal cell carcinoma developing after treatment of a basal cell carcinoma. *Journal of the American Academy of Dermatology, 28*(1), 22–28.

Moloney, F. J., Comber, H., O'Lorcain, P., O'Kelly, P., Conlon, P. J., & Murphy, G. M. (2006). A population-based study of skin cancer incidence and prevalence in renal transplant recipients. *The British Journal of Dermatology, Dermatology*(3), 498–504.

Rigel, D. S., Robinson, J. K., Ross, M., Friedman, R. J., Cockerell, C. J., & Lim, H.W. (Eds.). (2011). *Cancer of the skin>* (2nd ed.). Philadelphia, PA: Elsevier Saunders.

Rogers, H. W. (2009). A relative value unit-based cost comparison of treatment modalities for nonmelanoma skin cancer: effect of the loss of the Mohs multiple surgery reduction exemption. *Journal of the American Academy of Dermatology, 61*(1), 96–103.

Shepherd, V., Davidson, E. J., & Davies-Humphreys, J. (2005). Extramammary Paget's disease. *BJOG: An International Journal of Obstetrics & Gynaecology, 112*(3), 273.

Silverberg, M. J., Leyden, W., Warton, E. M., Quesenberry, C. P., Engels, E. A., Asgari, M. M. (2013). Infection status, immunodeficiency, and the incidence of non-melanoma skin cancer. *Journal of the National Cancer Institute*. doi: 10.1093/jnci/djs529. [First published online: January 4, 2013].

Silverman, M. K., Kopf, A. W., Bart, R. S., Grin, C. M., Levenstein, M. S. (1992). Recurrence rates of treated basal cell carcinomas. Part 3: Surgical excision. *The Journal of Dermatologic Surgery & Oncology, 18*(6), 471.

Miller, S. J. (2013). Staging cutaneous squamous cell carcinoma. *JAMA Dermatology, 149*(4), 472–474.

Tarantola, T. I., Vallow, L. A., Halyard, M. Y., Weenig, R. H., Warschaw, K. E, Grotz, T. E., ... Otley, C. C. (2013). Prognostic factors in Merkel cell carcinoma: analysis of 240 cases. *Journal of the American Academy of Dermatology, 68*(3), 425–432.

Ulrich C, Kanitakis J, Stockfleth E, & Euvrard S. (2008). Skin cancer in organ transplant recipients—where do we stand today? *American Journal of Transplantation, Transplantation*(11), 2192–2198.

van der Pols, J. C., Williams, G. M., Pandeya, N., Logan, V., & Green, A. C. (2006). Prolonged prevention of squamous cell carcinoma of the skin by regular sunscreen use. *Cancer Epidemiology, Biomarkers & Prevention, 15*(12), 2546–2548.

Wang, J. T., Palme, C. E., Morgan, G. J., Gebski, V., Wang, A. Y., & Veness, M. J. (2012). Predictors of outcomes in patients with cutaneous metastatic head and neck squamous cell carcinoma involving cervical lymph nodes: Improved survival with the addition of adjuvant radiotherapy. *Head and Neck, 34*,1524–1528.

Werlinger, K. D., Upton, G., & Moore, A.Y. (2002). Recurrence rates of primary nonmelanoma skin cancers treated by surgical excision compared to electrodesiccation-curettage in a private dermatologic practice. *Dermatologic Surgery, 28*, 1138–1142.

Young, J. L., Ward, K. C., & Ries, L. A. G. (2007). Cancer of rare sites. In: L. A. G. Ries, J. L. Young, G. E. Keel, M. P. Eisner, Y. D. Lin, M-J. Horner [Eds.], *SEER survival monograph: Cancer survival among adults: US SEER Program, 1988-2001, patient and tumor characteristics* (pp. 251–261). Bethesda, MD: National Cancer Institute. [NIH Pub. No. 07-6215].

CHAPTER 9

Superficial Bacterial Infections

Mary E. Nolen

Skin and soft tissue infection (SSTI) is a very common cause of patient presentation to primary care and the emergency department. SSTIs comprise nearly 20% of patient visits to dermatology providers. The normal skin of a healthy individual is naturally resistant to infection. The normal skin flora actually protect us from invasion of other organisms which vary by anatomic location. *Staphylococcus aureus,* a gram-positive organism, is usually found on the surface of exposed skin, while *Pseudomonas aeruginosa*, a gram-negative bacteria, occurs on the moist areas of axilla, groin, and web spaces.

Several elements, however, can upset the host–bacteria relationship and transform the status quo into an infectious state. The risk of pathogenesis is influenced by the virulence of the organism, the portal of entry, and the ability of the host to defend and respond to the presence of the organism.

Bacterial infections, also known as pyoderma of the skin, can manifest either as a primary cutaneous process, such as impetigo, or as a manifestation of a systemic infection such as toxic shock syndrome (TSS). This chapter will focus on the recognition and treatment of common SSTIs including those infections that have systemic involvement.

The clinician's ability to recognize and treat infections of the skin early in the course of the disease will insure that patients receive optimal antimicrobial therapy when indicated. Likewise, the ability to distinguish true infection from other inflammatory conditions will spare our patients the risk and expense of unnecessary medicines.

Treatment for bacterial infections often requires the use of antibiotics and other antimicrobial drugs. Proper use of this group of medicines will be discussed primarily as they pertain to dermatology. Alternative treatments will be suggested when possible to minimize the frequency of drug resistance.

ANTIBIOTIC SELECTION

Antibiotic selection is pivotal to the treatment of any bacterial infection, and the optimum choice is based on many factors. The individual pathogen and its susceptibility profile will largely determine the most appropriate antimicrobial. The mechanism of action (MOA) will determine whether the drug is bacteriostatic or bacteriocidal. In other words, you need to choose the right drug for the specific bug. In addition, drug interactions and adverse effects must be considered along with the patient's immune status, age, pregnancy state, and genetic predisposition. A history of drug allergy is essential when deciding treatment; however, many patients confuse true allergy with gastrointestinal upset, especially if they were advised to discontinue the drug. The degree of a penicillin allergy, for example, may not prohibit the use of cephalosporins if needed, so a careful and probing history is sometimes required.

The increase in drug resistance in the United States is in part the result of improper prescribing without bacteriologic information to support its use. Drugs can sometimes be eliminated altogether if other interventions such as incision and drainage and supportive measures are instituted. It is important to remember the old rule when prescribing medication: "Right drug, right dose, right duration, right patient and right time" (Dryden, Johnson, Ashiru-Oredope, & Sharland, 2011).These decisions demand that we as clinicians possess a thorough understanding of the available classes of drugs, their MOA, and effectiveness in various conditions as well as special circumstances in which they should not be used.

This section briefly reviews the common classes of antibiotics used effectively in dermatology for the treatment of SSTIs.

Topical Antibiotics

Drugs such as mupirocin (Bactroban), retapamulin (Altabax), neomycin, gentamycin, polymyxin, and bacitracin are often used in the treatment of superficial skin infections. The greatest drawback is their propensity for allergic contact dermatitis. Subsequently, most dermatologists advocate the use of white petrolatum only on surgical wounds and minor trauma. Topical antibiotics, however, have long been successful in the treatment of acne and rosacea (see chapter 4).

Systemic Antibiotics

These agents are classified by their potential to eradicate or inhibit the growth of the bacteria. Although they can be very effective, there is significant potential for adverse effects and drug interactions. The MOA will determine whether the drug is bacteriostatic or bacteriocidal and will therefore influence the course of treatment.

Penicillins

Penicillins are β-lactam antibiotics and are bacteriocidal agents. Their MOA is to inhibit bacterial cell wall synthesis by binding or destroying enzymes needed for cell growth. Dicloxacillin is highly effective against β-lactamase resistant-penicillin. Oxacillin, cloxacillin, and floxacillin are all used effectively for pyoderma caused by *Streptococcus pyogenes* or *Staphylococcus aureus*.

Cephalosporins

As with penicillins, cephalosporins inhibit the enzymes needed for cell wall formation and are bacteriocidal. They have been grouped by multiple generations based on their antimicrobial activity. The first generation (cephalexin, cefazolin, cephadroxil) is very effective against staphylococci and nonenterococcal streptococci. It is not usually effective against methicillin-resistant *S. aureus* (MRSA). The second generation (cefaclor, loracarbef, cephproxil, cefuroxime axetil) is less effective against gram-positive organisms and more effective against gram-negative organisms. The third generation (ceftriaxone, ceftizoxime, cefixime, cefoperazone) also has good gram-negative activity and especially good activity against *P. aeruginosa*.

Macrolides

While erythromycin was the first drug in this class, it has been outfavored by the newer macrolides because of its significant GI side effects and lack of activity against gram-negative organisms.

Clarithromycin, azithromycin, and dirithromycin are the newer macrolides. They are bacteriostatic and work by penetrating the cell walls of the bacteria. They then bind to the ribosome, inhibiting the RNA-dependent protein synthesis. Both clarithromycin and azithromycin have good activity against gram-positive *Staphylococcus* and *Streptococcus* and are also effective against atypical mycobacteria and toxoplasma gondii. They are used effectively in the treatment of pyodermas, abscesses, infected wounds, erysipelas, and ulcers.

β-Lactam/β-lactamase inhibitor combinations such as amoxicillin/clavulanate and ampicillin/sulbactam have good activity against MRSA, some *Klebsiella* species, *Haemophilus* species, *E. coli,* and *Proteus.* They are very useful in polymicrobial infections such as animal or human bites (see chapter 13).

Quinolones

The quinolones also have several generations of bacteriocidal agents. The second-generation drugs—ciprofloxacin and ofloxacin—are very effective against intracellular pathogens. They are the most effective drugs against gram-negative *P. aeruginosa.* The third generations—levofloxacin and moxifloxacin—have a very broad spectrum of action, including some atypical pathogens. Ciprofloxacin otic solution is useful in treating external otitis media. Diabetic foot ulcers, wounds, and interdigital toe-web infections are all improved with proper use of quinolones.

Tetracycline

The tetracycline family is widely used in dermatology more often for its anti-inflammatory rather than antimicrobial properties. They are bacteriostatic and have been more effective against gram-positive than gram-negative organisms. Many group A streptococci are resistant to tetracycline and it is not available in the United States at this time. Minocycline and doxycycline are widely used for acne and related disorders because of its effect on propionibacteria. Doxycycline is excreted through the GI tract and is the only tetracycline acceptable for use in renal failure. While highly effective for use in acne, photosensitivity is common and may prohibit use in individuals who work outdoors or spend significant time exposed to the sun.

Miscellaneous Drugs

Trimethoprim–sulfamethoxazole

This combination antimicrobial is effective against *S. aureus* and *S. pyogenes* but is not widely used because of its propensity to cause hypersensitivity reactions. It has found favor of late, however, in the treatment of MRSA infections. Trimethoprim–sulfamethoxazole (TMP–SMX) is contraindicated in patients taking methotrexate (interferes with folic acid synthesis) and warfarin (potentiates drug and increased risk of bleeding). Newer antibiotic agents such as linezolid and daptomycin are bacteriocidal and are very useful for severe soft tissue infections, including MRSA infections.

Discussion of the most common superficial bacterial infections will be divided into those caused by gram-positive and gram-negative organisms.

GRAM-POSITIVE BACTERIAL INFECTIONS

The two bacteria that most commonly cause skin infections are *S. aureus* and group A β-hemolytic streptococcus (GAS). *S. aureus* is present on all skin surfaces and is considered a normal part of skin flora. Streptococci, however, are secondary invaders and attack skin that is already traumatized, causing infections such as cellulitis.

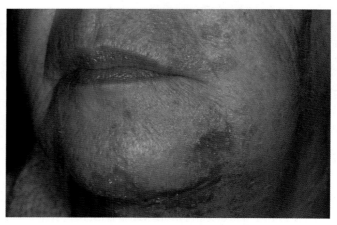

FIG. 9-1. Impetigo.

Infections caused by both of these organisms can range from a superficial skin infection to sepsis with multiorgan involvement.

Impetigo

Perhaps the most familiar and widely known infection of the skin is impetigo. This is a highly contagious, superficial skin infection usually found in children. Adults can also acquire it from direct skin-to-skin contact. It can be seen in two forms: nonbullous and bullous type.

Pathophysiology

Historically, *nonbullous impetigo* was caused almost exclusively by GAS. But today most cases are caused by *S. aureus* alone or in combination with GAS. *Bullous impetigo* is caused by strains of *S. aureus* that produce a toxin which results in the formation of blisters in the epidermis.

Clinical presentation

Nonbullous impetigo is the more common type and occurs primarily in children on the face (nose and mouth) and extremities. It usually begins as 2- to 4-mm erythematous macules that evolve into vesicles or pustules. Later, these lesions erode with the hallmark honey-colored crusts and surrounding erythema. These lesions tend to be asymptomatic, but itching and soreness may be mild. Systemic symptoms rarely occur (Figure 9-1).

Bullous impetigo is less common and tends to occur in neonates and children. It begins as small vesicles that later develop into large bullae. These blisters are flaccid, and the contents may be clear or cloudy (Figure 9-2A). The blisters break easily and develop a perimeter of scale which may measure up to 5 cm, but no crust or surrounding erythema is seen (Figure 9-2B). A crust may form, which, if removed, will reveal a moist, red base. There may be few or numerous lesions, and they may occur on any surface, but typical infections occur on the face, trunk, buttocks, and perineum.

Because of the presence of blisters, bullous impetigo is considered to be a localized form of staphylococcal scalded skin syndrome (SSSS; see chapter 6). The organism is thought to be harbored in the nose and then spread to normal skin.

Diagnostics

Impetigo is often diagnosed clinically, but if the diagnosis is in question, a culture may be obtained from beneath the crust or fluid of an intact blister. A positive culture for streptococcus may be useful in patients who are later suspected of poststreptococcal nephritis.

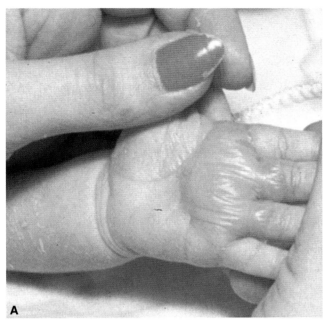

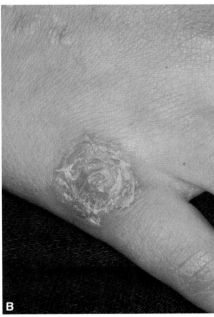

FIG. 9-2. **A:** Bullous impetigo. **B:** Bullous impetigo, dried with perimeter of scale but no erythema.

DIFFERENTIAL DIAGNOSIS Impetigo

Nonbullous Type
- Herpex simplex virus
- Insect bite
- Eczema or contact dermatitis
- Tinea
- Scabies
- Varicella

Bullous Type
- Allergic contact dermatitis
- Bullous insect bite
- Thermal burn
- Herpex simplex virus
- Autoimmune bullous dermatoses
- Bullous pemphigoid
- Bullous erythema multiforme
- Stevens–Johnson syndrome

Management

Impetigo is often treated successfully with topical 2% mupirocin (Bactroban, Centany) ointment applied three times daily until all the lesions have cleared. On occasion, if the lesions are few, it may resolve spontaneously. Topical retapamulin (Altabax) is also approved for uncomplicated skin infections caused by *S. aureus*. It is less effective and not approved for MRSA. Careful washing of the area with an antibacterial cleanser is suggested, whereas hydrogen peroxide is not recommended.

If the infection is widespread, or there are systemic symptoms, oral antibiotics are indicated. A 5- to 10-day course of dicloxacillin, amoxicillin clavulanate, or a cephalosporin such as cephalexin or cefadroxil will result in rapid clearing. Erythromycin is less effective and penicillin V is not indicated.

Prognosis and complications

Impetigo is a superficial infection and usually clears without scarring. Approximately 5% of nonbullous cases are caused by *S. pyogenes* and can be complicated with an acute poststreptococcal glomerulonephritis. Mupirocin ointment 1% may be indicated for use in the nose b.i.d. for up to 1 year.

Special considerations

Athletes engaged in a wide variety of sports are at greater risk of developing superficial bacterial infections, including MRSA infections. Treatment considerations for superficial bacterial infections in athletes must include removal from competition until cleared and the use of occlusive dressings during play (Table 9-1).

The National Federation of State High School Associations Regulations (2006) state:

- All suspect skin conditions require current, written documentation from provider stating the athlete's participation would not be harmful to an opponent.
- All coaches are to perform routine skin checks of their wrestlers and require them to seek medical attention if there is a suspect skin condition.
- Athletes must shower after each event, do not share towels or personal hygiene items, have all open wounds or abrasions evaluated by the coach or certified athletic trainer before each practice or competition, and use clean gear with each event or practice.

Referral and consultation

Most infections of this type are treated by the primary care or dermatology provider. Infections resistant to treatment or frequent recurrences may benefit from a consultation with dermatology or infectious disease for consideration of combination therapy and prophylaxis.

Patient education and follow-up

Because most impetigo occurs at a site of minor trauma, careful washing of the site with antibacterial cleanser is recommended for infection prevention. If all lesions resolve and no new ones occur, follow-up is not necessary. Failure to respond to treatment may indicate a resistant strain of organism and needs to be seen and cultured.

TABLE 9-1	NCAA Guidelines for Skin Infections and Return to Play		
CONDITION	**MINIMUM THERAPY DURATION**	**TYPE THERAPY**	**SPECIAL CONSIDERATION**
Bacterial Infections Impetigo Folliculitis Cellulitis* Furuncles Carbuncle	72 hr No new lesions 48 hr Covered w/ occlusive dressing No wet or draining lesions	Oral antibiotic >72 hr	Lesion dry and covered w/nonpermeable bandage Wash clothing, pads, headgear, and towels after every practice and competition Clean wrestling mats w/ 1% bleach after every use
Herpes gladiatorum Herpes whitlow Herpes zoster	All vesicles crusted, no symptoms > 72 hr Oral ABX 120 hr (5 days) No active lesions	Oral antivirals Acyclovir Famvir Valacyclovir	
Molluscum/warts	Immediately return to play after treatment	curetted or removed any method	Solitary lesions—covered w/ bio-occlusive dressing Warts on face and hands must be covered
Tinea corporis	72 hr	Topical antifungal	Wash w/ketoconazole shampoo; apply terbinafine or naftifine and cover with bio-occlusive dressing (OP site)
Scabies	Complete Tx Negative mineral oil prep	Topical	Must clean clothing and equipment
Lice	Complete Tx Re-examination shows no infestation	Topical	Clean clothing and equipment

*Incl. MRSA.
Adapted from NFHSA Sports Related Skin Infections Position Statement and Guidelines 2010

CLINICAL PEARLS

- Poststreptoccocal nephritis may occur 1 to 3 weeks after an acute episode of streptococcal impetigo but the incidence is low. If the infection is caused by specific strains of *Streptococcus*, the incidence of glomerulonephritis is increased. It occurs most commonly between the ages of 6 and 10 and is often asymptomatic.
- Strep infections have been an associated trigger for guttate psoriasis. This may in fact be the presenting sign and initial episode of the condition.

Folliculitis

Folliculitis is an inflammation of the hair follicle. It can be caused by infection, irritation, or physical injury. It may involve the superficial portion of the hair follicle or may be a deeper process.

Pathophysiology

Many infectious agents are responsible for folliculitis, including bacteria, fungus, and yeast. Folliculitis can also be a noninfectious process related to irritation from shaving, secondary to drug therapy (i.e., systemic corticosteroids), or it may be associated with the use of long-term antibiotics for acne. Diabetes and immunosuppression are important risk factors for folliculitis.

This section addresses bacterial folliculitis caused by common gram-positive organisms. Please see the gram-negative section for additional types.

Clinical presentation

Superficial folliculitis is usually caused by *S. aureus* and appears as an erythematous papule or pustule surrounding the hair. A deeper process may present initially as a red, tender nodule which may eventually develop a point in the center (Figure 9-3). Differential diagnosis may vary depending on location.

DIFFERENTIAL DIAGNOSIS Folliculitis

- Impetigo
- Fungal infection
- Candida folliculitis
- Herpes simplex virus
- Pseudofolliculitis barbae (face)
- Steroid acne (trunk)
- Keratosis pilaris (extremities)
- Perioral dermatitis (face)
- Scabies
- Insect bites

Diagnostics

It may be important to identify the specific etiology of the folliculitis so that appropriate treatment can be rendered. Culture and sensitivities should be done if there is a fresh pustule. The most effective way to culture is to pierce the pustule with a no. 11 blade, expose the contents, and transfer them to a culture swab. An alcohol swab can be used to wipe the skin initially; however, if the procedure is done correctly, the swab should not touch the skin, just the contents of the pustule. The purpose is to eliminate contamination of the culture by swabbing the skin. A KOH prep could also be done on the contents of a pustule to rule out fungus or yeast.

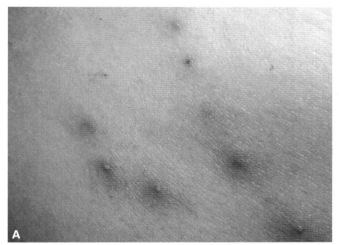

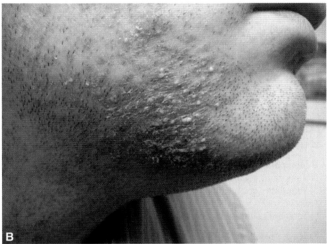

FIG. 9-3. A: Follicular pustules and rim of erythema. **B:** Folliculitis in the beard.

Management

Superficial infection may be treated successfully with antibacterial cleansers such as chlorhexidine (Hibiclens) and topical antibiotics such as 1% clindamycin solution or gel applied b.i.d. after washing. Systemic antibiotics may be needed if there is little response to topicals but should be prescribed based on the culture and sensitivities.

Prognosis and complications

Most superficial infections resolve without scarring. Some postinflammatory discoloration may persist for some times.

Patient education and follow-up

It is important that patients understand prevention of bacterial infections, including reinfection, is largely dependent on good personal hygiene. Patients should be advised to avoid sharing personal items such as razors and towels. Athletes must make sure they are following the NCAA guidelines for play.

Cellulitis and Erysipelas

Cellulitis is an infection of the deep dermis and subcutaneous tissue. Erysipelas involves the upper dermis and superficial lymphatics. Both of these conditions are common infections that result from invasion of bacteria at the site of trauma or surgical wound. Maceration of web spaces and cracks in the skin from tinea pedis create a very common portal of entry.

TABLE 9-2	Differential Diagnosis of Cellulitis and Erysipelas

ADULTS	
INFECTIOUS	**NONINFECTIOUS**
Erythema migrans	Gout
Toxic shock syndrome	Contact dermatitis
Necrotizing fasciitis	Stasis dermatitis
Gas gangrene	Bursitis
Herpes zoster	Insect bite
Tinea	Deep vein thrombosis
	Drug reaction
	Erythema nodosum
	Lymphedema
	Lipodermatosclerosis
	Granuloma faciale

CHILDREN	
Erythema migrans	Contact dermatitis
Toxic shock syndrome	Insect bite
Necrotizing fasciitis	Drug reaction
Tinea	

Pathophysiology

Cellulitis is generally seen in adults and caused by GAS. Cellulitis associated with furuncles, carbuncles, or abscesses is usually caused by *S. aureus*. In contrast, cellulitis that is diffuse or unassociated with a defined portal is most commonly caused by streptococcal species. Important clinical clues to other causes include physical activities, trauma, water contact, and animal, insect, or human bites. *Erysipelas* is usually caused by GAS and occurs in the young, the aged, and the immunocompromised.

Clinical presentation

Both cellulitis and erysipelas are characterized by erythema, warmth, pain, swelling, and tenderness. Cellulitis is often preceded by fever, chills, and malaise, and produces an ill-defined area of erythema most often on lower extremities and may be accompanied by purulent drainage or abscess formation (Figure 9-4A). Severe infections may present with vesicles, bulla, lymphangitis, and involvement of regional lymph nodes (Figure 9-4B). The presentation of cellulitis is almost always unilateral. If there is bilateral manifestations, or if it does not respond to antibiotic therapy, consider diagnoses such as stasis or contact dermatitis (Table 9-2).

Erysipelas, in contrast, produces a fiery-red, well-demarcated, raised plaque, with palpable borders often on the face or extremities. The buttock is also a frequent site. The onset is acute, spread is rapid, and may be accompanied by fever and chills (Figure 9-5).

Diagnostics

The diagnosis of cellulitis and erysipelas is generally made clinically. Diagnostics may be considered if the cellulitis is extensive, has purulent drainage, MRSA is suspected, the patient is immunocompromised, occurs in an unusual location, or is accompanied by signs and symptoms of systemic infection. If so, the following tests are recommended:

Laboratory studies. Wound culture and drug susceptibility tests if there is drainage or the portal of entry is clinically involved, blood

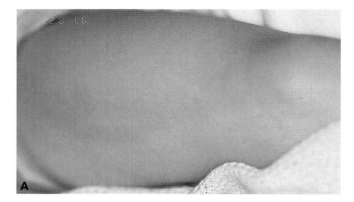

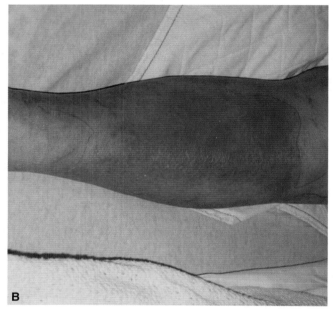

FIG. 9-4. **A:** Cellulitis of the knee, which developed at the site of a minor wound. The child presented with fever and lymphangitic streaking. **B:** Cellulitis.

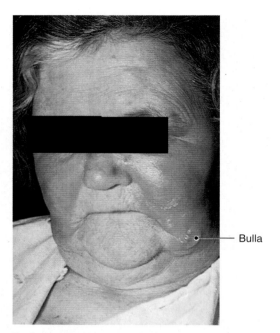

FIG. 9-5. Erysipelas. This patient has large, confluent erythematous plaques. A bulla is present near the angle of her jaw.

BOX 9-1   **Management of Uncomplicated Cellulitis**

Uncomplicated Cellulitis is Defined as:
Nonpurulent cellulitis
No exudates or abscess
No fever
No immunosuppression

Empiric Antimicrobial Treatment for β-Hemolytic Streptococci*
Cephalexin 250–500 mg q.i.d.
Dicloxacillin 500 mg q.i.d.
Clindamycin[†] 300–450 mg t.i.d.
Linezolid[†] 600 mg b.i.d.

---

* Cellulitis and erysipelas are usually caused by group A β-hemolytic streptococcus.
[†] Also has activity against CA-MRSA.
Adapted from Infectious Diseases Society of America (2011).

---

culture, complete blood cell count with differential, creatinine, bicarbonate, creatine phosphokinase, ASO titre, CRP, culture of needle aspiration, or punch biopsy specimens.

Hospitalization. If patients exhibit hypotension and/or an elevated creatinine level, low serum bicarbonate level, elevated creatine phosphokinase (2–3 times the upper limit), and C-reactive protein level >13 mg per L, hospitalization should be considered.

Surgical consultation for inspection, exploration, and/or drainage may be needed.

Radiology. Radiography is performed if osteomyelitis is suspected. An MRI or CT scan is taken to determine if deeper infection to muscle or fascia is present. Ultrasound can help to identify abscesses.

Management

Cellulitis not associated with abscess is usually treated with systemic antimicrobials against GAS or *S. aureus* for 10 days (Box 9-1). In addition, lower-leg skin care, including elevation, compression, and emollients, should be performed.

Referral and consultation

For patients who show signs of systemic illness, have facial edema, or do not respond to oral therapy, consultation with a dermatologist or infectious disease specialist is recommended.

Prognosis and complications

Cellulitis may be recurrent and each episode may cause lymphatic inflammation and lead to lymphedema. Identification and treatment of the portal of entry is essential to prevent recurrences.

Patient education and follow-up

Patients prescribed a regimen of systemic and topical antibiotic therapy should be reevaluated in 24 to 48 hours to assess their clinical response. Progression of infection, despite antibiotic therapy, could be due to an infection with resistant microbes or a deeper, more extensive process. Recurrent infections may also signify inadequate dosing of the antibiotic.

It is important to explain to patients that cellulitis generally occurs where there is a break in the skin barrier. Therefore, treating an underlying infection such as tinea pedis is paramount to prevent recurrences. Keeping the skin well hydrated with emollients after every shower will prevent dryness and cracking. Elevation and compression stockings are also encouraged to minimize edema.

Special considerations
Periorbital cellulitis
Cellulitis around the eye or involving the eyelid and periorbital area should be carefully investigated. Periorbital erythema and edema may be seen in both preseptal and true orbital cellulitis, and the clinician should be aware of the difference. In periorbital cellulitis, trauma to the eyelid may result in inflammation or infection and may involve the soft tissues around the eye. Although the swelling may be significant, the patient should not experience pain or limited movement of the eye. Periorbital cellulitis is generally treated adequately with antibiotics.

In contrast, orbital cellulitis is often the progression of an upper respiratory infection or sinusitis. The infection spreads beyond the orbital septum and may be the result of a tumor on the optic nerve. Orbital cellulitis is characterized by swelling of the conjunctiva, pain, and limited eye movement, and the pupil will often have a very sluggish reaction to light (afferent pupil). This condition has a high morbidity and generally necessitates emergent recognition, intravenous antibiotics, and/or surgical intervention (Figure 9-6).

Complicated Skin and Soft Tissue Infection

Management of complicated SSTI involves the presumption that MRSA may be the causative organism. This section will primarily discuss community-acquired (CA) MRSA. The presence of MRSA indicates that the oxacillin minimum inhibitory concentration (MIC) is > 4 μg per mL and therefore not able to suppress the growth of the organism.

The prevalence of MRSA has been increasing rapidly in both the hospital and community. It is relevant to this discussion because MRSA is the most common identifiable cause of SSTI. Risk factors for MRSA common to both populations include an underlying medical condition, recent use of antibiotics, recent trauma to the skin, foreign bodies that could be embedded in skin, exposure to contacts with the infection, and a history of MRSA infection.

Pathophysiology
We know that the organism *S. aureus* is very common in children and adults. The organism is not found in soil or water but lives in

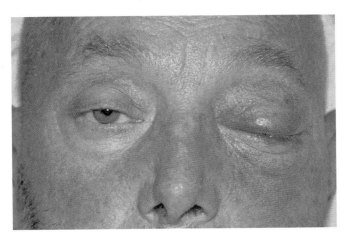

FIG. 9-6. Left orbital cellulitis with marked periorbital edema, erythema, and proptosis.

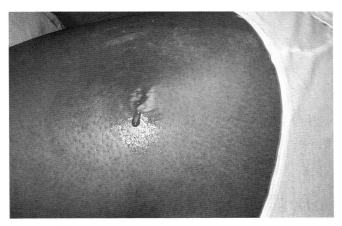

FIG. 9-7. MRSA infection.

the nose and on the skin. It is usually spread through skin-to-skin contact with an infected individual's skin or personal items such as razors or towels. The most common sources of infection are schools, dormitories, and athletic facilities.

Clinical presentation
Clinical presentation of the patient with CA-MRSA may range from superficial pustules, as seen in folliculitis, to large, fluctuant abscesses. The patient's general appearance is an important part of the presentation. The overall appearance of illness with fever, hypotension, and tachycardia as well as larger-than-usual areas of involvement should alert the clinician to the possibility of this type of infection. Cellulitis with or without drainage or abscess formation may be apparent (Figure 9-7). (See the discussion on abscess, furuncles, and carbuncles for further details.)

Diagnostics
The diagnostic procedures for CA-MRSA are the same as those indicated for cellulitis. In most cases, there is drainage, so wound culture must be performed. Immunocompromised patients who have failed previous treatment or who have had multiple recurrences should be cultured with sensitivities. Blood cultures are done if the patient is systemically ill (fever, hypotension, tachycardia, etc.).

DIFFERENTIAL DIAGNOSIS Community-acquired MRSA
• Skin and soft tissue infection
• Cellulitis
• Spider bite
• Impetigo
• Sepsis

Management
The management options for suspected MRSA in SSTI include drainage, antimicrobial therapy, wound care, patient education, and follow-up (Figure 9-8). Mild, superficial infections may be treated with topical agents alone. If there is a collection of purulent material, incision and drainage is recommended, and a culture must be sent for Gram staining and susceptibility testing.

If the infection is localized, incision and drainage may be sufficient treatment as long as the patient is a healthy individual with

Outpatient[†] management of skin and soft tissue infections in the era of community-associated MRSA[‡]

Patient presents with signs/symptoms of skin infection:
- Redness
- Swelling
- Warmth
- Pain/tenderness
- Complaint of "spider bite"

YES ▶

Is the lesion purulent (i.e., are <u>any</u> of the following signs present)?
- Fluctuance—palpable fluid-filled cavity, movable, compressible
- Yellow or white center
- Central point or "head"
- Draining pus
- Possible to aspirate pus with needle and syringe

NO ▶

Possible cellulitis without abscess:
- Provide antimicrobial therapy with coverage for *Streptococcus* spp. and/or other suspected pathogens
- Maintain close follow-up
- Consider adding coverage for MRSA (if not provided initially), if patient does not respond

YES

† For severe infections requiring inpatient management, consider consulting an infectious disease specialist.
‡ Visit **www.cdc.gov/mrsa** for more information.

1. Drain the lesion
2. Send wound drainage for culture and susceptibility testing
3. Advise patient on wound care and hygiene
4. Discuss follow-up plan with patient

Abbreviations:
I&D—incision and drainage
MRSA—methicillin-resistant *S. aureus*
SSTI—skin and soft tissue infection

If systemic symptoms, severe local symptoms, immunosuppression, or failure to respond to I&D, consider antimicrobial therapy with coverage for MRSA in addition to I&D. (See below for options)

Options for empiric outpatient antimicrobial treatment of SSTIs when MRSA is a consideration*

Drug name	Considerations	Precautions**
Clindamycin	■ FDA-approved to treat serious infections due to *S. aureus* ■ D-zone test should be performed to identify inducible clindamycin resistance in erythromycin-resistant isolates	■ *Clostridium difficile*-associated disease, while uncommon, may occur more frequently in association with clindamycin compared to other agents.
Tetracyclines ■ Doxycycline ■ Minocycline	■ Doxycycline is FDA-approved to treat *S. aureus* skin infections.	■ Not recommended during pregnancy. ■ Not recommended for children under the age of 8. ■ Activity against group A streptococcus, a common cause of cellulitis, unknown.
Trimethoprim-Sulfamethoxazole	■ Not FDA-approved to treat any staphylococcal infection	■ May not provide coverage for group A streptococcus, a common cause of cellulitis ■ Not recommended for women in the third trimester of pregnancy. ■ Not recommended for infants less than 2 months.
Rifampin	■ Use only in combination with other agents.	■ Drug–drug interaction are common.
Linezolid	■ Consultation with an infectious disease specialist is suggested. ■ FDA-approved to treat complicated skin infections, including those caused by MRSA.	■ Has been associated with myelosuppression, neuropathy and lactic acidosis during prolonged therapy.

- MRSA is resistant to all currently available beta-lactam agents (penicillins and cephalosporins)
- Fluoroquinolones (e.g., ciprofloxacin, levofloxacin) and macrolides (erythromycin, clarithromycin, azithromycine) are not optimal for treatment of MRSA SSTIs because resistance is common or may develop rapidly.

* Data from controlled clinical trials are needed to establish the comparative efficacy of these agents in treating MRSA SSTIs. Patients with signs and symptoms of severe illness should be treated as inpatients.
** Consult product labeling for a complete list of potential adverse effects associated with each agent.

Role of decolonization

Regimens intended to eliminate MRSA colonization should not be used in patients with active infections. Decolonization regimens may have a role in preventing recurrent infections, but more data are needed to establish their efficacy and to identify optimal regimens for use in community settings. *After treating active infections and reinforcing hygiene and appropriate wound care,* consider consultation with an infectious disease specialist regarding use of decolonization when there are recurrent infections in an individual patient or members of a household.

FIG. 9-8. CDC-recommended treatment of SSTI in the era of CA-MRSA.

TABLE 9-3	Management of Recurrent MRSA Infection			
PERSONAL HYGIENE	**ENVIRONMENTAL HYGIENE**	**DECOLONIZATION**	**LOWER EXTREMITY SKIN CARE**	
Wound care Cover draining wounds Hand hygiene after touching infected skin Avoid reusing/sharing personal items if active infection	Clean high-touch surfaces	Mupirocin twice daily × 5–10 days Consider dilute bleach baths: ¼ cup per ¼ tub (13 gallons) of water for 15 min, 2×/wk for 3 mo	Compression Elevation Emollients	

Adapted from Infectious Diseases Society of America. (2011).

uncomplicated skin lesions (<5 cm). Adjunct antimicrobial therapy is recommended under the following conditions:

- Skin lesions are severe or extensive
- Signs of systemic infection
- Associated with chronic illness
- Immunosuppression
- Extremes of age and involvement of the hands, face, or perineum (difficult-to-drain areas)
- Patient failure to respond to incision and drainage alone

Treatment should always consider local susceptibility patterns. The IDSA (Liu, 2011) recommends the following options for empiric treatment of purulent cellulitis/CA-MRSA in an adult:

- TMP-SMX DS, 1 to 2 tab b.i.d.
- Doxycycline, 100 mg b.i.d.
- Minocycline, 100 mg b.i.d.
- Clindamycin, 300 to 450 mg t.i.d.
- Linezolid, 600 mg b.i.d.

Special considerations

When MRSA is suspected in children, similar principles of treatment apply. If the lesion is fluctuant, incision and drainage may be sufficient. If the child is ill-appearing or febrile, adjuvant systemic therapy is recommended and includes clindamycin, TMP-SMX, and doxycycline if appropriate for children 8 years of age and older.

Empiric coverage for MRSA with oral antibiotics may not necessarily improve the outcome; however, it is thought to prevent recurrences. If the infection is severe, hospitalization and parenteral antibiotics such as vancomycin or clindamycin are indicated. MRSA infection is a reportable disease in some states.

Patient education and follow-up

Preventing recurrence is a priority when dealing with MRSA infections, and it requires the cooperation of the patient and family (Table 9-3). Prevention involves personal hygiene, which means covering wounds and eliminating exposure to others. Environmental hygiene requires cleaning high-touch areas in the home, including all areas that are touched by bare hands, such as doorknobs, toilet seats, and bathtubs. In some cases, if these two measures fail, eradication of the persistent organism may require decolonization. Otherwise, follow-up measures are the same as those used in cellulitis.

Referral and consultation

CA-MRSA can be difficult to eradicate if all members of the household do not cooperate. Repeated infections should be referred to an infectious disease specialist for consideration of decolonization.

Abscesses, Furuncles, and Carbuncles

Pathophysiology

An abscess is a walled-off collection of pus that may be sterile or the result of infection that can occur in any organ or tissue. Sterile abscess can arise as a response to a foreign body, an inflamed sebaceous cyst, or even an odontogenic sinus. A furuncle begins in a hair follicle, commonly associated with *S. aureus*, that extends deeper into subcutaneous tissue and may develop into an abscess. A carbuncle represents involvement of multiple inflamed abscesses arising in contiguous follicles and sinus tracts, forming a single mass.

Risk factors include contact with someone who has an infection caused by staph species, diabetes, any other skin condition (such as eczema) that may alter the skin barrier, and immunosuppression (Figure 9-9).

Clinical presentation

An abscess begins as a tender, red/erythematous nodule that eventually becomes fluctuant in the center with a prominent point (Figure 9-10). Spontaneous rupture and drainage can occur especially with pressure or friction. Once opened, the patient becomes at increased risk for infection usually by *S. aureus*. Abscesses extending into the subcutaneous area may not have an obvious point, and may be accompanied by fever, chills, and fatigue, and lymphadenopathy may be present.

Furuncles favor hair-bearing locations and tend to occur on the neck, axillae, and buttocks (Figure 9-11). Carbuncles are larger nodules and painful masses composed of multiple furuncles with several sinus openings (Figure 9-12).

DIFFERENTIAL DIAGNOSIS Abscesses, furuncles, and carbuncles

- Ruptured epidermoid or pilar cyst
- Cystic acne
- Hidradenitis suppurativa
- Primary immunodeficiency disease
- Atypical mycobacterial infection
- Primary and secondary immunodeficiency disease

Diagnostics

Skin abscesses can be caused by one or several pathogens, and in the era of MRSA, culture should be obtained.

Management

Incision and drainage is recommended for any fluctuant and localized lesion and is the CDC's treatment of choice for suspected CA-MRSA infections. In the absence of a culture-proven infection, the role of systemic antibiotics has been debated. If the wound is deep, a drain or gauze wick may be placed to keep the wound open and

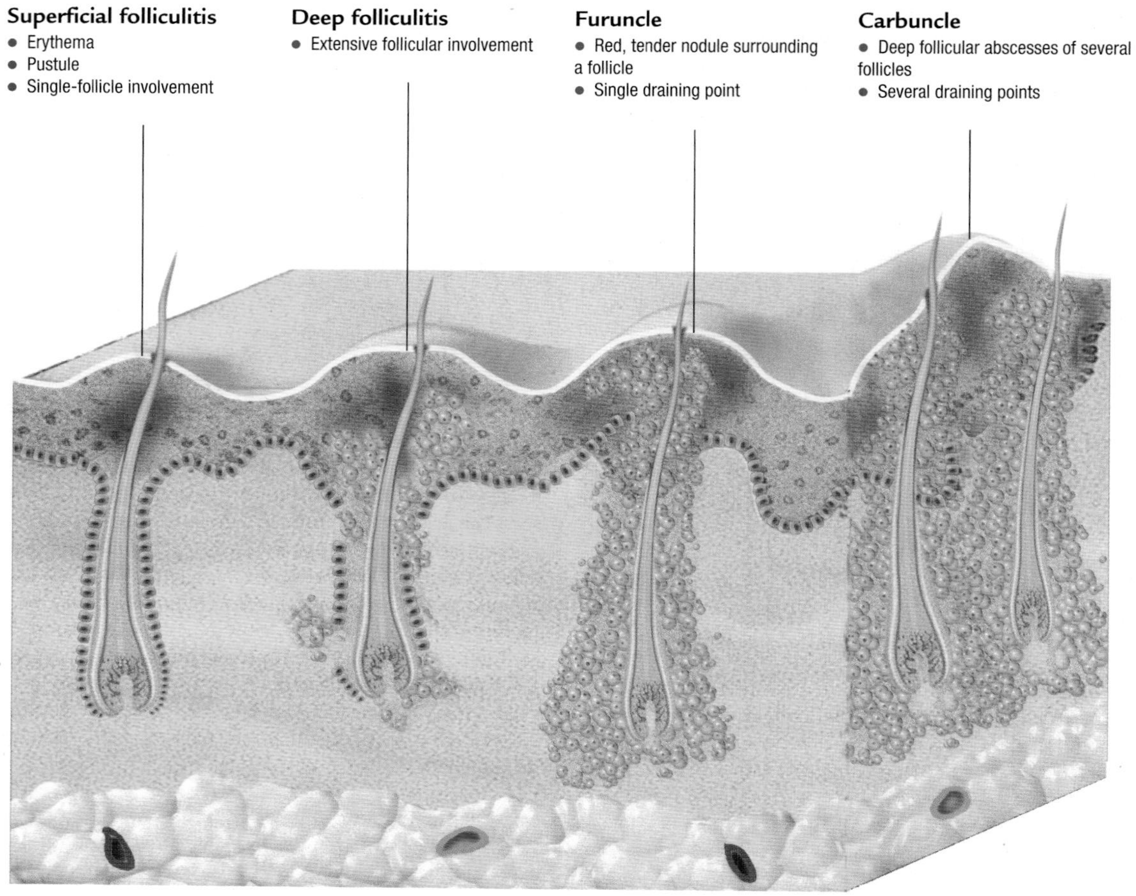

Superficial folliculitis
- Erythema
- Pustule
- Single-follicle involvement

Deep folliculitis
- Extensive follicular involvement

Furuncle
- Red, tender nodule surrounding a follicle
- Single draining point

Carbuncle
- Deep follicular abscesses of several follicles
- Several draining points

FIG. 9-9. Distinguishing folliculitis, furuncles, and carbuncles.

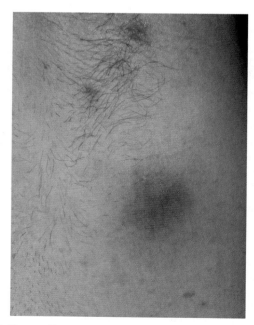

FIG. 9-10. Abscess. Note prominent central point.

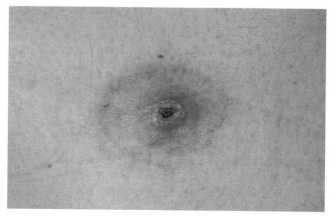

FIG. 9-11. Furuncle.

allow for continued drainage. Warm compresses will aid in healing and will help facilitate drainage.

Special considerations

Abscesses that develop on the central face, around the eyes and nose, are at increased risk for cavernous sinus thrombosis (CST),

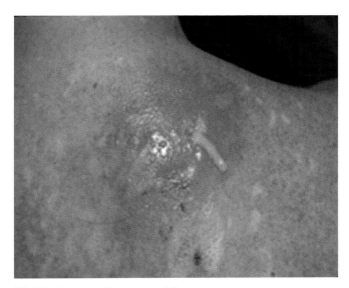

FIG. 9-12. Carbuncle. Note multiple follicular openings

which is associated with staphylococcal or streptococcal infections. Symptoms of CST include decrease or loss of vision, chemosis (the swelling of the *conjunctiva*), exophthalmus, headaches, and paralysis of the cranial nerves which course through the cavernous sinus. This infection is life-threatening and requires immediate treatment, which usually includes antibiotics and sometimes surgical intervention.

Prognosis and complications

Recurrent furunculosis is a hallmark of MRSA infection and the most common presentation; therefore, care must be taken to minimize autoinoculation and spread of infection to others. It is recommended that topical mupirocin be applied to the anterior nares daily for the first 5 days of every month. Frequent hand washing with antibacterial cleansers such as chlorhexidine (Hibiclens) and bleach baths (see chapter 3) are helpful to reduce the overall bacterial colonization. A reculture after 3 months can assess the effectiveness. It is unclear whether the use of systemic antibiotics reduces the risk of reinfection. If all simple abscesses are treated with systemic antibiotics, it is feared that there will be increased resistance to the drugs most needed to treat MRSA. Furuncles, and especially carbuncles, can be slow to heal and result in scarring.

Referral and consultation

A consult with an infectious disease specialist may be important for recurrent infections or for immunosuppressed individuals. Surgical consult with an ENT specialist should be obtained for suspicion of CST.

Patient education and follow-up

Same as for MRSA.

Toxic Shock Syndrome

TSS is a systemic, multiorgan disease that can involve the kidney, liver, muscle, and CNS as well as skin. Originally described in 1978 in a pediatric population, it gained the attention of the public and the medical community in 1980, when multiple cases were linked to the use of tampons in menstruating women. Most of the cases involved young Caucasian women aged 15 to 19 years. Over time, the proportion of cases related to tampon use decreased significantly, largely because super absorbent products, and products containing synthetic materials were removed from the market.

Pathophysiology

The causative organism identified at the time was a specific strain of *S. aureus* that produces a toxin known as TSS-1. In almost 90% of the cases, the toxin has been isolated, known as TSS toxin-1 (TSST-1). Today, most cases are a nonmenstruating type and may be related to other toxins produced by *S. aureus*, such as staphylococcal enterotoxins A, B, C, and D. These enterotoxins behave like superantigens and stimulate the T cells to release massive amounts of cytokines such as tumor necrosis factor α and β, interleukin 1 and 2, and interferon γ. These cytokines are responsible for inflammation and cause fever, rash, tissue injury, and shock.

Those individuals most at risk for developing TSS have been found to lack the antibody to TSST-1. In the general population, 70% to 80% of people possess the antibody present from birth to 6 months, and 90% to 95% of people have the antibody by age 40. Patients with clinical TSS are deficient in the TSST-1 antibody. This failure to produce the antibody may explain why some individuals relapse after the first episode.

Group A streptococcus (GAS) can also produce a TSS-like syndrome, which has several of the same clinical signs. GAS must be considered in the differential diagnosis, but it usually presents with severe pain and tenderness at a surgical site or site of trauma. The average age (20–50 years) is slightly older streptococcal TSS. SSTI is more common in streptococcal TSS.

Clinical presentation

The signs and symptoms of TSS occur rapidly in an otherwise healthy individual and may vary depending on the organ involved and the causative organism. Unlike staphylococcal TSS, streptococcal infection is usually accompanied by severe pain. Both conditions are marked by fever, hypotension, and systemic involvement. Where staphylococcal TSS produces a diffuse erythematous eruption, streptococcal TSS tends to have a soft tissue infection with erythema surrounding the wound. Renal involvement is common in both and usually presents with an elevated BUN. Providers are cautioned to include TSS in the differential diagnosis of fever and rash, even if all categories of symptoms are not present.

DIFFERENTIAL DIAGNOSIS Toxic shock syndrome
• Group A streptococcus
• Drug eruption
• Kawasaki disease
• Scarlet fever
• Viral exanthems
• Staphylococcal scalded skin syndrome
• Toxic epidermal necrolysis

Diagnostics

Diagnosis is based on clinical presentation using the CDC criteria (Box 9-2) The average age (20-50 years) is slightly older in strep TSS. Cultures should be obtained from mucosal and wound sites when possible. SSTI is common in streptococcal TSS; so inquire about recent surgical procedures or skin infections. Blood cultures have very low yield for the presence of *S. aureus*, but they may confirm the presence of other gram-positive or gram-negative organisms. Blood cultures are positive in streptococcal TSS, almost 50% of the time. Streptococcal TSS has a much higher mortality rate.

BOX 9-2 CDC Criteria for Toxic Shock Syndrome

Probable Case: laboratory findings and 4 of 5 clinical symptoms
Confirmed Case: laboratory findings and all 5 clinical symptoms

Clinical Symptoms:

- Fever >102
- Hypotension (systolic <90)
- Erythroderma (diffuse)
- Involvement of 3 organ systems (i.e., headache, muscle aches, mucous membrane hyperemia, nausea and vomiting, elevated liver enzymes, etc.)
- Desquamation, 1–2 wk after the rash (usually palms and soles)

Laboratory Findings:

- Blood and cerebrospinal fluid cultures—negative
- Serologies negative for Rocky Mountain spotted fever, leptospirosis, or measles

From Centers for Disease Control and Prevention National Notifiable Diseases Surveillance System (NNDSS). Toxic shock syndrome (other than Streptococcal) (TSS). *2011 Case Definition.*

Management

Box 9-3 lists steps in management of patients with TSS.

Referral and consultation

Patients suspected of TSS will likely be hospitalized. Consultation with an infectious disease specialist and a dermatologist are indicated.

Patient education and follow-up

Women are cautioned to change tampons regularly or every 8 hours and to alternate use of tampons and sanitary pads. Avoid the use of super absorbent tampons. If using sponge, cervical cap, or diaphragms, never leave one in longer than 24 hours, and wash with warm soapy water after each use. Promptly remove tampon or any vaginal insert at the first sign of fever or illness.

Necrotizing Fasciitis

Necrotizing fasciitis (NF) is a deep, life-threatening infection which not only affects the skin and soft tissue but also rapidly spreads to involve the fascia and muscle (Box 9-4). The lay public has coined it the "flesh-eating bacteria." Individuals at greater risk for contracting this infection include those with diabetes, hepatitis C infection, HIV infection and immunosuppression, alcoholism, history of injectable drug use, and recent surgical or traumatic wounds from burns or lacerations from childbirth and peripheral vascular disease. A recent history of varicella is considered a predisposing factor for NF. The use of NSAIDs has been implicated as well, because of the inhibition of neutrophil function, which leads to increased cytokine production and further development of inflammation. The disease is found in all age groups and affects men and women equally.

Pathophysiology

NF can be caused by either a mixture of organisms or one predominant organism. Type 1 NF is a mixed infection of aerobes and anaerobes, and often associated with surgery of the abdomen and bowel. Type 2 NF is generally GAS alone or in combination with other β-hemolytic streptococci. GAS and *S. aureus* may occur simultaneously. In communities with a high prevalence of CA-MRSA, this may also be a cause of NF.

BOX 9-3 Management of Toxic Shock Syndrome

Universal Recommendations

- IV fluid is essential to reverse hypotension.
- Drain and culture any wounds
- Examine and culture the vagina in menstrual and nonmenstrual TSS and remove and culture any object found (tampon, sponges)
- Explore any surgical wounds
- Antibiotics against staphylococcal infection are needed to eradicate the organism and reduce recurrences.
- Nasal culture, if positive, should be treated with mupirocin.
- Intravenously administered immunoglobulin and corticosteroid therapy may be useful if there is no response to other treatments.

The toxins released by these microbes cause occlusion of the blood vessels, which quickly progresses to necrosis of the involved tissue.

Clinical presentation

NF usually begins as a simple skin abrasion or insect bite, most commonly on the lower extremity of adults and the trunk of children. Pain may develop soon after with progressive, erythema, edema, cellulitis, and fever and may be mistaken for simple cellulitis. The area of redness expands rapidly and develops a dusky bluish coloration centrally. The pain is often exquisite and constant in the early phase, and is disproportionate to the appearance of the lesion, a hallmark characteristic. As the infection progresses, the skin becomes insensate from thrombosis of superficial blood vessels and destruction of superficial nerves. There may be diffuse swelling, and hemorrhagic blisters may form because of the occlusion of vessels. Crepitus in the tissue, caused by formation of gases from mixed bacteria, is pathognomonic and an ominous sign (Figure 9-13). Systemic symptoms develop with fever, nausea, anorexia, elevated WBC, confusion, and hypotension. Patients may present with a mixed picture of TSS and NF.

DIFFERENTIAL DIAGNOSIS Necrotizing fasciitis

- Cellulitis or other soft tissue infections
- Deep vein thrombosis
- Septic arthritis
- Warfarin necrosis
- Brown recluse spider bite
- Toxic shock syndrome

Diagnostics

Radiographic imaging can be useful in determining the depth of infection. Ultrasound may detect abscesses. Soft tissue x-ray, CT scan, and MRI may be helpful at visualizing gas formation along the fascial plane. Surgical exploration is necessary when the diagnosis is uncertain, infection is not responding to antibiotics, the local wound shows signs of necrosis, or there is a presence of gas in the tissue. Gram stain and culture of tissue should aid in determining the antibiotic choice.

BOX 9-4 Ominous Signs of Deep Soft Tissue Infection

Constitutional symptoms
Crepitus
Necrosis
Purpura
Pain disproportionate to the clinical signs
Rapid progression

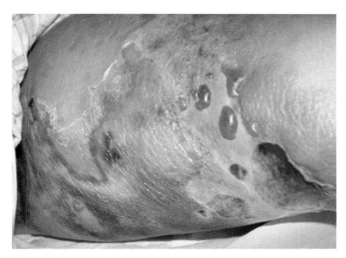

FIG. 9-13. Necrotizing fasciitis.

Management

Early and aggressive surgical intervention to debride all necrotic tissue in addition to broad-spectrum antibiotic therapy is the standard treatment. Debridement is continued until all healthy tissue is visible. This generally results in multiple surgical procedures over the course of several days. Skin grafting is often necessary if the wounds are extensive. Antibiotic therapy is empiric initially but modified based on the culture and gram stain. Broad-spectrum drugs effective against gram-positive, gram-negative, and anaerobic organisms are used. Carbapenems are used in conjunction with clindamycin for its antitoxin effect as well as agents against MRSA such as vancomycin, daptomycin, and linezolid. Patients with sensitivity to these drugs may be given fluoroquinolones plus metronidazole. IVIG may be helpful in severe GAS infections.

Prognosis and complications

NF has a high degree of mortality and is most closely associated with the development of streptococcal TSS. The hospital course and rehabilitation can take weeks and months. The loss of limb or amputation is very common, and organ failure is possible. Patients often are left with significant cosmetic disfigurement and disability due to the amount of muscle, soft tissue, and bones that is removed.

Referral and consultation

Suspicion of NF is a true emergency requiring patients be immediately transported to the nearest medical center. Immediate consultation with the surgeon is imperative.

Patient education and follow-up

After surviving an episode of NF, patients must be prepared for a long and extensive recovery. Care must be taken to avoid future trauma, to maintain meticulous personal hygiene, and to promptly treat any open wounds to avoid infection.

CLINICAL PEARLS

- The amount of pain is out of proportion to the apparent skin findings and while the pain is intense initially, the skin later becomes anesthetic.
- Watch for crepitus, rapidly progressing erythema, and the development of dusky color and hemorrhagic bullae centrally.
- Any suspicion of NF demands an emergency consultation with a surgeon.

GRAM-NEGATIVE BACTERIAL INFECTIONS

Gram-negative bacteria tend to live where the skin is warm and moist such as the axilla and groin and include such organisms as *Pseudomonas* and *Corynebacteria*.

Pseudomonas Folliculitis

The most common of the gram-negative infections is *P. aeruginosa* folliculitis, also known as "hot tub" folliculitis.

Pathophysiology

P. aeruginosa is an intestinal gram-negative rod commonly found in the anogenital and axillary regions. This bacterium thrives in warm, moist environments and feeds off the dead skin cells shed during the bath. Chlorine or bromine are generally added to the tub or pool water to kill the bacteria. If the chemical composition of the water is not correctly balanced, the bacteria will flourish and produce an annoying and uncomfortable eruption in most individuals.

Clinical presentation

In as little as 8 hours after exposure to a contaminated pool, red, urticarial papules and plaques may appear often with a pustular center on all skin surfaces except the head. This is often accompanied by a burning sensation and tends to be worse in the areas beneath the bathing suit. The eruption can be widespread but is self-limiting and resolves after 7 to 10 days, often with residual brownish discoloration (Figure 9-14).

DIFFERENTIAL DIAGNOSIS Pseudomonas folliculitis

- Gram-positive folliculitis
- Acne
- Candidiasis
- Miliaria
- Sea bather's eruption
- Insect bite
- Impetigo

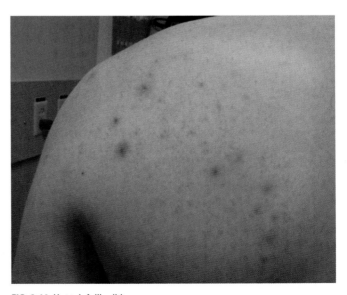

FIG. 9-14. Hot tub folliculitis.

Management

Often no treatment other than showering and removing the wet suit is needed. Sometimes topical clindamycin is prescribed twice daily. If it is resistant to topical treatment, ciprofloxacin 500 mg can be given twice daily for 7 days or less if the rash resolves.

Patient education and follow-up

Complete cleaning of the tub is part of the treatment and involves draining the water completely, cleaning the tub itself, and then making sure the proper ratio of chemicals is added to the fresh water. Be sure to notify the hotel or owner of the tub that this problem exists.

Erythrasma

Erythrasma is a common skin eruption that generally occurs in the skin folds. It is often misdiagnosed and can be a chronic problem for individuals.

Pathophysiology

The warmth, moisture, and darkness of intertriginous areas encourage the growth of the causative organism *Corynebacterium minutissimum*.

Clinical presentation

Erythrasma is usually asymptomatic. It can present as pink-to-brown, well-defined macules or patches with scale. It is commonly seen in the groin, axilla, inframammary area, and toe-web spaces, where maceration is common. It is often mistaken for tinea or candidiasis; however, there is no inflammation or advancing border (Figure 9-15A).

DIFFERENTIAL DIAGNOSIS: Erythrasma
• Tinea curis or pedis
• Psoriasis
• Atopic dermatitis
• Contact dermatitis
• Tinea versicolor

Diagnostics

The diagnosis of erythrasma is a clinical one made by observing a coral-red fluorescence on Wood light examination. The fluorescence is the result of porphyrins which are produced by the bacteria (Figure 9-15B). KOH prep will be negative, but it is often difficult to obtain scale for examination. (See chapter 24 for details on Wood light examination.)

Management

Topical treatment is usually sufficient. Washing with benzoyl peroxide followed by application of a topical antibiotic such as clindamycin or erythromycin should resolve the problem. Erythrasma is often mistreated first as a dermatophyte infection; so erythrasma should always be considered when topical antifungals fail to improve the condition.

Patient education and follow-up

Treatment should be complete after 4 weeks. If not, the patient should return for reevaluation and consideration of a different diagnosis or presence of a coinfection.

Interdigital Toe Infection

This is usually a mixed infection that often begins as tinea pedis. It is often associated with closed toe shoes (especially steel-toe) and is

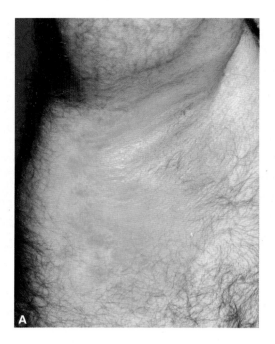

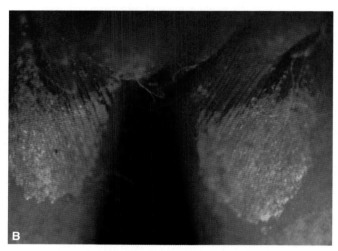

FIG. 9-15. A: Erythrasma. **B:** Coral-red fluorescence with Wood lamp shows erythrasma in the groin.

seen frequently in individuals who spend a lot of time engaged in physical activities, either occupationally or recreationally.

Initially, the dermatophyte infection may alter the continuity of the stratum corneum and allow for the invasion of multiple microbes. It is often associated with hyperhidrosis, which provides the perfect environment for gram-negative infection. *P. aeruginosa* is a common pathogen.

Clinical presentation

Peeling and cracking of the toe-web spaces may be the presenting sign. Increased moisture will lead to maceration, and sometimes the peeling extends to the plantar surface of the toes extending down to the metatarsal heads. If *P. aeruginosa* is involved, you may begin to see a greenish coloration to the skin of the web spaces (Figure 9-16). It is often accompanied by burning and pain rather than itch.

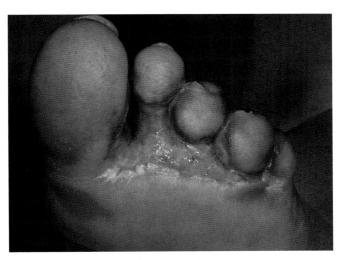

FIG. 9-16. Interdigital toe infection.

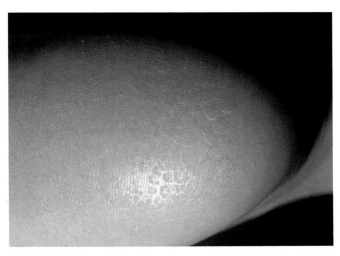

FIG. 9-17. Pitted keratolysis with erosions not reflecting light as does the intact skin.

DIFFERENTIAL DIAGNOSIS Interdigital toe infection

- Tinea pedis
- Erythrasma
- Intertrigo
- Impetigo
- Candida infection
- Hyperhidrosis

Diagnostics

Identification of the various organisms that may be present is necessary to achieve complete resolution. A KOH prep is helpful in identifying the presence of dermatophyte or yeast. A fungal culture will provide the specific organism. A bacterial culture should also be done to aid in the identification of organisms and selection of antimicrobials. A Wood light examination will help rule out erythrasma if there is no coral fluorescence. If the patient's immune status is in question, a complete blood count with differential should be ordered along with a blood glucose measurement.

Management

Excessive sweating is a major contributing factor to interdigital infection. This can be controlled by using antiperspirant products such as aluminum chloride 20%. This should be applied nightly with occlusion until the sweating is diminished and then continued on a regular basis to minimize moisture. A broad-spectrum topical antifungal such as econazole nitrate cream 1% or sertaconazole nitrate cream 2% should be prescribed for b.i.d. application. This drug is a good choice because of its antibacterial qualities as well. If *P. aeruginosa* is isolated, ciprofloxacin can be used.

Patient education and follow-up

Patients must be educated about the underlying cause of this condition. Encourage them to continue using the drying agents on a regular basis. Advise them to be aware of new or recurrent infections such as tinea pedis and encourage early interventions. If this is a severe case, you should see the patient back in 2 weeks. You may need to contact the patient before then to report on culture results if a change in treatment is needed. Otherwise a follow-up visit in 4 weeks is reasonable.

Pitted Keratolysis

This is a superficial bacterial infection that is confined to the stratum corneum. It presents a bizarre pattern which is often most apparent when the skin is wet such as after a bath or shower.

Pathophysiology

At least two organisms have been identified to be responsible for pitted keratolysis: *Kytococcus sedentarius* and *Dermatophilus congolensis*, both of which produce an enzyme that degrades the keratin and results in pitting of the stratum corneum.

Clinical presentation

Pitted keratolysis is most common on the weight-bearing areas of the feet and is often associated with hyperhidrosis. There are numerous small, punched-out depressions on the heel, the plantar surface of the toes, and over the metatarsal heads. There is no inflammation, and the infection is otherwise asymptomatic (Figure 9-17).

DIFFERENTIAL DIAGNOSIS Pitted keratolysis

- Warts

Diagnostics

These organisms are difficult to culture, and the diagnosis is generally made clinically. A biopsy of a superficial shave of the skin would reveal the filamentous organisms with a regular hematoxylin and eosin stain.

Management

Controlling the sweating is a large part of treatment. Aluminum chloride 20% (Drysol) can be applied at bedtime with occlusion nightly until the sweating stops and then periodically for maintenance. Benzoyl peroxide, as well as topical antibiotics such as erythromycin 2% solution and clindamycin 1% solution or gel, can be applied b.i.d..

Patient education and follow-up

Explaining the role of increased sweating will help the patient understand the need for keeping the feet dry. Advise with regard to early treatment if the symptoms recur.

BILLING CODES ICD-10

Cellulitis and erysipelas	A46.0
Cutaneous abscess	L02
Erythrasma	L08.1
Necrotizing fasciitis	M72.6
Impetigo	
Bullous	L01.03
Nonbullous	L01.01
Gram-negative toe-web infection	L01.1
Pseudomonas folliculitis	L73.9
Pitted keratolysis	L08.89
Toxic shock syndrome	A48.3

READINGS

Bolognia, J. L., Jorizzo, J. L., & Schaffer, J. V. (2012). *Dermatology* (3rd ed.). Philadelphia, PA: Elsevier Saunders.

Centers for Disease Control and Prevention. Mission critical: Preventing antibiotic resistance. http://www.cdc.gov/ncidod/dbmd/diseaseinfo/groupastreptococcal_g.htm

Chua, K., Laurent, F., Coombs, G., Grayson, L., & Howden, B. (2011). Not Community-Associated Methicillin-Resistant *Staphylococcus aureus* (CA-MRSA) A Clinician's Guide to Community MRSA—Its Evolving Antimicrobial Resistance and Implications for Therapy. *Clinical Infectious Diseases, 52*, 1–38.

Dryden, M., Johnson, A. P., Ashiru-Oredope, D., & Sharland, M. (2011). Using antibiotics responsibly: Right drug, right time, right dose, right duration. *The Journal of Antimicrobial Chemotherapy, 66*(11), 2441–2443.

Habif, T. (2010). *Clinical dermatology: A color guide to diagnosis and therapy* (5th ed.). China: Elsevier Inc.

Likness, L. P. (2011). Common dermatologic infections in athletes and return-to-play guidelines. *The Journal of the American Osteopathic Association, 111*(6), 373–379.

Liu, C., Bayer, A., Cosgrove, S., Daum, R., Friden, S., Gorwitz, R., Kaplan, S., Karchmer, A., Levine, D., Murray, B., Rybak, M., Taran, D., Chambers, H. *52*(3), 18–55.

National Federation of State High School Associations Sports Related Skin Infections Position Statement and Guidelines 2010.

Madaras-Kelly K., Remington R., Oliphant C., Sloan K., & Bearden, D. (2008). Efficacy of oral beta-lactam versus non-beta-lactam treatment of uncomplicated cellulite. *The American Journal Medicine, 121*(5), 419–425.

Stevens D., Bisno A., Chambers H., Everett E., Dellinger P., Goldstein E., & Gorbach, S. (2005). Practice Guidelines for the Diagnosis and Management of Skin and Soft Tissue Infection. *Clinical Infectious Diseases, 41*(10), 1373–1406.

Wolverton, S. (2013). *Comprehensive dermatologic drug therapy*. Philadelphia, PA: Elsevier Saunders.

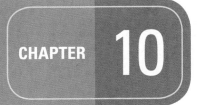

CHAPTER 10 — Viral Infections

Kelly Noska

Patients frequently present to primary care with viral infections, which can be challenging to diagnose because of their various clinical presentations. Viruses are a large group of submicroscopic infective agents and are separated into two main groups, the DNA and RNA virus types. Viruses can also be classified by their mode of transmission, for example, airborne viruses. This chapter will cover a broad range of viral skin diseases; however, the viral exanthems will be discussed in chapter 6, Pediatrics.

Structurally, viral particles (virion) contain a central core of genetic material (RNA or DNA) within a protein coat (capsid). Some viruses have an outer membrane, known as the envelope, which enables the virus to identify and bind to the host membrane. Viruses require living cells to grow and multiply. Infections occur when the virus introduces its own genetic material into the nucleus of a cell within the host. The host cell will then reproduce normally and will subsequently reproduce the newly introduced viral particles. These particles are then spread throughout the host and infection ensues. Treatment of viral infections depends on the structure of the virus and is aimed at stopping reproduction, not killing the virus, as is often seen in antibacterial therapy.

WARTS

Warts, or verruca, are one of the most common viral infections seen in primary care and affect approximately 7% to 10% of the population. They are small, benign growths caused by the human papilloma virus (HPV), a member of the papovavirus group. They are frustrating for both patients and providers as treatment is often tedious and long term.

Pathophysiology

The papovaviruses are double-stranded, naked (nonenveloped) DNA viruses and are characterized by their slow growth. These viruses typically infect the epithelia of the skin or mucosa, favoring certain locations such as the hands, feet, face, or genitalia. Over100 subtypes of HPV have been identified, and infections can be categorized as anogenital lesions (condyloma acuminatum or genital warts) and nongenital lesions (common warts or verruca). Anogenital warts will be discussed in chapter 21.

While warts themselves are not cancerous, some strains of HPV (usually ones not associated with warts) are oncogenic. Cutaneous warts can be spread through direct person-to-person skin contact or indirectly through contaminated surfaces and objects (e.g., swimming pools, showers). Autoinoculation of the virus from an existing lesion to adjacent skin is commonly seen on the hands in the interdigital and periungual areas. The risk of becoming infected will depend on the immune status of the exposed individual, the amount of virus present during exposure, and the nature of the contact.

Clinical Presentation

Common warts (verruca vulgaris)

Verruca vulgaris, also known as common warts, usually occurs in patients between the ages of 5 and 20 years. Only 15% occur after the age of 35 years. Common warts can be found anywhere on the body but are predominantly found on the hands, particularly the fingers and palms, where fissuring and bleeding can occur at times. A major risk factor is frequent immersion of hands in water; so they are frequently seen in food handlers. Lesions range in size from <1 mm to >1 cm, with the average size being around 5 mm. Typical morphology is a rough, skin-colored papule with a grayish surface that interrupts normal skin lines. The clinical presentation is so characteristic that "verrucous" is used as an adjective to describe the morphologic features of other dermatologic conditions with a similar appearance, such as a seborrheic keratosis.

It is thought that common warts on the body are spread by autoinoculation from the hands. Periungual warts, typically seen at the proximal and lateral nail folds, are often seen in patients who bite their nails (Figure 10-1).Warts may be seen in or around the mouth in these patients as well. Digitate or filiform warts, small (usually 1–3 mm) pedunculated skin-colored papules with multiple, small finger-like projections, can be seen on the face and scalp (Figure 10-2).

Flat warts (verruca plana)

Flat warts, also known as verruca plana, can affect children and young adults, typically present as multiple 2- to 4-mm flat-topped papules. Color can range from slightly erythematous or pink, or tan/brown on lighter skin, to darker brown or hyperpigmented on darker skin. These generally appear in crops on the face, neck, dorsal hands, wrists, elbows, or knees. Men who shave their faces, and women who shave their legs or underarms, can spread the virus and develop numerous flat warts at the site. This is frequently seen in atopic patients from scratching. The distribution is usually more linear (Figure 10-3). Fortunately, of all HPV types, flat warts have the highest rate of spontaneous remission.

Plantar warts (verruca plantaris)

Plantar warts, also known as verruca plantaris, typically present as hyperkeratotic, flesh-colored verrucous papules or plaques. It is common to see multiple lesions present at the same time. Size can range from <1 mm to >1 cm. Lesions may be mistaken for either a callus or a corn, due to their tendency to occur on the pressure points on the ball of the foot, particularly at the mid-metatarsal area. A callus is a circumscribed area of superficial hyperkeratosis, caused by repeated friction or pressure. A corn, or clavus, is a circumscribed thickening of the skin with a central translucent, hornlike core, also caused by repeated friction or pressure. If a callus is pared down, it will reveal normal-appearing skin underneath. If a corn is pared down, it will reveal a clear, horny core. This can be useful in determining diagnosis and treatment.

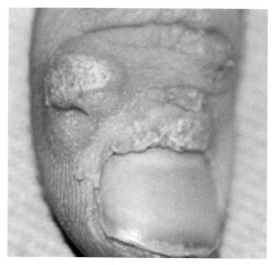

FIG. 10-1. Periungual warts.

Anogenital warts and condylomata acuminata

Genital warts are the most common sexually transmitted infection. The estimated lifetime risk for infection in sexually active adults can be as high as 80%. Genital HPV is closely linked with cancer of the cervix, glans penis, anus, and vulvovaginal area. There are more than 30 types of HPV associated with genital warts (see chapter 23) and at least 15 types that are oncogenic or high risk.

DIFFERENTIAL DIAGNOSIS Warts
• Seborrheic keratoses
• Acrochordons (skin tags)
• Clavus (corn) or callus
• Molluscum contagiosum (MC)
• Squamous cell carcinoma

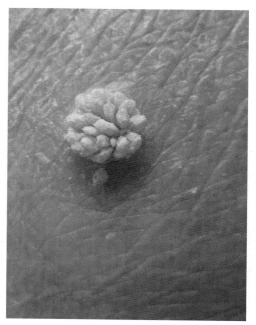

FIG. 10-2. Filiform wart.

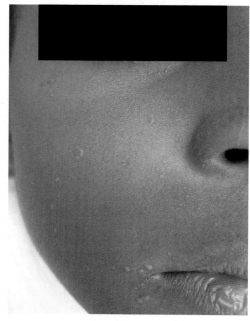

FIG. 10-3. Flat warts.

Diagnostics

Diagnosis is made on clinical appearance. Warts will always interrupt normal skin lines (dermatoglyphics; Figure 10-4), and usually, thrombosed capillaries can be seen (Figure 10-5). If not immediately apparent, a no. 15 blade can be used to lightly pare away hyperkeratotic debris from the surface of the lesion. When this is done, pinpoint black to red dots, which represent the thrombosed capillaries, will be revealed. This is considered a diagnostic sign and is not seen in other skin lesions with a similar clinical appearance.

Although seborrheic keratoses can have a very verrucous appearance, the presence of pseudohorn cysts (keratin deposits within the

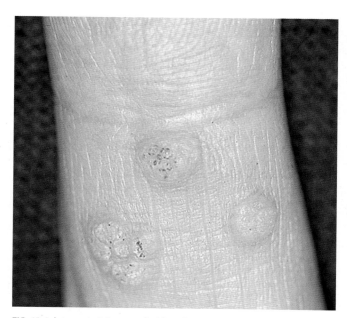

FIG. 10-4. Interrupted dermatoglyphics of warts.

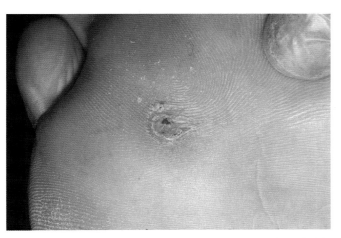

FIG. 10-5. Thrombosed capillaries after paring wart. This sign is pathognomonic.

thickened surface) on close examination can help to differentiate them from warts. Seborrheic keratoses are also often pigmented. Skin tags are soft, fleshy, pedunculated skin-colored papules that can have a clinical appearance similar to filiform wart, but will lack the characteristic finger-like projections on close examination.

A corn or clavus can commonly be mistaken for a wart because of its tendency to interrupt normal skin lines, but will not have the capillary dots when pared. Squamous cell carcinoma should be considered when lesions have irregular growth, ulceration, or are resistant to therapy, particularly when seen in sun-exposed areas or in immunosuppressed patients. Biopsy is not typically necessary, especially in nongenital lesions, but may be done in challenging cases to confirm the diagnosis.

Management

Warts are a benign skin condition, and spontaneously resolve in up to two thirds of patients, without treatment, within 1 to 2 years. Despite this, warts are a frequent reason for office visits and dermatology referrals. The majority of warts can be successfully treated in the primary care setting or even by the patient at home. The plan of care should be based on the clinical appearance, location, age, and the immune status of the patient. Clinicians should remember that verrucae do not necessarily need to be treated. Monitoring or no treatment is an acceptable option for the patient.

Treatment is indicated if the lesions are painful or interfere with function, and should be pursued before they multiply and while they are still small. Viruses cannot be seen, so even if the treated area appears normal, the virus may exist in the remaining tissues, and the wart may recur. All existing warts should be treated at the same time, if possible.

The goal of therapy is to remove the wart without leaving a scar. Current therapies are not wart specific, and the mechanisms of action in existing therapies are either destructive or immune-based. Therapies available are both over-the-counter and in-office treatment; both may take several weeks or months and recurrence is common. A Cochrane review of evidence-based studies showed that salicylic acid and cryotherapy are the two preferred treatment methods. Table 10-1 summarizes treatment options.

TABLE 10-1	First- and Second-line Treatment Options for Warts			
THERAPY	**ADVANTAGES**	**DISADVANTAGES**	**CONTRAINDICATIONS**	**COMMENTS**
First-line				
Salicylic acid (keratolytic)	Available over the counter, inexpensive, easy application, effective, including plantar warts or thick lesions, nonscarring	Macerates any skin where it is applied, reapplied if it gets wet, requires multiple applications, can cause tenderness	Peripheral neuropathy, peripheral artery disease, nonintact skin or erosions, pregnancy	Can be used in conjunction with cryotherapy
Cryotherapy (thermal destruction)	Effective in older children and adults, anesthesia is not necessary, great for warts on hands, safe in pregnancy and breastfeeding, fast, can treat multiple lesions and thick lesions	Painful, can result in hyper- or hypopigmentation especially on dark skin tones, caution should be used in the treatment of facial warts, requires multiple in-office treatment by clinician, which can be expensive and inconvenient	Cryoglobulinemia, cold agglutinins, cold urticaria	Treatment on fingers and toes (especially with freeze–thaw–freeze cycle) may cause hemorrhagic bullae which are benign, use caution on the digits and near nerves (severe pain and neuropathy), cautioned use in dark skin tones, treatment of periungual warts may result in nail deformity; see chapter 24 for instructions on use
No intervention	No cost or risk of pain or scarring, two thirds of warts spontaneously resolve within 1–2 years	Warts may grow or spread on self or transmission to others, psychosocial burden, pain, and bleeding especially on the hands and feet		Patient education regarding transmission and prevention of autoinoculation

(continued)

TABLE 10-1 First- and Second-line Treatment Options for Warts *(continued)*

THERAPY	ADVANTAGES	DISADVANTAGES	CONTRAINDICATIONS	COMMENTS
Second-line (not evidence-based)				
Duct tape (occlusive)	Inexpensive, easy to do at home, easy for children, pain-free	Can be difficult to keep tape on, effectiveness is uncertain		Cover with duct tape, leave on for 6 days, then soak and pare; leave uncovered overnight; then repeat cycle until resolved
Cimetidine (systemic immune modulator)	Available over the counter	Many possible drug interactions	See FDA recommendations	Mostly anecdotal reports
Cantharidin (blistering agent)	Painless at time of application, useful for multiple lesions and in young children, no scarring	In-office treatment only, blisters can cause discomfort, response varies, may need additional treatment with same or other modalities	Face or genital mucosa	Caution with use on digits, severe blistering can occur if applied incorrectly; see chapter 24 for instructions on use
Third-line: If no improvement with above therapies repeated over several months, consider referral to dermatology for more aggressive treatment				

Destructive therapies

Salicylic acid is generally first-line therapy and is available in liquid form, topical plasters, or patches and can be used by adults and children. It should be avoided in patients with peripheral neuropathy as the extent of tissue damage can go unnoticed and the risk for impaired healing may exist. The liquid forms come in two strengths, 17% (Occlusal HP, Duoplant, Compound W, Duofilm, and Wart-Off) and 27.5% (Virasal). These are used in children and on thinner warts in adults, allowing for easy application to multiple areas. However, lower-strength preparations may not be as effective in the treatment of thick or plantar warts. In these cases, more potent preparations containing 40% salicylic acid in plaster form (Mediplast or Duofilm patch) may be used. If treatment is performed in the office, a no.15 blade should be used by the clinician to pare down the thick keratotic layer prior to treatment in order to allow the medication to effectively penetrate to the infected tissue and hopefully shorten course of treatment.

Cryotherapy, using liquid nitrogen, is the most common in-office treatment of warts. This is useful in older children and adults, but poorly tolerated in young children because of the associated discomfort. Multiple treatments spaced about 2 to 4 weeks apart are typically required. Patients should also be instructed to use salicylic acid between treatments after the blister has resolved to aid in resolution.

Duct tape is a commonly used household remedy for warts; however, there is conflicting evidence to support its effectiveness. If desired, the silver brand of duct tape that is sticky enough to adhere to the skin is recommended. The goal is to keep the wart occluded with the duct tape as much of the time as possible and can be used in combination with salicylic acid for enhanced benefit.

Cantharidin liquid 0.7% is a topical destructive agent that is used by many providers in the office setting. Also known as cantharone, cantharidin is an extract of a blistering insect that is an effective treatment approach for children since the application process is pain-free. The patient can, however, develop pain when the treated sites evolve into blisters. Canthacur PS is a combination of cantharidin, podophyllin 5%, and salicylic acid 30%. This is a good choice for patients with multiple, thick plantar warts where deeper penetration is needed. Repeating treatments every 3 to 4 weeks may be required. Cantharidin is not currently approved by the U.S. Food and Drug Administration (FDA); however, it is on the FDA's proposed bulk substances list, which allows preparations containing cantharidin to be administered by providers in the office. See chapter 24 (Skills Section) for details on cantharidin application.

Immune-based therapies

There have been reports of the off-label use of oral cimetidine given in doses of 30 to 40 mg/kg/day being effective in the treatment of warts. This is thought to be due to its systemic immunomodulatory effects. Although this medication is available over the counter, caution should be used when recommending this treatment as there are multiple potential drug interactions associated with its use. The medication by itself is generally safe and well tolerated. Additional immune-based therapies, including topical agents and intralesional treatments, may be available for use by an experienced practitioner in a specialty setting.

Advanced therapies

Sometimes warts can be recalcitrant to common therapies. Advanced treatments or third-line therapies are available, but should be administered by an experienced dermatology provider. Other topical therapies are used effectively but are off label for use in the treatment of warts and include imiquimod cream, 5-fluorouracil, and squaric acid dibutylester. Surgical excision, ablative laser, curettage and desiccation, and snip or shave excision can be performed depending on patient circumstances and office setting. Some dermatology specialists use intralesional immunotherapy with candida antigen or bleomycin. These more aggressive therapies can have significantly higher risks for infection, scarring, and side effects, which should be discussed prior to the procedure with the patient.

Referral and Consultation

Patients with recurrent, recalcitrant, or clinically atypical lesions should be referred to a dermatologist for evaluation and treatment. For patients who do not respond to first- or second-line therapies, consider a referral to a dermatologist for more advanced treatment options.

Special Considerations

Immunosuppression. In general, warts of all types are more common and more difficult to treat in immunosuppressed patients. The clinical presentation may be different, making correct diagnosis of the lesion challenging. A referral to a dermatologist or for biopsy may be necessary.

Pediatrics: Treatment should be aimed at using the least painful methods and lowest potential for permanent side effects like scarring and dyschromia. More destructive methods should be reserved for the most difficult cases where scarring is not a consideration.

Pregnancy: Salicylic acid is a pregnancy category C medication and should not be used in pregnant patients due to the possibility of premature closure of the ductus arteriosus associated with its use. Cryotherapy is the treatment of choice in pregnancy.

Prognosis and Complications

Warts are self-limiting and will spontaneously resolve, most within 2 years. Warts that have been present for an extended period of time are less likely to resolve spontaneously. Emphasis should be placed on the fact that warts may take weeks to months to resolve, so that patients do not become discouraged and stop treating lesions at home prematurely. Also remind patients that recurrence is common and can be frustrating.

Patient Education and Follow-up

Education is particularly important for patients treating lesions at home. It is important to review with the patient that salicylic acid will destroy healthy skin as well as the wart, and that the medication should only be applied to the affected area and a few millimeters of surrounding skin to ensure complete treatment. Plain petrolatum can be applied to the normal skin surrounding the wart prior to treatment in order to prevent damage to normal skin.

Prior to treatment, it is also helpful to soak the area in warm water to help soften the skin and allow for better penetration of the medication. Plasters or patches are affixed to clean skin and kept dry for 2 to 3 days. The patch is then removed, the wart pared down with a nail file or pumice stone, and the process is repeated until the wart has resolved. It is important to instruct patients to follow these steps before reapplying the salicylic acid. It should be noted that whatever tool they are using at home to pare down the warts should be dedicated only for this purpose and should not be used elsewhere on the body, or by other members of the household to minimize autoinoculation or spreading of warts. Instruct the patient to use an electric shaver (not a razor) on warts in hair-bearing areas such as the face or legs. For plantar warts, avoid going barefoot through the house and disinfect the shower base with a diluted bleach solution after bathing. Be sure to wear sandals or shower shoes in public facilities or pools.

Follow-up is individualized and depends on the patient, the extent of the disease, and the treatment being utilized. If a wart is being treated by the practitioner within the office setting, reasonable follow-up is every 2 to 4 weeks.

MOLLUSCUM CONTAGIOSUM

MC is a self-limiting viral skin infection commonly seen in primary care. This challenging skin eruption can have tremendous psychosocial impact that drives patients to seek treatment for the infection. Patients, families, school and daycare facilities, and clinicians can become frustrated with attempts to eradicate MC.

Although MC is a common infection of childhood, it can occur in adolescents and adults. In adults, genital lesions are usually sexually transmitted. Anogenital lesions in children are usually spread through autoinoculation. Patient populations like those with atopic dermatitis or immunosuppression have a higher incidence of MC when compared to the general population.

Pathophysiology

MC is a large double-stranded DNA virus that consists of four closely related members of the poxvirus group. The virus contains unique genes that encode proteins and impairs the host's immune response and ability to fight the infection. MC is a localized, subacute viral infection of the epithelium that is spread by direct skin-to-skin contact, especially with wet or disrupted skin surfaces. Swimming or bathing with an infected person can increase the risk of transmission. It may also be spread by autoinoculation, sexual contact, shared clothing, and towels. The incubation period can range from 1 to 7 weeks.

Clinical Presentation

MC lesions typically present as 2- to 5-mm firm, skin-colored to pink, pearly dome-shaped papules with a central dell or umbilication (Figure 10-6). The dell may not be obvious but a soft white central core may be present. In children, the distribution may be generalized and can range from a few to more than 100 lesions. Common areas of involvement include the face, trunk, and extremities. Genital lesions can occur in up to 10% of childhood cases with widespread involvement. If the genitals are the only area affected, the possibility of sexual abuse should be considered.

Adults will typically have fewer than 20 MC lesions, commonly seen on the lower abdomen, upper thighs, and the penile shaft in men. Mucosal involvement is very uncommon; however, sexually transmitted lesions will occur in the anogenital region or pubis. In atopic patients, lesions will commonly occur in areas of dermatitis (Figure 10-7). Lesions seen in immunocompromised patients may be large, up to 1.5 cm, and known as *giant molluscum* or may be widespread with hundreds of lesions.

MC can spontaneously resolve in immunocompetent patients within about 2 months, and infection usually clears completely in several months. Lesions can become erythematous and swollen, which many believe is a sign of impending clinical resolution or the beginning of the end (BOTE) (Butala, Siefried, Weissler, 2013). Lesions may be pruritic or sometimes pustular. Molluscum dermatitis, a common phenomenon, is characterized by the

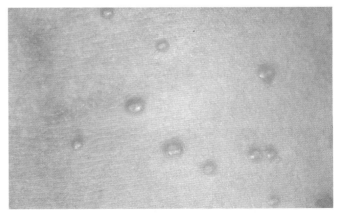

FIG. 10-6. Classic molluscum lesion.

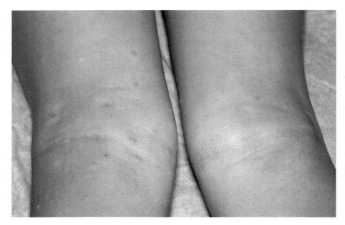

FIG. 10-7. Molluscum in atopic dermatitis.

development of eczematous patches or plaques surrounding the lesions. The dermatitis has been attributed to the localized reaction to the virus.

DIFFERENTIAL DIAGNOSES   Molluscum contagiosum
• Genital warts
• Folliculitis
• Keratosis pilaris
• Basal cell carcinoma
• Infectious processes such as cryptococcosis or histoplasmosis

Diagnostics

Diagnosis is clinically made by the characteristic appearance of the lesions. MC lacks the verrucous appearance of warts and presents as discrete lesions, whereas warts often coalesce into larger lesions. Solitary lesions or a giant molluscum that occurs on the face can be differentiated from basal cell carcinomas that typically present as a translucent skin-colored papule with telangiectasias and rolled borders.

Biopsy is not necessary but may be performed to confirm the diagnosis especially in the case of large lesions or extensive involvement. The virus itself cannot be cultured; however, bacterial culture may be needed if there is concern for secondary infection. If the central umbilication or dell is not obvious, a dermatoscope or magnifying lens may help identify the central core.

Confirmation can also be made in the office by gently curetting the white, central core from the lesion, placing it between two slides with a drop of potassium hydroxide (KOH). The slide is gently heated and then crushed with firm, twisting pressure. The contents from the central core contain most of the viral cells and can be directly examined with microscopy. *Molluscum bodies* appear as dark, round cells that disperse easily with slight pressure (Figure 10-8). Normal epithelial cells are flat, varied rectangular shapes, and tend to remain stuck together in sheets.

CLINICAL PEARLS
■ The central umbilication may not always be visible on clinical examination. Lightly spraying or touching the surface of the lesion with liquid nitrogen will often reveal this distinctive finding.
■ The umbilication will appear against the frozen white background and is a helpful diagnostic sign (Figure 10-9).

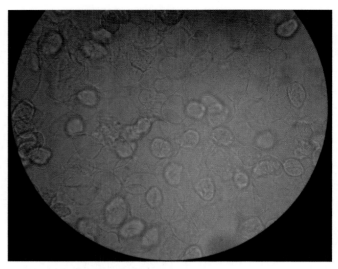

FIG. 10-8. Molluscum bodies on KOH prep.

Management

MC can ultimately resolve without any treatment. Therefore, the plan of care should be individualized to the patient. Consideration should be given to the patient's age, location of lesions, number of lesions, risk for scarring, risk for hyper- or hypopigmentation, and immune status. Treatment may be provided in order to prevent lesions from spreading to other areas on the body or transmission to others. All sexually transmitted lesions should be treated along with screening for other sexually transmitted infections. Further treatment indications include pruritus, secondary infection, surrounding dermatitis, or scarring.

Prior to treating MC, a full skin examination should be performed to identify any other lesions on the body. Incomplete treatment can result in autoinoculation and treatment failure. In cases where there is associated dermatitis or pruritus, the provider may consider treating the patient with a topical agent that will help to repair and maintain the epidermal barrier.

There are many additional treatment options available; however, a 2012 Cochrane review concluded that there is no evidence showing that one method is convincingly more effective than the others. Topical treatment is common and includes the use of cantharidin,

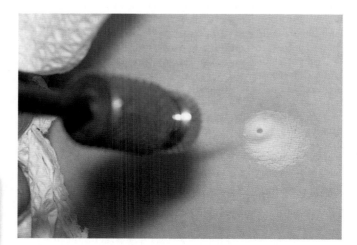

FIG. 10-9. Frozen molluscum. The central dell becomes apparent with light cryotherapy.

as discussed previously in the treatment of verruca. Since the application is painless, children are more cooperative, but painful blisters may follow application. Clinicians should consider testing 2 to 3 lesions initially to ensure that the patient does not have sensitivity to it.

Cryotherapy is a destructive method that can be used in primary care but has limitations due to the discomfort of the procedure, especially in children. Other therapies are geared toward removing the viral core of the MC. Curettage is a successful method used by experienced clinicians for treatment in children or adults with a limited number of lesions. Topical anesthetic cream (EMLA) can be applied 30 to 60 minutes prior to treatment to minimize the discomfort associated with the procedure. This method may also cause a small scar so the treatment site should be chosen carefully. Nicking the lesion with a no. 11 blade and sterile needle allows the removal of the central core and can be effective. Less invasive approaches include application of surgical or duct tape daily (after bathing) for 16 weeks, which can lead to a cure in up to 90% of children. Strong adhesives may cause a contact dermatitis.

Referral

In recalcitrant cases, generalized widespread lesions, or where immunosuppression is suspected or confirmed, referral to a dermatologist would be recommended. Treatment modalities that may be utilized in a dermatology setting include imiquimod, podophyllotoxin 0.5%, laser therapy, topical retinoids, trichloroacetic acid, and cidovir. Lesions located in the periocular region should be referred to an ophthalmologist for management.

Special Considerations

Immunosuppression: Patients may be referred to an infectious disease specialist for consideration of antiretroviral (ARV) therapy. Patients with extensive lesions should be tested for human immunodeficiency virus (HIV) and the possibility of other immune deficiency disorders should be considered.

Genital lesions: Should raise suspicion for other sexually transmitted infections.

Pregnancy: Curettage, cryotherapy, and incision with expression of the central core are all safe treatment options to use during pregnancy. *Podophyllin, podofilox, and imiquimod are all teratogenic and are contraindicated during pregnancy.*

Prognosis and Complications

MC is generally self-limiting and is not associated with malignancy. Complications include secondary infection and scarring as a result of treatment. In immunosuppressed patients, MC can be difficult to treat and may recur for years.

Patient Education and Follow-up

While it is not necessary to isolate the infected individuals, patients and parents of infected children should be educated on transmission-reducing methods. Children with MC should not be prevented from attending school or daycare. Lesions in areas that are likely to come in contact with others, such as those on the arms or legs, should be covered with clothing or a watertight bandage. Patient should be instructed to avoid scratching to prevent autoinoculation.

Infected children should not bathe with others, and towels should not be shared in order to prevent spread of infection. Sexual activity with affected individuals should be avoided until lesions are resolved. Condoms will not provide a barrier from areas commonly affected with MC. Patients with atopic dermatitis and a history of molluscum and/or flat warts can benefit from regular moisturizing with a preparation containing ceramides to protect the normal skin barrier and help prevent autoinoculation. The use of topical corticosteroids in these patients is controversial.

Follow-up and monitoring of patients with MC is dependent on the treatment modality used and the number of lesions on individual patients.

HERPES SIMPLEX VIRUS

Herpes simplex virus (HSV) is one of the most prevalent infections worldwide. It is estimated that about 90% of adults in the United States have HSV-1 antibodies. HSV infections are caused by two different human herpes virus types. HSV-1 is more prevalent than HSV-2 and is typically associated with oral herpes simplex infections (cold sores). HSV-2 is typically associated with genital herpes simplex infections. However, HSV-1 has been found in genital infections and HSV-2 in oral infections, presumably as a result of oral genital sexual contact, or autoinoculation. Genital HSV infections are discussed in chapter 21.

Pathophysiology

The human herpes virus is a double-stranded, linear DNA virus. HSV is a neurotropic virus that can be transmitted through respiratory droplets, direct contact with an active lesion, or contact with virus-containing fluid such as saliva or cervical secretions in patients with no evidence of active disease. The virus replicates at the site of inoculation and then travels along the dorsal root ganglion where it becomes dormant until reactivation. All persons infected with HSV-1 and HSV-2 infection are potentially infectious even if they have no clinical signs or symptoms. It has been estimated that up to 20% of adults may be shedding HSV at any given time. Individuals infected with one subtype of HSV can contract the other subtype. HSV infections which result in open sores will increase the risk of other infections, including HIV and sexually transmitted diseases.

HSV infection has two phases, the primary infection and the secondary phase. Most patients have no lesions or findings during the primary infection with HSV, when disease can only be detected by an elevated IgG antibody titer. During the primary infection, the virus becomes established in a nerve ganglion. When the patient has his/her first clinical lesion, this is usually a recurrence and represents the secondary phase. The risk of recurrence varies based on the virus type and site of infection. Various triggers can reactivate the virus and include, but are not limited to, sun exposure, stress, and physical trauma.

Clinical Presentation

Classic clinical presentation of HSV infection is characterized by grouped, uniform appearing vesicles on an erythematous base. These vesicles will then turn into pustules, umbilicate, and subsequently dry and form crusts on the skin, or exudate on mucous membranes. Presentation can vary based on factors such as anatomical location and immunosuppression. Clinical hallmarks of the latter include pain, an active vesicular border, and a scalloped periphery. Early vesicles may never be seen, lesions may appear as erosions or crusts, and presentation is often atypical in this population. The repeated appearance of a lesion at the same location should make the clinician suspicious for HSV.

Orolabial herpes

Although most patients have no lesions or findings during the primary infection with HSV-1, approximately 1% of patients will develop herpes gingivostomatitis. This presents as herpetic lesions on the oral mucosa, tongue, and tonsils, accompanied by flu-like symptoms. Oral lesions have an aphthous appearance with white or yellow exudate on a red base (Figure 10-10).Painful lesions can cause dehydration as a common complication. Patients can be acutely ill, and in severe cases may require treatment with intravenous antiviral therapy. If left untreated, symptoms can last approximately 1 to 2 weeks. Primary infection is usually associated with more constitutional symptoms, longer duration, and prolonged viral shedding when compared to recurrent episodes.

Recurrent orolabial herpes is primarily caused by HSV-1. This is commonly referred to as "fever blisters" or "cold sores." In many cases, there is a prodrome of tingling, itching, or burning that occurs 12 to 24 hours before cutaneous lesions appear. Clinical presentation consists of grouped vesicles over an erythematous base on the lips, commonly at the vermillion border (Figure 10-11). Lesions can also occur wherever the virus was inoculated or proliferated during the initial episode, such as inside the mouth, cheeks, eyelids, or earlobes. Vesicles evolve to form crusts within a few days. Other associated clinical symptoms can include local discomfort, headache, nasal congestion, and mild flu-like symptoms, including fever. Lymphadenopathy is frequent. Common triggers for orolabial herpes include UV exposure (especially UVB), surgical and dental procedures of the lips (including braces), stress, and other systemic viral infections.

Herpes gladiatorum

Herpes gladiatorum is the name given to the herpes infection which results from direct skin-to-skin exposure through contact sports. Wrestlers are especially at increased risk, and the condition can be a major problem during school tournaments and sports camps. It has been estimated that up to one third of wrestlers will become infected after a single match with an infected individual. Lesions will appear approximately 4 to 11 days after exposure and may be preceded by a 24-hour prodrome. Common sites of infection include the lateral neck, side of the face, forearm, and ocular region.

Herpetic whitlow

Whitlow is the term given to herpetic lesions that develop on the fingers and periungual area. This was a common clinical presentation in

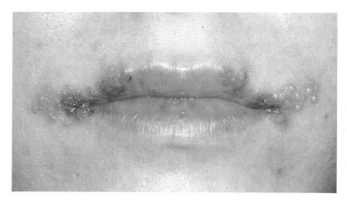

FIG. 10-11. Orolabial herpes.

health care workers and dentists prior to the introduction of universal precautions. It is no longer a common clinical presentation but is still seen, especially in children with orolabial herpes who autoinoculate by sucking their thumbs or biting their nails. Initial symptoms include tenderness and erythema of the nail fold or palmar surface with the development of deep-seated vesicles 24 to 48 hours after the prodrome (Figure 10-12).Presentation can vary from no visible vesicles to classic, grouped vesicles that may or may not form erosions.

Herpetic keratoconjunctivitis

Herpetic keratoconjunctivitis is the term given to describe HSV infections of the eye. Presentation can include unilateral conjunctivitis, blepharitis with vesicles on the lid, or punctate or marginal keratitis. Regional lymphadenopathy can also be seen. Recurrences are common and can lead to ocular ulcerations and corneal blindness. Patients should be immediately referred to an ophthalmologist.

Genital herpes

Genital herpes can be caused by either type of HSV, but primarily by HSV-2. Refer to chapter 21 for more detailed information on this topic.

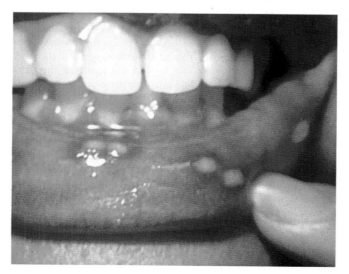

FIG. 10-10. Primary HSV infection. This patient has multiple erosions and gingivostomatitis.

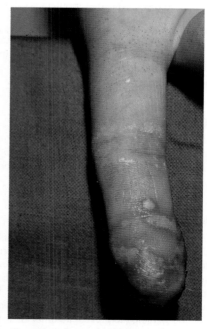

FIG. 10-12. Herpetic whitlow. Grouped pustules may be diagnosed as a bacterial infection. Recurrence at the same location is a clue to the diagnosis of HSV.

Eczema herpeticum

Eczema herpeticum is characterized by the acute development of herpetic lesions in sites of recent or active atopic dermatitis, occurring approximately 10 days after an exposure (Figure 10-13).There is associated lymphadenopathy and high fever. Secondary staphylococcal infection is a common associated clinical finding. Eczema herpeticum typically presents as a primary HSV infection, and recurrences are uncommon. The clinical course can range in presentation from mild to severe. Recurrent episodes are usually milder with fewer constitutional symptoms.

DIFFERENTIAL DIAGNOSES Herpes simplex virus

- Impetigo
- Aphthous ulcers
- Herpes zoster
- Herpetic whitlow
- Autoimmune blistering diseases

Diagnostics

Diagnosis can usually be made with a thorough history and physical examination. Impetigo, especially in children, may be mistaken for HSV. Vesicles appear straw colored and then crust in impetigo, and in HSV they follow a classic evolution from vesicles to umbilicated pustules to discrete crusts over an erythematous base. There is no prodrome of burning or tingling associated with impetigo.

Oral aphthae may be confused with HSV but typically appear on the anterior mouth and appear grayish in color. HSV typically manifests on the hard palate and attached gingiva, and is more erythematous. Herpes zoster is usually distinguished from HSV by the unilateral and dermatomal distribution. Herpetic whitlow is commonly confused with bacterial infections.

If confirmation of infection is required, viral culture can be performed preferably from early vesicular, crusted, eroded, or ulcerative lesions. It is considered a very specific and relatively rapid test. Positive results are often available in 48 to 72 hours. Sensitivity, however, may be as low as 25% to 50%. Only half of the true positives are available in 2 days. The rest may take 6 days or longer to be positive. In addition to culture, polymerase chain reaction (PCR) is also listed by the Centers for Disease Control and Prevention (CDC) as the preferred way to test for HSV infection as the assays are much more

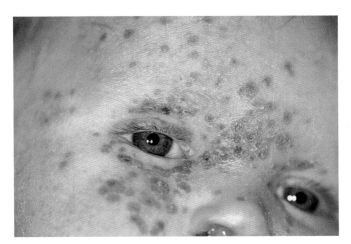

FIG. 10-13. Eczema herpeticum.

sensitive. In some cases, a biopsy may also be done and can detect viropathic changes and specific HSV antibodies. Serologic testing for diagnosis is generally not recommended.

CLINICAL PEARLS

- The repeated appearance of a lesion at the same location is an important clue for diagnosis of HSV.
- Any erosive mucocutaneous lesion in an immunocompromised patient should be considered HSV until proven otherwise.

Management

Management of HSV in the immunocompetent host is based on several factors, including the severity of the patient's symptoms, the presence of a primary or recurrent infection, site of the infection, and frequency with which the patient experiences recurrences. Careful consideration should be given to the patient's occupation, hobbies, and the cost of treatment.

Antiviral therapy used in the treatment of HSV is aimed at inhibiting DNA synthesis and include acyclovir, valacyclovir, and famciclovir. There are some differences between the medications.

Acyclovir

Acyclovir (Zovirax) is the most commonly used antiviral therapy in the world. It is the only FDA-approved drug in the treatment of HSV that can be used orally, topically, or intravenously. It is a pregnancy category B drug, is generally well tolerated, and is only contraindicated in patients with a hypersensitivity to the drug or any component of its formulation. It is not metabolized through the cytochrome P-450 pathway and therefore has very few interactions with other medications. Rare adverse effects include headache, nausea, and diarrhea. Acyclovir has the greatest in vitro activity against HSV-1 and HSV-2. However, it does not reduce the risk of recurrences over time.

In 2013, the FDA approved a new mucoadhesive buccal tablet (MBT) for use in immunocompetent individuals. It contains 50 mg of acyclovir, is indicated for recurrent orolabial herpes, and is a single-dose method. It should be used within 1 hour of the prodromal symptoms and before the appearance of clinical signs. The tablet is applied to the canine fossa, the area of the gum right above the incisor tooth, and will adhere to the gum. Please see package insert for complete instructions.

Valacyclovir and famciclovir

Valacyclovir (Valtrex) and famciclovir (Famvir) are both prodrugs. Valacyclovir is a prodrug of acyclovir, and famciclovir is a prodrug of penciclovir. Because of this, they have greater bioavailability and are dosed less frequently. The disadvantage is that they are also more expensive than acyclovir. Both drugs are pregnancy category B and have similar mechanism of action, pharmacokinetics, safety, and side effect profile as acyclovir. Indications for treatment in immunocompetent hosts are summarized according to clinical scenario. Table 10-2 lists specific dosing for antiviral medications for treatment of uncomplicated HSV in immunocompetent individuals 12 years of age and over.

Primary or initial infection

A symptomatic primary infection can have a duration of up to 2 weeks in untreated patients and can be complicated by systemic symptoms such as pharyngitis and odynophagia, which can result in dehydration. Treatment with oral antiviral therapy at the early stages of infection can help to shorten the duration of lesions, decrease the

TABLE 10-2	Oral Therapy for HSV Infections in Immunocompetent Patients
HSV INFECTION TYPE	**AGENTS AND DOSING**
Primary infection	Acyclovir: 400 mg t.i.d. for 10 days, or 200 mg 5 times daily for 10 days Valacyclovir: 1,000 mg b.i.d. for 10 days Famciclovir: 250 mg or 500 mg t.i.d. for 10 days
Initial recurrence	Acyclovir: 400 mg t.i.d. for 5 days Valacyclovir: 500 mg b.i.d. for 3 days Famciclovir: 125 mg b.i.d. for 5 days
Chronic suppression	Acyclovir: 400 mg b.i.d. Valacyclovir: 500 mg daily for <10 episodes/year, or 1,000 mg daily >10 HSV episodes/year Famciclovir: 250 mg b.i.d.
Episodic	Acyclovir: 200 mg or 400 mg taken 5 times daily for 5 days Valacyclovir: 2 g twice daily for 1 day Famciclovir: 750 mg twice daily for 1 day or 1,500 mg one single dose
Orolabial/herpes labialis	Acyclovir: (MBT) 50 mg single dose, use w/i 1 hr of prodrome Topicals: Docosanol 10% (Abreva); penciclovir 1% (Denavir); acyclovir 1% (Zovirax); acyclovir 5% and hydrocortisone 1% (Xerese) Oral famciclovir for recurrence: 1,500 mg as single dose Oral valacyclovir: 2 g and repeat in 12 hr

duration of odynophagia, reduce viral shedding, and lead to earlier cessation of fever. Initiation of antivirals should be within 72 hours clinical presentation in order to obtain the maximum benefit. Therapy is still considered when the patient is beyond the target 72-hour period but is continuing to develop new lesions or experiencing pain. Additionally, topical analgesics such as viscous lidocaine, benzocaine, and combination products may be used for painful lesions along with preparations that coat and protect lesions from irritants causing discomfort.

Recurrent infection

Patients will often have a recurrent infection that is minimally symptomatic and short in duration, making no treatment a perfectly acceptable option in this demographic.

The patient and clinician can decide on treatment of recurrences based on the individual frequency, severity, and associated clinical symptoms. There are multiple treatment strategies that may be used, including chronic suppression or episodic therapy.

Episodic treatment can be particularly helpful in patients who have infrequent recurrences and those who experience a distinct prodrome of symptoms. Oral antiviral therapy is started at the immediate onset of symptoms in order to reduce the duration and severity of outbreaks. Episodic treatment may also be used by patients prophylactically before planned exposure to an inciting trigger. Examples of this include patients who are about to undergo facial surgery, or those with anticipated excessive exposure to UV light (i.e., photodynamic therapy or natural sunlight).

Topical antiviral therapy, including topical acyclovir or penciclovir (Denavir), is used for episodic care. They are of modest benefit and require frequent application, up to five times per day. A combination product containing 5% acyclovir and 1% hydrocortisone (Xerese), applied 5 times a day for 5 days at the onset of symptoms, has been shown to be safe and effective in the treatment of early recurrent orolabial HSV. It reduces the frequency of both ulcerative and nonulcerative recurrences, and shortens the healing time when compared to topical acyclovir alone. Other topicals including benzalkonium chloride (Viroxyn) and docosanol (Abreva) may help to shorten healing time and duration of symptoms in some cases.

Chronic suppression therapy is useful for patients who have frequent (6 or more outbreaks per year) recurrences that are associated with systemic symptoms (erythema multiforme [discussed below], eczema herpeticum, or aseptic meningitis). Suppression therapy can also be used in patients who do not have specific prodromes and cannot accurately predict outbreaks. Although there are no specific guidelines on how long suppression therapy should be continued, the CDC recommends reassessing the need for ongoing therapy on a yearly basis. In many cases, the frequency of outbreaks decreases over time, and chronic suppression is eventually unnecessary. Caution the patient that there may be a risk of worsening outbreaks immediately following discontinuation. Antiviral therapy is considered safe for long-term use. Safety and efficacy have been documented among patients receiving chronic suppression therapy with acyclovir for as long as 6 years and with valacyclovir or famciclovir for 1 year.

Special Considerations

Athletes participating in contact sports, especially wrestlers, with a history of confirmed orolabial herpes should be on antiviral suppression therapy to decrease the risk of transmission to others. According to the NCAA rules, return to play requires all of the following:

- Oral antiviral medication (acyclovir, valacyclovir) for at least 5 days
- No new blisters or lesions for 72 hours
- Visible lesions must be covered with an impermeable dressing

Women frequently present with lesions of HSV on the buttocks. Assumption of recurrent episodes can be made if there is evidence of scarring or postinflammatory hyperpigmentation seen in the general area.

Immunocompromised and the elderly may have an atypical presentation, and be more severe, persistent, symptomatic, and resistant to therapy. Prophylactic systemic antiviral therapy is sometimes required in immunocompromised patients; however, antiviral resistance with prophylactic therapy can be a potential complication. In addition to immunocompromised patients, the elderly may also be at increased risk for infection and for major morbidity or mortality.

Neonates who are exposed at birth or who later show signs of HSV infection, as well as patients with *eczema herpeticum,* are considered a medical emergency and require hospitalization and IV antiviral therapy.

Prognosis and Complications

In healthy immunocompetent patients, primary HSV is typically a self-limiting condition and usually resolves within 2 weeks. Recurrent episodes respond well to treatment, but can vary in duration. Approximately 50% of cases of erythema multiforme are associated

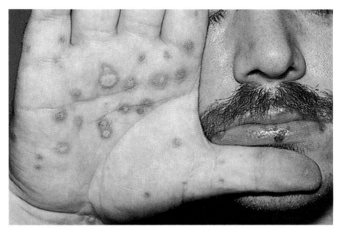

FIG. 10-14. HSV with erythema multiforme.

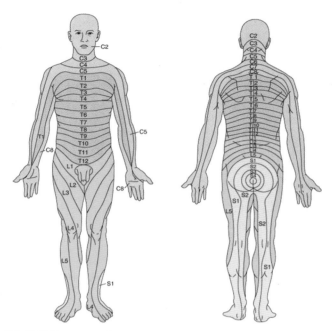

FIG. 10-15. Dermatome chart.

with a preceding HSV-1 or HSV-2 infection (Figure 10-14). Eczema herpeticum can be fatal in severe cases with associated *Staphylococcus aureus* septicemia, or viremia with infection of the internal organs. Other possible complications include herpes encephalitis, herpes pneumonia, aseptic meningitis, and herpes viremia. Herpes simplex infection has also been associated with Bell palsy.

Patient Education and Follow-up

Patients should be reassured and educated about the high prevalence of HSV to help reduce associated stigma. Education about prevention of disease transmission includes frequent hand washing and avoiding contact with immunocompromised individuals when they have active lesions. It is also important to discuss the chronicity of this infection. Patients with recurrent orolabial herpes should be educated about potential triggers, the effects of UV light, and the importance of sun protection to prevent outbreaks.

For primary infections and complicated cases, patients should be followed to insure resolution of lesions and systemic symptoms. In patients with uncomplicated recurrent disease, follow-up is on an as-needed basis.

HERPES ZOSTER

One out of three Americans will develop herpes zoster (VZV) or "shingles" during their lifetime. The unexpected skin eruption that may be accompanied by severe pain, burning, itching, and vesicles often prompts patients to seek health care from their primary care provider. Recognizing the signs and symptoms, which in some cases may be totally absent, is vital to early management to control the suffering and reduce complications from the infection. The incidence of VZV, as well as associated postherpetic neuralgia or PHN (discussed in Prognosis and Complications), dramatically increases with age. Before the age of 45, the incidence is less than 1 in 1,000 persons. In patients older than 75 years, the rate is more than four times greater and will occur in approximately 10% to 20% of the population.

Pathophysiology

VZV is caused by reactivation of the varicella virus in patients previously infected with chicken pox. The varicella virus enters the individual's dorsal root ganglia, where it remains latent in a process similar to HSV. The virus begins to replicate at some later time, traveling down the sensory nerve into the skin at the site of the associated dermatome (Figure 10-15).

VZV acquired from a patient with active varicella or zoster is rare. Zoster lesions do, however, contain high concentrations of the VZV that can be spread, presumably by the airborne route, and cause primary varicella in an exposed, susceptible individual.

Localized zoster is only contagious after the rash erupts and until the lesions crust. In general, zoster is less contagious than varicella. It is commonly thought that various factors play a role in the reactivation of the virus and include immunosuppression, medications, lymphoma, fatigue, stress, spinal surgery, radiation, and chemotherapy. Virus reactivation usually occurs only once in an individual's lifetime, and the incidence of a second reactivation in the same person is less than 5%.

Clinical Presentation

Cutaneous symptoms of VZV are usually preceded by a prodrome of one to several days of burning pain or itching in the affected area. Typically, a single dermatome is affected, but involvement may be seen in as many as three. Some patients may have up to 20 lesions outside the affected dermatome (Figure 10-16). The thoracic and lumbar dermatomes are the most frequently affected in VZV.

VZV characteristically presents as a unilateral group of vesicles, in a dermatomal distribution that does not cross the midline. Lesions will continue to erupt for several days, and may become pustular, hemorrhagic, necrotic, or bullous. After approximately 7 to 10 days, the lesions crust and are no longer considered infectious. The duration of lesions is dependent on the patient's age, severity of the eruption, and the presence of underlying immunosuppression. In rare cases, the patient may have pain in a dermatomal distribution, but no associated skin lesions ("zoster sine herpete"). In elderly patients, lesions may take up to 6 weeks or more to heal.

Disseminated herpes zoster

Disseminated VZV occurs when there are more than 20 lesions outside the affected dermatome. This phenomenon occurs chiefly

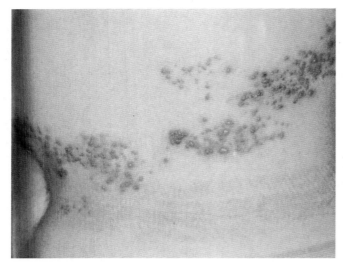

FIG. 10-16. Classic herpes zoster with fewer than 20 satellite lesions.

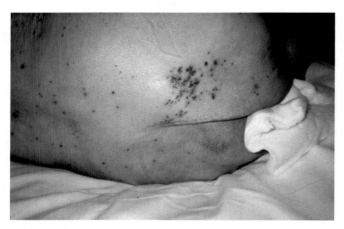

FIG. 10-17. Disseminated herpes zoster with more than 20 ungrouped satellite lesions. Note the initial dermatomal involvement on the buttock.

in elderly or debilitated individuals, especially in patients with lymphoreticular malignancy or acquired immunodeficiency syndrome (AIDS). The dermatomal lesions are sometimes hemorrhagic or gangrenous, and the outlying vesicles or bullae, which are usually not grouped, resemble varicella, and are often umbilicated or hemorrhagic (Figure 10-17). Involvement of the lungs and central nervous system may occur in the setting of disseminated zoster. Hospital admission should be initiated if this is suspected for careful evaluation, monitoring, and management.

Ophthalmic herpes zoster

Herpes zoster of the ophthalmic branch (V₁) of the trigeminal nerve (the fifth cranial nerve) is referred to as *ocular herpes zoster* or *herpes ophthalmicus or HZO*, and is a serious, sight-threatening condition. A prodrome of headache, malaise, and fever typically precedes a unilateral vesicular eruption along the trigeminal dermatome. Patients may also experience hyperemic conjunctivitis, episcleritis, and lid ptosis. Patients with suspected HZO require immediate evaluation by an ophthalmologist and treatment with systemic antiviral therapy. Approximately 50% of patients with HZO may develop

inflammation inside the eye or *uveitis*, which has an increased risk for complications of blindness, glaucoma, optic neuritis, encephalitis, hemiplegia, and acute retinal necrosis. Symptoms of uveitis include photosensitivity, pain, redness, and visual changes that occur about 1 to 3 weeks after the rash appears. The complications of HZO can be reduced from 50% to 20% to 30% with effective antiviral therapy started in the earliest stages. Ocular lesions of zoster and their complications tend to recur, sometimes as long as 10 years after the zoster episode.

> **DIFFERENTIAL DIAGNOSES** Herpes zoster
> - Herpes simplex
> - Contact dermatitis
> - Conjunctivitis

Diagnostics

Diagnosis is typically made based on the clinical appearance. HZO should be suspected in patients who develop vesicular lesions on the side and tip of the nose. This finding is known as the Hutchinson sign, and is associated with a high risk of HZO (Figure 10-18). The unilateral and dermatomal distribution of herpes zoster can help distinguish it from HSV. HSV lesions tend to be more uniform, and vesicles associated with shingles tend to vary in size. HSV is a recurrent condition, and herpes zoster typically only occurs once. Careful history taking can help to differentiate between the two. Herpes zoster of the hand can be particularly confusing and misdiagnosed as a contact dermatitis (e.g., poison ivy).

In circumstances where patients have an atypical presentation or diagnostic confirmation is required, viral culture may be sent. Additional testing is available and includes PCR testing and direct fluorescent antibody (DFA) testing; PCR can be used to detect VZV DNA rapidly and sensitively in properly collected skin lesion specimens. However, PCR testing for VZV is not available in all settings.

DFA staining is performed on a scraping from the base of the lesion. This test is rapid, and specific, but less sensitive, than PCR.

Management

The goal of therapy in the treatment of VZV is aimed at the following:

- Lessening the severity and duration of pain associated with the acute infection
- Promoting rapid healing of skin lesions
- Preventing new lesion formation
- Decreasing viral shedding
- Preventing the long-term complication of PHN

As in the treatment of HSV, the antivirals approved for the treatment of acute VZV infection include oral acyclovir, valacyclovir, and famciclovir. Oral antiviral therapy should be prescribed at the onset of symptoms and has been proven to decrease the duration of skin lesions, reduce acute pain, and decrease the incidence of PHN. Valacyclovir has proven to be more effective than acyclovir at decreasing the incidence of PHN and zoster associated acute neuritis. Oral antiviral treatment includes acyclovir 800 mg 5 times daily for 7 to 10 days; valacyclovir 1,000 mg t.i.d. for 7 to 10 days; and famciclovir 500 mg t.i.d. for 7 days.

It is highly recommended that primary care clinicians collaborate with ophthalmologist to manage HZO and determine the appropriate use of topical or systemic steroid therapy.

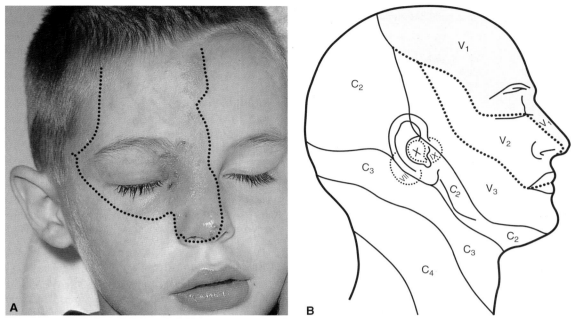

FIG. 10-18. **A:** Hutchinson sign. **B:** Note the involvement of the V_1 branch of the trigeminal nerve.

Special Considerations

The vast majority of patients have no underlying illnesses; however, for patients who experience one or more recurrences, or those who have longer than expected duration of symptoms, immunosuppression should be suspected. There is an increased incidence of VZV and PHN in the geriatric population. It occurs less frequently in children and may occur during pregnancy.

Pregnancy. Although pregnant women with maternal varicella are at risk for having babies with congenital varicella, maternal herpes zoster infection has not been associated with this complication. Transmission of herpes zoster to the fetus during pregnancy is rare. All of the aforementioned antivirals used in the treatment of herpes zoster are pregnancy category B and considered safe for use.

Pregnant women who have not been previously infected or vaccinated for chicken pox should be cautioned that exposure to someone with herpes zoster could cause a varicella infection. Susceptible women are at risk for developing a severe illness with varicella infection during pregnancy, and 10% to 20% of those may develop varicella pneumonia, which can be associated with significant maternal morbidity and mortality. Also, women who experience maternal varicella infection may have increased risk of fetal abnormalities and babies who develop herpes zoster during infancy. Women without evidence of immunity to varicella who have been exposed to the virus are advised to receive varicella-zoster immune globulin (VZIG) preferably within 72 to 96 hours after exposure.

Prognosis and Complications

The most common complications associated with VZV seen in primary care include PHN and secondary infection.

Scarring and postinflammatory hyper- or hypopigmentation is more common in elderly and immunosuppressed patients and correlate with the severity of the initial eruption. Other complications, including uveitis and keratitis, meningitis, motor neuropathy, and herpes zoster oticus (Ramsay Hunt syndrome—triad of ipsilateral facial paralysis, ear pain, and vesicles in the auditory canal and

auricle), have also been reported. All of these are less common than PHN and secondary infection.

The immunocompetent patients should experience complete resolution within 14 to 21 days.

Post herpetic neuralgia

PHN can affect approximately 10% to 15% of patients with herpes zoster. It is characterized by persistent pain lasting 4 or more months beyond the initial onset of cutaneous lesions. PHN can be divided into three different types:

- Constant, monotonous, usually burning or deep, aching pain
- Shooting, lancinating, or neuritic pain
- Triggered pain which is manifested as allodynia or hyperalgesia (increased sensitivity to pain)

PHN can be difficult to control especially in patients over 60 years old, who account for approximately 50% of the cases. Severe acute neuritis, severe rash, or history of prodromal symptoms can also increase the risk for development of PHN. Symptoms can range in severity from trivial to debilitating. Tricyclic antidepressants (TCA) such as amitriptyline 25 mg can be given at bedtime and are considered first-line therapy in the treatment of PHN. Lidoderm patch, gabapentin, and long-acting opiates may also be used. In some cases, symptoms are so severe that patients require referral to a pain clinic. Early intervention is optimal to minimize risk.

Zostavax

The zoster vaccine, Zostavax, is a live attenuated virus vaccine that is available for all eligible patients. See Box 10-1 for a summary of the indications and contraindications for Zostavax. There are some circumstances where vaccinating a patient who is immunocompromised may be warranted. For these patients, a heat-inactivated vaccine does exist and has been used. Although it will likely be less effective, it is a safer alternative than a live virus vaccine.

Zoster vaccination is not recommended for persons of any age who have received varicella vaccine. There is no specific time that you must wait after having shingles before receiving the shingles vaccine. The decision on when to get vaccinated should be made with your health care provider. Generally, a person should make sure that the shingles rash has disappeared before getting vaccinated.

Patient Education and Follow-up

Patients should be educated about disease transmission and instructed to avoid contact with susceptible persons at high risk for developing severe varicella in the household and occupational settings, until lesions are crusted. In addition, patients who are at high risk for developing VZV, especially the elderly, should be informed about how to recognize the signs and symptoms to aid with early detection and treatment. It is the provider's responsibility to counsel patients about the indications and encourage them to get the vaccine.

Follow-up is based on the duration and severity of symptoms and should be individualized for each patient.

ACUTE HUMAN IMMUNODEFICIENCY VIRUS

The Human Immunodeficiency Virus (HIV) has existed in the United States since at least the mid- to late 1970s and is believed to have originated from chimpanzees in West Africa. The Joint United Nations Programme on HIV/AIDS (UNAIDS) reports that about 33.3 million people worldwide are infected with HIV. Of the infected, about 22.5 million are inhabitants of sub-Saharan Africa.

As of this writing, the CDC 2011 surveillance report is the most current estimate of HIV infection in the United States. It was estimated that 1.2 million persons were living with HIV. Between 2008 and 2011, the actual number of new HIV cases remained fairly stable, with a small decrease among women. The highest burden for disease continues among African Americans and men who have sex with men (MSM) between the ages of 13 to 29.

According to the CDC, the majority of the economic burden of HIV in the United States comes from the medical care calculated to cost $379,668 for an individual with HIV in 2010.

Pathophysiology

HIV is a retrovirus and therefore carries a positive-stranded RNA and a DNA polymerase enzyme called reverse transcriptase. Once the virus attaches to the protein receptor site on the $CD4^+$ T lymphocyte, reverse transcriptase converts the viral RNA to DNA and becomes part of the host genome. New viral particles are then produced during normal cellular division, and the $CD4^+$ T lymphocytes are destroyed. A repetitive cycle of immune activation and reinfection leads to a progressive immunodeficiency, known as Autoimmune Deficiency Syndrome (AIDS), and eventually death (Figure 10-19).

Clinical Presentation

The skin findings in HIV can be classified into three broad categories: infections, pruritic eruptions, and neoplasms. This chapter will focus primarily on the pruritic eruptions, and the neoplasm Kaposi sarcoma (KS). There are multiple other skin conditions seen in HIV, with muco-cutaneous symptoms occurring in about 90% of patients affected by the virus. Although most of the skin conditions associated with the infection are not pathognomonic for HIV, they can provide important clues regarding immune status and underlying disease. This underscores the important role of the healthcare providers in the early detection, initiation of treatment, and prevention of disease related complications.

Primary infection/acute retroviral syndrome

The incubation period after initial infection is estimated to be approximately 3 to 6 weeks. Temporary flu-like symptoms, known as acute retroviral syndrome (ARS), are characterized by fever, myalgias, arthralgias, pharyngitis, and a diffuse, polymorphic erythematous, maculopapular eruption on the trunk (50%–70%) (Figure 10-20). Roseola-like or morbilliform lesions can appear on the upper body or face, and papulosquamous lesions on the palms and soles. Mucocutaneous lesions that appear similar to but larger than oral apthae may also be present.

Acutely infected patients are highly contagious during this stage of infection because the concentration of virus in plasma and genital secretions is extremely high. The skin eruption typically resolves spontaneously within 4 to 5 days, and systemic symptoms will spontaneously resolve within days to weeks, but in some cases may last up to 10 weeks. Seroconversion may take place within 1 week to 3 months, and there is a subsequent dramatic decline in viremia. The CD4+ T cells remain at a normal level of more than 500 per mm³, and the patient is without symptoms.

HIV-associated pruritus

HIV-associated pruritus is typically associated with a papular eruption which may be follicular or nonfollicular.

Follicular eruptions

Eosinophilic folliculitis (EF) is the most common pruritic follicular eruption seen in HIV; however, since the introduction of highly active retroviral therapy (HAART), it has become less common. It typically manifests in patients with a helper T-cell count below 250 cells per mL. Clinically, patients present with urticarial, follicular papules on the upper trunk, face, scalp, neck, which extend down the midline of the back to the lumbar region. Figure 10-21. Lesions

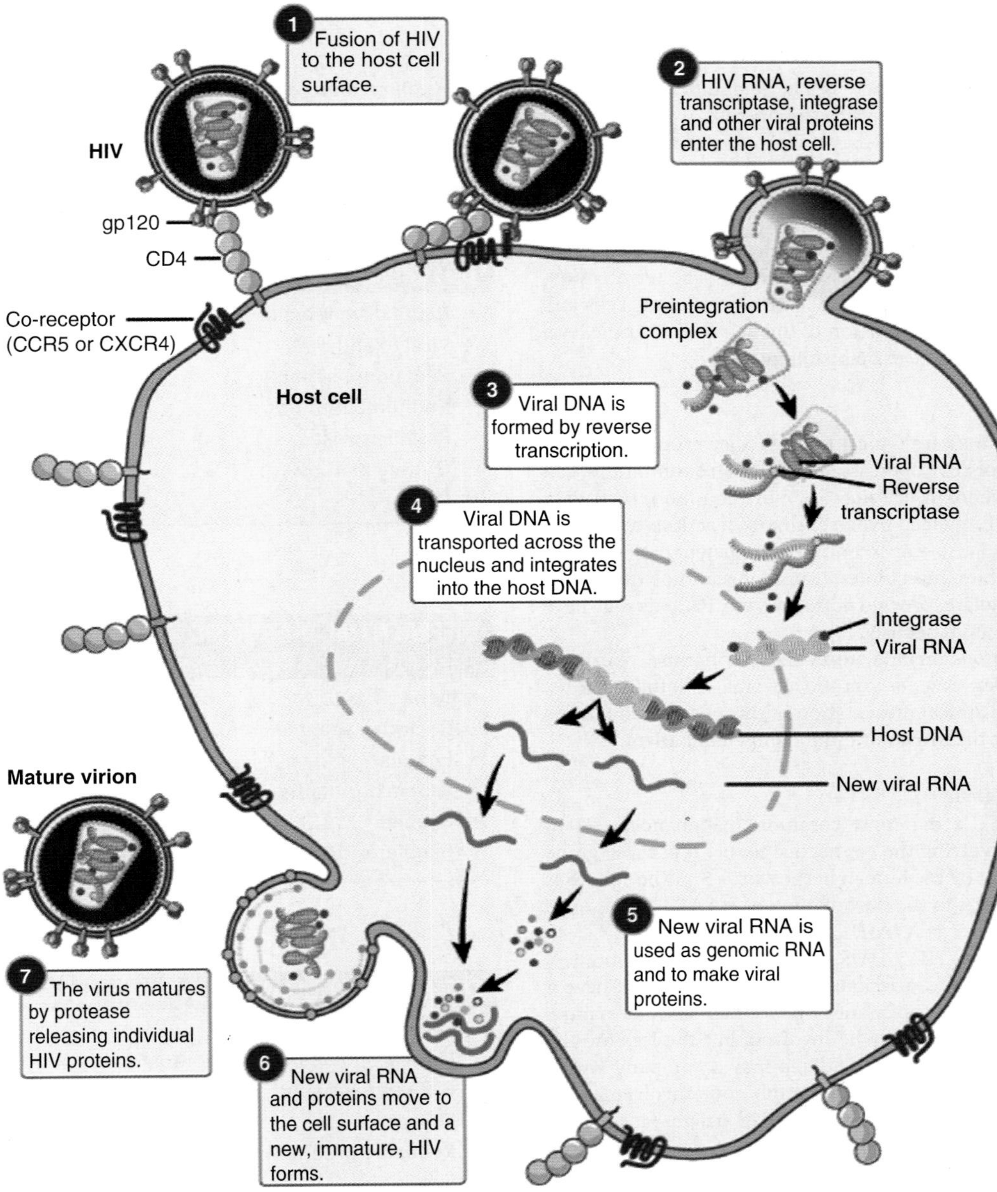

1 Fusion of HIV to the host cell surface.
2 HIV RNA, reverse transcriptase, integrase and other viral proteins enter the host cell.
HIV
gp120
CD4
Co-receptor (CCR5 or CXCR4)
Host cell
Preintegration complex
3 Viral DNA is formed by reverse transcription.
Viral RNA
Reverse transcriptase
4 Viral DNA is transported across the nucleus and integrates into the host DNA.
Integrase
Viral RNA
Host DNA
New viral RNA
Mature virion
5 New viral RNA is used as genomic RNA and to make viral proteins.
7 The virus matures by protease releasing individual HIV proteins.
6 New viral RNA and proteins move to the cell surface and a new, immature, HIV forms.

FIG. 10-19. HIV virus replication cycle.

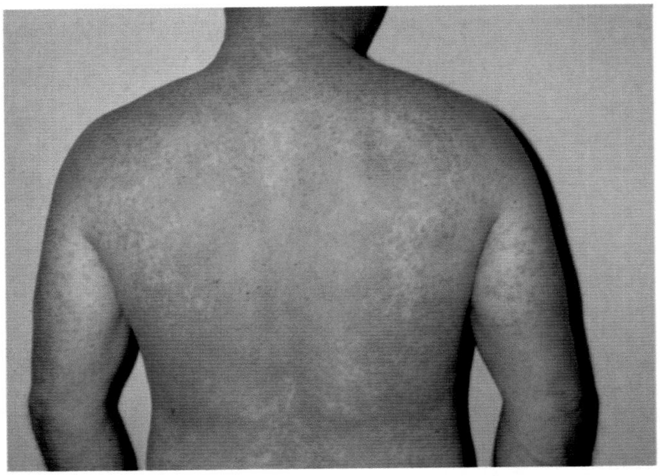

FIG. 10-20. Primary HIV infection. Acute HIV infection with associated morbilliform rash.

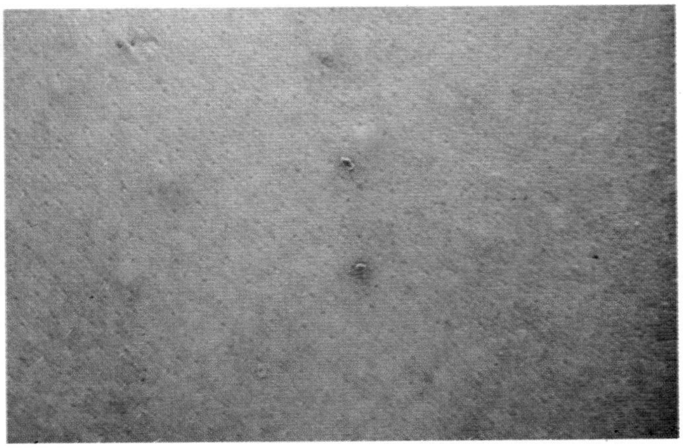

FIG. 10-21. HIV-associated EF.

typically occur in areas where there is a large number of sebaceous glands. Pustular lesions are rare since the pruritus is so severe that lesions become excoriated before they can progress to form pustules.

EF has a characteristic presentation of intense, intractable pruritus. The eruption has varying degrees of severity, and may spontaneously clear, only to flare unpredictably. A peripheral eosinophilia may be present and the serum IgE level may be elevated in about 25% to 50% of patients with HIV-associated EF. The term *eosinophilic folliculitis* arises from the presence of mononuclear cells and eosinophils around the upper portion of the hair follicle at the level of the sebaceous gland and seen on histology.

Nonfollicular eruptions

Hypersensitivity reactions are typical nonfollicular eruptions resulting from insect bites or arthropod assaults. These are commonly seen in temperate areas where insect bites are more common, such as in sub-Saharan Africa. Enhanced hypersensitivity reactions are simply a more exuberant response seen in immunocompetent patients. This can be seen with scabies, insect bites, transient acantholytic dermatosis, granuloma annulare, prurigo nodularis, etc. Patients may have multiple eruptions simultaneously.

Eczematous eruptions include atopic-like dermatitis, seborrheic dermatitis, nummular eczema, xerotic eczema, photodermatitis, and drug eruptions. Clinical presentation in this population may be much more dramatic than in an immunocompetent patient.

HIV-associated neoplasia

Kaposi Sarcoma (KS) is the most common malignancy seen in patients with HIV, involving the connective tissue. It is a low-grade vascular tumor caused by the human herpes virus 8. Although KS is not as common now due to the introduction of HAART, it was once considered a harbinger of HIV/AIDS.

KS in patients with HIV/AIDS often presents with numerous, symmetrical, widespread lesions. Papules and plaques have a purplish-brown or reddish appearance due to their vascular nature. Any mucocutaneous surface may be involved, but the legs are the most common area affected (90%). Edema may accompany lower-leg lesions, and can be associated with lymph node involvement in the inguinal area. It may also involve the hard palate, face, trunk, palms, soles, and penis (Figure 10-22A, B). KS can metastasize to other organs such as the lungs or gastrointestinal tract.

Not all patients with KS have HIV infections. Organ transplant recipients who are immunosuppressed are at an increased risk for

KS. Another more classic form of KS is typically seen in elderly Mediterranean men (especially Italian and Jewish descent) and has different clinical features. In classic KS, asymptomatic pink macules grow to become red to brown papules.

DIFFERENTIAL DIAGNOSIS Acute retroviral syndrome

- Acute drug reaction
- Viral exanthems
- Secondary syphilis
- Erythema multiform
- Pityriasis rosea
- Guttate psoriasis
- Urticaria

DIFFERENTIAL DIAGNOSIS HIV-associated eosinophilic folliculitis

- Acne
- Bacterial, yeast, steroid folliculitis
- Pustular psoriasis
- Atopic dermatitis
- Scabies
- Papular urticaria and drug eruption

DIFFERENTIAL DIAGNOSIS Kaposi sarcoma

- Dermatofibroma
- Dermatofibrosarcoma protuberans
- Bacillary angiomatosis
- Purpura
- Pyogenic granuloma
- Insect bites
- Nevi

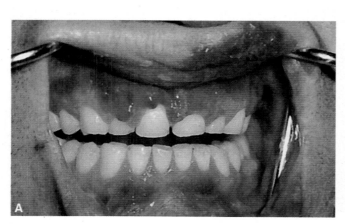
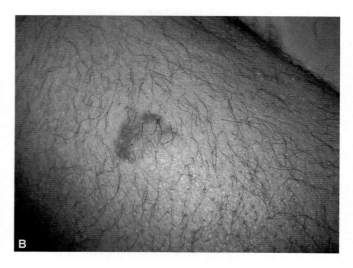

FIG. 10-22. Kaposi sarcoma.

Diagnostics

The goal of HIV testing is the early identification of individuals in the highly infectious phase of acute HIV infection. The current HIV diagnostic algorithm consists of a repeatedly reactive immunoassay (IA), followed by a confirmatory test, such as the Western blot (WB) or indirect immunofluorescence assay (IFA). Because current laboratory IAs detect HIV infection earlier than supplemental tests, reactive IA results and negative supplemental test results, very early in the course of HIV infection, have been erroneously interpreted as negative. The current laboratory diagnostic algorithm for HIV cannot detect acute infections and misclassifies approximately 60% of HIV-2 infections as HIV-1, based on HIV-1 WB results.

The CDC and many health departments recognize this problem and have proposed a new diagnostic algorithm which replaces the WB with an HIV-1/HIV-2 antibody differentiation assay as the supplemental test and includes an RNA test to resolve the dilemma created by a reactive IA and a negative supplemental test result if that should occur.

In retrospective studies, this algorithm performed better than the WB at identifying HIV-antibody-positive persons, detecting acute HIV-1 infections, and diagnosing unsuspected HIV-2 infections.

Management

Health care providers and public health officials should work to ensure that (1) sexually active, HIV-negative MSM are tested for HIV at least annually (providers may recommend more frequent testing, e.g., every 3 to 6 months); (2) HIV-negative MSM who engage in unprotected sex receive risk-reduction interventions; and (3) HIV-positive MSM receive HIV care, treatment, and prevention services. Reducing the burden of HIV among MSM is fundamental to reducing HIV infection in this country. The CDC website (www.cdc.gov) should be consulted for the latest recommendation.

Prophylaxis

Pre-Exposure (PrEP) is a new HIV prevention method, in which people who do not have HIV are treated with a daily dose of antiviral medications. When used consistently, PrEP has been shown to reduce the risk of HIV infection among adult men and women at very high risk for HIV infection through sex or injection of drugs.

Post-Exposure (PEP) is the use of antiretroviral drugs (ARV) drugs after a single high-risk event to stop HIV replication and spread throughout the body. PEP must be started as soon as possible to be effective—and always within 3 days of a possible exposure.

Follicular eruptions

EF is initially treated with topical corticosteroids and antihistamines. If the patient fails to respond, phototherapy (UVB or PUVA) or itraconazole (200 mg twice a day) may be effective. In some patients, repeated applications of permethrin (every other night for up to 6 weeks) may be of benefit. The use of permethrin is aimed at treating *Demodex* mites, which may be a trigger of this condition. Isotretinoin is also effective, often after a few months, in a dose of about 0.5 to 1 mg/kg/day. HAART may lead to a flare of EF, but usually resolves. Treatment of the nonfollicular eruptions is determined by the diagnosis and is similar to the treatment of these same dermatoses in persons without HIV infection.

Nonfollicular eruptions

Hypersensitivity and eczematous reactions can be treated with the traditional remedies of antihistamines, emollients, and topical corticosteroids.

Kaposi sarcoma

Treatment of KS is not curative, but can provide resolution of symptoms in most patients. The initiation of HAART has resulted in the involution of the lesions within 6 months in 50% of cases. This should be the initial management in most patients with mild-to-moderate disease (fewer than 50 lesions, and fewer than 10 new lesions/month). Other modalities of treatment are dependent on the CD4 cell count, as well as the number and extent of the lesions. Chemotherapy may be used intralesionally or systemically. Radiation, laser, and cryotherapy have all been used effectively, but the patient should be cautioned that the lesions may return.

CLINICAL PEARL

- Extreme worsening or sudden development of severe seborrheic dermatitis or psoriasis may be a presenting sign of HIV infection.
- The diagnosis of HIV should be suspected in any at-risk individual with the correct constellation of symptoms, prolonged or recalcitrant infections of unknown cause.

Referral

Patients with acute HIV infection should be referred immediately to an HIV clinical care provider to maximize treatment modalities and to help prevent the transmission of disease to others. There are many HIV clinics that have improved access and affordability of care for patients with HIV; however, they may be regionally located, which can be challenging for some patients. Referral to an infectious disease specialist, immunologist, oncologist, surgeon, and/or dermatologist should be considered as needed based on the clinical course and the provider's comfort level with specific therapies. Some patients require referral for specific behavioral interventions (e.g., a substance abuse program), mental health disorders (e.g., depression), or emotional distress. Diagnosis of an STD in an HIV-infected person indicates ongoing or recurrent high-risk behavior and should prompt referral for counseling. Management of infants, children, and adolescents who are known or suspected to be infected with HIV requires referral to physicians familiar with the manifestations and treatment of pediatric HIV infection.

Special Considerations

Pregnancy. According to the NIH, women in the United States should be tested for HIV infection as early during pregnancy as possible. A second test during the third trimester, preferably at <36 weeks gestation, should be considered, and is recommended for women known to be at high risk for acquiring HIV. Rapid HIV antibody testing at the time of labor or delivery should be performed on women with undocumented HIV status, and intrapartum ARV prophylaxis should be initiated in those who test positive. Breastfeeding should be avoided until results are available.

Prognosis

The cutaneous manifestations associated with primary HIV infection and ARS usually resolve spontaneously without treatment. Current HAART therapy helps to maintain a strong immune system, slow progression of HIV infection and transmission and reduces patient risk for secondary infections, which is the leading cause of death for patients with AIDs.

The initiation of HAART has resulted in the involution of Kaposi lesions within 6 months in 50% of cases. The overall prognosis of

KS depends largely on the initial clinical presentation, the presence or absence of nodal involvement, and histologic pattern. In both the immunosuppressed and the classic type of KS, the malignancy is slow growing and usually stays localized but does have a risk for metastasis.

Patient Education and Follow-up

Nonjudgmental prevention counseling and a review of methods and behaviors that lead to transmission should be initiated in any at-risk individual or persons seeking HIV testing. Patients on HAART should be educated on the importance of taking all medications as prescribed. Drug resistance can develop, especially in patients who are noncompliant with medications, and is the most common cause of treatment failure. Patients infected with HIV should also be educated about the importance of monitoring for any signs and symptoms of disease progression or associated complications and instructed to seek prompt care as necessary.

Patient monitoring and follow-up should be determined based on the patient's clinical status. Regular health screening every 3 to 4 months should include a thorough physical examination, complete review of systems, age-appropriate screening exams, CD4 counts, and viral load evaluation.

BILLING CODES ICD-10

Herpes simplex virus	B00.9
Herpes zoster without complications	B02.9
Herpes zoster ophthalmicus	B02.39
Human immunodeficiency virus	B20
Kaposi sarcoma, skin	C46.0
Molluscum contagiosum	B08.1
Wart, flat	B07.8
Wart, plantar	B07.0
Wart, viral	B07.9

READINGS

Butala, N., Siegfried, E., & Weissler, A. (2013). Molluscum BOTE sign: A predictor of imminent resolution. *Pediatrics. 131*(5), e1650–e1653.

Bolognia, J. L., Jorizzo, J. L., & Rapini, R. P. (2012). Cutaneous manifestations of HIV, human papillomaviruses, human herpesvirus and other viral diseases. *In Dermatology* (3rd ed., pp. 1285-1343). China: Elsevier Saunders.

Catron, T., & Hern, H. G. (2008). Herpes zoster ophthalmicus. *The Western Journal of Emergency Medicine, 9*(3), 174–176.

Habif, T. P. (2010). Warts, herpes simplex, and other viral infections. In *Clinical dermatology: A color guide to diagnosis and therapy* (5th ed., pp. 455–490). China: Mosby Elsevier.

CDC. (2010, December 17). Sexually transmitted diseases treatment guidelines. *Morbidity and Mortality Weekly Report Recommendations and Reports, 59*(12).

CDC. (2013, November 29). HIV testing and risk behaviors among gay, bisexual, and other men who have sex with men—US. *Morbidity and Mortality Weekly Report Recommendations and Reports, 62*(47), 958–962.

Hull, C. M., & Brunton, S. (2010). The role of topical 5% acyclovir and 1% hydrocortisone cream (Xerese™) in the treatment of recurrent herpes simplex labialis. *Journal of Postgraduate Medicine, 122*(5), 1–6.

Ivyanskiy, I., & Thomsen, S. F. (2013). Cutaneous viral disease in HIV infection [Review]. *Skinmed: Dermatology for the clinician, 11*(1), 33–37.

James, W. D., Berger, T. G., & Elston, D. M. (2011). Viral diseases. In *Andrews' diseases of the skin: Clinical dermatology* (11th ed., pp. 361–413). China: Mosby Elsevier.

Klein, R. S. (2012). Treatment of herpes simplex virus type 1 infection in immunocompetent patients. In: UpToDate, Post TW (Ed), UpToDate, Waltham, MA. (Accessed on May 19, 2013.)

Kwok, C. S., Gibbs, S., Bennett, C., Holland, R., & Abbott, R. (2012, September 12). Topical treatments for skin warts. *Cochrane Review. The Cochrane Library.org.*

Riley, L. E. (2013, July 29). Varicella-zoster virus infection in pregnancy. *UpToDate. com.*

Stulberg, D. L., & Hutchinson, A. G. (2003, March 15). Molluscum contagiosum and warts. *American Family Physician, 67*(6), 1233–1240.

Van Der Wouden, Johannes et al. (2012). Interventions for cutaneous molluscum contagiosum. *Cochrane Review, Vol 4. The Cochrane Library.org. American Family Physician, 67*(6), 1233–1240

Wolverton, S. E. (2012). *Comprehensive dermatologic drug therapy* (4th ed.). Philadelphia, PA: Saunders Elsevier.

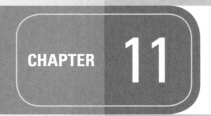

CHAPTER 11 Benign Neoplasms

Kathleen Haycraft

Practitioners must be familiar with the normal before they are capable of identifying the abnormal. Essential dermatology knowledge and skills are imperative to diagnose benign lesions and to prevent both over diagnoses and misdiagnoses. Proper evaluation and diagnosis of any lesion can be key to identifying underlying systemic disease.

Patients often seek advice from their primary care provider for the evaluation and treatment of skin lesions. Some are concerned about malignancy, while others are distressed by their cosmetic appearance or symptoms. This chapter addresses benign neoplasms that are common. Despite reassurance that they are benign, many patients wish to have these lesions removed. The desire to treat benign lesions needs to be balanced with the potential for undesirable cosmetic outcomes.

The management and follow-up care for most benign neoplasms are similar unless noted otherwise in the topic discussion. Diagnosis of common neoplasms is usually a clinical one unless there are any suspicious features concerning to the clinician. If a biopsy is indicated, the appropriate technique should be selected based on the type, number, and location of the lesions. Once a diagnosis is made, management options should be discussed in detail with the patient. Clinicians should consider many variables about the patient and disease when performing elective procedures to remove lesions.

Patient education regarding benign lesions is always important and should emphasize the signs and symptoms of skin cancer, including sudden changes or the development of abnormal features. Symptoms of sudden and irregular growth, ulceration, pain, bleeding, or red or blue color changes should prompt the clinician to reevaluate the lesion and perform a biopsy as indicated. Although most diagnoses and management of benign lesions can be done by primary care, collaboration or consultation with a dermatologist may be considered. Clinicians who are unsure of the diagnosis, have difficulties with biopsy interpretation, or are inexperienced in procedural skills for treatment or removal should make a referral to a dermatologist.

SEBORRHEIC KERATOSIS

Seborrheic keratosis (SK) is the most common benign cutaneous tumor. They are associated with senescence and have some genetic correlation. Synonyms include seborrheic verruca and senile warts. The plural of SK is seborrheic keratoses.

Most individuals will have at least one SK in their lifetime. Seborrheic keratoses occur at any age; however, the frequency increases in the mid- to later decades of life. They are one of the most common reasons that prompt individuals to seek evaluation for a suspicious skin lesion. There is no gender preference and reduced prevalence in darker skin. SK may occur after an erythrodermic drug eruption, erythrodermic psoriasis, or exfoliative erythroderma.

Pathophysiology

The exact cause of SK is not known. Although frequently referred to as "wart-like lesions," SKs are not related to a virus. They have been linked to mutations in the FGFR3 and P13K genes. Changes occur in the epidermis and are associated with histologic evidence of proliferation of the basal keratinocytes with associated apoptosis.

Clinical Presentation

SKs have a wide range of appearances and can occur anywhere on the body. They are primarily distributed on the face, chest, back, and arms. The color of SKs can range from tan to dark brown or even black, which can mimic the appearance of melanoma. The most common history and presentation is a slow-growing, waxy, and rough-textured plaque that crumbles. Older generations often referred to them as "barnacles" as they can sometimes be scraped off. In the early stages of development, the lesion may be small and smooth, whereas in the later stages, SKs may become elevated, enlarged, and darker in color. Some have a wart-like appearance due to the presence of keratin that deposits, called horny pearls or pseudocysts. Typically, SKs are asymptomatic but can become extremely pruritic and irritated, especially in areas of friction such as the inframammary folds or the bra area.

Due to the variety of clinical presentations, it can be difficult to differentiate an SK from a benign wart or malignant nodular melanoma. Therefore, careful examination of SKs is important so that benign lesions are not unnecessarily biopsied and possible malignant neoplasms are not overlooked. In some rare cases, melanoma can arise in an established SK. The patient may report a new onset of itching, bleeding, pain, or color changes, which should not be disregarded even if the lesion has been present for years.

It can be helpful to use an otoscope or dermatoscope to gain a closer visual examination of the lesion. Subtypes of SKs can have classic features that provide diagnostic clues (Figure 11-1).

- *Dermatosis papulosa nigra* is a subtype of SK that occurs in skin of color, primarily on the face and at an earlier age. The dark brown papules vary in size from pinpoint to a few millimeters.
- *Stucco keratoses* (barnacles) are subtypes of SK that are numerous light brown to white in color scaly papules that are distributed on the tibia, ankle, and feet. Stucco keratoses have an appearance of being "stuck on." They are more frequent in Caucasians and exacerbated by excessive UVR exposure.
- *Pigmented SKs* occur as the proliferating keratinocytes trigger neighboring melanocytes, resulting in increased melanin in the SK and resultant darker appearance.
- *Reticulated SKs* are seen on sun-exposed skin and visibly have a variation in color and ridge patterns. They have been postulated to develop from solar lentigo.
- *Cerebriform SKs* appear to have sulci and ridges similar to the brain.
- *Multiple SKs* may interfere with the examiner's ability to identify underlying cutaneous malignancies.

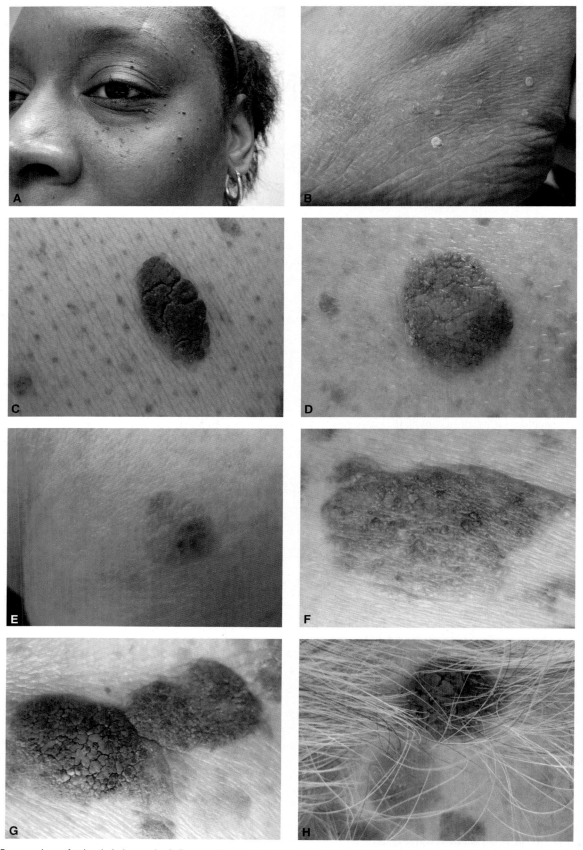

FIG. 11-1. Presentations of seborrheic keratosis. **A:** Dermatosis papulosa nigra. **B:** Stucco keratoses commonly found on the ankle. **C:** Pigmented seborrheic keratosis. **D:** Cerebriform seborrheic keratosis. **E:** Reticulated seborrheic keratosis. **F:** Pseudocysts or horny pearls of seborrheic keratosis. **G:** Dark brown to black seborrheic keratosis often concerning patients for skin cancer. **H:** Seborrheic keratosis of the scalp can appear differently due to the hair follicles.

- Actinic keratosis
- Basal cell carcinoma (especially pigmented)
- Squamous cell skin carcinoma
- Melanoma
- Wart
- Intradermal nevus
- Sebaceous nevus
- Prurigo nodularis
- Acrochordon/skin tag

Management

SKs are benign and do not require treatment. Patients may request treatment for cosmetic reasons or for symptomatic relief from pruritus, irritation, or tenderness. The preferred method is cryotherapy for smaller and thinner lesions. Patients should be warned that SKs may need more than one treatment and can recur. Care must be taken as aggressive cryotherapy may result in hypopigmentation or scar that can appear more disfiguring than the SK. Thicker or larger SKs may be handled more easily with shave excision. Ammonium lactate and α-hydroxy acids have been shown to reduce the appearance of SKs.

Prognosis and Complications

SK can be disfiguring, especially if they involve the face or large and dark lesions. Their appearance can make individuals self-conscious, lower their self-esteem, and be perceived as a sign of aging. Complications occur if a malignancy is missed or treatment is overly overaggressive. Patients who "pick" at their lesions may develop secondary infections.

The *Leser–Trélat* sign is a rare but sudden eruption of numerous SKs that precedes, accompanies, or follows an underlying malignancy (Figure 11-2). There is no evidence to support this phenomenon, yet most clinicians consider it to be a reliable indicator. Until definitive data can support or reject *Leser–Trélat*, primary care providers should ensure that the patient has completed age–appropriate screening examinations and other diagnostics indicated from the patient history and physical.

SEBACEOUS HYPERPLASIA

Pathophysiology

Enlarging sebaceous hyperplasia (SH) is a common disorder of middle-aged adults where the sebaceous gland is enlarged. Histologically, there is an increased number of basal cell and superficial

sebaceous lobules surrounding a dilated pore or follicle. They are thought to be related to levels of circulating androgens, yet studies do not support a gender preference. Other variables include excessive sun exposure or other forms of radiation. SH has a higher incidence with aging, in transplant patients, and in pregnancy. Immunosuppressed patients treated with cyclosporine are also at increased risk for developing SH.

Clinical Presentation

SHs usually present as soft, yellowish, 2- to 3-mm papules occurring as single or multiple lesions on the face (predominately nose, cheeks, and forehead). Lesions have a central dell (umbilication) surrounded by "crown vessels" (Figure 11-3). The vessels occur in an organized manner on the outer rim and not in the dell. This is compared to the erratic pattern blood vessel usually found across the center of a basal cell carcinoma. The lesions are soft to palpation in contrast to basal cell carcinoma, which tends to be firmer with erratic pattern of telangiectasia across the central area. Some individuals state that they express the lesion's contents upon squeezing.

- Acrochordon
- Benign nevi
- Acne
- Basal cell carcinoma
- Milia
- Wart or molluscum
- Sebaceous adenoma
- Sarcoidosis
- Syringomas
- Trichoepithelioma
- Xanthoma

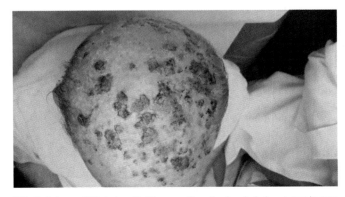

FIG. 11-2. Leser–Trélat sign. Sudden eruption of seborrheic keratoses in man diagnosed with genitourinary cancer.

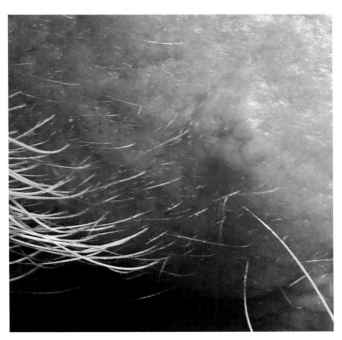

FIG. 11-3. Sebaceous hyperplasia with central dell and crown of jewels outer border.

Management

In most cases, SHs do not need to be treated. If they are widespread, disfiguring, or diffuse, several therapies may be implemented. It is important to note that the lesions will frequently recur after discontinuation of therapy. Isotretinoin should only be used by experienced dermatology practitioners who are knowledgeable about the medication and registered with *iPLEDGE*, the federally monitored information and restricted distribution program. Phototherapy (with combined use of 5-aminolevulinic acid or PUVA) can be helpful in some cases. All of the above treatments are considered off label and will not likely be covered by health insurance.

A wide variety of destructive agents may be utilized, including phototherapy, laser treatment, cryotherapy, cauterization or electrodesiccation, topical chemical treatments (bichloracetic acid or trichloroacetic acid), and shave excision. Destruction of SHs may result in atrophic or ice pick scarring or changes in pigmentation (transient or permanent) that may be less desirable than the original lesion.

Special Considerations

SH can occur in newborns and is not a cause for alarm. Oral retinoids and tazarotene should not be used in childbearing females without the necessary birth control methods and monitoring through *iPLEDGE*. Both are category X in pregnancy.

SYRINGOMA

Pathophysiology

A syringoma is a benign adnexal (eccrine sweat gland) tumor located in the superficial dermis with numerous ducts embedded in a sclerotic stroma.

Clinical Presentation

Syringomas present as flesh-colored, translucent, or yellow papules. There are several subtypes, but most are small (often 1–3 mm) papules located on the eyelids, axilla, umbilicus, or vulva. Syringomas are more common in women and have an onset around puberty (Figure 11-4). Most are asymptomatic, but patients may report pruritus. Patients can be distressed by their appearance and seek treatment for cosmesis.

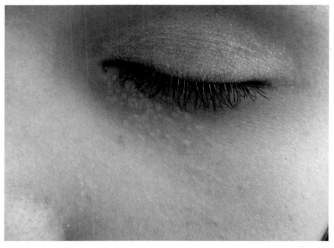

FIG. 11-4. Syringomas on a young woman distressed by their appearance.

DIFFERENTIAL DIAGNOSIS Syringoma
• Basal cell carcinoma
• Cutaneous tuberculosis
• Sarcoidosis
• Granuloma annulare
• Microcystic adnexal carcinoma
• Milia
• Sebaceous hyperplasia
• Steatocystoma
• Trichoepithelioma
• Xanthelasma

Management

Treatment is not necessary for these benign tumors. If requested for cosmetic enhancement, modalities to treat syringomas may include scissor excision, electrodesiccation, electrocautery, laser, cryotherapy, trichloroacetic acid, dermabrasion, topical retinoids, and oral isotretinoin (not FDA approved). The size, location, and number will influence the type of modality employed.

Clinicians should heed a word of caution if attempting to treat syringomas prominently located on the patient's face, often close to the lid margin. Remember, if the syringoma is visibly obvious, so will any resulting scar, abnormal pigmentation, or complication that results from your treatment. As always, an experienced clinician in the procedure should perform treatment of benign lesions for cosmetic purposes. Preauthorization for the procedure with the patient's insurance company is advised as coverage for the procedure varies significantly.

Prognosis and Complications

Syringomas are benign, but in rare instances, they are associated with Brooke–Spiegler syndrome and Down syndrome. Syringomas of the scalp can produce scarring alopecia. These lesions may affect self-esteem and body image, especially at puberty.

SKIN TAGS

Acrochordon, also called skin tag or fibroepithelial polyp, are benign but annoying lesions that frequently prompt patients to come to your office. Everyone hates the appearance and feeling of skin tags! The plural form is acrochordia.

Pathophysiology

Histologically, skin tags are a fibrovascular papule covered by normal epidermis. Skin tags have been linked to HPV types 6 and 11; however, it is not known if this is pathogenic or opportunistic. Nearly half of the population has skin tags. They are uncommon in children and increase with age. There may be some familial predispositions. They have a predilection for females more than males, and are significantly increased in the morbidly obese and patients with metabolic disorders.

Clinical Presentation

Skin tags are small, soft, pedunculated (atop an elongated stalk) papules that favor the skin folds. They are commonly located in areas of friction including the neckline, axilla, inframammary and inguinal

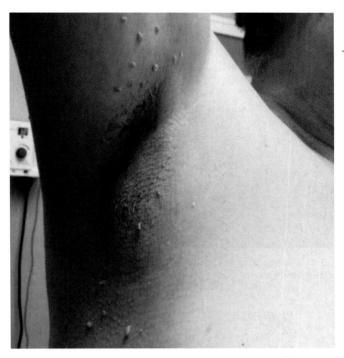

FIG. 11-5. Skin tags or acrochordons commonly found in areas of friction.

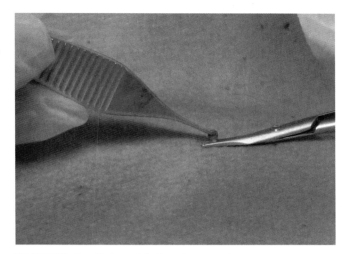

FIG. 11-6. Clipping skin tags at the base for removal.

folds, and eyelids. They may be hyperpigmented or flesh color and vary in size from 1 to 8 mm. Secondary changes include inflammation, hemorrhagic crust from trauma or friction, and necrosis from torsion (Figure 11-5).

DIFFERENTIAL DIAGNOSIS Skin tags

- Neurofibroma
- Melanomas (may develop at the base)
- Premalignant fibroepithelial tumor (Pinkus tumor)
- Seborrheic keratoses
- Verruca, genital and nongenital

Diagnostics

The diagnosis of skin tags is a clinical one. Biopsy may be indicated if there are any suspicious features. Additionally, if multiple tags are present, a thorough history and physical should be performed to rule out any underlying metabolic abnormalities. Practitioners excising skin tags should be cautioned against discarding the tissue (skin tag) without sending it to pathology. While it may be an additional cost to the patient, the clinician should ensure that they have not overlooked a malignancy.

Management

Skin tags do not require treatment but can be removed if pruritic, painful, or irritated. Management modalities include electrodesiccation, scissor excision (clipping), ligation, and cryotherapy (Figure 11-6). Over-the-counter products containing salicylic, retinoic, or carbolic acid, coal tar, and "natural" ingredients are available. Popular do-it-yourself products promoted on the internet and television entice patients to use homeopathic or "quick" fixes for patients tired of living with these ugly lesions. Ligation of a skin tag, by tying it at the base with string or dental floss, is an old-fashioned

remedy. Patients sometimes use an abrasive tool or body scrub to exfoliate the papules when they are small. Brave patients tired of the lesions have been known to use nail clippers or scissors and cut them off themselves. Often these treatments result in only partial resolution, severely inflamed lesions, or secondary infections, which prompts the patient to visit your office for complete resolution.

Prognosis and Complications

Although they are benign, skin tags can become symptomatic, including irritation, pain, and bleeding usually from clothing, jewelry, or necklace. Torsion sometimes occurs and results in necrosis, with the papule turning black and falling off. Most importantly, misdiagnosis of a skin tag could be melanoma and basal cell carcinoma.

FIBROUS PAPULES
Pathophysiology

Fibrous papules are a harmless type of angiofibroma without a known cause. Histologically, there is fibrosis surrounding blood vessels or adnexa. Some consider it a type of nevus.

Clinical Presentation

Fibrous papules are firm, dome-shaped papules that usually occur on the lower portion of the nose and occasionally on other areas of the face (Figure 11-7). They are almost always a solitary lesion but occasionally present as multiple papules on the face. Fibrous papules are flesh, red, or pink color and may have hair protruding from the lesion. Clinically, they can be difficult to differentiate from an early basal cell carcinoma. Multiple fibrous papules or angiofibromas in a butterfly distribution of the face may be a clinical manifestation of tuberous sclerosis and prompt further evaluation.

DIFFERENTIAL DIAGNOSIS Fibrous papules

- Basal cell carcinoma
- Melanocytic nevus
- Ruptured hair follicle

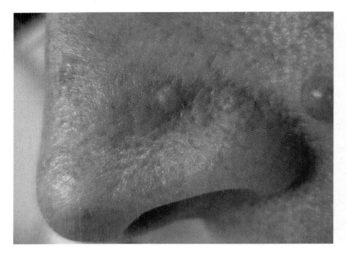

FIG. 11-7. Fibrous papule on the nose.

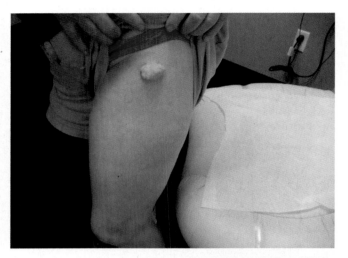

FIG. 11-8. A large pedunculated fibroepithelial polyp that looks very similar to a large neurofibroma.

Management

Treatment is not necessary for these fibrous papules, but may be performed for symptomatic or cosmetic reasons. Curettage or shave removal can be considered, but may result in a scar and the lesion may recur. Excision may also be performed and has better cosmesis and less likelihood of recurrence.

Prognosis and Complications

If treated, patients should be advised regarding scars and recurrence.

NEUROFIBROMA
Pathophysiology

The cell of origin of neurofibromas has not been isolated. Perineural fibroblasts synthesize collagen and create a network that wraps around the nerves and associated Schwann cells. There are two types of neurofibromatosis associated neurofibromas, which are discussed in chapter 6.

Clinical Presentation

In adults, solitary neurofibromas are soft fleshy papules that are usually flesh color to pinkish white. They can vary in size from a few millimeters to centimeters (Figure 11-8). Button-holing may be present (pressure with your finger may invaginate the lesion). Multiple neurofibromas presented in childhood should be evaluated for neurofibromatosis (Figure 11-9).

Management

When one or two lesions are present, they are usually spontaneous lesions without systemic significance. Treatment may be considered if a neurofibroma is symptomatic or is cosmetically undesirable. Surgical excision and CO_2 laser may yield the best results. Shave excisions can leave large scars and a higher risk for recurrence.

Prognosis and Complications

Rarely, neurofibromas may cause itching or pain. Isolated lesions are not a cause for concern if no other abnormalities are found.

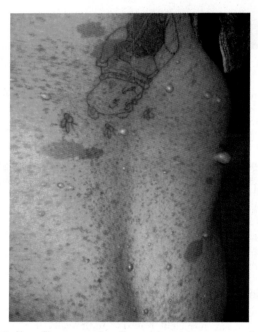

FIG. 11-9. Neurofibromas and café au lait patches on a patient with neurofibromatosis.

PRURIGO NODULARIS

"Picker's nodules" (PN) or Hyde nodules, are benign lesions that can be one of the most challenging skin conditions for clinicians to manage. Considered by most to be a neurodermatitis, PN has a higher incidence in patients with atopic dermatitis, HIV, hepatic disease, anemia, renal disease, celiac disease, insect bites, stress, and lymphoproliferative disease.

Pathophysiology

PN is the result of repeated scratching or rubbing of the skin, henceforth the name. Firm nodules are characterized by hyperkeratosis of the epidermis and hypertrophy of the dermal nerve fibers. PN can be associated with systemic disease, disc disease, post CVA, and psychiatric illness. Therefore, an appropriate history and physical may be indicated.

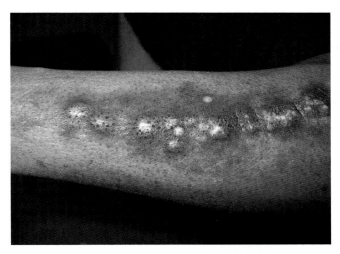

FIG. 11-10. Prurigo nodularis usually found on the extensor surfaces, sometimes developing a linear distribution.

Clinical Presentation

Solitary or multiple nodules are symmetrically distributed and favor the extremities. Lesions are firm, reddish-purple, and vary in size from pea-sized to larger. As the lesions progress, they may coalesce or become fissured, appear verruciform, or have linear distribution (Figure 11-10). Although the lesions may be asymptomatic, paroxysmal pruritus can range from mild to severe.

DIFFERENTIAL DIAGNOSIS Prurigo nodularis
• Squamous cell carcinoma
• Basal cell carcinoma
• Dermatofibroma
• Lichen simplex chronicus
• Sarcoidosis

Diagnostics

If the patient's history and physical examination are normal, no workup is indicated. If the patient's history and examination are suspicious for underlying diseases associated with PN, further serologies should be considered.

Management

The chronicity of PN, scarring, and disfigurement, combined with the psychological variables of these lesions, make treatment very difficult and resistant to many modalities. Furthermore, there is very little evidence to guide care. Corticosteroids are first-line treatment for PN and should be high or moderate potency, and used under occlusion. An Unna boot can be used to increase corticosteroid penetration through occlusion and provide a barrier to impede scratching. Corticosteroid-impregnated tape can be helpful as it adheres to the lesion for an extended period of time.

Repeated intralesional corticosteroid therapy may be effective in some patients, but can result in abnormal pigmentation and atrophy. Cryotherapy can soften the lesions and may be used adjunctively with other treatments.

Other topical agents include capsaicin 0.025% or 0.075%, which relieves pruritus by interfering with neuropeptides in the sensory nerve pathways. However, the cream must be applied three to six times daily and commonly causes erythema and burning. Off-label use of topicals including vitamin D_3, calcipotriene, or tacrolimus ointment has been utilized with some varying degree of success.

If topicals fail to control pruritus associated with PN, clinicians should consider adjunctive therapy with antihistamines, which may need to be prescribed at high doses (see chapter 19). Symptoms may necessitate progression to systemic therapy, which has been shown to be effective in PN, including possible underlying neurodermatoses and psychodermatoses. First-line systemic agents include gabapentin, SSRIs, and naltrexone.

In severe disease, the primary care provider should refer management of PN to experienced dermatologists. Systemic therapy with cyclosporine has had good results but includes high risk for cardiovascular, renal, and metabolic side effects. Thalidomide has been effective but commonly results in an intolerable peripheral neuropathy. Case reports of newer-generation thalidomide, lenalidomide, has shown some effectiveness with less neurotoxicity. None of these pharmacologic therapies are FDA approved treatments for PN and lack randomized controlled studies. If PN is due to neurotic excoriations, antidepressants or referral to a psychiatric clinician may be warranted.

DERMATOFIBROMA

Pathophysiology

Dermatofibromas (DFs), also called superficial benign histiocytomas, are round soft tissue nodules composed of spindle cells that are haphazardly arranged and extend deep into the fat. The etiology is unknown; however, they are associated with minor or repeated trauma to the skin (i.e., insect bite, nick in the skin, etc.). There is an increased incidence in women (this may be related to shaving legs). Multiple DFs (>6) have been associated with underlying diseases like systemic lupus erythematosus, myasthenia, AIDS, and internal malignancy.

Clinical Presentation

A DF usually develops as a solitary nodule on an extremity. The patient may or may not remember a previous insult (e.g., an insect bite, shaving). They are usually asymptomatic, but occasionally may be pruritic or extremely tender. They appear as a small, firm, exophytic papule or macule on the lower extremities of adults. Some patients may have multiple lesions, which help support the diagnosis. They may be flesh, tan, or purple-brown color. Hypertrophy of the overlying epidermis may exist. DFs characteristically have a "dimple" or Fitzpatrick sign that occurs when placing lateral pressure with the thumb and forefinger (Figure 11-11).

DIFFERENTIAL DIAGNOSIS Dermatofibromas
• Dysplastic nevus
• Basal cell carcinoma
• Blue nevus
• HIV cutaneous lesions
• Cutaneous T-cell lymphoma
• Merkel cell carcinoma
• Keloid/hypertrophic scar
• Keratoacanthoma
• Melanoma
• Melanocytic nevus
• Prurigo nodularis
• Spitz nevus

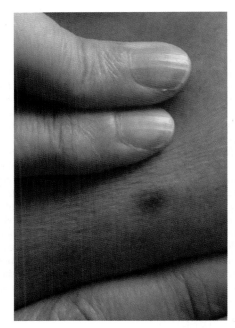

FIG. 11-11. The dimple sign helps diagnose a dermatofibroma.

Management

Treatment is not usually indicated for a DF. Patients may request removal for cosmetic reasons or because the DF causes itching or irritation. Steroid injections and cryotherapy have had limited success. When surgical excision is considered, clinicians experienced in removing DFs understand the importance of excising the reticular dermis to avoid recurrence.

Prognosis and Complications

Patients may be assured that these are benign lesions. Most complications exist due to improper diagnosis or aggressive treatment. The clinician and patient should identify the initial cause of the DF, as continued trauma or irritation (scratching or picking) at the excision site may result in a similar or worse lesion. This should be discussed in detail with the patient before excision is performed. Spontaneous regression with resultant postinflammatory pigmentation rarely occurs. Even though these DFs are benign, the overlying epidermis has a slightly increased risk for the development of basal cell carcinoma.

CORNS AND CALLUSES
Pathophysiology

Corns and calluses are the result of recurrent friction and pressure that produce hyperkeratosis.

Clinical Presentation

The appearance and location of a corn differs from that of a callus. Both are thick, scaly papules and plaques that appear yellowish or gray color. They are benign lesions but can become tender or painful. Calluses occur due to pressure, friction, or irritation and usually on the palmar aspects of hands and plantar surface of the feet. Poorly fitting shoes can cause callus on toes, while high-heeled

shoes create a pressure point on the ball of women's feet, causing a callus. Deformities, like bunions, can cause pressure points resulting in calluses over the first metatarsal (Figure 11-12). Individuals performing heavy lifting or pulling may have thick calluses on their palms. Those engaged in repetitive motions involving their hands or fingers can have locations with chronic friction causing calluses. Corns resulting from chronic pressure can form on plantar and dorsal aspects of the feet and toes (Figure 11-13). They can be in linear arrangement.

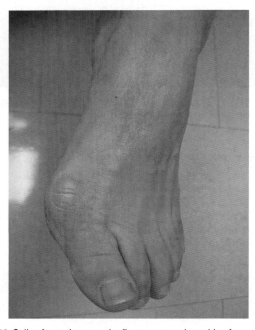

FIG. 11-12. Callus formation over the first metatarsal resulting from a bunion.

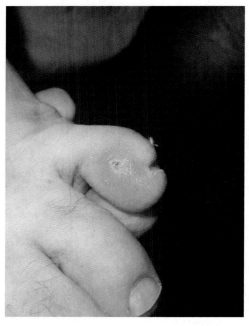

FIG. 11-13. Corns develop from pressure points on the feet and toes.

- Warts
- Squamous cell carcinoma

Diagnostics

Corns occur at specific pressure points, whereas calluses occur over a broad area of skin. Corns and calluses may be confused as warts but lack the black pinpoint vessels and disruption of the skin lines typical in warts. Paring the lesion can be helpful when looking for underlying vessels.

Management

Corns and calluses do not need treatment unless they create pain. The initial approach should begin with reducing pressure or friction to the area by using proper-fitting shoes, lower-heeled shoes, gloves or socks, and by a change in mechanics (writing style). Over-the-counter salicylic acid can slowly thin the lesion and can be used in combination with abrasion/exfoliation measure. Keratolytics like urea 40 % (in a variety of vehicles) can be effective. Paring the corn or callus to remove the excess skin can help relieve tenderness. Surgical excision is rarely indicated.

KELOIDS AND HYPERTROPHIC SCARS

Pathophysiology

A keloid is scar tissue initially composed of type 3 collagen that is later replaced by the proliferation of type 1 collagen. Keloids contain thicker collagen fibers that are tightly packed together. Hypertrophic scars exhibit randomly organized collagen in modules of fibroblasts and small vessels. Young adults between 10 and 30 years old are at higher risk for keloids associated with tattooing, ear piercing, acne, vaccination sites, and pseudofolliculitis barbae. Older adults can develop extensive keloid scarring after major surgical procedures. African Americans and Asians are at higher risk and a lower risk for Caucasians. There is a familial tendency.

Clinical Presentation

Clinicians often use the term *keloid and hypertrophic scars* interchangeably. But careful examination of the lesion can distinguish the two. Hypertrophic scars present as thickened scar tissue that remains within the borders of the original injury (Figure 11-14). Keloids, in comparison, appear as an exuberant amount of scar that extends beyond the border of the original injury or laceration (Figure 11-15). They may be a rubbery or firm nodule with a smooth surface. Brown or reddish hyperpigmentation can occur. Keloids can occur anywhere, but the most common sites are ear lobes, arms, and over the clavicle. Keloids may originate from a minor point of trauma such as an inflamed papule, like those seen in acne. Pruritus, pain, and cosmetic concerns can prompt patients to seek treatment.

- Dermatofibroma
- Xanthogranuloma
- Chronic folliculitis
- Sebaceous cysts

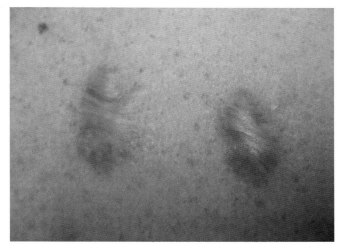

FIG. 11-14. Hypertrophic are thickened scars that do not exceed the wound border.

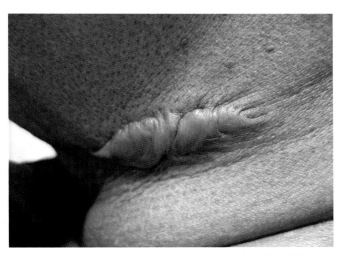

FIG. 11-15. Exuberant scar tissue in a keloid extends beyond the initial wound border.

Management

The goals for management of keloids are to address and prevent disfigurement, relieve pruritus and tenderness, and maintain function. The treatment of choice is intralesional injection of corticosteroids (triamcinolone) directly into the site, reducing the risk for systemic effects. Lesions are usually injected every 4 to 8 weeks for a maximum of 6 months. Clinicians should ensure that there are no signs of bacterial, viral, or fungal infections in the area. The patient should be advised of the risks for atrophy, abnormal pigmentation, telangiectasia, hypertrichosis, and impaired wound healing. Systemic effects are usually minimal but still need to be considered, especially if serial treatments are planned. The technique of the clinician can have a significant impact on the effectiveness or side effects.

Keloids that are large, bulky, or located in cosmetically sensitive areas may need a more aggressive approach. Surgical excision may be considered but requires pre- and postoperative intralesional steroids. Radiation therapy has also been effective after surgical de-bulking of keloid tissue. Silicone sheeting and cryosurgery may be an adjunctive therapy. Laser treatment has had variable degrees of success in reducing the size, color, and skin texture of keloid and hypertrophic scars. The off-label use of imiquimod has been used postoperatively to prevent keloids/hypertrophic scars in patients with a history of keloids. Many of these modalities may be combined to optimize patient outcomes.

Special Considerations

Ear piercing in infants, toddlers, and young children can result in keloids and hypertrophic scars. Open heart surgery patients can develop keloids or hypertrophic scars during the postoperative period. In severe cases, keloid scarring can create pain and restrict chest wall expansion that requires treatment.

Prognosis and Complications

Patients with a history of keloid scarring have a high risk of recurrence after any injury or procedure. In addition to disfigurement, keloids can cause restriction of mobility and function in the surrounding area. Patients should understand the long course of treatment required and the possibility that the lesion may not resolve or may spontaneously recur.

Referral and Consultation

Management of keloids should be referred to dermatology. Additional consults with a plastic surgeon and a radiation therapist may be necessary.

Patient Education and Follow-up

Patients should be educated to protect keloids and hypertrophic scars from UVR, which can cause hyperpigmentation. Simply covering it with band-aids before sun exposure will help.

CHONDRODERMATITIS NODULARIS CHRONICA HELICIS

Pathophysiology

Chondrodermatitis nodularis chronica helicis (CNH) is an inflammatory condition of the helix. Ears have a modest blood supply and very little subcutaneous tissue for cushioning. This predisposes the ear to ischemia from pressure and friction. Most cases occur in mature males in their later years and favor the ear that they sleep on. Sixty percent of lesions involve the right ear. CNH presents less often in females and typically involves their antihelix. Multiple nodules may occur, but it is not a malignant process.

Clinical Presentation

CNH is a chronic inflammatory nodule (sometimes multiple) that develops on the helix or antihelix of the ear. They can become erythematous and tender. Occasionally, the nodules may develop scale or crust with underlying shallow central erosion. This can be attributed to the chronicity of the condition or the frequent removal (picking) of the scale by the patient. These lesions can mimic hypertrophic actinic keratosis that can occur on the highly exposed UVR areas of the face and especially the ear. However, it can be helpful to remember that more solar damage occurs on the left side (the driver's side), whereas most CNH occur on the right ear. This is not absolute but may be helpful in assessing these lesions for potential malignancy.

DIFFERENTIAL DIAGNOSIS Chondrodermatitis nodularis chronica helicis
• Actinic keratosis
• Squamous cell carcinoma
• Basal cell carcinoma

Diagnostics

Clinicians may assess the lesion and patient behaviors to favor the diagnosis of CNH. Conservative therapy may be prescribed and a plan for short-term follow-up to assess the response should be made. If there is no improvement with treatment, a shave biopsy may be diagnostic as well as curative.

Management

Conservative treatment includes emollients to the ear, especially before bedtime, to reduce friction that causes inflammation. Moderate-to high-potency topical corticosteroids can also help reduce inflammation. A change in sleep position or use of an ear pillow (a doughnut pillow) can relieve the pressure and friction to the helix and antihelix to promote healing. Patients with intense sun exposure can benefit from broad-brimmed hats and sun avoidance to reduce irritation or risk of skin cancer.

Shave excisions can be helpful to remove the inflammatory nodule and allow a pathological examination to rule out cancer. Electrodesiccation, intralesional corticosteroids, cryotherapy, and laser therapy have also demonstrated some success.

EPIDERMOID CYST

Pathophysiology

An epidermoid cyst develops from excess keratin plugging the pilosebaceous unit in the epidermis. The term *sebaceous cyst* is often used interchangeably but is a misnomer as the contents of the cyst are keratin and not sebum. Other synonyms include epidermal inclusion cyst, keratin cyst, and infundibular cyst. The fatty, white, cheesy material found in the cyst is composed of keratin and not sebum. They may develop from chronic trauma or inflammation. There is no racial predilection, but there is male gender preference. They tend to occur in the third or fourth decade of life. Hereditary causes include Gardner syndrome and basal cell nevus syndrome. They may occur as a result of deep penetrating injuries.

Clinical Presentation

An epidermoid cyst presents as a compressible nodule that ranges from 5 mm to 2 cm. They have a predilection for the face, back, scalp, ears, upper arms, scrotum, and chest. Epidermal cysts can be flesh, yellow, or white in color with a smooth surface due to the outward pressure from the contents (Figure 11-16). A central punctum is often obvious, and the cyst is freely movable over underlying tissue. Since the cyst is slow growing, it is typically asymptomatic. It may grow large, develop erythema and tenderness, and spontaneously rupture. *Pilar cysts* are a type of epidermoid cyst that occurs on the scalp. The thicker, fibrous capsule of keratin tends to be smoother and can make excision of an intact cyst easier.

DIFFERENTIAL DIAGNOSIS Epidermoid cyst
• Abscess
• Lipoma
• Steatocystoma multiplex

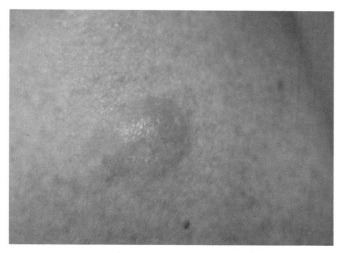

FIG. 11-16. Epidermoid cysts are soft yellow nodules.

Diagnostics

Epidermoid cysts are commonly a clinical diagnosis and do not require biopsy. If there is any doubt, an easy diagnostic is to prep the top of the cyst and make a small incision with a no. 11 scalpel. Expression of keratin will confirm the diagnosis and reduce the size of the cyst.

Management

Small epidermoid cysts do not require treatment and may even go unnoticed. Patients often self-treat by expressing the cyst themselves and report a foul odor from the thick, curd-like contents. The epidermoid cyst can be reduced without surgical intervention with a simple incision and drainage allowing for the contents to be gently expressed (Figure 11-17). Ruptured cysts are often misdiagnosed as infection but can easily be cultured.

Larger, symptomatic, infected, or cosmetically undesirable cysts can be excised or drained. Surgical treatment includes elliptical or punch excision. Care should be taken to remove the cyst wall and reduce the dead space with closure. Although epidermoid cysts are typically sterile, some clinicians prefer to incise and drain (I&D) inflamed lesions and treat with antibiotics before surgical excision. Firmer pilar cysts originate in the hair follicle, but treatment is the same.

Special Considerations

It is rare for epidermoid cysts to occur before puberty. Early onset may suggest the clinician consider an alternative diagnosis. Multiple epidermoid cysts may be associated with the actinic comedones in Favre–Racouchot syndrome more common in middle-aged Caucasians.

Prognosis and Complications

Multiple or large epidermoid cysts can be cosmetically undesirable and may affect the patient's self-esteem. Secondary infection can occur especially with chronic manipulation by the patient. Proper excision techniques usually prevent reoccurrence; however, under the best of circumstances, the lesion may regrow. Scarring is the biggest risk for surgical excision, and abnormal pigmentation of the overlying skin can occur if the cyst is chronically inflamed or ruptured. Skin cancers rarely occur at the site of the cyst.

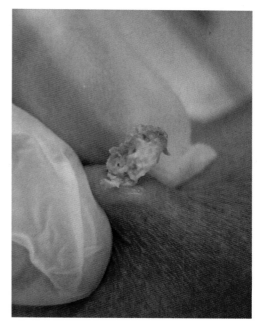

FIG. 11-17. A simple I&D of epidermoid cyst can reduce the size and expel odorous, thick white keratin.

MILIA/MILIUM

Milia are small keratin filled sebaceous cysts that occur commonly on the face and round the eyes. Congenital milia are common in newborns and can be seen on the palate (Epstein pearls) as well as the face. Acquired milia also occur in both genders during adulthood. Secondary milia may occur after trauma (e.g., dermabrasion, sunburns, tattoos, radiotherapy, skin grafts, etc.) or skin conditions like contact dermatitis, autoimmune blistering diseases, and porphyria cutanea tarda.

Clinical Presentation

Milia are asymptomatic, 1- to 2-mm domed-shaped papules. They are yellowish to pearly white color. The common distribution is the face especially the periorbital region (Figure 11-18). Also found near the nasal ala, milia may mimic small acne lesions. Secondary milia can occur anywhere on the body with noted trauma or disease.

DIFFERENTIAL DIAGNOSIS Milia
• Acne vulgaris
• Syringoma
• Trichoepithelioma
• Favre–Racouchot syndrome (older patients)

Management

Milia are harmless and do not require treatment. However, if distressed by the cosmetic appearance of the lesion, patients may try to express the lesions themselves or seek medical treatment. Simple extraction includes superficially piercing (no. 11 blade or needle) the milia and gently expressing the petite keratin ball. There is no need for anesthesia, and bleeding is scant, if any. In

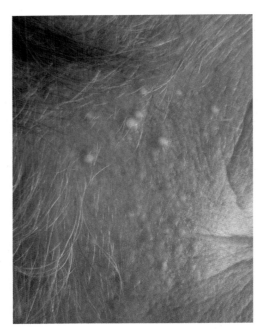

FIG. 11-18. Milia.

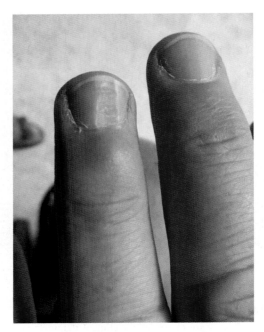

FIG. 11-19. Digital myxoid cyst causing deformity of nail plate.

the presence of numerous milia, other treatment modalities can be used and include laser, electrodesiccation, and dermabrasion. Off-label use of topical retinoids, oral retinoids, and minocycline are used for eruptive milia. Secondary milia are usually recalcitrant to therapy.

Special Considerations

Parents should be reassured that milia in an infant are benign and will resolve spontaneously.

DIGITAL MYXOID CYST
Pathophysiology

Digital myxoid cysts (DMCs), also called digital mucous cysts, are benign tumors that accumulate mucin. They are the most common cyst/tumor of the hand. It is thought to be caused by abnormal degenerative changes in the connective tissue and has been associated with osteoarthritis of the joint near the lesion. Others have suggested that they develop in areas of high friction or trauma. It is more uncommon, but DMCs can occur near the nail plate or on the toes. The onset of DMCs is after the fifth decade and is more common in women.

Clinical Presentation

Located on the dorsal aspect of a finger, over the distal interphalangeal joints, many believe that DMCs communicate with the underlying joint. They are classically a solitary, dome-shaped papule that is usually translucent or flesh color (Figure 11-19). The lesion is firm but fluctuant and is fixed. Smaller lesions may be unsightly but asymptomatic. However, if the nodule grows, the DMC may become painful, especially with movement of the joint. A DMC located near the nail may cause a deformity or groove in the nail plate.

DIFFERENTIAL DIAGNOSIS Digital myxoid cyst

- Xanthoma
- Rheumatoid nodule

Management

Often patients will attempt to open the lesion and get a clear or gelatinous drainage, only to have the lesion recur. A sinus tract communicating with the underlying joint must also be treated if the lesion is to resolve. Compresses and topical corticosteroids may provide symptomatic relief of a smaller lesion. Larger DMCs that are painful or limit function may be treated by surgical excision, I&D, cryotherapy, intralesional corticosteroids, and laser ablation. Clinicians experienced in treating DMCs are mindful about the risk for infection to the underlying joint space and recurrence.

Prognosis and Complications

Left untreated, DMCs may continue to grow and result in pain and limited mobility. Even with surgical treatment, there is a high incidence of recurrence. DMCs can cause deformity, arthritic pain, edema, and limitations in function. Complications secondary to treatment can include tendon or nerve injury, septic joint, scarring, and deformity.

Referral and Consultation

Many primary care and dermatology providers refer patients with DMC to orthopedic surgeons so that the joint space can be properly treated.

LIPOMAS

Lipomas are benign tumors in the subcutaneous layer of the skin found in approximately 1% of the adult population. Lesions contain encapsulated adipose tissue. The onset is usually during or after the fourth decade of life and rarely occurs in children. Multiple lipomas are associated with Madelung disease, Dercum disease, and Gardner syndrome. Some anti-HIV protease drugs have been known to cause lipomas. There is also an increased incidence in patients with family members who have lipomas. That differs from familial lipoma syndrome, which is a genetic disorder where young adults present with hundreds of lipomas.

Clinical Presentation

Lipomas can be found anywhere on the body, but are most common on the trunk and extremities. They can occur as isolated or multiple lesions in a wide range of sizes. Palpation of a lipoma will yield a soft, mobile tumor demonstrating the "slippage sign" (gently slide fingers off the edge of the tumor). They grow slowly and are typically asymptomatic. Patients may report pain with pressure on the lesion or with movement.

DIFFERENTIAL DIAGNOSIS Lipoma

- Sebaceous cysts
- Liposarcoma
- Lymph nodes

Management

Lipomas are benign, but elective treatment may be performed by surgical excision, liposuction, or the injection of agents that trigger lipolysis (not FDA approved).

Referral and Consultation

Patients need to be referred for evaluation if the lipoma is larger than 5 cm, grows rapidly, becomes infected, or is increasingly painful. Large lipomas on the frontalis are deep in the muscle and are difficult to remove. Any lipomas in the midsacral region should be referred for neurologic evaluation as they may be associated with serious spinal cord lesions.

XANTHOMA/XANTHELASMA

Pathophysiology

Xanthomas develop from a deposition of lipids in the skin. They are yellowish in color due to the yellow color of cholesterol. Genetic defects in lipid metabolism, endocrinopathies (i.e., hypothyroidism, diabetes), systemic disease (renal failure, cirrhosis, malignancies), and medications (retinoids, corticosteroids, estrogens) can cause dyslipidemia that can cause xanthomas. Hypertriglyceridemias are characteristically associated with eruptive xanthomas, while hypercholesterolemia is associated with all the other types. Onset of these lesions occurs after age 50 years and is uncommon in children.

Clinical Presentation

Xanthomas can occur anywhere on the body and can range from a few millimeters near the eyes to plaques on the trunk and extremities. When a xanthoma occurs near the eyelid, it is referred to as xanthelasma. They appear as soft, flat, yellowish, well-demarcated papules/plaques usually located near the inner canthus (Figure 11-20). In contrast, eruptive xanthomas are red-brown papules that erupt all over the body, favoring the extensor aspects of the extremities and buttocks.

DIFFERENTIAL DIAGNOSIS Xanthoma

- Amyloidosis
- Sarcoidosis
- Necrobiosis lipoidica

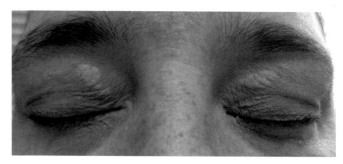

FIG. 11-20. Xanthelasmas are most often caused by a defect in lipid metabolism.

Diagnostics

Xanthelasma located near the eyelids are usually a clinical diagnosis. However, xanthomas on the trunk and extremities or those with atypical presentation can be biopsied for confirmation. Primary care providers should do a complete history, physical examination, and fasting lipids on patients diagnosed with xanthelasma. Age-appropriate screening examinations should be completed to rule out any underlying malignancies.

Management

The goal of treatment of xanthomas is geared toward evaluation and management of an underlying dyslipidemia to reduce the risk of cardiovascular disease. Targeted management should address the underlying cause or removal of offending medication. After serum cholesterol and triglyceride levels are controlled, development of new xanthomas may be significantly reduced. However, the initial lesions may remain. Cosmetic treatments may include laser therapy, trichloroacetic acid, and electrodesiccation near the eyes but should only be attempted by very skilled clinicians.

Patient Education and Follow-up

Dyslipidemia associated with xanthoma requires preventative education, lifestyle modification, and routine monitoring with primary care providers.

MUCOCELE

Pathophysiology

Mucoceles are benign, mucous-filled cysts of the oral mucosa. It is a swelling of the connective tissue and retention of mucin due to a ruptured salivary gland. The peak incidence of mucoceles occurs between ages 20 and 30 years.

Clinical Presentation

The papules/nodules may vary in size from a few millimeters to a centimeter and may be accompanied by mild inflammation. The most common location is the lower lip caused by trauma from biting the lip or an aphthous ulcer that preceded the papule (Figure 11-21). Palpation reveals a smooth, fluctuant to semifirm papule that is painless. They have a slight bluish or translucent color.

DIFFERENTIAL DIAGNOSIS Mucocele

- Parotid duct cyst
- Dermoid cyst (floor of the mouth)
- Hemangioma

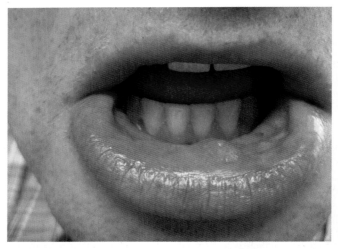

FIG. 11-21. Mucocele commonly found on the inside of the lower lip.

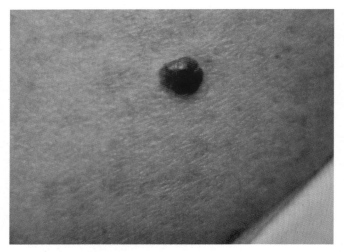

FIG. 11-22. Cherry angioma.

Diagnostics

Solitary lesions that are characteristic of a mucocele are usually not biopsied. Similar to epidermoid cyst, piercing the mucocele to express the gelatinous contents can be diagnostic.

Management

While many resolve on their own, some may require surgical excision or laser therapy.

Referral and Consultation

Patients suspected of mucoceles secondary to lip biting may be referred to their dentist for evaluation.

CHERRY ANGIOMAS

Pathophysiology

One of the most common vascular neoplasms, cherry angiomas are begin papules that characteristically erupt in the third to fourth decade. Synonyms include senile angiomas, sessile angiomas, and de Morgan spots. They can increase during pregnancy and involute during postpartum. Lesions evolve from a proliferation of capillaries that create papules ranging from 3 to 5 mm.

Clinical Presentation

Cherry angiomas may begin as bright red pinpoint macules resembling petechiae. They do not blanch and are not symptomatic. They slowly develop into red papules without obvious telangiectasis. Cherry angiomas are usually found on trunk and sometimes on the extremities, and may increase in size and number with age (Figure 11-22). They can also occur on the scalp, which can scare the patient. Angiomas associated with hyperkeratosis of the overlying epidermis are referred to as angiokeratomas. Their most common distribution is the scrotum (Fordyce spots) and vulva.

DIFFERENTIAL DIAGNOSIS Cherry angioma

- Insect bites
- Amelanotic melanoma

Management

Cherry angiomas are benign and usually asymptomatic. Many patients may request treatment for cosmetic reasons. The lesions may be removed by scissor excision, electrodesiccation, laser, or curettage and typically do not result in scarring.

Special Considerations

In children, cherry angiomas may be confused with a developing infantile hemangioma. Blue rubber bleb nevus syndrome should be suspected if multiple compressible dark blue papules appear especially on the mucous membranes. Immediate referral to a dermatologist is essential.

VENOUS LAKE

Pathophysiology

Venous lakes (phlebectases) are dilated venules caused by solar damage to the vessel and dermal elastic tissue.

Clinical Presentation

Appearing as dark blue compressible macules (and sometimes patches), venous lakes develop in areas of heavy solar damage. Venous lakes are most frequently distributed on the lips, face, neck, hands, and ears in patients over 50 years old (Figure 11-23A). The lesions will blanch when compressed and return to the blue color within seconds to minutes (Figure 11-23B). If traumatized, a venous lake can bleed excessively, causing the patient anxiety. Otherwise, they are asymptomatic.

DIFFERENTIAL DIAGNOSIS Venous lake

- Solar lentigo
- Melanoma
- Blue nevus
- Basal cell carcinoma

Diagnostics

If symptomatic or suspicious for malignancy, a shave or punch biopsy should be performed. Experienced clinicians expect an increased risk for bleeding from the procedure and are prepared to manage it.

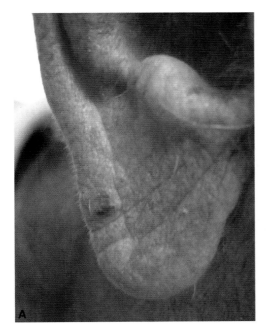
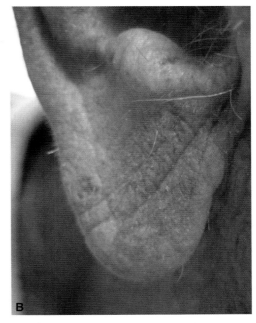

FIG. 11-23. **A:** Venous lake commonly found on the ears. **B:** When compressed, the lesion will blanch initially, then return to the blue-purple color within seconds.

Management

Treatment may include electrodesiccation, excision, laser, and cryosurgery. They may be difficult to differentiate from a melanoma and warrant biopsy. Any vascular lesion that develops rapidly should be referred to a dermatology practitioner.

PYOGENIC GRANULOMA

Pathophysiology

The pathogenesis of pyogenic granulomas (PGs) is unknown. They are acquired vascular overgrowths thought to be stimulated by trauma that results in an inflammatory and hyperplastic reaction. Synonyms are eruptive hemangioma and granulation tissue-type hemangioma. PGs are common in children and young adults, and there is a slightly increased incidence during pregnancy.

Clinical Presentation

PG presents as a solitary, rapidly growing dome-shaped vascular lesion that may follow trauma. These lesions are friable and prone to bleeding. Although most are red or pink with a moist shiny surface, some can be a darker brown with hemorrhagic crust. The most characteristic feature of a PG is a "collarette" at the base of the lesion (Figure 11-24). PGs typically occur on the face, arms, hands, and fingers. The patient may report a history of the lesion bleeding repeatedly or excessively.

DIFFERENTIAL DIAGNOSIS Pyogenic granuloma
• Cherry angioma
• Basal cell carcinoma
• Amelanotic melanoma
• Spitz nevus
• Glomus tumor

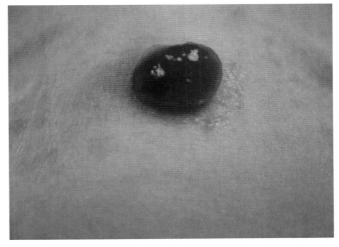

FIG. 11-24. Pyogenic granulomas are easily traumatized, causing bleeding.

Diagnostics

Experienced practitioners with strong dermatology knowledge and skills may make a clinical diagnosis. However, a biopsy may be necessary when the clinical presentation, distribution, or occurrence is questionable. Since there are several potential malignancies in the differential, biopsy for cure and diagnosis may be prudent.

Management

Small PGs may spontaneously regress. Large or symptomatic lesions can be excised (biopsied) but can recur. Excision usually requires cautery or electrodesiccation of the lesion at base for destruction of the culprit vessels. Imiquimod under occlusion has been successful in some cases (not FDA approved); however, the mechanism of action is unknown. Vascular laser therapy is helpful for recurrent lesions, and oral steroids have been used to treat giant PGs that recur.

Special Considerations

PGs during pregnancy can be monitored and may involute after delivery. Spitz nevus and PG both have an increased incidence in childhood and share the common characteristics of a sudden-onset, solitary red/pink papule, and frequent occurrence on the face and extremities. While PGs are benign, Spitz nevi do have risk of spitzoid melanoma, which can lead to higher morbidity if it is incorrectly diagnosed (see chapter 7). Referral to a dermatology practitioner is *highly* suggested.

Prognosis and Complications

Recurrence is possible but is not common if excised properly. A small scar will likely result from an excision. Misdiagnoses of melanoma or spitzoid melanoma are the greatest risk.

CLINICAL PEARLS

- Make sure the patient is aware of adequate healing time especially in advance of important events.
- For optimal patient outcomes, experienced dermatology practitioners should perform elective treatments of benign lesions.
- Advise the patient that all procedures have the potential risk for scarring, abnormal pigmentation, and complications such as secondary infections, which can result in poor cosmesis. Explain that the procedure outcomes may be less desirable than the original lesion.
- Before treating multiple lesions in a cosmetically sensitive site, test one lesion in the least obvious area to assess the patient response and perceived cosmesis.
- Always evaluate patient comorbidities that may impact or impede healing.
- Patients may request that seemingly benign lesions that are excised *not* be sent to pathology in order to reduce cost. However, clinicians should ALWAYS send excised specimens (including skin tags) to pathology.
- In general, punch or excisional removal usually has better cosmesis than shave technique.
- Excessive hyfrecation or cautery can result in scarring and damage to surrounding tissues.
- Cryotherapy can result in significant abnormal pigmentation and scars.
- If using Monsel's solution (ferric subsulfate) or silver nitrate applicators for hemostasis for a procedure, there is a small risk of tattoo or abnormal pigmentation from the iron and silver, respectively.

BILLING CODES ICD-10

Cherry angioma	D18.0
Chondrodermatitis nodularis chronica helicis	H61.009
Corns and calluses	L84
Digital myxoid cyst	M71.2–M71.3
Epidermoid cyst	L72.1
Fibrous papule	D10.6
Keloid, hypertrophic scar	L91.0
Lipoma	D17.910
Milia	L72.8
Mucocele	K11.6
Neurofibroma	L23.9
Prurigo nodularis	L28.1
Pyogenic granuloma	10L98.0
Sebaceous hyperplasia	L85.9
Seborrheic keratosis	L82.1
Destruction of benign lesions (CPT)	
1 lesion	17000
2 to 15 lesions	17003
> 15 lesions	17004
Skin tag	L91.8
Syringoma	D23.9
Venous lake (phlebectasis)	D18
Xanthoma	E78.2

READINGS

Bolognia, J. L., Jorizzo, J. L., & Shaffer, J. V. (2012). *Dermatology: 2-Volume set: Expert consult premium edition* (3rd ed.). Philadelphia, PA: Saunders.

Fitzpatrick, J. E., Morelli, J. G. (2011). *Dermatology secrets plus* (4th ed.). Philadelphia, PA: Mosby.

Fostini, A. C., Girolomoni, G., & Tessari, G. (2013). Prurigo nodularis: An update on etiopathogenesis and therapy. *The Journal of Dermatological Treatment, 24*(6), 458–462.

Habif, T. B. (2009). *Clinical dermatology* (5th ed.). Philadelphia, PA: Mosby.

James, W. D., Berge, T., & Elston, D. (2011). *Andrews' diseases of the skin* (11th ed.). Philadelphia, PA: Saunders.

CHAPTER 12

Superficial Fungal Infections

Janice T. Chussil

There are two categories of cutaneous fungal infections, or mycoses, dermatophytes and *Candida*, and other endogenous yeasts. Superficial infections involve the stratum corneum of skin as well as hair, nails and mucous membranes, whereas deeper fungal infections involve the dermis and subcutaneous tissue. The clinical presentation of fungal infections varies depending on the type of fungus, location, and immunologic response of the host. Most mycoses seen in primary care and dermatology are superficial infections. And although they are referred to as "superficial," if left untreated, they can become debilitating, develop secondary bacterial infections, and spread to other parts of the body or to close contacts. This chapter begins with an introduction to the diagnostic tests and treatment therapies before the discussion of diseases. Clinicians should be vigilant in developing a differential diagnosis, selecting appropriate diagnostic tests, and considering safe and effective therapy.

DIAGNOSTICS

Clinical presentation, along with laboratory findings, should be used to diagnose tinea since it can mimic many other skin diseases. Selection of the diagnostic test is based on access, cost, time, and value of pathogen identification. It should be noted, however, that the value of any fungal examination is only as good as the quality of the specimen submitted for analysis. The appropriate sampling techniques, advantages, and disadvantages for available fungal tests are provided in chapter 24.

- *Direct microscopy or KOH* preparation is the easiest and most cost-effective test available to clinicians regardless of the practice setting. Scrapings are obtained from the skin, hair, or nails to confirm the presence or absence of hyphae or spores. KOH does not identify the species of dermatophyte.
- *Fungal culture* is the gold standard for the definitive diagnosis of a fungal infection. It can be sent to a laboratory to provide further diagnostic confirmation, including the specific genus and species of the organism. This is important since some nondermatophyte molds and *Candida* species can look like dermatophytes under the microscope but will not respond to dermatophyte treatment. Analysis may take 2 to 6 weeks and can be costlier to the patient. This test should be considered for tinea infections that are recurrant or recalcitrant to conventional treatment modalities.
- *Dermatopathology* performed on a punch biopsy specimen may be helpful if the KOH preparation and/or culture fails to confirm your diagnosis or if you are considering other differential diagnoses. Specimens should be sent for routine histology, including periodic acid–Schiff (PAS), which is used to demonstrate fungal elements. Distal nail clippings can also be sent for histology and can help differentiate onychomycosis from psoriasis.
- *Wood's light* examination can be useful in evaluating specific fungal and bacterial infections. In tinea capitis, only the hair from hosts infected by *Microsporum canis* or *M. audouinii* will fluoresce blue-green, compared with *Trichophyton tonsurans* and other species that do not fluoresce. In tinea versicolor, the affected skin will appear yellow-green, and bacterial infections such as erythrasma, caused by *Corynebacterium minutissimum*, fluoresce a bright coral red.
- *Dermatophyte testing media* (DTM) is a convenient and low-cost in-office test in which clinicians inoculate media with a sample of the skin, hair, or nails. After 7 to 14 days of incubation at room temperature, dermatophytes cause a change in the pH and indicate their presence by changing the medium to a red color. DTM does not identify the species and can have false positives from contaminated samples (some molds, yeasts, and bacteria) or media left for more than 14 days.

ANTIFUNGAL AGENTS

Topicals

Because dermatophytes are limited to the epidermis, topical antifungals are effective and the first-line therapy for most superficial fungal infections. Topical antifungals have very little systemic absorption, resulting in low risk for adverse events or drug interactions. The most common side effects reported are symptoms of irritant or allergic contact dermatitis. Many topical antifungals are now available by prescription and over the counter. Selection of the most appropriate agent should be based on the suspected (or cultured) causative organism, severity, body surface area, comorbidities, cost, location(s) of infection, and potential for secondary infection. Severe or recalcitrant dermatophyte infections may require systemic treatment, with associated increased risk for side effects, drug interactions, and complications.

Topical antifungals used for the treatment of mucocutaneous infections belong to one of four classes: polyenes, imidazoles, allylamines/benzylamines, and others (Table 12-1). *Polyenes* are fungistatic agents effective against *Candida* but not dermatophytes or *Pityrosporum*. *Azoles* are also fungistatic but possess antibacterial as well as anti-inflammatory properties, and are used for dermatophyte, *Candida*, endogenous yeast, and secondary bacterial infections. The *allylamine/benzylamine* group has a broader spectrum of antifungal activity and can be both fungistatic and fungicidal. They are the drug of choice for dermatophytes, but relatively weak against *Candida*. Other topical antifungals include ciclopirox, which has a unique mode of action and structure and is fungistatic, fungicidal, and anti-inflammatory. It is effective against tinea pedis, tinea corporis, tinea versicolor, and candidiasis. Ciclopirox nail lacquer 8% is the only Food and Drug Administration (FDA)-approved topical for onychomycosis since it can penetrate the nail plate.

TABLE 12-1 Comparing Effectiveness of Topical Antifungals on Types of Organisms

	PREGNANCY CATEGORY	DERMATOPHYTE	YEAST	GRAM + BACTERIA	GRAM – BACTERIA	ANTI-INFLAMMATORY	ADVANTAGES
POLYENES fungistatic							
Nystatin	CA (pastilles)	0	++++				
AZOLES fungistatic							
Miconazole 2%	C	+	+++				
Clotrimazole 1%	B	+	+++				
Ketoconazole 2%	C	+	+++	++		++	Anti-inflammatory effect in seb dermcomparable to hydrocortisone
Oxiconazole 1%	B	+	+++				Vehicle great for hyperkeratotic soles and interdigital infections
Econazole 1%	C	+	+++	+	+	+	
Sertaconazole 2%	C	+	+++	++			
ALLYLAMINES fungistatic and fungicidal							
Naftifine 1%	B	+	+			+++	
Terbinafine 1%	B	+++	+			+++	
BENZYLAMINE fungicidal							
Butenafine 1%	B	++++	++			+++	
OTHER AGENTS							
Ciclopirox 1%	B	++	++++ (C. albicans)	+++	+++	+++	Penetrates nail plate
Selenium sulfide 2.5%	C		+++ (only Pityrosporum)				Effective in follicular epithelium

0, no effect or activity against specific organism; +, mildly effective activity; ++, moderately effective; +++, strongly effective; ++++, most effective.

Systemics

Griseofulvin was the first systemic antifungal used for the treatment of superficial fungal infections of the hair, skin, and nails. Although effective, newer agents have improved bioavailability and absorption, resulting in greater efficacy and shorter duration of therapy. The most common oral antifungals include terbinafine (Lamisil) from the allylamine group, and fluconazole (Diflucan) and itraconazole (Sporanox) both from the azole group. Newer antifungals reach the layers of the stratum corneum faster and are retained longer, resulting in higher cure rates, compared with that of griseofulvin.

Antifungals also vary in their detectable levels present in the eccrine or sweat glands. Itraconazole can be detected in the eccrine sweat glands within 24 hours and is excreted into the sebum, which explains why it is commonly used off-label for tinea versicolor.

Systemic treatment for onychomycoses is also advantageous as terbinafine stays in the nail for about 30 weeks after therapy, while fluconazole (off-label) and itraconazole continue for 6 and 12 months, respectively. So once therapy is completed, drug levels remain present in the toenails and fingernails to improve the mycotic cure rate.

When considering oral antifungal therapy, a careful review of the patient's comorbidities, as well as medications, is critical. Metabolism of antifungals occurs through the cytochrome P450 system and therefore can affect the metabolism of the antifungal or patient's other medications. Patients with liver or renal disease and the elderly may not be good candidates for oral antifungal therapy. Patient lifestyle, including use of alcohol, should be discussed, as well as the need for monitoring. The risk of interactions, adverse events, monitoring, and contraindications are listed in Table 12-2.

| TABLE 12-2 | Systemic Antifungal Agents for Treatment of Superficial Cutaneous Fungal Infections | | | |

DRUG	INDICATIONS	SIDE EFFECTS	INTERACTIONS & MONITORING	CONTRAINDICATION & CAUTION
Griseofulvin (pregnancy category C)	Adults: 500 mg daily (except tinea pedis & onychomycosis, 1 g daily)	Usually well tolerated but may have: rash, hives, headache, fatigue, GI upset, diarrhea, photosensitivity	CYP3A4 inducer (decrease levels): OCPs, warfarin, and cyclosporine increases alcohol levels	Pregnancy (or intent) Avoid: alcohol use
	Peds: Microsize: 10–15 mg/kg/day given daily or b.i.d. or 125–250 mg for 30 to 50 lb and 250–500 mg for >50 lb Ultramicrosize: 3–5 mg/kg/day given daily or b.i.d. or 125–187.5 mg for 35–60 lb and 187.5–375 for >60 lb Off-label use by experts: commonly use microsize at 20–25 mg/kg/day and ultramicrosize at 10–15 mg/kg/day Improved absorption with fatty meal Duration Capitis: 4–6 wk; corporis: 2–4 wk; pedis: 4–8 wk; cruris and barbae: till clear; fingernail: 4 mo; and toenails: 6 mo		Monitor: baseline CBC, BUN/Cr, LFTs Repeat 6 wk	Contraindicated in liver failure or porphyria
Terbinafine (pregnancy category B)	Adults: 250 mg daily Onychomycosis: fingernails for 6 wk and toenails for 12 wk Off-label use: tinea corporis, pedis, capitis, barbae, and candidiasis	Headache, GI upset, visual disturbance, rash, hives, elevated LFTs	Inhibits metabolism of drugs using CYP2D6	Caution with hepatic and renal disease
	Peds: Lamisil granules for capitis (>4 yr old): 125 mg/day for <25 kg; 187.5 mg/day for 25–35 kg; and 250 mg/day for >35 lb for 2–4 wk		Drug interactions: TCAs, antidepressants, SSRIs, b-blockers, warfarin, cyclosporine, rifampin, cimetidine, caffeine, theophylline	Avoid if history of lupus
			Monitor: baseline LFTs, CBC, BUN, Cr; repeat in 6 wk; more often if symptoms or immunosuppressed	
Fluconazole (pregnancy category C)	Adults: 150–200 mg Vulvovaginal candidiasis: 150 mg as a single dose only. If recurrent, 150 mg weekly Oropharyngeal candidiasis: 200 mg. Take 2 orally on the first day, then one daily for 2 wk	Headache, GI upset, abdominal pain, rash, diarrhea	Inhibits metabolism of drugs using CYP2C9	Caution if renal or hepatic disease QT prolongation Arrhythmic condition
	Peds: Oropharyngeal candidiasis (6 mo and older): 6 mg/kg/day orally on day one, followed by 3 mg/kg/day for 2 wk		Monitor: baseline LFTs Repeat in one month	Contraindicated in severe liver disease

(continued)

TABLE 12-2 Systemic Antifungal Agents for Treatment of Superficial Cutaneous Fungal Infections *(continued)*

DRUG	INDICATIONS	SIDE EFFECTS	INTERACTIONS & MONITORING	CONTRAINDICATION & CAUTION
Itraconazole (pregnancy category C)	**Adults** Onychomycosis: Toenails and/or fingernails—continuous 200 mg daily for 12 wk Fingernails only—*pulsed therapy*, take 200 mg b.i.d. for 1 wk, then off 3 wk. Repeat 1–2 times	GI upset, abdominal pain, diarrhea, constipation, decreased appetite, rash, pruritus, headache, dizziness, elevated LFTs	Inhibits metabolism of drugs using CYP3A4	Patients with ventricular dysfunction or congestive heart failure
	Peds: Off-label use only Improved absorption with food, especially acidic foods		Caution: use H₂ blockers and PPIs, calcium channel blockers, lovastatin, simvastatin, ergot alkaloids	Contraindicated in chronic renal failure
			Monitor: baseline LFTs. Repeat/month Less risk of elevated LFTs with pulse therapy	

Note: In 2013, the FDA advised limited use of systemic ketoconazole in view of liver injury, adrenal gland problems, and drug interactions. Oral ketoconazole should not be used for mucocutaneous infections or first-line treatment for any mycotic infection unless it is life-threatening or alternative therapy is not tolerated or available. There are many off-label uses of systemic antifungals that can be safe and effective treatments for dermatophyte and yeast infections. Primary care providers should understand the risks, benefits, and efficacy of off-labeled prescribing, or refer recalcitrant or severe cases to dermatology.

This text will not review the systemic use of ketoconazole (azole) as its use in dermatology has become very limited. Historically, oral ketoconazole (Nizoral) has been used off-label for many years for treatment of benign mucocutaneous infections such as tinea versicolor. In 2013, the FDA warned that oral ketoconazole should not be used for dermatophyte infections or as first-line treatment for any mycotic infection in view of the risk of liver injury, adrenal problems, and drug interactions. Thus far, these risks have not been associated with topical ketoconazole, which continues to be FDA indicated for treatment of dandruff, candidiasis of the skin, tinea versicolor or *Pityrosporum*, seborrheic dermatitis, and tinea infections.

DERMATOPHYTES

Pathophysiology

Dermatophytes are a group of fungi comprising three genera: *Trichophyton*, *Microsporum*, and *Epidermophyton*. Dermatophyte infections are commonly called *tinea* or *ringworm*, given their annular or serpiginous border in the presenting lesions. Some patients misunderstand and worry that there may actually be worms in their skin; so it is advantageous to teach patients about the true etiology. Unlike *Candida*, dermatophytes can survive only in the stratum corneum (top layer) of the skin, hair, and nails, and not on mucosal surfaces such as the mouth or vaginal mucosa. Subtypes of tinea are classified by the area of the body infected or the pathogen responsible for the infection.

The majority of tinea infections are caused by *T. rubrum*, with the exception of tinea capitis. *T. tonsurans* is the most common causative organism of capitis in the United States, while *M. canis* is the most common worldwide. Transmission occurs from direct contact with an infected host, which may be human to human (anthropophilic), animal to human (zoophilic), or soil to human (geophilic). Dermatophytes can survive on exfoliated skin or hair, and live on moist surfaces in the environment such as showers or pools, bedding, clothing, combs, and hats for 12 to 15 months. Once exposed, the incubation time to symptoms is usually 1 to 2 weeks. Clinicians should keep this in mind when dealing with community outbreaks of tinea.

Generally, tinea occurs in the adolescent and adult population, except for tinea capitis, seen mostly in children between the ages of 3 and 7 years. Healthy people may become infected, but there are several host and environmental factors that predispose someone to dermatophyte infections. People on topical and systemic corticosteroids or with suppressed immune systems are more susceptible. Crowded living conditions, poor hygiene, high humidity, athletes in contact sports (i.e., wrestling), or close contact with infected persons, animal, or soil can increase one's risk for infection. Studies suggest that individuals may have a genetic predisposition to particular strains of dermatophytes among members of the same household.

Subtypes of Tinea

Tinea pedis

Athlete's foot or tinea pedis is the most common disease affecting the feet and toes. It can present with a variety of symptoms depending on the causative organism and may include pruritus, inflammation, scale, vesicles, bullae, or may sometimes be asymptomatic. The most common pathogens are *T. rubrum*, *T. mentagrophytes*, and *E. floccosum*. Tinea pedis is transmitted by direct contact with contaminated shoes or socks, showers, locker rooms, and pool surfaces, where the organism can thrive. It is very contagious and can lead to household outbreaks or recurrence of the infection. Chronic tinea pedis can lead to fungal infections of the toenails, secondary bacterial infections, or entry of organisms that can cause cellulitis of the lower legs. These disease complications are important to consider in the management of diabetic, immunocompromised, and elderly patients. There are four types of tinea pedis affecting the feet and toes:

- *Moccasin* type involves one or both heels, soles, and lateral borders of the foot, presenting as well-demarcated hyperkeratosis, fine white scale, and erythema (Figure 12-1). The pathogens are commonly *T. rubrum* or *E. floccosum*. This type is chronic and very recalcitrant to therapy.

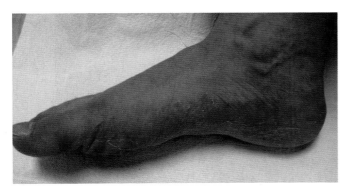

FIG. 12-1. Mocassin-type tinea pedis.

- *Interdigital* type involves infection of the web spaces and can cause very different symptoms of erythema and scaliness, or maceration and fissures. The third and fourth web spaces are most commonly involved and are at risk to develop a secondary bacterial infection (Figure 12-2). Obtaining a KOH from the macerated area can be difficult and may require bacterial cultures. The causative organisms are usually *T. rubrum*, *T. mentagrophytes*, and *E. floccosum*.
- *Inflammatory/vesicular* involves a vesicular or bullous eruption often caused by *T. mentagrophytes* and involves the medial aspect of the foot (Figure 12-3).
- *Ulcerative* type presents with erosions or ulcers in the web spaces. *T. rubrum*, *T. mentagrophytes*, and *E. floccosum* are common pathogens, with frequent secondary bacterial infections in diabetic or immunocompromised patients.

DIFFERENTIAL DIAGNOSIS Tinea pedis

- Psoriasis
- Dermatitis (contact and dyshidrotic)
- Pitted keratolysis
- Bacterial infections
- Erythrasma
- Bullous disease

Management
Hyperkeratosis, which may accompany tinea pedis, should be treated with a keratolytic agent to allow for better penetration of the

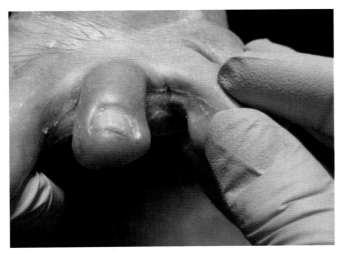

FIG. 12-2. Interdigital tinea pedis with maceration.

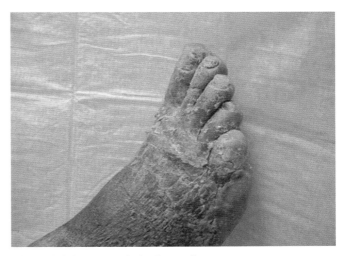

FIG. 12-3. Inflammatory vesicular tinea pedis.

antifungal as it softens and thins the keratin layer. Topical preparations such as lactic acid, ammonium lactate, or salicylic acid are available in a variety of formulations as both prescription and over-the-counter treatment. If vesicles are present, Burow solution (13% aluminum acetate) can be used for anti-itch, astringent, and antibacterial properties. It is available over the counter, both as *Domeboro* or generic, and is applied as wet compresses four times daily. Topical antifungals should be applied immediately following the compresses for maximum penetration.

Interdigital maceration can be treated with aluminum chloride hexahydrate 20% (Drysol, Hypercare) twice daily to provide an antibacterial and drying effect. The broad-spectrum activity of the topical azoles, especially econazole and sertaconazole, is a good choice for interdigital maceration often involving secondary bacterial infections. Moisture-wicking socks or a change in socks or shoes midday can help decrease prolonged periods of moisture of the feet.

Systemic antifungals are often necessary for extensive moccasin-type tinea pedis or when topical treatment has failed. Terbinafine and itraconazole are more effective than griseofulvin in the treatment of tinea pedis.

Tinea cruris
Often referred to as "jock itch," tinea cruris is a dermatophyte infection of the groin but may also affect inner thighs and buttocks, and presents with well-demarcated erythematous or tan plaques with raised scaly borders or advancing edge (Figure 12-4). There may be vesicles present on the border with severe inflammation and pruritus as a complaint. Clinicians should also inspect the feet of patients diagnosed with cruris as spores can be transmitted when patients are putting on their underwear. It is helpful to have patients put on their socks first before putting on their underwear.

DIFFERENTIAL DIAGNOSIS Tinea cruris

- Erythrasma
- Inverse psoriasis
- Seborrheic dermatitis
- Intertrigo
- Candidiasis
- Hailey–Hailey disease

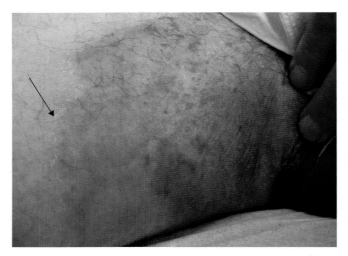

FIG. 12-4. Tinea cruris. Advancing border with scale (*arrow*).

Management

Tinea cruris responds to any of the topical antifungals, with the allylamines being more effective. Antifungals should be applied for 2 to 4 weeks until clear, and then one week longer. In a culture proven tinea, if the infection does not clear within the expected time period, treatment should be changed to another class of topical antifungal or to a systemic agent. Eruptions not responding to therapy should prompt a KOH test and culture if these had not been done or a reconsideration of the diagnosis of tinea.

Tinea corporis

Ringworm or tinea corporis is a dermatophyte infection (*T. rubrum* most common pathogen) involving areas of the trunk and extremities, not including the groin and palms. It presents as pruritic, erythematous, scaly macules or papules that expand outward to form classic annular or arciform lesions with a raised and sometimes a vesicular advancing border (Figure 12-5). The central area flattens and turns from red to brown as the border broadens. The lesions may fuse, producing large gyrate patterns, and include large body surface areas (Figures 12-6 and 12-7).

A clinical variant of tinea corporis is Majocchi granuloma, and involves the invasion of the dermatophyte into the hair follicles.

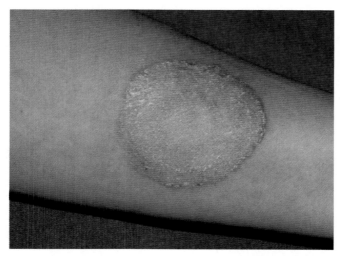

FIG. 12-5. Tinea corporis. The scaly border is potassium hydroxide positive.

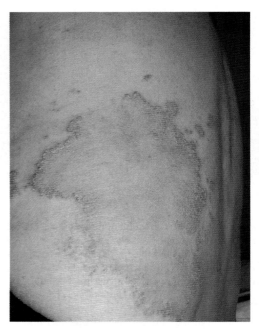

FIG. 12-6. Tinea corporis with gyrate lesions forming.

The characteristic lesions are erythematous, perifollicular papules and pustules. It commonly occurs on the legs of young women from shaving, but can be seen in men and children in other hair-bearing areas. Immunocompromised patients may have a more nodular presentation.

DIFFERENTIAL DIAGNOSIS Tinea corporis
• Dermatitis (nummular, atopic, contact, etc.)
• Psoriasis
• Pityriasis rosea
• Tinea versicolor
• Annular erythemas
• Subacute lupus erythematosus
• Granuloma annulare
• Mycosis fungoides

Management

Tinea involving small body surface areas usually responds quickly to topical therapy, especially from the newer agents in the allylamine and benzylamine groups. Systemic antifungals should be considered if the patient is immunocompromised, eruption involves large body surface areas, tinea is not responsive to topical therapy, or dermatophyte infection is a Majocchi granuloma. Terbinafine is a good agent for systemic therapy and is well tolerated by both children and adults. A topical antifungal may be used in conjunction with oral therapy. Skin eruptions diagnosed as tinea corporis that do not respond to antifungals, or are recurrent, should be reevaluated (Figure 12-7).

Tinea manuum

Tinea manuum is a dermatophyte infection of the dorsal hand, palm, or interdigital spaces. Because of the lack of sebaceous glands on the palm, it can have two different clinical presentations. Patients with palmar involvement have symptoms similar to those of moccasin-type tinea pedis, with erythema, hyperkeratosis, and fine scaling in

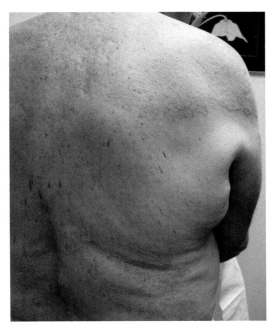

FIG. 12-7. Tinea corporis large, diffuse areas. Includes differential diagnosis eczema, CTCL mycosis fungoides, dermatomyositis, and psoriasis.

palmar creases. Patients often think their hand is just very dry and have no idea it is an infection. You may find patients with "two feet, one hand" syndrome, with tinea presenting in both feet and one hand—usually the hand/fingers that pick their feet or toenail fissures (Figure 12-8). Tinea manuum on the dorsum of the hand has a more annular presentation similar to tinea corporis. For this reason, it is important to examine the dorsum of the hands and feet, as well as the nails that may be involved.

DIFFERENTIAL DIAGNOSIS Tinea manuum

- Dermatitis
- Dyshidrotic eczema
- Psoriasis
- Scabies
- Lichen simplex chronicus

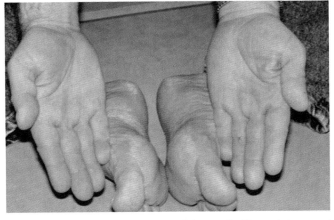

FIG. 12-8. "Two feet, one hand" variant of tinea pedis. The scale is present on one hand only.

Management
Topicals alone may not be effective for tinea manuum because of the thickness of the stratum corneum. There are no treatment guidelines for tinea manuum; consequently, clinicians typically follow treatment recommendations for tinea pedis using terbinafine and itraconazole. Systemic antifungals should be considered for recurrent or nonresponsive infections.

Tinea faciei
Dermatophyte infections of the glabrous (non-hair-bearing) skin of the face are called tinea faciei. It is commonly misdiagnosed as the lesions are not always classic annular plaques. The infection may be the result of autoinoculation from the patient's tinea pedis or corporis. Often, tinea faciei presents with mild erythema with some fine scales and can be photosensitive. Clinicians may treat it with topical corticosteroids for an eczematous condition transforming it into tinea incognito. A KOH test and/or biopsy can differentiate it from cutaneous lupus, eczema, seborrheic dermatitis, polymorphic light eruption, and psoriasis.

Tinea barbae
Tinea barbae affects the hair follicles of the beard and mustache area and occurs mostly in adolescents and men. Superficial tinea barbae presents as classic annular plaques, similar to tinea corporis, as both are caused by *T. rubrum*. Even though it is the same pathogen, the presentation of barbae is more severe and inflammatory. Deep follicular tinea barbae is less common and can be acquired from zoophilic dermatophytes such as *T. verrucosum* and *T. mentagrophytes*. It occurs in farmers and is usually acquired from contact with the hide of cattle. Alopecia and regional lymphadenopathy can be present.

DIFFERENTIAL DIAGNOSIS Tinea barbae

- Bacterial folliculitis
- Furuncle
- HSV/VZV
- Acne
- Rosacea

Management
Once diagnosed, tinea faciei responds well to topical antifungals. Because of the follicular involvement, treatment of tinea barbae usually requires oral antifungals for 2 to 4 weeks. Terbinafine is the drug of choice along with topical antifungals. The patient should be cautioned that shaving could hasten the resolution of the infection or cause more spread of the dermatophytes.

Tinea capitis
Tinea capitis is a fungal infection of the scalp and hair, and commonly occurs in children in low socioeconomic and crowded living conditions. Spores can be transmitted by hairbrushes, combs, hats, and furniture. Tinea capitis is classified as either ectothrix or endothrix infections that manifest with a variety of symptoms. Most tinea capitis present with alopecia, but may have scale, pruritus, papules, and pustules (Figure 12-9). When these symptoms are presented along with tender lymphadenopathy, the clinician should have a high index of suspicion for tinea capitis. Inflammation may be mild to severe and depends on the pathogen, host's immune system, partial treatment, and possible secondary bacterial infections.

Endothrix (infection on inside of hair shaft) caused by *T. tonsurans* is responsible for 90% to 95% of tinea capitis in the

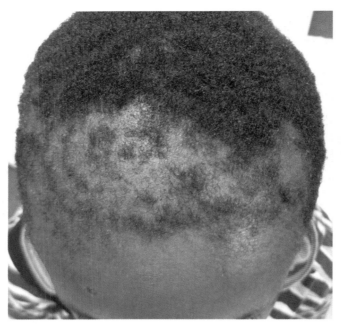

FIG. 12-9. Tinea capitis with patchy alopecia. May also have papules, scale, and erythema.

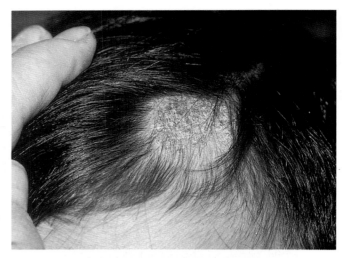

FIG. 12-11. Tinea capitis "gray patch type." Note alopecia with broken-off hairs close to scalp surface. Microsporum canis was found on culture, and the area fluoresced green with a Wood's lamp.

Other symptoms can include low-grade fever, malaise, and alopecia. Sequelae such as scarring and permanent hair loss may occur in severe infections.

United States. Patients have patchy alopecia (also called "black dot" tinea), with noninflammatory scaliness, and black dots where hair is broken off at the follicular orifice (Figure 12-10). Ectothrix (infection on outside of the hair shaft) is less common and called "gray patch" tinea capitis. *M. canis* is usually the causative organism, presenting as partial alopecia with short broken-off hairs close to the surface of the scalp (Figure 12-11). A Wood's lamp will make *M. canis* fluoresce green, compared with *T. tonsurans*, which does not.

One third of children with tinea capitis develop a kerion that presents as a tender boggy plaque, with pustules that sometimes form a serum crust (Figure 12-12). Clinicians may mistakenly suspect a bacterial infection and treat the patient with antibiotics. Conversely, the kerion is a host's exuberant immune response to the fungus and is often accompanied by cervical and/or occipital lymphadenopathy.

DIFFERENTIAL DIAGNOSIS Tinea capitis

- Seborrheic dermatitis
- Psoriasis
- Dermatitis
- Pyoderma
- Folliculitis decalvans
- Trichotillomania
- Alopecia areata
- Discoid lupus

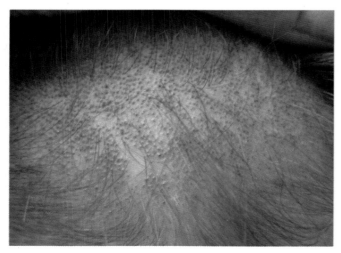

FIG. 12-10. Tinea capitis "black dot" characteristic presentation with *T. tonsurans*.

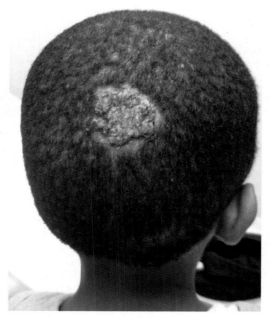

FIG. 12-12. Kerion in patient with tinea capitis.

Management

Tinea capitis requires treatment with systemic antifungals. Selection of the antifungal should be based on the causative organism, tolerability, availability and cost, and side effects. Griseofulvin has been the gold standard for tinea capitis and is inexpensive and well tolerated, with few side effects. A 6-week course of griseofulvin is the most effective antifungal treatment against tinea caused by *Microsporum* species. However, treatment duration should continue for two additional weeks after the symptoms have resolved. Infections from *M. canis* typically require a longer treatment period than do those from *T. tonsurans*. Studies show that off-label use of terbinafine therapy for *Trichophyton* species has a better cure rate and shorter duration of therapy. Table 12-2 shows dosages and duration of treatment of tinea capitis with oral antifungals. Off-label use of terbinafine, fluconazole, and itraconazole in dermatology has been safe and effective. Clinicians should refer patients with severe or recalcitrant cases to dermatology.

Management of patients with kerions should also include a bacterial culture and consideration of antibiotics as appropriate. Although there are no studies to support it, dermatology practitioners often treat severe kerions with oral prednisone (0.05 to 1 mg/kg/day) for 10 to 14 days to help reduce the inflammatory response and pain.

Household members of patients with tinea capitis should be screened for dermatophytes in an effort to reduce the risk of transmission and reinfection. Off-label use of ketoconazole 2%, selenium sulfide 2.5%, and ciclopirox 1% shampoos is a common adjunctive treatment to reduce spores in the patient's household members.

ASSOCIATED SKIN FINDINGS

Id Reaction

An *id* reaction, also called autoeczematization and dermatophytids, is an acute cutaneous reaction to a dermatophyte. Manifestations include a disseminated, erythematous maculopapular or vesicular eruption which may be pruritic. It occurs 1 to 2 weeks following the primary infection. It appears distant to the tinea and can involve the arms, legs, and trunk. The eruption will clear when the tinea has been treated, although topical steroids may help relieve some of the symptoms.

Tinea Incognito

This is a confusing diagnosis that occurs when a dermatophyte is treated with a topical corticosteroid because it is misdiagnosed as eczema or other type of dermatitis. Tinea, when treated with corticosteroids, may lose its characteristic scaly annular and defined border. Instead it may have diffuse erythema with or without scale, papules, or pustules. If you suspect a tinea incognito, have the patient stop the corticosteroid. Scale should recur within a few days, and a KOH test is performed. If positive, then the patient is treated accordingly.

CANDIDIASIS INFECTION

Pathophysiology

Candida albicans is the most virulent of the yeasts and is responsible for most mucocutaneous infections. This organism is a normal component of flora in the mouth, gastrointestinal tract, and vaginal mucosa. A variety of factors such as skin maceration, antibiotics, oral contraceptives, diabetes, and immunosuppression may alter the local environment and cause the proliferation of *C. albicans* sufficient to become pathogenic. Candidiasis, that is, any fungal infection caused by a *Candida* species, is typically diagnosed based on clinical presentation.

Oral candidiasis

Oral candidiasis or thrush presents with white plaques on the tongue, buccal mucosa, soft palate, and pharynx. Adherent plaques can be scraped off with a tongue blade to reveal a bright red mucosal surface (Figure 12-13). Thrush occurs mostly in infants, but patients who are immunocompromised, diabetic, or on antibiotic or corticosteroid therapy (i.e., asthma inhalers) are at greater risk. Symptoms may include burning and pain with eating, diminished taste, erythema, and erosions. The yeast may extend to the corners of the patient's mouth (*angular cheilitis* or *perlèche*), causing fissures and erythema, and increasing the risk for secondary bacterial infection usually by a staphylococcal species (Figure 12-14). Perlèche may occur independent of oral thrush and is seen in patients with poor-fitting dentures, excessive drooling or salivation, thumb sucking, or lip licking. Deep marionette lines extending down the chin may also become inflamed and eroded.

DIFFERENTIAL DIAGNOSIS Oral candidiasis

- Oral hairy leukoplakia
- Geographic or hairy tongue
- Lichen planus
- Stomatitis
- Vitamin B$_5$ deficiency

Management

Management of oral candidiasis should begin by identifying the predisposing factors and correcting them. Good oral hygiene and mouth rinses after using steroid inhalers can reduce the recurrence. Immunosuppressed patients and patients on cancer treatment may need prophylaxis for chronic infections. Topical antifungals are used to treat most oral candidiasis. Nystatin suspension, commonly prescribed as a "swish and swallow," is more effective in infants than in adults. The suspension can be easily administered with a dropper in the infant's mouth between the buccal mucosa and tongue. Clotrimazole troches (medicinal lozenges that dissolve slowly in the mouth)

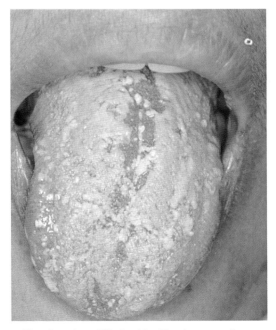

FIG. 12-13. Thrush, oral candidiasis with white plaques easily removed with gauze.

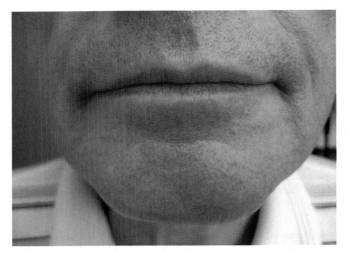

FIG. 12-14. Perlèche in corners of mouth.

are very effective in adults. For severe cases or recurrent infections, fluconazole is the most commonly used systemic, but requires caution by the prescriber in view of the numerous drug interactions (Table 12-2). Consultation with infectious disease experts may be necessary for immunosuppressed patients, as systemic antifungals such as itraconazole, voriconazole, posaconazole, and amphotericin B may be necessary. Reinfection can be reduced by sanitizing infected surfaces of infant's bottles and nipples and treating infected nipples of breastfeeding mothers. Perlèche is treated with topical azole creams and antibacterials as appropriate.

Intertriginous candidiasis

Candidiasis of the skin folds presents with erythematous moist plaques with satellite pustules and papules in inframammary, axilla, groin, perineum, and gluteal folds (Figures 12-15 and 12-16). Interdigital involvement of the fingers and toes usually has more maceration, erythema, and erosion. *Intertrigo* should be mentioned here, as it can often mimic fungal infections. Intertrigo is a chronic inflammatory dermatosis with fine fissures and erythema involving the inframammary, axillary, umbilical, gluteal, and inguinal folds (Figure 12-17). It is not an infection but is due to chronic, friction, and moisture usually

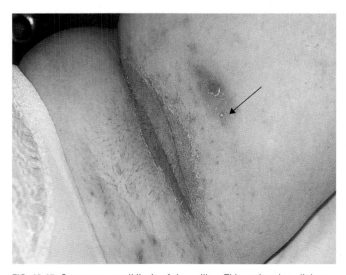

FIG. 12-15. Cutaneous candidiasis of the axillae. This patient has diabetes. Note the satellite pustules.

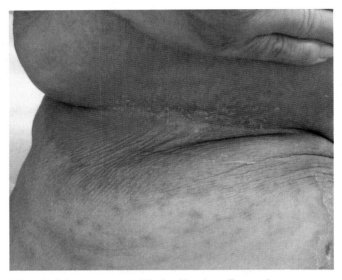

FIG. 12-16. Inframammary candidiasis with red satellite papules.

in obese patients. Conversely, intertriginous candidiasis presents with erythematous, well-demarcated plaques, which may progress to maceration, oozing and erosions, and fissures.

Cultures may be necessary to differentiate candidiasis from other dermatoses, but key clinical findings may provide helpful clues for differential diagnoses. Tinea cruris is not typically macerated and usually has bilateral involvement of the inguinal folds but not the scrotum. The erythema from intertrigo usually extends equally onto the thigh and groin and includes fissures, compared with candidiasis, which usually has extensive involvement, including the scrotum, and has satellite papules and pustules. Inverse psoriasis is not usually scaly and will commonly affect more than one intertriginous area such as the axillae, inframammary folds, gluteal folds, and inguinal folds.

DIFFERENTIAL DIAGNOSIS Intertriginous candidiasis
• Intertrigo
• Inverse psoriasis
• Erythrasma
• Tinea
• Streptococcal infection
• Folliculitis
• Contact dermatitis

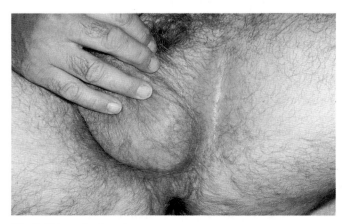

FIG. 12-17. Intertrigo in groin.

Management

Topical azole antifungals are effective but must be accompanied by treatment to keep the areas dry. Application of Burow's compresses to moist areas for 20 minutes prior to applying the antifungal can be helpful. Creams should be rubbed in well to prevent excess moisture, or the use of a lotion may be preferred. Patients should be instructed to carefully dry skin folds after showering. Use of a hair dryer can be helpful, especially when the skin is macerated, and can also reduce transmission of spores with a contaminated bath towel. If unresponsive to topical antifungals, oral itraconazole or fluconazole should be used to clear the infection and then maintained with topicals.

The goal of therapy for intertrigo is to keep the area dry, which is a difficult task, especially under the breast and inguinal folds. After gently washing with a cleanser and patting the skin dry, barrier products such as zinc oxide can reduce friction and "seal" the skin from excessive moisture. Newer products, such as fabric impregnated with silver (Interdry), reduce the friction and odor, along with absorbing moisture and suppressing yeast, fungal, and bacterial growth.

Candida balanitis

Balanitis occurs most often in older uncircumcised males and causes erythema, tender papules or pustules, white exudate, and edema on the glans penis (Figure 12-18). The cause of candida balanitis is usually poor hygiene, and the infection occurs more frequently in men who have had vaginal or anal intercourse with an infected partner. Recurrent infections can lead to phimosis or the inability to retract the foreskin due to scarring and edema.

DIFFERENTIAL DIAGNOSIS Candida balanitis

- Eczema
- Psoriasis
- Lichen planus
- Lichen sclerosis

Management

Good hygiene is necessary for resolution of balanitis, and most infections resolve completely after circumcision. Treatment should include a topical azole cream twice daily until the infection is cleared or a one-time dose of fluconazole (150 mg) along with prevention of reinfection. Culture for bacteria can be taken if suspected, or the infection can be treated with topical bacitracin or mupirocin. If phimosis or meatal stenosis occurs, consult a urologist.

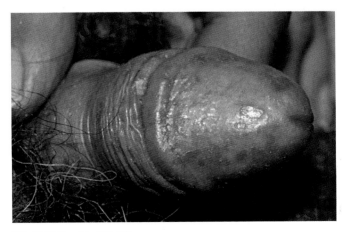

FIG. 12-18. Candida balanitis.

Vulvovaginal candidiasis

Most women, at some time in their lives, have experienced the excruciating pruritus, burning, and discharge of a vulvovaginal candidiasis (VVC) infection. Symptoms can also include erythema, edema, dysuria, dyspareunia, and sometimes satellite papules and vesicles that can extend from the vagina and surrounding area. More than 90% of the infections are caused by *C. albicans*, which is an opportunistic pathogen that occurs when the normal flora of the vagina is disrupted. The imbalance and infection can be triggered by a recent antibiotic therapy, diabetes, sexual partner with infection, change in hormones (HRT, tamoxifen therapy, pregnancy, and possibly oral contraceptives), tight-fitting or synthetic clothing, and immunosuppression.

Management

With the availability of low-cost, over-the-counter yeast treatments, many women self-treat before even seeing their primary care provider. This can be convenient in resolving the problem, but can also delay the diagnosis and treatment of sexually transmitted infections, resistant yeast other than *C. albicans*, or recurrent VVC that needs a different therapy. Diagnosis can be made from a simple KOH slide from the vaginal secretions but must be more than 1 week after the patient has used vaginal antifungal treatment. Fungal cultures can be sent if there is any doubt, and bacterial cultures are not useful.

The Centers for Disease Control and Prevention recommends the classification and treatment of VVC as simple or complicated (Table 12-3). Topical antifungal creams and vaginal tablets or suppositories are very safe and effective. Several imidazoles—miconazole, clotrimazole, and butoconazole—are available over the counter and may be used for 1 day to 1 week. Prescription econazole (not available in the United States) and terconazole are available in 3- to 7-day doses. Patients with severe or recurrent infections that do not resolve should be evaluated for underlying disease. Pruritus can be relieved with cool compresses to the perineum and use of the topical antifungals on the outside of the vagina.

Diaper candidiasis

See chapter 6.

PITYROSPORUM

Pathophysiology

The endogenous yeast *Pityrosporum orbiculare*, previously called *Malassezia furfur*, is a normal component of skin flora and most prevalent in areas of the body with increased sebaceous activity. An overgrowth of *Pityrosporum* is responsible for both tinea versicolor and pityrosporum folliculitis. Because it is an overgrowth of normal flora, these infections are not contagious to others. Exogenous factors such as excess heat and humidity, hyperhidrosis, pregnancy, oral contraceptives, systemic steroids, immunosuppression, or genetic predisposition can promote proliferation of the organism in the stratum corneum. Tinea versicolor can be chronic and last for years because of genetic predisposition, recurrences, or inadequate treatment.

Tinea versicolor

This eruption is usually asymptomatic but sometimes can be mildly pruritic. It presents with sharply marginated hypopigmented, round macules and plaques with a fine scale on the upper trunk and neck. It is more evident in the summer as infected skin does not tan and creates a greater contrast on the affected area. Lesions may appear pink/brown in Caucasians, while it can appear as hypopigmented or hyperpigmented in patients with darker skin. It symmetrically involves the upper arms, abdomen, and neck (Figures 12-19 and 12-20). The diagnosis is made on clinical presentation, but a KOH prep will show budding fungal spores and short hyphae (often called

TABLE 12-3 Classification and Treatment of Vulvovaginal Candidiasis (VCC)

	UNCOMPLICATED VCC	COMPLICATED VCC
Characteristics	Sporadic/infrequent occurrence	Recurrent (more than 4 times/yr)
	Mild-to-moderate symptoms	Severe symptoms
	Likely pathogen *C. albicans*	Not likely *C. albicans*
	Immunocompetent	Immunocompromised
Treatment	*Intravaginal**	*Intravaginal**
	Azoles for 1–7 days	Azoles for 7–14 days
	Butoconazole 2% cream for 4 days	Clotrimazole 1% cream for 14 days
	Clotrimazole 1% cream for 7 days	Miconazole 2% cream for 17 days
	Miconazole 2% cream for 7days	Terconazole cream for 7–14 days
	Miconazole vaginal suppositories	*Oral*
	100 mg for 7 days	Fluconazole 150 mg—two doses 72 hr apart
	200 mg for 3 days	**For azole-resistant *Candida***
	1,200 mg for 1 day	Terconazole vaginal cream 7–14 days
	Terconazole 0.4% cream for 7 days	Boric acid vaginal tablets[†] 600 mg for 14 days
	Terconazole 0.8% cream for 3 days	
	Terconazole suppository for 3 days	
	Nystatin vaginal tablet for 14 days	
	Oral	
	Diflucan 150 mg PO one time only	

*Vaginal tablets and creams applied each night before bedtime.
[†]Boric acid vaginal tablets are toxic if ingested.

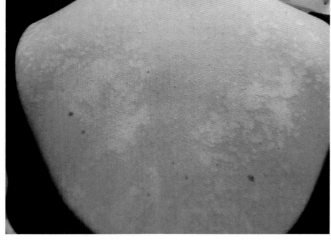

FIG. 12-19. Tinea versicolor with hypopigmented papules, fine scale.

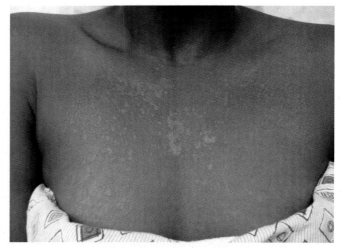

FIG. 12-20. Tinea versicolor with hypopigmented scaly macules in dark skin.

DIFFERENTIAL DIAGNOSIS Tinea versicolor

- Vitiligo
- Pityriasis alba
- Guttate psoriasis
- Hypopigmented mycosis fungoides
- Pityriasis rosea
- Eczema

"spaghetti and meatballs"). Clinicians should consider a skin biopsy for infections unresponsive to treatment.

Management

There are several treatment options based on the extent and location of the tinea. Recurrences are common; so a maintenance therapy is recommended. Topical antifungal creams or lotions are used if small reachable areas are involved, and should be applied for at least 2 weeks. It can take weeks to months for the abnormal pigmentation to resolve after the yeast has been treated. Many times the patient's neck, chest, and arms have been exposed to UVR and tanned, except the macules and patches of tinea versicolor do not darken and create a dichromic appearance. Ketoconazole shampoo 2% applied like a lotion to wet skin is highly effective when used for 3 to 14 consecutive days. Apply the shampoo from the neck to the thighs and allow it to dry for up to 15 minutes, then rinse off in the shower. Selenium sulfide lotion 2.5% can be used in the same manner but for 7 to 14 consecutive days. To prevent recurrences, the shampoo or lotion should be used once a week as maintenance therapy during summer and once a month during winter. Systemic antifungals are used off-label for cases that are extensive, unresponsive to topicals, or show frequent recurrences. Treatment can be with fluconazole (300 mg), given once a week for 1 to 4 weeks, or with itraconazole 200 mg, once daily for 5 to 7 days, or alternate dosing of 100 mg daily for 2 weeks. Griseofulvin and oral terbinafine are not effective. Historically, oral ketoconazole has been effective. In spite of this, clinicians should heed caution, with recent FDA warnings against the use of oral ketoconazole for most mucocutaneous fungal infections (Table 12-2).

Pityrosporum folliculitis

Pityrosporum folliculitis is due to an infection of the hair follicle and causes inflammation. Key predisposing factors include occlusion, oily skin, humidity, diabetes mellitus, and recent treatment with systemic broad-spectrum antibiotics or corticosteroids. Pityrosporum folliculitis presents with erythematous and sometimes pruritic perifollicular papules and pustules on upper back, chest, upper arms, and neck (Figure 12-21). It is often seen in young women and is easily misdiagnosed as acne. Simple diagnostic tests such as a KOH prep can help clinicians differentiate acne from pityrosporum folliculitis and help determine management.

DIFFERENTIAL DIAGNOSIS Pityrosporum folliculitis

- Acne
- Grover disease
- Sterile or bacterial folliculitis
- Eosinophilic folliculitis

Management

Pityrosporum folliculitis responds well to treatment with topical antifungals such as selenium sulfide 2.5% or ketoconazole 2% used two or three times a week as a body wash to the affected areas. Oral antifungals can also be used if necessary.

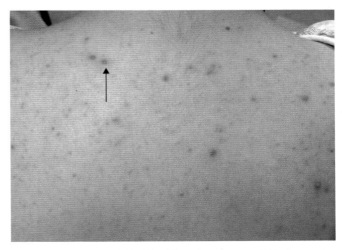

FIG. 12-21. Pityrosporum folliculitis with erythematous, perifollicular papules and pustules (*arrow*).

NAIL INFECTIONS

Fungal infections of the nails are commonly caused by dermatophytes, but may also be caused by yeast and/or molds, and bacteria. Toenails have a higher rate of infection than do fingernails, and the infections occur in both adults and children. Predisposing factors include trauma to the nail bed or fold (hangnails, injuries, trimming cuticles during manicure), increased age, peripheral vascular disease, immunocompromised and diabetic patients, and concomitant tinea infection of the skin. Since most dystrophic nails are often mistaken for fungal infections, diagnoses should be confirmed with direct microscopy or fungal culture.

Dermatophytes

Infections of the nails caused by dermatophytes are called onychomycosis or tinea unguium. There are three subtypes that correlate to anatomical aspect of nail involvement.

Distal/lateral subungual onychomycosis

Distal/lateral subungual onychomycosis (DLSO) is the most common nail infection, the majority of which is caused by *T. rubrum*. Dermatophytes invade the distal area of the nail bed, causing a yellow or white nail that thickens and lifts at the distal nail bed. Subungual debris can collect, and the nail crumbles or chips off (Figure 12-22).

Superficial white onychomycosis

Superficial white onychomycosis (SO) is a superficial invasion of the dorsal surface with *T. mentagrophytes* and *T. interdigitale* as the common pathogens. SO usually occurs in conjunction with bullous tinea pedis. Characteristics include a powdery white dry nail surface that stays attached to the nail bed (Figure 12-23).

Proximal subungual onychomycosis

Proximal subungual onychomycosis (PSO) starts at the proximal nail fold area and migrates to the underlying matrix and nail plate, causing separation from the nail plate. Hyperkeratotic white debris accumulates in proximal nail plate and obscures the lunula. *T. rubrum* and *Fusarium* species are usually the causative pathogens. Patients with PSO should be evaluated for compromised immune system.

Candida

Candida infections of the nails are associated with chronic paronychia (infection of the nail fold or cuticle) or excessive water exposure. Nails may have a varied appearance of green, yellow, black, or white with transverse ridging. Distal or lateral onycholysis (separation of the nail plate and bed) with yellow or white color occurs without this association (Figure 12-24). Nail plate involvement occurs only in immunocompromised states. In chronic candida paronychia, there is separation of the cuticle from the nail plate together with edema, erythema, and tenderness of the proximal nail fold.

Management

The management approach to nail infections may include systemic antifungals, topical therapies, or both. Although systemic antifungals have the highest cure rates for dermatophyte and *Candida* infections, the choice of treatment will depend on the age of the patient, comorbidities, extent of nail involvement, and the patient's current medications. If only one or two nails are involved with limited disease, topical ciclopirox may be a good choice. Ciclopirox nail lacquer 8% is the only FDA-approved topical for adults and children older than 12 years, for the treatment of onychomycosis. It should be considered as the first choice for patients on medications that may interact with systemic antifungals and/or patients with liver disease. Use of a keratolytic agent on thick nails before initiating therapy will aid in the absorption of the lacquer. It is helpful to warn patients that the treatment is a slow process (especially toenails) that takes months.

When several nails are involved or there are moderate-to-severe nail changes, systemic antifungals are preferred if circumstances are appropriate. Oral terbinafine has fewer drug interactions, higher cure rate, and longer time for relapse than does itraconazole, which affects the levels of several drugs in the blood. Recommended dosage and duration of therapy using oral antifungals are detailed in Table 12-2. To prevent recurrences after the nail infection has cleared, ciclopirox nail lacquer 8% or antifungal gels or creams can be applied to the nails two to three times a week.

Onychomycosis in children is less common and should prompt a discussion between the clinician and parents about considering the risks versus benefits of systemic therapy. Griseofulvin is the only FDA-approved systemic treatment for onychomycosis, but requires an extended therapy of 4 to 6 months, with limited effectiveness. Dermatology clinicians will use other agents like fluconazole,

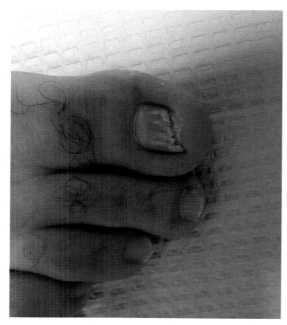

FIG. 12-22. Distal subungual onychomycosis.

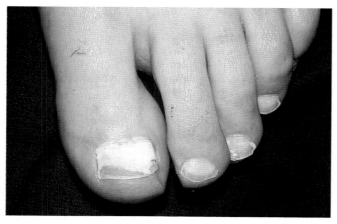

FIG. 12-23. Superficial white onychomycosis.

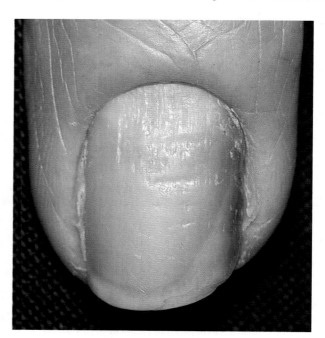

FIG. 12-24. Chronic paronychia. Note the swelling of the proximal nail fold, the loss of the cuticle, and the dystrophy of the nail plate.

terbinafine, and itraconazole off-label because of the shorter duration of treatment and greater efficacy.

There is limited evidence for the growing popularity of laser treatments for toenail fungus. It provides an alternative for patients who do not want to take or apply medications. Commercial providers report that laser therapy either kills the fungus or inhibits its growth. Treatments take about 45 minutes for 10 toes, and patients will need one to four treatments. The cost is $750 to $1,500 for the course of treatment and is not covered by insurance. Once the nails are cured, the infection can still recur; so preventative measures will still need to be taken.

SPECIAL CONSIDERATIONS

Pregnancy

Women of childbearing age who are treated with griseofulvin should be advised to use a backup birth control method if they are also taking oral contraceptives, as it can lower the efficacy. Terbinafine is FDA pregnancy category B and is the preferred drug of choice *if* the patient must be treated with a systemic antifungal before delivery. Diagnosis and management options should be discussed with the patient's OB/GYN before instituting therapy. Other systemic antifungals—itraconazole, fluconazole, and griseofulvin—are category C. There are several topical antifungals available, both by prescription and over the counter, that are FDA pregnancy category B and should be considered first (Table 12-1).

Geriatrics

Elderly patients who have thick nails or who cannot take systemic antifungals because of possible drug interactions should have their nails trimmed regularly and thinned by podiatry. Thick nails can cause pressure and pain and impede ambulation. Ciclopirox nail lacquer offers a relatively safe therapy for nail infections caused by dermatophytes. If systemic antifungals are used, clinicians may need to consider appropriate dosage adjustments.

Pediatrics

Although most systemic antifungals are relatively safe and effective in children, few are FDA approved for treatment of dermatophytes in children. Hence, primary care clinicians should consider referring patients with severe or recalcitrant infections to dermatology. If swallowing pills is an issue, terbinafine is available in tablets that can be crushed and Lamisil granules (packets) for mixture. Parents can crush griseofulvin tablets or use oral suspension (shaken well before administering); both should be given with a high-fat meal for better absorption. Ciclopirox nail lacquer can be used in children 12 years and older and offers a good alternative to systemics.

CLINICAL PEARLS

- If one class of antifungals is not effective in a culture-proven mycosis, switch to another class or consider a systemic antifungal.
- Select the appropriate vehicle for application of topical antifungals. Use creams in dry areas, gels, powders, or sprays in moist areas, and lotions or gels for hairy or large areas.
- Avoid combination antifungal/steroid creams; they contain high-potency steroids, which are *not* recommended for children and can cause striae.
- If feet and nails are infected, both must be treated to avoid reinfections.
- Tinea pedis is commonly transmitted to the groin; so both areas should be examined.

REFERRAL AND CONSULTATION

If you are unsure of the diagnosis or if the patient is not responding to treatment, consider repeat KOH test, fungal and bacterial cultures, a skin biopsy, and/or referral to dermatology. Podiatry is helpful in maintaining nail growth and foot health, especially in diabetics.

PATIENT EDUCATION

Have the patient apply the topicals until the skin is clear and then for at least 1 week longer. Remind patients that fungal infections have a high rate of recurrence and may need a prescribed maintenance plan. Precautions should be taken to prevent the recurrence of tinea pedis: wash your feet daily and dry them well (especially between the toes), avoid tight footwear, wear sandals or shoes that breathe in warm weather, apply absorbent powder such as Zeasorb to feet, and wear cotton or synthetic socks and change them when they become moist. To prevent tinea pedis from spreading to the groin, instruct the patient to put on their socks before underwear. And discuss the realistic expectations of resolution of fingernails in 6 months and toenails in 9 months.

FOLLOW-UP

Patients should return in 2 to 4 weeks to evaluate response to treatment. If the skin infection is not responding, additional or repeated diagnostics should be considered. Repeat culture or test for cure, after symptoms are resolved. When using systemic antifungals, clinicians should monitor serum studies, as indicated in Table 12-2.

BILLING CODES ICD-10

Candidiasis	B37.0
Dermatophytosis	B35.0-B36
Genital candidiasis	B37.3/B37.4
Mucocutaneous candidiasis	B37.7
Oropharyngeal candidiasis	B38.0
Superficial fungal infection	B36
Tinea barbae	B35.0
Tinea capitis	B35.0
Tinea corporis	B35.4
Tinea cruris	B35.6
Tinea pedis	B35.2
Tinea versicolor	B36.0

READINGS

Bellsyer, E. S., Khan, S. M., & Torgerson, D. J. (2012). Oral treatments for fungal infections of the skin of the foot. *Cochrane Database of Systematic Reviews, 10,* CD003584.

Bolognia, J. L., Jorizzo, J. L., & Rapini, R. P. (2012). *Dermatology* (3rd ed.). Spain: Mosby Elsevier.

Crawford, F., & Hollis, S. (2009). *Topical treatments for fungal infections of the skin and nails of the foot.* (Review) Copyright © 2009. The Cochrane Collaboration. Published by John Wiley & Sons, Ltd.

Gonzalez, U., Seaton, T., Bergus, G., Jacobson, J., & Martínez-Monzón, C. (2012). Systemic antifungal therapy for tinea capitis in children. *Cochrane Database Syst Rev.* 2007 Oct 17;(4):CD004685.

Gupta, A. K., & Drummond-Main, C. (2013). Meta-analysis of randomized, controlled trials comparing particular doses of griseofulvin and terbinafine for the treatment of tinea capitis. *Pediatric Dermatology, 30*(1), 1–6.

Habif, T. P. (2010). *Clinical dermatology: A color guide to diagnosis and therapy* (5th ed.). Philadelphia, PA: Mosby.

Paller, A.S., & Mancini, A.J. (2011). *Hurwitz clinical pediatric dermatology* (4th ed.). New York, NY: Elsevier.

Scott, T.D. (2011). Procedure primer: The potassium hydroxide preparation. *Journal of the Dermatology Nurses' Association, 3*(5), 304–305.

Wolverton, S. E. (2013). *Comprehensive dermatologic drug therapy* (3rd ed.). New York, NY: Elsevier.

13 Infestations, Stings, and Bites

Melissa E. Cyr

Insect infestations, stings, and bites are quite prevalent throughout the world. Infestations occurring in indoor dwellings and insects living in temperate climates can cause problematic bites throughout the year, and may produce a vast array of clinical manifestations. Human and animal bites occur less frequently; however, they still have the potential to produce significant morbidity and mortality.

SCABIES

Scabies is a highly contagious, common parasitic infection, characterized by intense itching and superficial burrows. It is caused by the microscopic mite *Sarcoptes scabiei*. Scabies infections affect both males and females of all socioeconomic and ethnic groups. Transmission most often occurs through direct skin-to-skin contact, with a higher incidence occurring through prolonged contact within households or neighborhoods. For this reason, outbreaks are common in extended-care facilities, prisons, child care facilities, and schools. Less frequently, the mite is transmitted by indirect contact through fomites, and can live for up to 3 days on inanimate objects like bedding or clothing.

Pathophysiology

The adult mite that affects humans is female, approximately 0.3 to 0.4 mm long, and has a flattened, oval body with four pairs of legs (Figure 13-1). The infestation begins when the fertilized female mite burrows into the skin and moves linearly beneath the most superficial layer of the epidermis (stratum corneum), depositing eggs and fecal pellets (scybala) along the way. These deposited eggs hatch, and within several weeks, larvae grow into adult mites, capable of reproducing and perpetuating the infestation cycle.

After approximately 1 month, an allergic reaction (delayed-type IV hypersensitivity reaction) occurs in response to the mites, eggs, and scybala, transforming the initial, minor, localized itching into severe and widespread pruritus. Subsequent scabies infections in a sensitized individual can produce generalized pruritus more rapidly because of this hypersensitivity response.

Clinical Presentation

The clinical presentation varies based on the type and location of lesions. Symptoms begin insidiously and are often mistaken for skin conditions such as dermatitis. Widespread pruritus is common, and severe nocturnal pruritus is the hallmark characteristic of scabies infection. Light pink curved or linear burrows, occasionally seen with a black dot on one end representing the mite, are pathognomic but not always seen. Scratching the area can destroy burrows (Figure 13-2), displace mites, and promote the spread of mites to other locations on the body.

Older children and adults commonly present with red papules and vesicles that can be seen in the finger webs, wrists, lateral aspects of feet and hands, waist, axillae, buttocks, penis, and scrotum (Figure 13-3). Infants and small children may develop pustules on the palms and soles, and in some cases the head and neck. A good rule of thumb is to always suspect scabies on men with pruritic papules on the scrotum or penis (diaper area for children) or nipple region in women. Nodules on the trunk and axillae may erupt as a result of the host's exuberant immune response to the scabies.

Crusted (Norwegian) scabies

Crusted scabies (also called hyperkeratotic or Norwegian) is severe and less common than general scabies infection. Patients at risk are the immunocompromised, elderly, and/or mentally or physically disabled. Compromised immunity, along with decreased itch sensation, leads to the infestations of hundreds to millions of mites. These patients classically present with asymptomatic, hyperkeratotic crusting on the palms and soles, thickened (dystrophic) nails, thick crusts and gray scales on the trunk and extremities, and verrucous

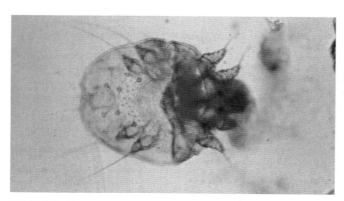

FIG. 13-1. Scabies mite.

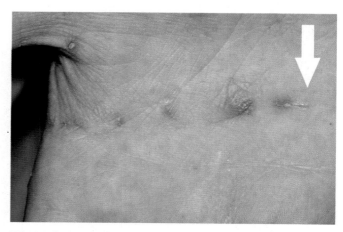

FIG. 13-2. Scabies linear rash.

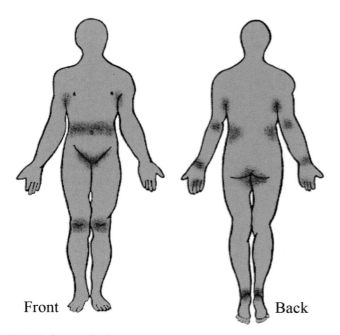

Front   Back

FIG. 13-3. Scabies distribution.

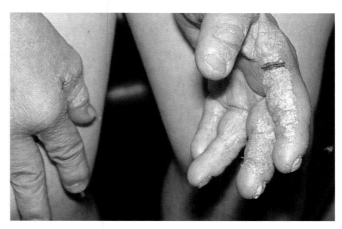

FIG. 13-4. Norwegian scabies.

(wart-like) growths in areas of trauma (Figure 13-4). Hair loss may also be present. Mites involved in crusted scabies are not more virulent than those found in traditional scabies infection; they are present in massive numbers. Individuals infected are highly contagious and therefore require quick and aggressive medical treatment.

DIFFERENTIAL DIAGNOSIS Scabies

- Pruritus (generalized or prolonged)
- Dermatitis
- ID reaction
- Folliculitis
- Psoriasis (crusted scabies)
- Arthropod bites (i.e., bedbugs)
- Dermatitis herpetiformis
- Varicella
- Bullous pemphigoid (urticarial phase)

Diagnostics

The diagnosis of scabies may be based on clinical suspicion. A definitive diagnosis is often made through identification of mites, feces (scybala), eggs, or egg casings under microscopy by performing a mineral oil mount (see chapter 24: Mineral Oil Prep).

Management

Management of scabies requires both pharmacologic treatment and environmental eradication. Topical permethrin 5% cream is the treatment of choice (Table 13-1). Many of the topical treatments available are generally effective after one application; however, a second treatment after 1 week is common. Several second-line therapies are available, including topical sulfur 10% lotion and crotamiton 10% lotion, which has a higher failure rate of 40%.

Warning: Lindane 1% topical application, once considered the treatment of choice, is now FDA approved only for use in individuals

who failed appropriate doses of other approved therapies or are intolerant to other treatments, in view of its neurotoxic side effects. In 2009, the American Academy of Pediatrics recommended that lindane not be used for children even as a second-line therapy. The state of California banned the use of lindane because of its reported neurotoxicity and environmental hazards.

Oral ivermectin, an antihelminthic agent, has been used off label for effective treatment of scabies with concurrent use of a topical scabicide. Ivermectin tablets, available in 3 mg, are dosed 200 μg per kg and may be repeated in 2 weeks. It should not be used in children under 5 years of age. Ivermectin is very effective in scabies epidemic and immunocompromised patients. Treatment for Norwegian scabies may require 200 μg per kg dose on days 1, 2, 8, 9, 15 and further doses on days 22 and 29, if severe.

Patients should be instructed on the appropriate application of topical scabicides. It is important to bathe prior to application, which is generally recommended at bedtime. Ensure fingernails are trimmed and clean. Apply topical scabicide to all skin from the neck down, ensuring all skin folds are treated, including finger and toe webs, under the fingernails, axillae, umbilicus, and the anal and vaginal clefts. Inadequate coverage is the primary cause of treatment failure. In infants, covering their hands with mittens helps prevent removal and ingestion of the product. If infection of the face or scalp is suspected, such as the case with infants or crusted scabies, also treat the skin above the neck, avoiding the eyes and mucous membranes. If the scabicide is washed off or removed prior to the required treatment duration, reapply more.

Once the recommended application time has lapsed, the patient may wash off the topical scabicide using soap and warm water. It is important to stress that only clean towels, clothing, and linens should be used to decrease reexposure. Members of the same household, including intimate contacts, should be treated empirically with topical scabicides at the same time as the infected patient. All clothing, bedding, and towels in contact with infected skin must be washed and dried on the hottest possible settings. Items unable to be washed may be sealed in a plastic bag for at least 1 week. Floors and chairs should be cleaned and vacuumed, while pets do not require treatment. Children may return to school and adults to work the day after treatment. Schools and workplaces may require a written statement from the patient's health care provider.

Crusted scabies is more challenging to treat because of the thick, hyperkeratotic scale, making it difficult for topicals to penetrate and kill thousands of mites. Combination therapy with topical permethrin and oral ivermectin is frequently used. Despite treatment with scabicides, inflamed pustules, erosions, and crusts may occur

TABLE 13-1 Prescribed Medications for Treatment of Scabies

MEDICATION	ADULT NONCRUSTED	ADULT CRUSTED	PEDIATRIC NONCRUSTED	PEDIATRIC CRUSTED	SPECIAL INFORMATION
Permethrin 5% cream (Rx)	Apply × 1, may repeat in 7 days if live mites still present; rinse after 12 hr	Apply q.d. × 7 days, then 2×/wk until cured; rinse after 12 hr (recommend use w/ oral ivermectin)	>2 m: Apply × 1, may repeat in 14 days if live mites still present; rinse after 8–12 hr	>2 m: Apply QD ×7 days, then 2×/wk until cured	Pregnancy category: B Lactation: Probably safe Diminished sensitivity has been documented Apply neck down, w/special attention to the nails and umbilicus
Lindane 1% lotion (Rx)	Apply 30 mL 1% lotion ×1 (maximum 60-mL dose for larger adults; rinse off after 8–12 hr	Not indicated	1 mo–5 yr: Apply ×1 (max: 15 mL); rinse off after 8–12 hr >6 yr: Apply ×1 (max: 30 mL); rinse off after 8–12 hr	FDA approved but **not recommended** for use on open, crusted skin Must try other agents first	**Black-Box Warnings** Pregnancy category: C Lactation: Probably safe Contraindicated in seizure disorder Neurotoxicity NOT first line treatment Do not retreat Do not apply on open wounds Banned in some geographic areas Apply neck down, w/special attention to the nails & umbilicus
Ivermectin 3-mg tablets (Rx)	0.2 mg/kg PO ×1 (may repeat in 2 wk if symptoms persist)	0.2 mg/kg PO ×1 on days 1, 2, 8, 9, 15 (may also give on days 22 & 29 for severe cases; use with topical scabicide)	Not FDA approved	Not FDA approved	Pregnancy category: C Lactation: Safety unknown Give on an empty stomach

secondary to scratching. Pruritus associated with hypersensitivity to mites can last for up to 2 to 4 weeks after effective treatment.

Special Considerations

Pediatrics: Infants have widespread skin involvement more often than adults with a different distribution and presentation. Delay in diagnosis is often the result of treating other diagnoses of pruritus, such as eczema. Infants and children may present with more scaly papules and vesicles especially in occluded areas such as the axillae and diaper region. Involvement of the face and scalp (especially the occipital area) are seen more frequently in children than in adults. Application of permethrin to infants more than 2 months old should include the scalp, head, neck, trunk, and extremities. Parents should be given careful instruction to avoid the eyes. Make sure that the permethrin is applied to the palms and soles, interdigital areas, umbilicus, folds of skin (inguinal, neck, axillary, etc.), and periungual areas. The use of lindane in infants is not recommended in view of increased risk for toxicity. Acropustulosisofinfancy (API) is associated with scabies infection, and presents with itchy vesicles or pustules on the palms and soles in children up to age 3 years (Figure 13-5). Symptoms usually occur after a history of scabies infection and are usually misdiagnosed as a recurrence. These findings represent an allergic response to the scabies mite and not a current infection. There are no burrows seen in API. However, clinicians should be prudent and perform a mineral prep to ensure the child has not been reinfected. Specific treatment of API is often not warranted, unless lesions are extremely pruritic. With appropriate scabies treatment, pustules will flatten gradually and resolve over a few months.

Pregnancy: There are no adverse effects of scabies in pregnancy; however, treatment options for scabies during pregnancy should be limited to topical permethrin (pregnancy category B). Ivermectin and lindane are not recommended for use in pregnancy.

Geriatrics and immunosuppression: The initial presentation of scabies in the elderly or immunosuppressed patient very often yields fewer cutaneous lesions than younger or otherwise healthy adults, and is more consistent with nonspecific dry, scaly skin that may have several nodules. Severe pruritus, however, is often still observed. In these

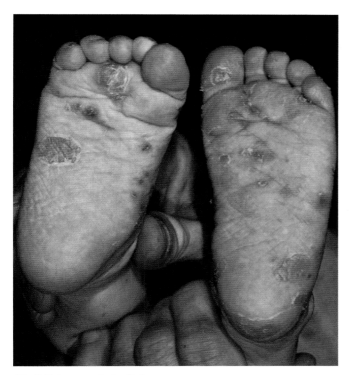

FIG. 13-5. Acropustulosis of infancy.

populations, the face and scalp may also be involved. As mentioned previously, Norwegian or crusted scabies is seen increasingly in these populations. Transmission of scabies is greatest in those living in close contact, and through sharing clothing and bedding. Assisted care personnel or facility administration should be notified so that other residents may be screened and measures taken to avoid an outbreak.

CLINICAL PEARL

Inflammatory nodules on the genitals are considered scabies until proven otherwise, so always examine the genitals in suspected scabies cases.

Prognosis and Complications

Patients with scabies infections have an excellent prognosis with proper treatment. Postscabetic pruritus, associated with a hypersensitivity response, is common and may persist for weeks after treatment, despite scabies eradication. Properly treated patients should begin to show steady improvement in pruritus after about 2 to 3 weeks. Symptoms are typically managed with oral antihistamines (e.g., cetirizine, loratadine, or hydroxyzine) and topical corticosteroids. Short courses of oral corticosteroids are generally reserved for severe and intractable cases.

Secondary infections caused by *Staphylococcus aureus* or *Streptococcus pyogenes* may occur. Antibiotic use should be considered as indicated.

Referral and Consultation

Referral to dermatologist or an infectious disease specialist may be considered if the patient shows no improvement with sufficient treatment after 3 to 4 weeks. Consultation may be considered earlier in patients who are immunosuppressed with disseminated infection. A skin biopsy may be attained if the diagnosis is questionable or no response to treatment.

Patient Education and Follow-up

Patient education is an important step to successfully treating scabies infection. Patients should be educated not only on application technique of antiparasitic medication but also on household management of inanimate objects since mites can live up to 3 days off a human host. The Centers for Disease Control and Prevention (CDC) has up-to-date information on prevention, control, and institutional spread. Patients can be reassured that after full treatment they are able to return to school and work and resume normal social interactions.

PEDICULOSIS

Pediculosis, commonly known as lice, is a contagious type of parasite that feeds on human blood. Infestation occurs through close personal contact, as well as through inanimate objects, such as brushes, combs, hats, clothing, and bedding. Lice infestations have become an increasing problem throughout the world, and usually occur with crowded living conditions or poor hygiene. In endemic areas, body lice are capable of transmitting infectious diseases such as typhus, relapsing fever, and trench fever.

Pathophysiology

Lice are parasites that live on the skin of their host. They feed on human blood approximately five times per day by piercing the host's skin and injecting saliva, causing a pruritic response. Without feeding, adult lice are able to live off of a human host for approximately 10 days, and up to 3 weeks as eggs or nits. Some experts use the term *eggs* to describe the container for a developing louse nymph and refer to 'nits' as the empty egg casing, whereas other experts refer to "eggs" and "nits" interchangeably; the latter reference is the context to which it will be referred to in this text.

Lice are small (<2 mm or about the size of a sesame seed), flat, and wingless insects that crawl and do not hop or fly. After feeding, they appear on human skin as characteristic rust-colored flecks. Pets cannot transmit human lice infestations, as these lice affect humans only.

Clinical Presentation

Head lice

Pediculus humanus capitis, or head lice infestation, can affect any part of the scalp, with accompanied dermatitis commonly seen on the occipital scalp, neck, and behind the ears (Figure 13-6). Nits are attached to the base of the hair with a glue-like substance secreted by the louse, within approximately 3 to 4 mm of the scalp. Occasionally, eyelash involvement occurs, presenting with redness and localized edema. Pediatric patients and their caregivers or household members have the highest prevalence of head lice, and girls are affected more than boys. It is seen across all ethnicities, but notably less in African Americans. After approximately 3 to 8 months of infestation, sensitization to lice can cause pruritus and posterior cervical adenopathy. Subsequent scratching of the scalp increases patient risk for bacterial infection, inflammation, pustules, and crusting.

Body lice

Caused by *Pediculus corporis*, body lice is an uncommon parasitic infestation associated with poor hygiene and the spread of infectious diseases. They do not live directly on the body; rather, they reside and lay their eggs in seams of clothing and return to the skin surface to feed only, making direct visualization for diagnosis difficult. Like head lice, hypersensitivity occurs over time, leading to pruritus and risks of secondary bacterial infection.

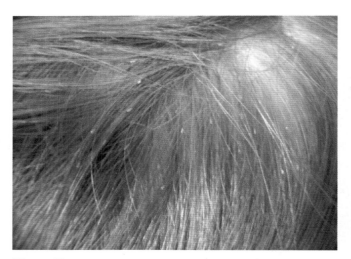

FIG. 13-6. Nits.

Pubic lice

Pediculus pubis or pubic lice received its nickname "crabs" based on its short, broad body with large front claws resembling a crab (Figure 13-7). Pubic lice are highly contagious, and sexual exposure with an infected partner yields a high rate of transmission. These patients are therefore more likely to be at increased risk for coinfection with other sexually transmitted disease. Pubic hair is the most common site of infestation; however, heavy infestation may occur in the perianal, proximal thigh, abdominal, axillae, and facial hair. Pruritus is a common symptom, along with a crawling sensation in affected areas. Inflammation and adenopathy can occur with regional infestation.

DIFFERENTIAL DIAGNOSIS Pediculosis

- Psoriasis
- Dermatophyte infection
- Seborrheic dermatitis
- Contact dermatitis
- Folliculitis
- Drug reactions
- Delusions of parasitosis
- Arthropod bites or other parasitic infestations, such as scabies
- Systemic causes of generalized pruritus

Diagnostics

Scalp and pubic lice are easier to diagnose through direct visualization, or with the aid of a magnifying glass. According to the American Academy of Pediatrics, the gold standard diagnosis is observing a live, moving louse on the scalp or pubic area; however, this is difficult as they move quickly and try to avoid light (Frankowski & Bocchini, 2010). A fine-toothed "nit" comb may be utilized to aid in diagnosis by combing the hair with teeth touching the scalp in a downward pattern near the crown to remove nits and live lice. In general, the closer the nits are to the scalp, the more recent the infection. However, the presence of nits may not indicate active infestation, as they may be retained on the shafts of hair for months after successful treatment. Dandruff or other hair debris may be easily misdiagnosed for nits or egg casings; however, generally hair debris is not as tightly adhered to the hair shaft as are nits. Utilizing a

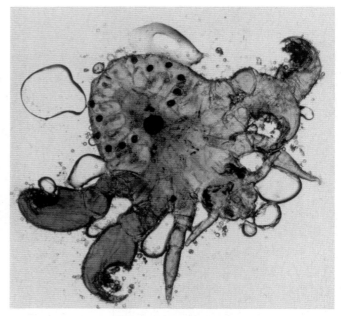

FIG. 13-7. Crab louse.

Wood's lamp may facilitate diagnosis as nits containing an unborn louse fluoresce white and empty nits fluoresce gray. Body lice may also be visualized on seams of clothing and may actually be seen crawling.

Management

To avoid overtreatment and risks, treatment for pediculosis should only be initiated when a skilled professional has made a definitive diagnosis. Treatment of lice and nits must include both topical therapy and environmental control measures. Unfortunately, the availability of over-the-counter topical antipediculide medications, along with improper diagnosis, has led to documented resistance in the United States to all topical medications used to treat lice, including permethrin, pyrethrin, and lindane. The choice of topical is predicated on the clinician's awareness of resistance in their communities. Pediculicides treat both lice and nits, and should be reapplied after 1 week. Patients using pediculicides on their hair should rinse off over a sink and not a shower, to reduce skin exposure.

Treatment for head and pubic lice is similar (Table 13-2). Various nonmedical methods of management are discussed under "Patient Education" below. The CDC recommends environmental treatment measures for cases of body lice, which include removing infested clothing and laundering with hot water (at least 130°F). Medical treatment and improved hygiene practice will usually resolve infestations. Clinicians should consider prophylactic treatment of household contacts, including sexual partners.

There are many traditional therapies that are not evidence-based or required to meet FDA approval, but are commonly used by patients and some providers. The application of a dilute white vinegar solution to the hair is used to soften the "cement" of the nit on the shaft and has been reported to make nit removal easier. During outbreaks at schools and daycare, many parents apply a thick, occlusive substance (petrolatum, mayonnaise, olive oil) to children's hair in an effort to smother the nit and prevent nit adherence to the hair shaft. Wet combing may be performed at home using a high-quality, commercially available nit comb, as an alternative to or in addition to topical pesticide medications.

TABLE 13-2	Medication Options for Pediculosis Capitis and Pubis			
MEDICATION	**CAPITIS (DAY 1 & 8)**	**PUBIS (DAY 1 & 8)**	**SPECIAL INFORMATION**	**EFFICACY**
Permethrin 1% cream/lotion (OTC)	Topical application for 10 min to clean, dry hair	Topical application for 10 min to clean, dry hair	None	*Capitis:* Poor–fair *Pubis:* Fair
Permethrin 5% cream (Rx)	Topical overnight application to clean, dry hair	Topical application for 8–12 hr	Approved for use ≥/2 mo of age Pregnancy category: B	*Capitis:* Poor–fair *Pubis:* Good
Lindane 1% shampoo (Rx)	Topical application for 4 min to clean, dry hair, then add water to lather and rinse	Topical application for 4 min to clean, dry hair, then add water to lather and rinse	Potential CNS toxicity Not recommended for infants or breast feeding Pregnancy category: C	*Capitis:* Poor–fair *Pubis:* Poor
Spinosad 0.9% cream (Rx)	Topical application for 10 min to dry hair	Not FDA approved	Approved for use ≥/4 yr of age Pregnancy category: B	*Capitis:* Poor–fair
Benzyl 5% alcohol lotion (Rx)	Topical application for 10 min to dry hair	Not FDA approved	Approved for use ≥/6 mo of age Pregnancy category: B	*Capitis:* Poor–fair
Ivermectin 0.5% lotion (Rx)	Topical application for 10 min to dry hair	Not FDA approved	Approved for use ≥/6 mo of age Pregnancy category: C	Not available
Ivermectin 3-mg tablets (Rx)	Adults: 0.2 mg/kg PO Q10 days × 2 doses Pediatric: Not FDA approved for lice	Adults: 0.25 mg/kg PO Q10 days × 2 doses Pediatric: Not FDA approved for lice	Give on an empty stomach Potential CNS toxicity Not recommended in breastfeeding Pregnancy category: C	*Capitis:* Poor–fair *Pubis:* Excellent

Adapted from Bolognia, J. L., Jorizzo, J. L., & Schaffer, J. V. (2012). *Dermatology* (3rd ed.). Philadelphia, PA: Elsevier Saunders.

And even more drastic measures include shaving or cutting their children's hair in an effort to eradicate the lice infestation. Parents can become frustrated and embarrassed by lice infestation, and are anxious to reach a quick resolution. Shaving or cutting a child's hair is not recommended as there can be associated psychological implications, especially in young girls.

Special Considerations

Pediatrics: School nurses play an important role by screening pediatric populations for infestations and providing education to reduce transmission. Valuable public health measures may be implemented if an outbreak is suspected, such as storing clothing (e.g., hats and scarves) separately. Some schools may implement "no nit" policies, requiring students to refrain from school based on the presence of nits alone. The American Public Health Association does not support this practice because the presence of nits alone does not make the child contagious. In some school districts, students may return to school after completing wet combing or appropriate insecticide. According to the American Academy of Pediatrics (2010), however, diagnosing a child with active head lice means it is likely the child has been infested for at least 1 month by the time it is discovered, and therefore poses little risk to other students from infestation; students are encouraged to attend classes, but maintain distance from other students until adequately treated. Eyelash infestation with head and pubic lice is seen primarily in the pediatric population and may cause secondary complications, such as infection or eye lid dermatitis. Presence of pubic lice infestation of the eyelashes or eyebrows may be a sign of possible sexual abuse.

Pregnancy: During pregnancy, pharmacological treatment options are limited. Special attention should be made when selecting an appropriate treatment. Table 13-2 lists options available for treatment during pregnancy, and other, nonpharmacological methods may also be utilized, as described under Management.

Geriatrics: There are no special considerations for elderly patients.

Prognosis and Complications

Prognosis is excellent since symptoms should completely resolve with successful treatment. Potential complications may include secondary bacterial infection from scratching, or hypersensitivity reaction. Large, live, moving lice suggest reinfestation, whereas lice of different sizes suggest treatment resistance, and patients should be reevaluated.

Referral and Consultation

Similar to scabies, recalcitrant cases should be reevaluated for the correct diagnosis. Patients who are immunosuppressed or have disseminated symptoms may be referred to a dermatologist or infectious disease specialist.

Patient Education and Follow-up

Environmental measures are important to treat lice and control outbreaks. Carpeting, mattresses, car seat, and furniture should be vacuumed. Bedding and clothing, including hats, should be laundered on a weekly basis. Brushes and combs should be washed in hot water (>130°F) or thrown away. A fine-toothed comb should be used once weekly for several weeks after treatment to confirm successful treatment. There are various commercial businesses and salons that provide lice and nit removal services, which may be an option to patients who do not feel comfortable with or are otherwise unable to perform their own combing treatments.

Follow-up is not generally warranted unless the patient experiences continued symptoms despite adequate treatment, or if they develop any complications such as a secondary bacterial infection.

TICK BITES

Ticks are nonvenomous, bloodsucking, external parasites which can harbor various infectious diseases. There are two distinct classifications of ticks: soft-bodied ticks (Argasidae) and hard-bodied ticks (Ixodidae). Hard-bodied ticks are vectors for more serious infectious diseases; they feed on their hosts much longer (up to 10 days) and are generally much more difficult to remove. Ticks feed by first using their curved, sharp mouth parts to bite and then secrete a glue-like substance to help adhere to their host. The bite itself is often painless and can go unnoticed, especially if in an inconspicuous area. Ticks generally wait on bushes and tall grass for a host to pass by, or are transmitted by pets bringing ticks into the home. Lyme disease and Rocky Mountain spotted fever (RMSF) are the two most common tick-borne infectious diseases in the United States.

Lyme Disease

Lyme disease, caused by *Borrelia burgdorferi* in the United States, is a bacterial spirochete infection transmitted through deer ticks (*Ixodes scapularis*), and is the most common tick-borne disease in the

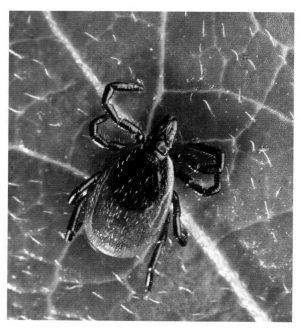

FIG. 13-8. Adult deer tick.

United States and Europe (Figure 13-8). White-tailed deer, white-footed mice, as well as other mammals and birds, are important disease reservoir hosts on which these ticks feed during their 2-year life cycle (Figure 13-9). Deer ticks in the United States are also responsible for the transmission of at least three different species of *Borrelia*, babesiosis, and human granulocytic anaplasmosis.

Lyme disease has been reported all across the country, particularly in and around coastal New England, including Massachusetts, Rhode Island, and Connecticut; other coastal states including New York, New Jersey, Delaware, Maryland, and Pennsylvania; and Minnesota

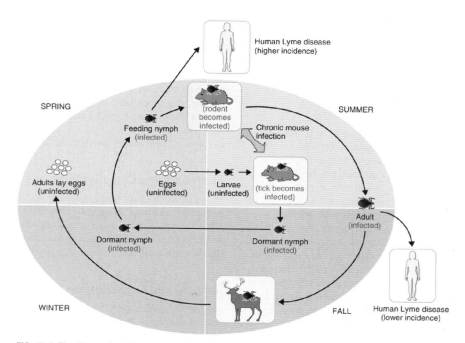

FIG. 13-9. The life cycle of *I. scapularis* (deer tick). Deer ticks are the arthropod vectors that transmit the spirochete *B. burgdorferi* to humans, causing Lyme disease.

TABLE 13-3	Physical Characteristics of *I. scapularis*
Nymph	Tiny and round
	Often compared to a poppy seed in size and appearance
Adult	Approximately 3 mm in length
	Four pairs of legs
	Color ranging from primarily black to orange-reddish depending on sex
Engorged	Large, globular-shaped abdomen
	The abdomen will be a light grayish-blue color

and Wisconsin. While infection may occur at any time of year, risk is highest during the summer or early fall due to increased tick exposure. Aside from living in endemic areas, individuals who have outdoor hobbies, such as hiking or camping, or an outdoor occupation, such as forest rangers, are at highest risk. Children are also at high risk because of increased outdoor activity.

Pathophysiology

The deer ticks' life cycle evolves from larvae, to nymphs, to adulthood. Tick size and appearance may provide helpful clinical clues for the experienced clinician to distinguish this from other arthropod or other tick bites (Table 13-3). Both nymphal and adult ticks are capable of transmitting infection. Figure 13-10 shows hard ticks capable of transmitting disease in the United States, including *I. scapularis*, associated with the transmission of Lyme disease; *Dermacentor variabilis*, associated with the transmission of RMSF; and *Amblyomma americanum*, associated with the transmission of human granulocytic ehrlichiosis, tularemia, and Southern tick-associated rash illness, or STARI, which is not covered in this text. Feeding ticks are firmly attached to the skin (Figure 13-11). If the tick is small and walking

on the skin surface, it is incapable of transmitting Lyme disease. The presence of an engorged tick embedded in the skin, or once it has detached after feeding, yields a higher risk of disease transmission. The duration of the tick's attachment is important when evaluating the risk of disease. Transmission of the disease rarely occurs within the first 48 hours of attachment in unengorged ticks (Hu, 2013). Time recollection may be difficult for patients while eliciting history, so it is often helpful to ask about all recent possible exposures.

Clinical presentation

Early detection of Lyme disease can be a challenge since only about 30% of patients have a known bite. Symptoms can be very subtle and often attributed to a brief viral illness, never suspecting a tick-borne illness.

Lyme disease may be localized to the skin or may involve multiple organs such as the joints, heart, and nervous system depending on the stage of infection. The three stages of infection discussed here are summarized in Table 13-4.

> **CLINICAL PEARL**
>
> Lyme disease is an important differential diagnosis for patients presenting in the summer with flu-like symptoms and no cough.

DIFFERENTIAL DIAGNOSIS Lyme disease

- Other tick-borne diseases
- Meningitis
- Joint disorders
- Dementia or delirium
- Chronic fatigue syndrome or fibromyalgia
- Cellulitis
- Contact dermatitis
- Granuloma annulare
- Heart block
- Systemic lupus erythematosus

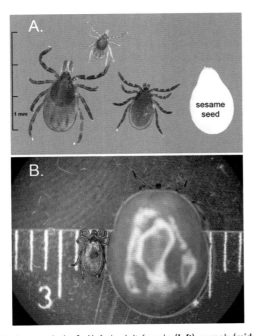

FIG. 13-10. *I. scapularis.* **A:** Unfed adult female **(left)**, nymph **(middle)**, and adult male **(right)**. **B:** Unfed **(left)** and fully engorged adult female **(right)**.

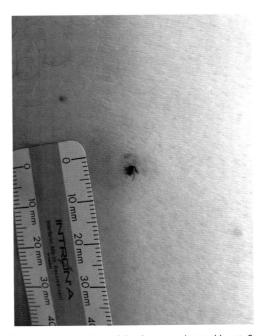

FIG. 13-11. Embedded deer tick almost undetectable at 2 mm before engorgement.

TABLE 13-4	Stages of Lyme Disease and Clinical Manifestations	
STAGE	**ONSET**	**CLINICAL MANIFESTATIONS**
Early localized infection	3–30 days after bite	Initially erythematous papule with central punctum
		Erythema migrans (EM): ring-shaped, migrating, flat erythematous rash (Figure 13-13), may spread beyond site of bite
		EM not always present
		Rash fades in 3–4 wk
		Flu-like symptoms may be experienced
		Excellent prognosis with treatment
Early disseminated infection	1–9 mo after tick bite	Includes cardiac, neurologic, and musculoskeletal manifestations
		Cardiac manifestations: pericarditis, AV node block, and mild left ventricular dysfunction
		Neurologic disease: meningitis, facial palsy, mild encephalitis with confusion, radiculoneuritis, mononeuritis multiplex, ataxia, and myelitis
		Good prognosis with appropriate treatment
Persistent/late infection	Months to years after the bite	Arthritis > neurologic manifestations
		Arthritic joint involvement: intermittent and persistent arthritis
		Chronic neuroborreliosis (Lyme-associated neurologic manifestations): rare
		Neurologic findings: cognitive changes, spinal pain, and distal paresthesias
		Post–Lyme disease syndrome: small subset of patients who experience subjective symptoms despite treatment

TABLE 13-5	Diagnostics in Lyme Disease
Serologic testing (Figure 13-14)	IgM antibodies to *B. burgdorferi* typically appear within 1–2 wk following clinical manifestations
	IgG antibodies typically appear 2–6 wk following clinical manifestations
	There is no indication to perform serum testing at time of bite
	False-positive ELISA titer levels may occur in the presence of other disease (e.g., infectious mononucleosis, RMSF, and syphilis) Prior subclinical Lyme infections may also produce false-positive results
Tick PCR testing	Routine testing of ticks for *B. burgdorferi* is not recommended since results should not direct clinical management
	If the tick was not attached >36 hr, prophylaxis is not indicated, even if the tick tests positive for disease
	If the tick was attached >36 hr, prophylaxis should be given as soon as possible, without awaiting results of PCR testing

Adapted from Hu, L. (2013). Evaluation of a tick bite for possible Lyme disease. In: J. Mitty (Ed.), *UpToDate*.

Diagnostics

Laboratory testing becomes important to aid in the diagnosis of Lyme disease, especially in patients who do not present with erythema migrans, or when there is no clear history of tick bite (Table 13-5, Figures 13-12 and 13-13). If serologic testing is performed, it is recommended to wait 4 to 6 weeks after the tick bite to avoid false-negative or false-positive results. Treatment should not be delayed while waiting for laboratory testing if clinical disease is suspected.

Management

The primary step in the management of tick bites is tick removal, covered in detail under "Patient Education" below. Patient anxiety may be increased after a tick bite especially in endemic areas, which

may result in overtreatment. Prophylaxis may be considered if the patient meets all of the appropriate criteria described in Box 13-1. Patients who do not meet all of the criteria or do not receive prophylaxis should be monitored for the development of clinical manifestations of Lyme disease.

Pharmacologic treatment of Lyme disease depends on the stage and clinical manifestations (Box 13-1). Patients requiring treatment for prophylaxis or early localized cutaneous disease may be safely managed in the primary care setting. Involvement with an appropriate specialist (e.g., cardiologist, neurologist, rheumatologist, or infectious disease specialist) is recommended once the disease advances and is affecting other organ systems. A subset of patients may experience transient, usually self-limiting worsening during the first 24 hours of treatment, and many experience

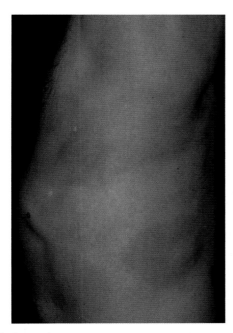

FIG. 13-12. Erythema migrans.

flu-like symptoms, such as fever, chills, myalgias, headache, tachycardia, or hyperventilation, described as the Jarisch–Herxheimer reaction.

Special considerations

Pediatrics: Children are at increased risk for contracting Lyme disease due to increased outdoor exposure. After playing outdoors, especially in endemic areas, parents should examine children for any ticks and remove them promptly. Doxycycline, which is primarily used to treat Lyme disease, is only appropriate for use in children older than 8 years.

BOX 13-1 | Pharmacologic Treatment of Lyme Disease

Criteria:
- Identification of deer tick (nymphal or adult)
- Tick attached ≥/36 hours (if time unavailable, if engorged)
- Resides in or traveled to endemic area
- It is within 72 hr of tick removal
- Doxycycline is not contraindicated*

Prophylaxis—if *all* of the above criteria are met

Adults: Doxycycline* 200 mg PO × 1

Children ≥ 8 years: 4 mg/kg PO × 1 (to maximum dose of 200 mg)

Early Lyme Disease

Adults: Doxycycline* 100 mg PO b.i.d. × 14–21 days; or amoxicillin/clavulanate 500 mg PO t.i.d. × 14–21 days; or cefuroxime/axetil 500 mg PO b.i.d. × 14–21 days

Children ≥8 years: Doxycycline 1–2 mg/kg b.i.d. × 14–21 days; amoxicillin/clavulanate 50 mg/kg PO divided t.i.d. × 14–21 days; cefuroxime axetil 30 mg/kg PO divided b.i.d. × 14–21 days

---

* Doxycycline is a relative contraindication in pregnant women and children under 8 years. The clinician should carefully weigh the risks.

Adapted from Wormser, G. P., Dattwyler, R. J., Shapiro, E. D., Halperin, J. J., Steere, A. C., Klempner, M. S., . . . Nadelman, R. B. (2006). IDSA Guidelines: The clinical assessment, treatment, and prevention of lyme disease, human granulocytic anaplasmosis, and babesiosis: Clinical Practice Guidelines by the Infectious Diseases Society of America. *Clinical Infectious Diseases*, 43(1), 1089–1134.

Pregnancy: Doxycycline, the primary treatment for Lyme disease, is not appropriate for use during pregnancy or breastfeeding. Pregnant women who contract Lyme disease should be treated promptly and thoroughly using appropriate medications, such as amoxicillin with clavulanate, to reduce the risk of transplacental migration of *B. burgdorferi* spirochetes to the fetus.

Geriatrics: Some of the clinical manifestations of early disseminated and late/persistent infection may mimic age-related changes, such

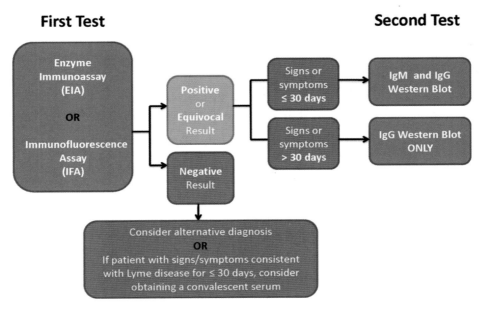

FIG. 13-13. Two-tiered testing for Lyme disease.

as ataxia, mild cognitive declining, or arthritis, resulting in delayed diagnosis and treatment.

Prognosis and complications
Adequate treatment of early Lyme disease is generally quite effective, with rare complications, and an overall good prognosis. The potential for multisystem involvement and subsequent higher risk of morbidity are associated with late-stage disease. Complications in later stages include acute and late neurologic complications, arthritic joint complications, cardiac complications, and post–Lyme disease syndrome.

According to the CDC, approximately 10% to 20% of patients who have been successfully treated for Lyme disease will have on-going symptoms, such as arthralgias, myalgias, or fatigue, which may last up to 6 months. These ongoing symptoms are described as Posttreatment Lyme disease syndrome (PTLDS). There is debate on the etiology of PTLDS; however, studies have shown that prolonged treatment of these symptoms with antibiotics are associated with worse outcomes and are not helpful in treating symptoms of PTLDS. Consideration of other etiologies which may be causing these symptoms, such as chronic fatigue syndrome or fibromyalgia, should be entertained in patients who have ongoing signs of PTLDS beyond 6 months with adequate treatment.

Referral and consultation
Consultation is rarely required in patients with early disease who are treated effectively. Despite appropriate treatment, patients with persistent symptoms should be considered for consultation with the appropriate specialist based on their continued symptoms (e.g., rheumatology, neurology, or cardiology). Patients who present with advanced disease, or those who fail to respond to recommended treatment, should be sent to infectious disease for further evaluation and treatment.

Patient education and follow-up
Discuss the general signs and symptoms of Lyme disease with patients who have experienced a tick bite, especially those in endemic areas, with instructions to notify their provider immediately with any signs or symptoms of early disease.

Patients should be educated on disease prevention. Tick repellents such as N, N-diethyl-meta-toluamide (DEET) and protective clothing, such as long sleeves and pants tucked into socks, help prevent tick bites when outdoors. Patients should be educated to check their skin, including the scalp, carefully after spending time outdoors to detect and remove ticks as soon as possible.

Tick removal: To avoid touching the tick, use tweezers, forceps, or gloved fingers to grasp the tick as close to the skin surface as possible, then apply constant, steady pressure pulling straight up, without twisting or jerking for 3 to 4 minutes until the tick slowly backs out (Figure 13-14). Take care not to squeeze, puncture, or crush the tick. If mouthparts remain embedded, do not attempt to retrieve them; they are typically expelled spontaneously. Consumer devices are available, which safely remove ticks (e.g., tick off or tick nipper). It is important that patients disinfect the skin thoroughly after removing the tick and wash their hands to help reduce disease transmission. Other methods often tried include petroleum jelly, nail polish, a flame or heat source, or isopropyl alcohol; however, these methods are not generally successful to induce the tick. The CDC offers further patient information.

Rocky Mountain Spotted Fever
RMSF is caused by *Rickettsiae rickettsii*, and is primarily spread by the American dog tick and the Rocky Mountain wood tick (both

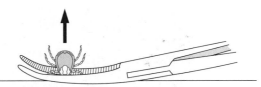

FIG. 13-14. Tick removal.

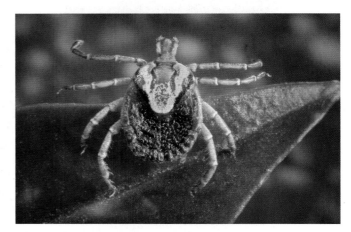

FIG. 13-15. Female cayenne tick, known vector for *R. rickettsii*.

Dermacentor species) (Figure 13-15). Although RMSF first got its name because of its observation in Montana, it has been reported in many areas of the United States, Canada, Central and South America. Five states account for over 60% of reported infections: Oklahoma, Tennessee, North Carolina, Arkansas, and Missouri (CDC, 2012).

Pathophysiology
The highest incidence of RMSF infection occurs between late spring and early fall, when the *Dermacentor* species ticks are most active. Ticks are both a reservoir and vector for the disease, and primarily transmit the organism to their hosts through saliva while blood feeding. Ticks must be attached for approximately 24 hours to transmit the bacteria. Adult ticks prefer to feed off medium-sized mammals, including pets, helping bring infected ticks into close contact with humans. Larvae and nymphal ticks generally prefer to feed on smaller mammals, such as rodents.

Clinical presentation
Symptoms start abruptly sometime between 3 and 21 days after the bite. The classic clinical triad associated with RMSF is rash, fever, and a history of tick bite. Fever is a vague symptom, and because tick bites may go unnoticed, RMSF is often a diagnostic challenge during initial disease. Earliest symptoms are often nonspecific and include headache, fever, myalgias, nausea, vomiting, and anorexia.

Several days after these initial symptoms present, subtle, nonpruritic, pink macules develop on the extremities, often including the palms and soles, before moving inward toward the trunk (Figure 13-16). Over the next several days, the rash may become papular, petechial, nonblanching, and red. Rocky Mountain spotless fever occurs less frequently, and refers to a subset of patients who never develop the rash. Patients with RMSF often require hospitalization. Later-stage infection involves multiple organ systems, including the lungs, gastrointestinal system, central nervous system, and the kidneys.

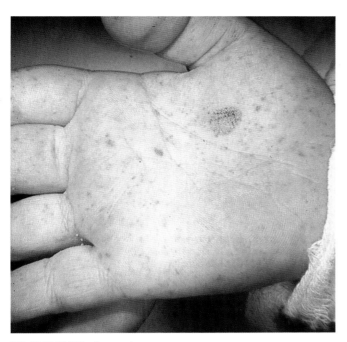

FIG. 13-16. RMSF palmar rash.

DIFFERENTIAL DIAGNOSIS Rocky Mountain spotted fever

- Nonspecific viral or bacterial infection
- Other rickettsial infections
- Meningitis
- Vasculitis and purpuric conditions
- Syphilis
- Bronchitis or pneumonia
- Measles, (rubella or rubeola)
- Dengue fever or malaria
- Hepatitis
- Infectious mononucleosis
- Kawasaki disease

Diagnostics

Diagnosis during initial disease is attained through a detailed history and evaluation of clinical manifestations. Treatment should begin as soon as possible, preferably before day 5 of the illness. Laboratory rickettsiae confirmation may take up to 2 weeks, during which time treatment should begin. According to the CDC, the gold standard for serologic testing at this time is the indirect immuno fluorescence assay (IFA) with *R. rickettsii* antigen. It is important to remember that IgG and IgM levels may remain elevated for months after infection. Other serum laboratory testing includes complete blood count (CBC) and complete metabolic panel (CMP). Expected laboratory findings in RMSF include normal-to-low leukocytes, low platelets, elevated AST/ALT, low sodium, and elevated BUN. Clinicians living in endemic areas should possess a high degree of clinical suspicion when evaluating patients.

Management

Despite the advent of antibiotics, which has substantially reduced morbidity and mortality rates, RMSF continues to be a very serious and potentially fatal infectious disease requiring prompt recognition and treatment. Once diagnosis is clinically suspected, treatment should be initiated. Doxycycline is the drug of choice for the treatment of RMSF in all ages and is often trialed in patients with a suspected diagnosis of

RMSF. Failure to respond to therapy indicates diagnosis is less likely. Adults (except in pregnancy or lactation) should be treated with doxycycline 100 mg PO b.i.d. until there is no fever plus 2 to 3 additional days. Therapy usually takes approximately 1 week, or up to 2 weeks in critically ill patients. Doxycycline may be administered intravenously for more critically ill patients unable to take the oral preparation.

Special considerations

Pediatrics: Children aged 5 to 9 years have the highest incidence of disease and develop the associated rash more rapidly than adults. Although tetracyclines are generally avoided in children under 8 because of the risk of tooth staining, doxycycline is the drug of choice for RMSF (2 mg/kg PO b.i.d.), given the risks versus benefit consideration. Despite the risks of tooth staining, doxycycline is the drug of choice for treatment of RMSF.

Pregnancy: Pregnant patients should be referred and managed by an infectious disease specialist since tetracyclines are contraindicated during pregnancy due to teratogenicity. If considering rickettsiae testing, a false-positive result may occur during pregnancy, especially during the third trimester.

Geriatrics: Advanced age is a risk factor associated with increased morbidity and mortality in RMSF infection.

Prognosis and complications

Mortality rate with treatment is 3% to 7%, and without treatment may exceed 30%. Early diagnosis and treatment generally yields the best chance of favorable outcome. Male gender, older age, and underlying systemic diseases generally increase the risk of fatality. African Americans have been linked with higher morbidity rates due to the difficulty detecting the rash in dark skin, delaying diagnosis and treatment. Complications of RMSF are similar to other generally severe diseases requiring prolonged hospitalizations, including paralysis, hearing loss, movement disorders, speech disorders, bowel and bladder incontinence, amputations, and death.

Referral and consultation

Patients may require hospitalization and evaluation by infectious disease specialists, especially if patients are high-risk, pregnant, elderly or have underlying conditions.

Patient education and follow-up

See Patient Education under Lyme Disease for tick bite prevention and removal information. No follow-up after tick bite or a successfully treated early localized disease is necessary. Patients with later stages of infection present with increased mortality and should have regular follow-up with pertinent specialists until clinical manifestations have completely resolved.

BEDBUGS

Bedbugs are parasitic insects found worldwide, whose presence has been documented for thousands of years. *Cimex lectularius* refers to the common bedbug seen in temperate climates, and *Cimex hemipterus* is found primarily in warmer climates; both feed on human blood. High rates of infestation occur in homeless shelters and refugee camps. Rates of infestation in developed countries have increased dramatically over the past decade, due to increased international travel, increased immigration from developing countries, and increased resistance to, as well as bans on, particular insecticides. They are thought to be suspected vectors for certain infectious diseases, such as hepatitis B and Chagas disease. Bedbugs are for the most part nocturnal and have an affinity for warm areas, particularly near or around beds or bedding.

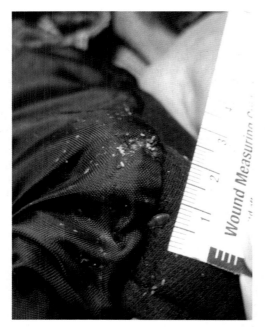

FIG. 13-17. Adult bedbugs with nymphs and eggs in the seams of a coat.

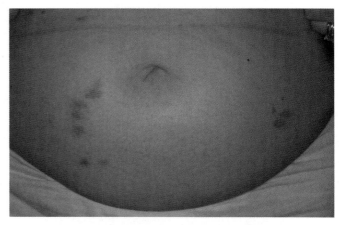

FIG. 13-18. Bedbug bites are often arranged in linear patterns or groups and referred to as "breakfast, lunch, and dinner".

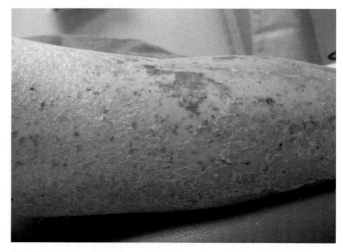

FIG. 13-19. Leukocytoclastic vasculitis secondary to chronic bedbug bites.

Pathophysiology

Bedbugs are reddish-brown insects with a flattened, oval-shaped body. They have a segmented abdomen and a retroverted mouthpiece optimized for sucking blood. They measure 5 to 7 mm in size, with males measuring smaller than females. Bedbugs have a very short life cycle and become fully adult and capable of reproducing in only 3 weeks, which explains the rapid increase in numbers. They generally hide in seams and folds of luggage, sheets, mattresses, clothing, and furniture (Figure 13-17). Bedbugs emerge from hiding at night to feed, and their bites generally go unnoticed. Clinical manifestations from bites occur due to a hypersensitivity response to the salivary proteins injected during feedings.

Clinical Presentation

Generally, bedbug bites present as edematous and erythematous papules, which are often quite pruritic. Occasionally, bites are vesicular or urticarial, and a central, hemorrhagic punctum may be observed. Bites classically appear in a "breakfast, lunch, and dinner" linear pattern, which represents the linear journey of the bug through the night (Figure 13-18). Bites may also be observed in a scattered distribution and are generally located on areas exposed during sleep, such as the arms, legs, waist, head, neck, and shoulders. The degree of response to the bites, as well as clinical appearance, is highly individualized and depends on one's degree of sensitization and reaction to saliva proteins. Reaction to bites may take several days to weeks to manifest. Figure 13-19 shows leukocytoclastic vasculitis, which is a more severe reaction secondary to chronic bedbug bites.

DIFFERENTIAL DIAGNOSIS Bedbugs

- Drug eruptions
- Dermatitis herpetiformis
- Other insect bites (i.e., scabies)
- Delusions of parasitosis

Diagnostics

The diagnosis of bedbugs is primarily achieved through a detailed history and clinical findings. Patients will often seek medical attention for unexplained pruritic lesions and expect a definitive diagnosis of bedbugs or not. Laboratory diagnostics are not generally used in formulating the diagnosis. Furthermore, skin biopsy may direct the diagnosis toward an arthropod bite, but would not specifically identify the offending insect.

Management

Management of clinical symptoms varies based on the extent of involvement and degree of severity. Treatment of minimally symptomatic patients is aimed at preventing secondary infections from scratching. Pruritus may be treated with topical or oral corticosteroids, or with antihistamines (e.g., cetirizine, loratadine, or hydroxyzine). Secondary infection may be treated with antibiotics. Severe cases may require administration of epinephrine. Patients with a history of asthma may experience an exacerbation of symptoms thought to be associated with bedbug excrement.

Environmental control is essential to adequately treating bedbugs and reducing the risks of transmission. The U.S. Environmental Protection Agency (EPA) has compiled their top 10 tips for the treatment and eradication of bedbugs (Box 13-2). Eradication has

BOX 13-2   Top Ten Bedbug Tips

1. Make sure you really have bedbugs, not fleas or ticks or other insects.
2. Don't panic: Treatment is difficult, but it is not impossible.
3. Think through your treatment options—don't immediately reach for the spray can: Consider an integrated pest management approach, which may reduce or eliminate the need for use of pesticides.
4. Reduce the number of hiding places: Clean up the clutter in your home.
5. Frequently wash and heat-dry your bed linens, bed spreads, and clothing that touches the floor to reduce bedbug populations.
6. Do-it-yourself; freezing is not usually reliable for bedbug control.
7. High temperatures can kill bedbugs.
8. Don't pass your bedbugs on to others.
9. Reduce populations to reduce bites
10. Turn to professionals, if needed.

generally been accomplished with insecticides such as permethrin or dichlorvos. Recent recommendations include removal by mechanical means such as vacuums. High heat (130°F) can also be successful at killing them. Cracks and crevices in headboards and walls around sleeping areas should also be inspected and treated appropriately.

Prognosis and Complications

Bedbug bites yield an overall excellent prognosis. Complications include possible secondary bacterial infections from scratching, hypersensitivity reactions, and considerable emotional stress. Immunosuppressed patients may have a slightly increased risk of contracting hepatitis B or Chagas disease with exposure. Bedbug bites are rarely fatal, but could occur due to anaphylaxis.

Referral and Consultation

Referral to dermatologist may be considered if the patient shows no improvement with sufficient treatment after 6 to 8 weeks, or may be considered earlier if the diagnosis is uncertain.

Patient Education and Follow-up

Prevention should be emphasized because eradication of bedbugs is difficult, often requiring the assistance of professional exterminators experienced in bedbug termination. Their small bodies and ability to go without feeding for long periods of time make them easily transportable in the seams and folds of luggage, bedding, clothing, and furniture. The best way to prevent bedbugs is to regularly inspect these items for signs of infestation, including the presence of bedbugs or their exoskeletons in the folds of mattresses or bedding. The smell of a sweet, musty odor, or rusty-colored blood spots on mattresses and bedding from blood-filled excrements are also indications of infestation. The EPA and CDC provide valuable information on bedbugs and offer several helpful tips for dealing with and eradicating these infestations.

Follow-up is not warranted unless patients continue to be symptomatic or develop complications, such as secondary bacterial infection.

SPIDER BITES

Spiders are generally not aggressive arthropods, and bite only in self-defense. They are carnivorous with short fangs, often too short to penetrate human skin. Spider bites are frequently over diagnosed by clinicians as patients often present with other similar appearing conditions claiming to have been bitten by a spider. However, spider bites are not often noticed at the time of occurrence, making precise diagnosis more difficult. Of all the spiders in the United States, only the black widow and brown recluse spiders are capable of producing severe reactions.

The black widow spider, or *Latrodectus mactans*, is a female spider that attained its name because they attack and consume male partners after mating. Although there are several other widow spiders throughout the world, this section will focus on the black widow spider as it is the most common one seen in the United States.

Black widow spiders are black, shiny, and have a fat abdomen resembling a grape. They have red hourglass-shaped markings ranging from one to two red triangles, spots, or irregular blotches on the ventral surface of their abdomen (Figure 13-20). Adult females can grow up to 3 to 4 cm long and contain powerful neurotoxic venom. Although more prevalent in the South, black widows can be found in every state, with the exception of Alaska. These shy spiders generally dwell in garages, barns, or outdoors around homes in garden equipment, tools, or woodpiles. They generally only migrate indoors during cold weather or if attracted by other insect infestations in the home.

Brown recluse spiders, or *Loxosceles reclusus*, are typically difficult to identify. Common nicknames of the brown recluse include the fiddleback spider or violin spider, because of the violin-patterned markings found on the dorsum of some spiders. They are a nonaggressive spider and native to the United States. They are generally limited to the Midwest, South, and West, and are often encountered in homes since they populate and thrive around humans. Brown recluse spiders often inhabit dark, dry, and generally undisturbed areas such as closets, garages, woodpiles, and sheds. Human contact generally occurs when these areas are disturbed or the spiders feel threatened by someone putting on clothing where the spider is hiding. Brown recluse spiders range from cream-colored to dark-brown or blackish gray, and may range from 6 to 20 mm in size (Figure 13-21).

Pathophysiology

Venom from the black widow spiders contains some of the most potent neurotoxins, affecting the victim's nervous system. Individuals

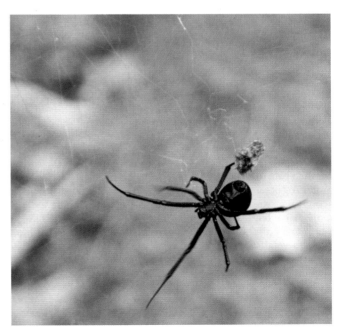

FIG. 13-20 Black widow spider.

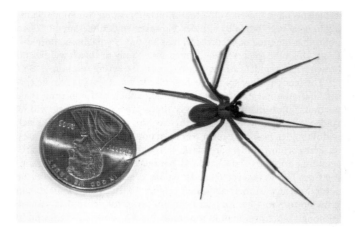

FIG. 13-21. Brown recluse spider.

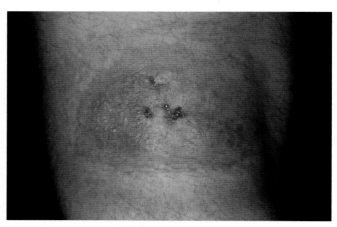

FIG. 13-22. Spider bite.

react to the toxin differently. It may be localized or be a severe reaction. The brown recluse spider venom contains enzymes that cause localized tissue necrosis. It also triggers immune responses that can either be localized or, in some cases, result in anaphylaxis.

Clinical Presentation

Black widow spider bite
Patients present reporting a recent history of doing yard work, spending time outdoors, cleaning their garage, or other activities which may account for their exposure. Bites can range from asymptomatic to a sharp, stinging sensation. Bites typically occur on the extremities, and most often, the lower extremities. Based on their genus, the term *latrodectism* is used to describe both the local and systemic manifestations of black widow bites. Bites typically appear as blanched, circular macules with a central punctum and peripheral erythema, whereas other bites present with more edema and induration (Figure 13-22). Unlike bites of the brown recluse, these bites do not become necrotic and rarely develop secondary infections.

Between 20 minutes and 2 hours after the bite, systemic manifestations begin to develop. These symptoms are often pronounced and may include headache, nausea, anxiety, tachypnea, localized or extensive diaphoresis and painful muscle spasms, and severe abdominal pain with abdominal wall rigidity.

Brown recluse bite
Brown recluse spider bites are often not initially felt, and generally occur while a patient is dressing as the spider resides in their clothing. They are found on the trunk, upper extremities, or thighs, and rarely on the face and hands. Many bites present as a minor, erythematous plaque without wound necrosis, and occasionally with two puncture marks. Localized cutaneous symptoms such as itchiness and pain occur after a few hours. As these spiders are capable of producing potentially deadly venom, even a small exposure can have serious risks, such as cutaneous necrosis. Central pallor develops in more severe bites after several hours. After a few days, the bite expands to a progressively enlarging, necrotic ulcer with eschar measuring several centimeters, and results in sloughing of tissue. The expansion typically stops after 10 days, and tends to heal by second intention with rare scarring.

Generalized symptoms develop over several days, can be quite severe, and are more common in children. Nausea and vomiting, rash, fever, myalgias, and arthralgias may occur. Rarely hemolysis, disseminated intravascular coagulation, thrombocytopenia, and even death can result.

DIFFERENTIAL DIAGNOSIS Spider bite

Black widow spider bite
- Rabies
- Tetanus
- Myocardial ischemia or infarction
- Acute surgical abdomen
- Necrotizing fasciitis

Brown recluse spider bite:
- Trauma
- Infection (i.e., streptococcal, staphylococcal, or deep fungal infection—community-acquired methicillin-resistant *Staphylococcal aureus* infection is more prevalent than spider bite)
- Other spider or insect bites
- Pyoderma gangrenosum
- Ulcers associated with arterial or venous insufficiency

Diagnostics

Diagnosing a spider bite can be challenging to the clinician, as frequently the bite is not felt or observed. The diagnosis is often made clinically, and is only considered definitive if the patient observed a spider inflicting the bite and that spider was collected and identified by an expert entomologist (Vetter, Swanson, & White, 2013).

Laboratory testing is nonspecific and yields little assistance in formulating the diagnosis. In patients who are experiencing severe systemic symptoms, abnormal laboratory results may include abnormal liver enzymes, elevated white blood cell count, increased serum creatine phosphokinase, and glucose levels. Differential diagnoses should always be entertained when making the diagnosis.

If a skin biopsy or hair sample is attained at the site of the bite up to 3 to 4 days after the bite, the *Loxosceles* venom may be detected through various methods of testing not widely available at this time (Bolognia, Jorizzo, & Schaffer, 2012). Differential diagnoses should always be entertained in the absence of definitive observation.

Management

Black widow spider bite
The application of ice to the site is recommended immediately after the bite to help promote vasoconstriction and reduce the spread of venom. Cleanse the site with mild soap and water, and elevate

the affected extremity. In mild, localized bites, oral analgesics may be administered to help control pain. Administer a tetanus booster vaccination if indicated. The majority of patients will only develop localized reactions; however, patients who have moderate-to-severe systemic envenomation symptoms will require hospital evaluation. In hospitalized patients, parenteral analgesics, benzodiazepines (i.e., lorazepam or diazepam), and/or calcium gluconate may be administered to control painful muscle spasms.

Black widow antivenins are available in endemic areas, and administration may be considered in collaboration with a medical toxicologist or physician experienced in managing widow spider bites. Indications to use antivenin may include patients' age, patients who are pregnant, have underlying cardiac disease, severe pain and muscle spasms despite other treatment, hemodynamic instability, or respiratory distress. Administration needs to occur in a monitored, critical care setting by experienced providers because its use has been linked to severe anaphylaxis, serum sickness, and death. Bites have high mortality, however, low morbidity, which is a reason why antivenin is not routinely administered.

Brown recluse bite

Management varies based on the severity of the bite. Conservative treatment is generally recommended, as most bites are mild and rarely progress into systemic manifestations. Localized wound care is important; bites should be cleaned with mild soap and water and treated with rest, ice, and elevation. Bites should be monitored for the development of necrosis and secondary bacterial infection. Oral antibiotics used to treat cellulitis (See chapter 9) should be implemented if there are signs or symptoms of infection. Dapsone is an antileukocytic antibiotic often administered in brown recluse bites to prevent or decrease necrosis in wounds with a progressing, dusky center. It is important to screen patients for G6PD deficiency prior to administration of dapsone because of the risks for hemolytic anemia. Antivenin is not widely available in the United States, but often prescribed for more severe variants of recluse spider bites found in South America. Surgical debridement is discouraged until the eschar can be removed 6 to 10 weeks after the bite. Any patient with a brown recluse bite who is experiencing systemic manifestations such as myalgias, arthralgias, rash, or fever should be evaluated in an emergency department setting, and may require intravenous hydration, steroids, and hospitalization.

Special Considerations

Children, the elderly, and immunosuppressed individuals are more susceptible to systemic illness with envenomation. Infants who have experienced a black widow bite may have a generalized erythematous skin reaction, and may be inconsolable. Antivenin administration should be considered in patients less than 16 years of age, greater than 60 years of age, and those who are pregnant. Brown recluse bites occurring during pregnancy are not associated with increased adverse risks to the mother or fetus.

Prognosis and Complications

Bites are generally mild and heal supportively without scarring after several weeks. Secondary bacterial infections are rare in black widow spider bites, but if present, may be managed with oral antibiotics. Other rare complications include hematuria, compartment syndrome, rhabdomyolysis, toxic epidermal necrolysis, cardiomyopathy, pulmonary edema, priapism, and intestinal ileus. Death is uncommon.

Referral and Consultation

Any patients exhibiting signs of worsening or systemic envenomation should be evaluated in the emergency room, especially the high-risk populations noted above. If antivenomation is needed, regional poison control centers or the Department of Public Health may be contacted for further antivenin information.

Consultation with a plastic surgeon or wound specialist may be necessary since patients with large, complicated wounds and/or delayed wound healing may require skin grafting or other interventions. Hospitalization for close observation and laboratory monitoring is recommended for all patients exhibiting signs of systemic envenomation or rapidly enlarging wounds.

Patient Education and Follow-up

Wound care instructions should be provided to any patient with these spider bites. The signs and symptoms of secondary wound infection and progressive skin necrosis should also be discussed. Patients who have received antivenin should be informed of the signs of serum sickness, which may develop several weeks after administration, and include rash, malaise, fever, and arthralgias. Patients should be informed to seek treatment immediately with the development of any of these symptoms.

Measures aimed to prevent bites are not always helpful, but may include insecticides and traps administered by pest control services, shaking out clothing and shoes before use, wearing gloves and long sleeves while working outdoors, modifying beds to avoid unnecessary ruffles or crevices, and avoiding underbed storages.

Patients who have received antivenin should be monitored for signs of serum sickness, which may develop up to 2 to 3 weeks after administration. Patients should be followed daily after the brown recluse spider bite for wound checks until the wound has stabilized and begins to improve. During the first 72 hours after the bite, a urinalysis should be performed daily to check for hematuria, and a CBC should be performed to monitor for thrombocytopenia (Arnold, 2012).

DOG, CAT, AND HUMAN BITES

Dog and cat bites are among the most common bite injuries encountered. Dog bites account for 60% to 90% of all animal bites, followed by cat bites (5%–20%), then rodent bites (2%–3%) (Endom, 2013). Although human bites generally occur less frequently than animal bites, they often harbor more pathogens than do animals and have a higher incidence of serious infections and complications. The spectrum of injury ranges from minor injuries which heal with conservative therapy, to severe and disfiguring injuries which can be fatal.

Pathophysiology

Both aerobic and anaerobic bacteria are involved in dog and cat bites, combined with the patient's own skin flora. The most common pathogen involved in both dog and cat bites is *Pasteuerella* species, followed by *Staphylococci* and *Streptococci* (Endom, 2013). Rabies infection in dogs is common in underdeveloped nations, but is generally not problematic in the United States due to strict vaccination laws. Because of their long, sharp, and deeply piercing teeth, cat bites are more frequently associated with anaerobic bacteria, such as *Fusobacterium*, *Porphyromonas*, *Prevotella*, and *Bacteroides*.

Both aerobic and anaerobic bacteria infect human bite wounds, and are typically pathogens that are found in oral and skin flora. These include *Eikenella corrodens* (gram-negative anaerobe), group A *Streptococcus* (aerobic gram-positive cocci), and *Haemophilus* species.

Clinical Presentation

Dog bites

Dog bites may range from minor wounds to quite severe and potentially fatal injuries. Crush and avulsion injuries are the most commonly seen injuries associated with dog bites, due to their strong jaws and rounded teeth. The head and neck are common sites of injury in infants and young children. Extremities, particularly the dominant hand, are the most frequent sites in adults. Fatalities, although rare, typically involve uncontrolled infection in deep lacerated and puncture wounds, and internal organ crush injuries affecting deeper structures such as nerves, tendons, bone, muscles, and vasculature.

Cat bites

The upper extremities are the primary location of cat bites. The anatomical design of a cat's sharp and slender teeth frequently produces deep puncture wounds, resulting in damage to underlying structures, including bones or joints which can become infected. For information on cat scratches, please refer to the section on "cat-scratch fever."

Human bites

A variety of human bites are observed; however, the most common types are clenched-fist injuries, or fight bites. Bites on the hand, are at particularly high risk for cellulitis, joint sepsis, and osteomyelitis because of the close proximity of the underlying structures. Other bites seen are chomping injuries, which tend to be closed injuries; bites involving the ears or nose, which may involve loss of tissue and structure; and puncture wounds. Often an erythematous arcuate or oval-shaped area with or without bruising is observed at the site of injury.

> **DIFFERENTIAL DIAGNOSIS** Dog, cat, and human bites
>
> - Patients are often able to provide an appropriate history.
> - Varying causative bacterial agents should be considered when providing empirical prophylaxis or treating subsequent bacterial infection.

Diagnostics

Cultures are generally of limited value after acute injury, but may help if the patient is not responding to treatment with broad-spectrum antibiotics after several days to weeks. Radiographic evaluation should be considered, especially in bites involving underlying joints or bones, to ensure there are no fractures or joint space penetration. CT scans may be necessary for more severe bites which may involve underlying organs, such as those occurring in young children.

Management

Most acute bite wounds are treated in the emergency department. Primary care clinicians may still encounter less severe acute bites, follow-up care after the emergency department, or bites with secondary bacterial infection. A thorough examination, including a motor-sensory evaluation, is a vital step in the management of bite victims. Determination of the extent of injury, appropriate diagnostics, and subsequent management must be tailored for each situation. Superficial, minor-appearing bites may occlude crush or deep-seated injuries, such as lacerated tendons or vasculature, osseous or joint involvement, or organ injuries. Some areas require notification of dog bites to local animal control or local law enforcement.

Wound care

Patients are often initially evaluated in the emergency department after acute bite injury; however, minor wounds may be managed successfully in the primary care setting. It is essential to refer patients to an appropriate specialist, such as plastics or general surgery, for high-risk wounds, including, but not limited to, deep puncture wounds; if there are underlying injuries, such as fractures or nerve damage; large wounds with loss of tissue; or wounds involving higher risk or increasingly cosmetic areas, such as overlying joints or body structures, the hands, or face.

Cleaning the site with high pressure, saline irrigation after injury greatly reduces bacterial count and is the cornerstone of wound management. This can be achieved by using a 10-mL syringe with an 18-guage angiocatheter attached, taking care to avoid further trauma from accidental injection. Debridement of devitalized tissue and clots may help prevent infection and promote quicker healing, with care not to debride underlying, healthy tissue. Surgical wound closure after an acute bite is controversial. Delayed wound closure, or healing with secondary intention, should be considered in wounds that clinically appear infected, puncture wounds or those more than 24 hours old, whereas low-risk wounds less than 8 hours old may be considered for closure (Presutti, 2001). Minor or low-risk wounds being followed in the primary care setting should be evaluated again after 24 to 48 hours. The patient should be instructed in general wound care and monitoring for signs and symptoms of infection.

Immunization

Immunization with the tetanus immunoglobulin or vaccine booster may be considered based on the patient's vaccination history. Anti-rabies treatment may still be considered if the animal's rabies status cannot be confirmed. This treatment is generally reserved for wild animals such as bats, raccoons, or skunks, and done in consultation with the local Department of Public Health.

Antibiotics

Prophylactic administration of broad-spectrum antibiotics is controversial. Low-risk wounds such as shallow, nonpuncture wounds generally do not warrant prophylactic antibiotic administration, and can be monitored for the development of infection. Higher-risk wounds such as cat bites, massive crush injuries, bites involving the hand, deep wounds, and those occurring in immunosuppressed individuals should receive prophylaxis with a broad-spectrum antibiotic. If the patient still presents with an infected wound after 3 to 5 days of prophylactic antibiotics, a full 10-day course (or longer) of antibiotics is indicated. See Table 13-6 for treatment recommendations. Wound cultures generally are not performed in acute bite wounds as they generally do not yield helpful treatment information. Cultures should, however, be considered if patients do not respond to prescribed antibiotic therapy.

Special Considerations

Pediatrics: Animal bites resulting in death are more prevalent in infants and small children, accounting for 10 to 20 deaths per year in the United States (Endom, 2013). Young children often and unknowingly may provoke the animal with their uninhibited behavior, resulting in bites.

Pregnancy: There are no special considerations aside from limited antibiotic treatment options during pregnancy.

Geriatrics and Immunocompromise: Immunocompromised patients, such as those with HIV, asplenia, kidney or hepatic disease, or the

TABLE 13-6	Oral Antibiotics Used in Dog, Cat, and Human Bites	
TYPE OF BITE	**FIRST-LINE TREATMENT**	**ALTERNATIVES**
Dog Bites	Amoxicillin-clavulanate §B	Doxycycline (§D/±) Clindamycin + fluoroquinolone(§C) Clindamycin + trimethoprim-sulfamethoxazole (§D)
Cat Bites	Amoxicillin-clavulanate §B	Doxycycline (§D/±) Clindamycin + trimethoprim-sulfamethoxazole (§D) Cefuroxime (§B)
Human Bites	Amoxicillin-clavulanate §B	Clindamycin + fluoroquinolone(§C) Clindamycin + trimethoprim-sulfamethoxazole (§D) Penicillin + 1st-generation cephalosporin (§B)

§B, pregnancy category B; §C, pregnancy category C; §D, pregnancy category D; ±, not appropriate in pediatrics under age 8

elderly, are at higher risk for serious, life-threatening infection after an animal bite due to compromised immunity. HIV and Hepatitis B prophylaxis should be considered when treating human bite wounds.

Prognosis and Complications

Patients heal favorably after bites without complication. Bites involving the hand generally yield higher risks including septic arthritis or osteomyelitis. These patients may experience residual disability and complications if they fail to seek treatment. Patients may initially ignore wounds and present later with pain, edema, or purulent drainage, and subsequently have an increasingly complicated course. Hospitalization is occasionally warranted in healthy patients who have been treated with suboptimal antibiotic therapy fever, rapidly evolving cellulitis, sepsis, hemodynamic instability, immunosuppression, and crush injuries. Other potential complications include cosmetic deformities and loss of limb.

Referral and Consultation

Extensive wounds require acute evaluation in the emergency department. Based on the location and severity of the wound, general, plastic, orthopedic, or neurosurgeons may be consulted. Bite wounds involving the hand resulting in decreased or loss function will require evaluation by a hand surgeon. Local public health departments should be notified of all animal bites when there is a question of rabies exposure for guidance with prophylaxis. Law enforcement and animal control may also become involved for safety.

Patient Education and Follow-up

Patients should be instructed on how to care for their wound, including frequency of cleansing and dressing. Education about the risks of infection despite adequate wound care is also important. Patients should be informed to look for and report erythema, edema, fluctuance, and purulent drainage. Infection should be reported promptly to initiate appropriate antibiotic treatment.

In-office reevaluation after a high-risk bite is generally within 24 hours and a low-risk bite within 48 hours. Follow-up is highly individualized based on the location and type of wound with consideration of the patient's underlying comorbidities. Follow-up is aimed at ensuring the wound is healing without complications such as infection or disability.

CAT-SCRATCH DISEASE

Cat-scratch disease (CSD), also known as cat-scratch fever, is typically a self-limiting, benign, infectious disease caused by bacteria *Bartonella henselae*. Adults rarely exhibit symptoms of the disease; children and immunocompromised patients are most often affected. Transmission has rarely been associated without known trauma.

Pathophysiology

B. henselae is a gram-negative bacillus carried by otherwise healthy cats. Cats typically contract the disease from other affected cats via the cat flea, with a small portion of domestic cats and up to half of all stray cats carrying the bacterium in their blood. Cats under the age of one are generally at higher risk of carrying the bacterium due to flea infestation. Most cases occur during the fall or winter.

Clinical Presentation

In classic CSD, patients will present with a nonpruritic, red papule appearing at the site of inoculation approximately 3 to 5 days weeks after a cat bite or scratch. Scratches most often occur on the upper extremities or face. This lesion evolves over the course of a few days into a vesicle, then dries into a crust. Skin manifestations may go unnoticed, and upon resolution, the lesion typically heals leaving a depressed scar, much like a chicken pox scar. After approximately 1 to 2 weeks following exposure, unilateral regional lymphadenopathy develops and, in some patients, flu-like symptoms, including fever, chills, headaches, fatigue, anorexia, backache, and/or abdominal pain. Severe cases may present with splenomegaly. CSD is often a self-limiting condition, but lymphadenopathy may persist for several months.

DIFFERENTIAL DIAGNOSIS Cat-scratch disease

Infectious
- Viral (cytomegalovirus, Epstein–Barr virus)
- Bacterial (Nocardia, LGV)
- Fungal

Noninfectious
- Sarcoidosis
- Pyogenic granuloma

Malignant neoplasms
- Kaposi's sarcoma

Diagnostics

Diagnosis is typically suspected after the patient presents with a primary cutaneous granulomatous lesion with regional lymphadenopathy, and exposure to a cat within the past 1 to 2 weeks. Serum indirect immunofluorescence assay (IFA) and enzyme-linked immunoassay (ELISA) testing may be performed to detect serum antibodies to *B. henselae*. Skin or lymph node biopsy may be performed, but is not routinely suggested.

Management

Because CSD is often self-limited, it generally requires no treatment. Antipyretic treatment is recommended in febrile patients. Antibiotic treatment should be considered in immunocompetent patients with systemic illness, or immunosuppressed patients, and comanagement with an infectious disease specialist is strongly recommended. Antibiotic treatment aimed at gram-negative bacterial coverage may be employed in severe cases and includes azithromycin, doxycycline, rifampin, clarithromycin, ciprofloxacin, gentamicin, or trimethoprim/sulfamethoxazole. These agents are considered to be effective in decreasing lymph node size, but do not alter the duration of the disease.

Special Considerations

Pediatrics: Children are more often affected by CSD than healthy adults, but still generally have favorable outcomes. Treatment with doxycycline should be avoided in children less than 8 years old.

Pregnancy: During pregnancy, azithromycin is used as a first-line treatment option for CSD.

Immunocompromised: Immunocompromised patients have the highest risk of developing systemic manifestations with a poor prognostic outcome after infection with CSD. Multiple complications may occur (see "Prognosis and Complications" below). Aggressive antibiotic therapy is indicated to reduce morbidity and mortality, and consultation with an infectious disease specialist is strongly recommended.

Prognosis and Complications

CSD generally has a favorable prognosis, and resolves spontaneously most of the time. Complications and morbidity occur most frequently in immunocompromised patients and include neurologic, vascular, skin, ocular and hepatic disorders.

Referral and Consultation

Referral or consultation to an infectious disease specialist should be considered in immunocompetent patients manifesting complications, in all immunosuppressed patients, or in instances of diagnostic uncertainty. Other specialists may be indicated based on disease manifestations.

Patient Education and Follow-up

Patients should be educated that pet quarantine or euthanasia is not necessary since the transmissibility of the organism from cats is transient. Teaching children to handle pets gently to avoid scratches or bites may reduce transmission. Avoidance of stray cats and regular flea treatments administered by their pet's veterinarian may reduce infection rates. Infected cats may be treated by their veterinarian with doxycycline; however, this may not decrease risk of transmission to humans. Patients may be directed to the CDC website.

Follow-up is generally not necessary as this is often a self-limiting disease. Patients with systemic complications or immunosuppression should be followed closely until disease is successfully treated.

BILLING CODES ICD-10

Brown recluse spider bite	E905
Cat bite	E906
Cat-scratch disease	A28.1
Dog bite	E906.0
Human bite (accidental)	E928.3
Human bite (assault)	E968.7
Lyme disease	A69.2
Pediculosis capitis	B85.0
Pediculosis corporis	B85.1
Pediculosis pubis	B85.2
Rocky Mountain spotted fever	A77.0
Scabies/Norwegian scabies	B-86

READINGS

Arnold, T. C. (2012, July 30). Brown recluse spider envenomation. In: J. Alcock (Ed.), *Medscape Reference*. Retrieved from http://emedicine.medscape.com/article/772295-overview

Bolognia, J. L., Jorizzo, J. L., & Schaffer, J. V. (2012). *Dermatology* (3rd ed.). Philadelphia, PA: Elsevier Saunders.

Centers for Disease Control and Prevention. (2010, March 25). *HIV transmission*. Retrieved June 15, 2013, from Department of Health and Human Services: http://www.cdc.gov/hiv/resources/qa/transmission.htm

Endom, E. E. (2013). *Initial management of animal and human bites*. In: J. F. Wiley (Ed.), UpToDate. Retrieved from http://www.uptodate.com/home/index.html

Frankowski, B. L., Bocchini, J. A., & Council on School Health and Committee on Infectious Disease. (2010). Head lice. *Pediatrics, 126*(2), 392–403.

Habif, T. P. (2010). *Clinical dermatology: A color guide to diagnosis and therapy* (5th ed.). St. Louis, MO: Mosby.

Hu, L. (2013). Evaluation of a tick bite for possible Lyme disease. In: J. Mitty (Ed.), *UpToDate*.

McCroskey, A. L., & Rosh, A. J. (2012, June 12). Scabies in emergency medicine. In R. E. O'Connor (Ed.), *Medscape Reference*. Medscape Reference: http://emedicine.medscape.com/article/785873-overview

Presutti, J. R. (2001, April 15). Prevention and treatment of dog bites. *American Family Physician, 63*(8), 1567–1573.

Vetter, R. S., Swanson, D. L., & White J. (2013). Bites of widow spiders. In: J. F. Wiley (Ed.), *UpToDate*. Retrieved from http://www.uptodate.com/home/index.html

CHAPTER 14

Disorders of Hair and Nails

Niki Bryn

Hair and nails are important appendages of the skin for both protection and self-esteem. In addition to protecting us and providing tactile sensations, our hair and nails can provide valuable clues to localized disorders and systemic disease. In the 21st century, there is a thriving industry dedicated to the enhancement of these otherwise ordinary appendages. While the process of enriching our hair and adorning our nails can be beneficial in the short run, long-term use of certain products can have their own deleterious effects. This chapter will review various hair and skin abnormalities, and will demonstrate some important information that can be obtained if the keen observer knows where to look.

DISORDERS OF HAIR

Disorders involving hair loss or excess have significant social and psychological implications for men and women. Hair styles and hair care can communicate much about a person, and diseases of the hair can have a significant impact on one's self-esteem. Understanding the anatomy and growth cycle of hair is fundamental to understanding the causes of hair growth abnormalities. In this section, we will discuss how to recognize disorders involving both hair loss and hair excess. Reduced eyelash growth is discussed in chapter 23.

Types of Hair

Hair follicles differentiate and produce three different types of hair: lanugo, vellus, and terminal hairs. Around the 12th week, the embryo develops *lanugo* hair, which is short, soft, and nonpigmented, over the entire body. This immature hair is shed about 1 month before birth and is replaced with vellus and terminal hairs. *Vellus* hair is relatively nonpigmented and is not associated with a sebaceous gland. *Terminal* hairs cover the head and often arms, legs, and other parts of the body and are associated with sebaceous glands.

Hair has two separate structures that work together, the follicle and the hair shaft. The inferior portion of the follicle includes the hair bulb and the dermal papillae from which the hair shaft is formed and is rooted in the subcutaneous fat. The emerging hair shaft consists of an outer cuticle which is tightly compacted to support the cortex, and the interior of the follicle with rapidly dividing and growing cells. Melanocytes in the hair bulb give the cortex its color. Each hair shaft has a tapered tip, and the hair is lubricated by the sebum produced by the sebaceous gland (Figure 14-1).

Hair Growth Cycle

The cycle of hair growth has three phases: anagen, catagen, and telogen. The *anagen* phase is the growth phase, which occurs when the cells in the bulb and the dermal papilla are actively dividing and forming a new hair shaft. Normally, 90% to 95% of hairs are in the anagen phase, which can last 2 to 6 years and enables some to achieve hair of extraordinary lengths. The anagen phase, which is genetically determined, is longest on the scalp and much shorter on other areas such as eyelashes and brows.

The *catagen* phase is a short transitional phase lasting a few days to weeks, with only a few hairs (<1%) at any given time. During this phase, the hair bulb goes through an involution and the outer sheath shrinks and detaches from the follicle but attaches to the hair shaft to develop a tighter club hair. The inferior portion of the hair shaft detaches from the dermal papilla, comes to rest at the level of the erector pili muscle, and is eventually pushed out. The dermal papilla rests under the hair follicle bulge before it starts to reform a new hair shaft.

The *telogen* phase is the resting phase and lasts 2 to 3 months, accounting for the average loss of 50 to 100 hairs daily. In many animals, telogen and shedding are seasonal but in humans it is random (Figure 14-2).

HAIR LOSS

Alopecia, or hair loss, can be divided into two main categories: scarring (cicatricial) and nonscarring (noncicatricial). Nonscarring *alopecia* is seen more commonly and comprises patchy hair loss, thinning, or shedding without any scarring features. Scarring alopecia is less common and associated with an inflammatory or infectious etiology. It is characterized by an area of complete destruction of the follicles with resulting scar formation. The hair loss is most often permanent and irreversible. Each of these categories can be further divided into diffuse or localized (patchy) hair loss. These four characteristics of alopecia are important clues for an accurate assessment and differential diagnoses (Table 14-1).

As with most medical problems, a good assessment of a patient with the complaint of hair loss begins with a complete history and physical examination. History alone is sometimes sufficient to determine the diagnosis, especially in nonscarring alopecia (Table 14-2). A physical examination should begin by assessing the entire scalp surface and the hair shaft. Other hair-bearing areas, such as eyebrows, eyelashes, beard and moustache, axillae, genitals, and extremities, should be inspected if indicated. As mentioned, specific characteristics of the alopecia can guide the clinician to develop a differential diagnoses and appropriate diagnostics. There are a few diagnostics needed in the evaluation of any hair loss (Box 14-1).

NONSCARRING ALOPECIA—DIFFUSE
Male Pattern Hair Loss

Patterned hair loss in men (MPHL) is viewed by some as inevitable and tolerable, while others find it unacceptable. MPHL is the most common cause of alopecia in men, with the highest prevalence in Caucasian males, having an onset before age 50, but usually showing signs of thinning before the age of 30 years. There is higher incidence of benign prostatic hypertrophy in patients with MPHL.

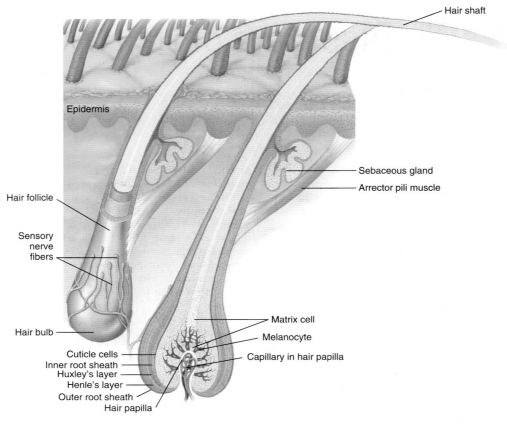

FIG. 14-1. Anatomy of hair.

Hair Growth Cyle

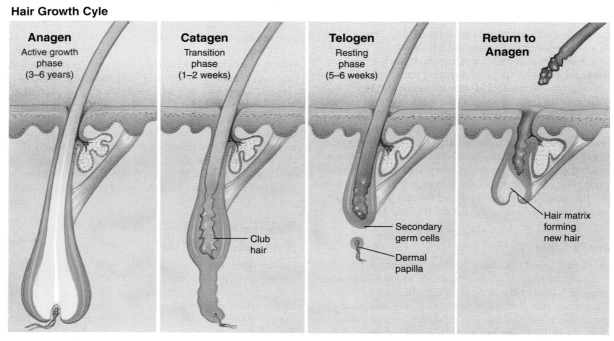

FIG. 14-2. Hair growth cycle.

TABLE 14-1	Characteristics of Alopecia for Differential Diagnosis	
TYPE	**DIFFUSE**	**PATCHY/FOCAL**
Nonscarring	Androgenetic alopecia (thinning) Telogen effluvium (shedding) Anagen effluvium	AA Trichotillomania Tinea capitis or infection*
Scarring	Lichen planopilaris Chronic cutaneous lupus erythematosus Dissecting cellulitis	Discoid lupus CCCA Acne keloidalis Traction alopecia

*If not treated early, can result in scarring alopecia.

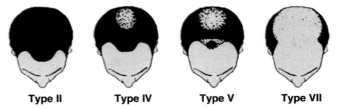

Type II   **Type IV**   **Type V**   **Type VII**

FIG. 14-3. Hamilton–Norward classification of male pattern baldness.

Pathophysiology

MPHL is caused by a genetically predetermined influence of androgens on hair follicles. Normally, 5α-reductase converts testosterone to the more potent dihydrotestosterone and increases scalp and beard growth in the male adolescent. Later in life, however, the dihydrotestosterone binds to the androgen receptor in the follicle, causing a shortening of the anagen cycle and miniaturization of hair follicles. The result is finer, shorter, and fewer hairs that can ultimately lead to baldness.

Clinical presentation

Most often it is not difficult to diagnose MPHL. Hair thinning and loss usually occur in the "M" distribution, affecting the bilateral temples and crown. These are considered the androgen-sensitive hair follicles. MPHL may be partial or complete and usually spares the sides and back. The Hamilton–Norwood classification is used to document and monitor the extent of hair loss. Seborrheic dermatitis is also commonly seen (Figure 14-3).

DIFFERENTIAL DIAGNOSIS Male pattern hair loss

- Alopecia areata (diffuse)
- Telogen or anagen effluvium

Management

MPHL is a cosmetic concern where both medical and surgical treatments are available. Determining how aggressive your patient wants to be is important when suggesting therapies. Medical therapies do not cure, but instead slow the progression and promote a thicker hair shaft. They also cannot grow hair on bald areas void of hair follicle. Minoxidil 2% and 5% topical solutions have been used for many years, however. Oral minoxidil was originally used as an antihypertensive drug for vasodilatory effects. But it also increases the anagen cycle and decreases miniaturization. Good results have been achieved using the 5% solution b.i.d. but will not achieve noticeable results for many months, and it must be continued for the long term. Minoxidil is applied to the entire affected area (dry scalp) twice daily and should remain on for at least 1 hour. When applied at night, it should be 2 hours before bedtime to prevent transfer of the product to the pillowcase. Touching the face during sleep could result in an increase of facial hair. The most common side effect is irritation and itching. It is more efficacious in young males with new onset of hair loss on the vertex and less effective in bitemporal loss.

Greater success has been seen with finasteride, a 5α-reductase antagonist, which blocks the conversion of testosterone to dihydrotestosterone, slowing the binding to androgen receptors and therefore slowing miniaturization. It is approved for use in males aged 18 years and older, dosed at 1 mg per day, and must be given for 3 to 6 months before success is determined. It is successful 70% to 80% of the time and should be continued indefinitely. Although there is no supporting evidence, many men use both oral and topical therapies concurrently. Patients should be advised that finasteride may decrease their libido or cause impotence and issues with ejaculation. Most symptoms subside upon discontinuance of the drug.

TABLE 14-2	Evaluation of Hair Loss: History	
PERSONAL HISTORY	**MEDICAL HISTORY**	**FAMILY HISTORY**
Ask the patient: • When did you first notice hair loss? • When did your hair last seem normal? • Was it sudden or gradual? • Is hair falling out (and seen in the drain or brush) or do you notice thinning (not as thick)? • Is the hair loss diffuse or patchy? • Is it only on the scalp or in other areas? • Any recent trauma, physical, or emotional? If yes, when did this occur? • What treatments have you tried? • Detailed inquiry about: • Hair care, products, styling • Use of tools (hot combs), relaxers or dyes, heat, use of extensions or weaves, and styling that pulls or binds (corn rows, ponytails, etc.)	List medications, especially new medications • Consider undeclared use of anabolic cortico steroids • Corticosteroids is one word use of prescription or over-the-counter herbs or supplements • Recent illness, surgeries, anesthesia, weight loss (diets) • Thyroid disease • Ob/gyn issues: menstrual irregularities, infertility • Skin conditions: acne, hirsutism, etc.	Balding male or female family members Thyroid disease

---

BOX 14-1 | **Important Findings in Patients with Hair Loss**

Physical Examination
- Location and pattern of hair loss
- Diffuse or localized
- Complete loss or thinning
- Hair texture, length, and color
- Presence of scarring
- Presence of erythema, pustules, scale, or abnormal pigmentation
- Nail findings
- Acne or hirsutism
- Patient affect and behaviors (i.e., anxiety)

Diagnostics (if indicated)
Part Width Test
Performed with the patient's head tipped forward, begin by parting the hair on the frontal scalp with a comb (if available) or the wooden end of a cotton-tipped applicator. Observe the width of the part and then compare the part width of the crown with many parallel parts on the temporal areas and occipital areas. Check to see if the part width is consistent in all sections.

Hair Pull Test
Consists of grasping 20 or so hairs on the crown. Pull gently but with enough pressure to tent the scalp and slide the fingers along the hair shafts distally to pull some hairs out. Examine the bulbs of the extracted hairs with a magnifier. Telogen hairs will appear as white bulbs at the end of the shaft. Fewer than six bulbs is considered normal (5%–10%). This may need to be repeated on two to three additional areas.

Punch Biopsy
Aids in the diagnosis of scarring alopecias. Indicated if the diagnosis is uncertain, the patient has multiple characteristics or failure to respond to treatment. A 4-mm (not any smaller) punch biopsy should be performed on the scalp area affected and close to the active edge of the scalp area. Be sure to get a sample of hair follicles and punch deep enough to get subcutaneous tissue where the bulb of anagen hairs will be located. Many clinicians will send two specimens, with one indicated for vertical sectioning, allowing for a good examination of the hair bulb. The specimen should be labeled for hair evaluation. Avoid specimens from the bitemporal area, which normally have some miniaturized hairs.

Laboratory Diagnostics
- Not often necessary but are guided by specific differential diagnoses.
- Fungal cultures can help to confirm tinea.
- Serologies help identify underlying disease causing alopecia: complete blood count and ferritin (iron-deficiency anemia); RPR (syphilis); antinuclear antibodies (autoimmune diseases); and TSH, T_4, and thyroid antibodies (hypothyroidism).
- In women, serum testosterone (free and total), DHEAS, and prolactin levels (if galactorrhea is present).
- Additional hormonal studies should be done in the presence of menstrual irregularities or hormonal abnormalities.

Surgical treatments include hair transplantation and scalp reduction. These are generally available through dermatology surgeons or plastic surgeons skilled in this fine art. Hair weaves are noninvasive techniques that use real hair to form a matrix which is then attached to the remaining short hairs. These treatments are commercially available through hair restorative groups or persons skilled in the process of creating wigs. Patients should be careful to avoid any harsh treatments on the hair or scalp and treat any scalp conditions like seborrheic dermatitis.

Female Pattern Hair Loss

Patterned hair loss in women (FPHL) is not as well understood as its male counterpart, but it is thought to be primarily genetic with at least one first-degree male relative with androgenic hair loss. It is a diffuse and nonscarring process. The onset for women is during their 20s or late 40s and can be perimenopausal. A common presenting complaint is "I can see my scalp" or "I am getting a sunburn on my scalp."

Pathophysiology
Because the pathogenesis of FPHL is not well understood, the term *androgenetic* is no longer accurate, although still often used. There is little evidence to support the theory that androgen levels were increased; furthermore, most women with FPHL lack any other signs of hyperandrogenism. Estrogen protects against hair loss and therefore FPHL is seen to some degree in all women who are postmenopausal.

Clinical presentation
The presenting complaint by patients is usually for generalized hair loss or thinning, while on examination hair changes are most visible on the crown. Excess shedding is not a symptom; lack of growth leading to thinning is the problem. The part width is increased when compared to the temporal and occipital areas and is often described as a Christmas tree pattern (Figure 14-4). There can be significant miniaturization and thinning of the crown, but the frontal border of hair is always preserved (Figure 14-5).

DIFFERENTIAL DIAGNOSIS Female pattern hair loss
- Telogen effluvium (acute and chronic)
- Diffuse alopecia areata

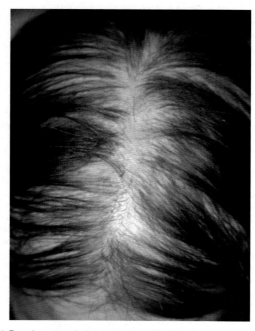

FIG. 14-4. Female pattern hair loss begins with widening central part and diffuse thinning.

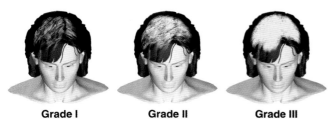

| Grade I | Grade II | Grade III |

FIG. 14-5. Ludwig classification of female pattern hair loss. Note the retention of the frontal hairline despite the increasing severity of hair loss.

Management

The only Food and Drug Administration (FDA)-approved treatment for FPHL is minoxidil 2% solution. Many clinicians start with a 2% solution twice daily to minimize side effects and increase to a 5% solution (off-label) if there has been no improvement after 6 months. The 5% preparation of minoxidil is more effective but also has higher risk of hypertrichosis on the malar prominences and forehead. The application and side effects are the same as with men. Most women with FPHL do not have hyperandrogenism; therefore, use of antiandrogens is neither indicated nor supported by any evidence. However, clinicians sometimes treat FPHL with oral contraceptives, spironolactone, or finasteride based on some anecdotal reports of success. Minoxidil is contraindicated in pregnancy and lactation.

Cosmetic aids such as powdered dyes or lotions can camouflage the scalp, making the hair loss less obvious. Wigs are often used in addition to hair extensions and weaves. Surgical therapies are available.

Referral and consultation

If DHEAS or testosterone levels are elevated and abnormal, a referral to an endocrinologist may be necessary.

Prognosis and complications

FPHL is a lifelong problem that does not have physical complications, but can have a significant psychosocial impact on patients.

Patient education and follow-up

Follow-up is generally not needed, and patients can continue use of Minoxidil indefinitely. However, sudden changes or rapidly advancing alopecia should prompt a reevaluation with the clinician.

Telogen Effluvium

Telogen effluvium (TE) is a nonscarring, diffuse hair loss, which causes women significant psychological stress. It is commonly seen in both primary care and dermatology offices.

Pathophysiology

TE occurs when there is an alteration in the hair growth cycle, primarily anagen and telogen phases. It is usually acute, but there are some cases of chronic TE occuring in middle-aged women. TE can be triggered by a significant emotional event or physical trauma in a patient's life. This can include illness, fever, hospitalization, surgery, childbirth, death of a loved one, or divorce. The growth cycle of the anagen hair is abruptly terminated, and a large number of follicles advance to the telogen phase. The result is shedding hairs at a higher than normal rate. In most cases of TE, less than half of the follicles are affected.

Medications that can cause TE include warfarin, isotretinoin, β-blockers, and ace inhibitors. It is not necessary to discontinue these medications as the hair growth cycle will eventually adjust itself back to normal. Discontinuing estrogen therapy or oral contraceptives can also cause a transient TE, and restarting therapy is not necessary.

Clinical presentation

Examination of a scalp with TE does not reveal noticeable abnormalities. There should be no erythema or scale and typically no areas of complete loss. Oftentimes, the density of the hair appears normal to the examiner, yet the patient gives a history of a significant change. Patients complain, "I am losing my hair" or "I am noticing a lot of hair in the shower drain." The key is that patients report increased shedding. These patients begin to shampoo less often in hope of preserving hair. They fail to realize that the average number of hairs lost daily is more evident on days they shampoo.

DIFFERENTIAL DIAGNOSIS Telogen effluvium

- Female pattern hair loss
- Diffuse alopecia areata

Diagnostics

It takes approximately 100 days for hairs to shed; therefore, the diagnosis of TE depends on the chronology of events and symptoms. The precipitating event is usually identified and precedes the hair loss by approximately 3 to 4 months. The shedding continues for about 1 to 2 months but may last 4 to 6 months before it subsides.

The Hair Pull Test can be performed to directly evaluate the hairs. If the test is positive, it confirms TE. A negative test would be found in patients with FPHL and MPHL. A test with more than 70% to 80% telogens should prompt the clinician to investigate an underlying metabolic or drug-associated etiology. Lack of regrowth in a timely manner should prompt the clinician to exclude other diseases like iron-deficiency anemia and endocrinopathies.

Management

No treatment is required for TE except patience and time. On occasion, patients can be quite anxious and request some form of treatment. For these individuals, minoxidil 2% or 5% can be recommended with all the same considerations as discussed above. The effectiveness is difficult to ascertain as the very nature of the condition will improve despite treatment. Recognition and treatment of triggering events is very important.

Prognosis and complications

TE is self-limiting and will resolve spontaneously. It can recur and sometimes become chronic. New hairs may not have the thickness or texture of the original hair.

Patient education and follow-up

Reassurance and psychological support is vital. In TE, patients are relieved to know that the condition will resolve and will not result in permanent balding. Patients should be advised that although they feel that they have less hair, they have the same number of hair follicles and hair shafts as before. Patient follow-up is only necessary if there is no resolution in the anticipated time frame discussed above.

Anagen Effluvium

Anagen effluvium is the sudden loss of hair, either partial or complete. The most common cause is chemotherapy, radiation, and, rarely, severe emotional or physical trauma. In this process, the rapidly dividing cells of the matrix are affected, leaving hair shafts that are narrowed, weakened, and easily broken. The hairs are shed in unison, about

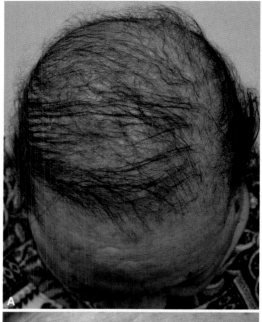

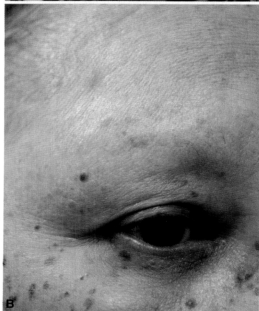

FIG. 14-6. Anagen effluvium is the sudden and complete loss of hair, usually occurring 2 to 3 weeks after chemotherapy. The scalp, eyebrows, or eyelashes can be affected. Regrowth occurs after therapy is discontinued, but the texture and color may be different.

2 weeks after the chemotherapy. After the chemotherapy or drug is discontinued, hair growth resumes. Occasionally, hair texture and color are different than pretreatment. Topical minoxidil can shorten the time of baldness by an average of 50 days, aiding in faster regrowth of hair once chemotherapy has been discontinued (Figure 14-6).

NONSCARRING ALOPECIA—LOCALIZED

Alopecia Areata

Alopecia areata (AA) is a total loss of hair at a specific site. Men and women are affected equally and age of onset can vary, but the first

occurrence of AA is usually before the age of 20 years in 60% of cases. AA is thought to occur secondarily to another autoimmune or T-cell-mediated disease such as thyroid disease, atopy, vitiligo, and lupus erythematosus.

Pathophysiology

The cause of AA is unknown but is believed to have a genetic predisposition with an environmental trigger. In the area of hair loss, the follicles have entered the telogen phase. As a result, the hair shaft is poorly formed and breaks at the scalp. However, the follicle remains intact.

Clinical presentation

Patients present with the complaint of a sudden "bald spot." The loss of hair may be preceded by a feeling of itching or burning. *Areata* means circumscribed areas with distinct borders, which in AA begin as round 1 to 4 cm areas of spot loss. The involved skin is normal in color and smooth, without scarring, scale, or erythema. Hairs on the periphery of the area break at the surface and resemble an "exclamation point" because of a narrow proximal end, widening into the thicker distal shaft (Figure 14-7).

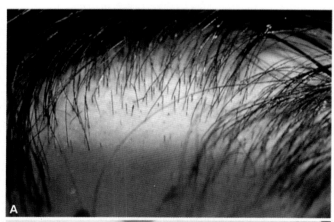

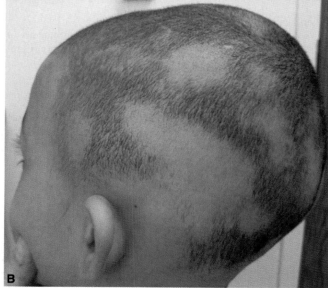

FIG. 14-7. **A:** Well-circumscribed patch of alopecia. "Exclamation" hairs (tapering at the proximal end with "!" appearance) are noted at the periphery. Typically, this condition responds to intralesional corticosteroids. **B:** AA in children can appear similar to tinea capitis (noninflammatory), which should be considered in the differential diagnosis.

AA is most common on the scalp but sometimes affects the beard, eyelashes, eyebrows—places that should entertain a possible diagnosis of trichotillomania. A pattern of hair loss surrounding the head like a band is referred to as an *ophiasis* pattern. Complete loss of hair on the scalp is termed *alopecia totalis*, while the loss of hair on the entire body, including eyelashes and eyebrows, is referred to as *alopecia universalis*. Be sure to check the nails, as nail changes are present in about 20% of AA patients. Proximal nail shedding, longitudinal ridging, and pitting have been observed.

> **DIFFERENTIAL DIAGNOSIS** Alopecia areata
> - Tinea capitis
> - Trichotillomania
> - Androgenic alopecia
> - Pseudopelade
> - Syphilis
> - Telogen effluvium

Diagnostics

AA is often a clinical diagnosis supported by the presence of exclamation-point hairs. Further diagnostic testing is usually not indicated. However, clinicians should have a high index of suspicion if the history and physical indicate a possible associated autoimmune disease.

If the diagnosis is uncertain, punch biopsies may be performed. Fungal culture and lymphatic examination can rule out tinea. Failure to grow back may warrant consideration of trichotillomania.

Management

Although regrowth can be spontaneous, timing is unpredictable. Treatment does not affect the course of the disease nor does it prevent new areas of loss. The goal of treatment is to stimulate regrowth in affected areas. Treatment depends on age, location, extent of hair loss, and the length of time the alopecia has persisted. Small areas will regrow, and treatment may not be necessary. Often, the areas of regrowth will present as white hairs, which may be a temporary or permanent change in hair color.

Treatment is not necessary but may be requested by the patient. Mid- to high-potency topical corticosteroids (TCS) twice daily should be effective within 3 months. Topical minoxidil 2% to 5% can be used as monotherapy or in combination with the TCS. Intralesional triamcinolone 10 mg per mL diluted 1:1 with lidocaine or normal saline can be effective for limited areas to stimulate new hair growth (Figure 14-8). Injections can be repeated every 4 to 6 weeks for 3 months. If the AA is in the beard area, the concentration of triamcinolone should be reduced to 2.5% to 5% per mL. Clinicians performing these injections should be experienced and the patient advised of the risks and side effects of atrophy, telangiectasias, and abnormal pigmentation.

Referral and consultation

If a topical or intralesional corticosteroid has been used over a 2- to 3-month period without improvement, or if the hair loss involves large areas, referral to a dermatologist is essential to confirm the diagnosis and consider other treatment options. Topical therapy with anthralin (a tar derivative), diphenylcyclopropenone (DCHP), or squaric acid (which are not widely available) has been used effectively by experienced dermatologists. Psoralen plus UVA and excimer laser have reported good results. Consultation with a reputable wig maker may be helpful. Psychological counseling may be helpful to patients in dealing with this skin disease.

Prognosis and complications

Hair regrowth commonly occurs within 1 to 3 months, and total hair regrowth is seen most of the time. The hairs may be the original color or they may be fine and white initially, but their presence on a follow-up examination can be encouraging for the patient. Alopecia totalis, universalis, and ophiasis pattern have a poor prognosis for regrowth. Associated autoimmune disorders may be discovered as the result of the patient's presentation of AA.

Patient education and follow-up

AA can be emotionally devastating for patients especially teens and young adults. Hair loss in odd patterns, the unpredictability of the course of the disease, and concerns for regrowth will contribute to the psychological impact. The National Alopecia Areata Foundation provides information and is support for both patients and providers.

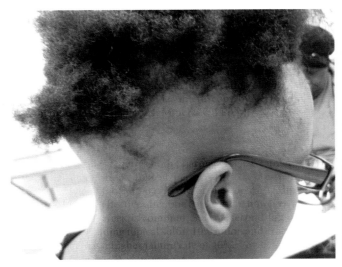 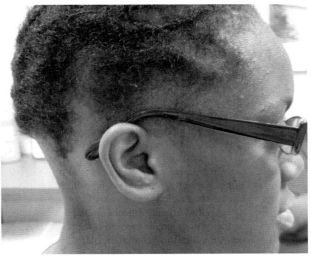

FIG. 14-8. Ophiasis pattern AA, a band-like distribution around the scalp. It usually has a poor prognosis for hair growth. In this 14-year-old African American girl, improvement was seen after two intralesional injections of triamcinolone, 6 weeks apart.

Trichotillomania

Trichotillomania is the repeated pulling or twisting of hair until it is extracted, creating noticeable spot loss. It is seen in children, adolescents and adults, and is more common in females.

Pathophysiology

This is a self-induced impulse control disorder. Trauma from twisting or rubbing results in hair loss by extraction. It is associated with depressive or anxiety conditions or may be a habit or tic. The act of pulling hair provides a sense of relief, satisfaction, or pleasure to the patient. Often an observer such as a parent or teacher will report the behavior; however, the behavior may not be seen if the child does it only in private or at bedtime.

Clinical presentation

The hallmark sign of trichotillomania is an area of hair loss with irregular borders and hairs of various lengths present at the same time. This distinguishes it from AA where there is complete loss of hair at the site. It is commonly seen in the easily-reached frontoparietal region of the scalp and should always be suspected when there is hair loss of the eyebrows or eyelashes. There is no inflammation or scarring present (Figure 14-9).

DIFFERENTIAL DIAGNOSIS Trichotillomania

- Tinea capitis
- Alopecia areata

Diagnostics

Direct examination of the hairs under a microscope will usually reveal a normal tapered end. A skin biopsy will show that the majority of the hairs are in anagen or growing phase and not in telogen, differentiating it from TE.

Management

Pharmacotherapy with antianxiety and antidepressant medications has been used with some success in the past. Recently, *N*-acetylcysteine (an amino acid) has been shown to be effective at decreasing this compulsive behavior. Referral for psychological evaluation and behavioral modification is key to the treatment of trichotillomania.

Traction Alopecia

Traction alopecia is caused by prolonged stress or pulling on an area of the scalp usually by hair styles such as braids, ponytails, hot combs, hair straighteners, or rollers. The change is usually temporary unless the traction is continued after the initial symptoms and then permanent scarring changes may occur.

Clinical presentation

The involved areas of alopecia are usually on the periphery, most commonly the frontal scalp. Loss of hair occurs slowly and with broken or vellus hairs seen at the site. Examination of the scalp is usually normal in the early process but some evidence of inflammation, papules or pustules, and broken hairs may be present. Over time, follicular loss and scarring occur (Figure 14-10).

DIFFERENTIAL DIAGNOSIS Traction alopecia

- Alopecia areata
- Telogen effluvium
- Chemical breakage

Diagnostics

In most cases, testing is not necessary.

Management

Awareness of the causative action usually results in a change in style or hair care regime. Avoidance of any traction or chemical stress on hair is advised.

Special considerations

Pediatrics. The early terminal hairs present on the back of the infant's head are shed at 3 to 4 months of age. This is often thought to be related to rubbing but is in fact a natural and expected occurrence.

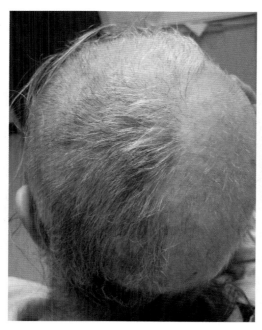

FIG. 14-9. Trichotillomania is characterized by irregular-shaped patches of hair loss along with varied lengths of remaining hairs.

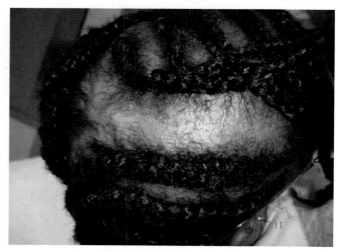

FIG. 14-10. Traction alopecia caused by the pulling or traction associated with hair styles like corn rows.

SCARRING ALOPECIA—LOCALIZED

The *primary* scarring (cicatricial) alopecias represent a series of conditions that usually involve a significant inflammatory process that targets the hair follicle and results in the complete destruction of the follicles, scarring in the reticular dermis, and permanent hair loss. Categorizing these conditions is often confusing, and there is considerable overlap. *Secondary* scarring alopecias are the result of a disease process unrelated to the follicle but which ultimately results in follicular destruction and hair loss. Examples of secondary scarring alopecia are chronic infections, deep burns, and radiation dermatitis. In this section, however, we will only discuss the primary scarring alopecias.

Discoid Lupus Erythematosus

Discoid lupus erythematosus (DLE), also known as chronic cutaneous lupus erythematosus, is an inflammatory process which results in scarring of the affected areas. It is slightly more common in African American women and occurs between the ages of 20 and 45, with peak occurrence in the fourth decade.

Pathophysiology

While there is more known about systemic lupus erythematosus (SLE) as an autoimmune disorder, DLE is less well understood. It is thought to occur in genetically predisposed individuals; however, the genetic connection is unclear. Ultraviolet light exposure and trauma are thought to be precipitating factors. A heat-shock protein is then induced within keratinocytes, leading to the destruction of the epidermal cells.

Clinical presentation

DLE is usually localized but can produce generalized lesions. It is commonly seen on the face, scalp, ears, and upper trunk. Early lesions are erythematous papules evolving into well-demarcated plaques with adherent scale. The scale penetrates the follicles and if lifted, reveals the characteristic spines on the undersurface which is said to resemble a carpet tack, the hallmark sign of DLE. Plugging of the follicles is also a characteristic finding on the scalp and is often seen in the conchal bowl of the ear. Areas of involvement may also exhibit telangiectasia and central hypopigmentation with peripheral hyperpigmentation. Without treatment, the disease progresses to cause a scarring alopecia and can be widespread and disfiguring (Figure 14-11).

DIFFERENTIAL DIAGNOSIS Discoid lupus erythematosus

- Pseudopelade
- Lichen planopilaris

Diagnostics

Antinuclear antibody testing is usually done to rule out systemic disease but is negative most of the time. Skin biopsy is usually confirmatory and demonstrates hyperkeratosis, follicular plugging, and a lymphocytic infiltrate.

Management

Initial treatment of DLE consists of complete UV light protection and use of broad-spectrum sunscreens at all times. Lesions require a high-potency TCS such as clobetasol ointment 0.05% and should be used in early lesions to minimize inflammation and scarring. Patients should be cautioned about additional atrophy. Intralesional injections of triamcinolone at concentrations of 3 to 5 mg per mL can be used on the scalp. If newer lesions continue to occur or existing ones continue to be active, systemic treatment may be used. Hydroxychloroquine

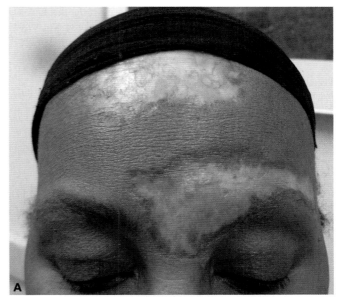
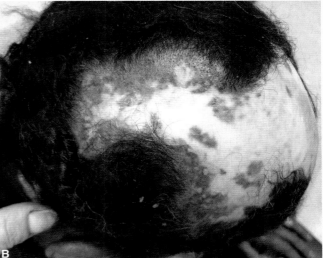

FIG. 14-11. **A:** Discoid lupus erythematosus. Scarring (permanent) alopecia and red scaly atrophic plaques are seen on the crown of the scalp. **B:** Depigmented atrophic plaques with hyperpigmented borders are typical of "burnt out" inactive discoid lupus; these changes are permanent.

can be initiated under the new 2011 testing guidelines. The American Academy of Ophthalmology has revised these guidelines to include a baseline examination within the first year of hydroxychloroquine use and again in 5 years in a nonrisk individual. Individuals at high risk for developing maculopathy should continue to have annual screening. CBC, LFTs, and G6PD are performed before initiating hydroxychloroquine use and annually thereafter.

Referral and consultation

Referral to a rheumatologist is recommended if the patients have symptoms of SLE or if the clinician has any suspicion of systemic disease. Patients with DLE should be referred to a dermatology specialist to confirm diagnosis and management.

Prognosis and complications

DLE is usually limited to the skin. The incidence of developing SLE has been estimated to be 5% to 10%, with some newer evidence that this occurs in approximately 16% of cases. The most significant complication of DLE is the depigmentation, scarring, and alopecia, which are permanent. Repigmentation can occur sometimes after treatment but is less likely when there is scarring or destruction of hair follicles.

Patient education and follow-up

If cutaneous lesions of DLE remain active, follow-up visits at 4- to 6-week intervals are recommended. Patients should be advised to return if they develop any systemic symptoms. Routine follow-up depends on the drug therapy.

Central Centrifugal Scarring Alopecia

Central centrifugal scarring alopecia (CCCA) is a progressive, scarring alopecia generally seen in African American women, although it has been reported in men. CCCA has been referred to as "hot comb alopecia," "follicular degeneration syndrome," "pseudopelade," "folliculitis decalvans," and "tufted folliculitis." There is a suspected association between CCCA and development of diabetes mellitus but there is no evidence to support it at this time.

Pathophysiology

The cause of CCCA is multifactorial and the condition occurs in all races. Certain hair care practices have been identified and are associated with an increased risk for CCCA: heat (hot combs, flat irons, or hair relaxers), chemical treatments, and hair stylings that use traction.

Clinical presentation

Hair breakage is often an initial sign and is commonly seen with the use of chemical hair products. CCCA exhibits hair loss at the crown initially and remains most severe on the crown or vertex of the scalp, gradually expanding in a centrifugal fashion. The affected scalp may appear smooth and shiny and in some areas, a few short, brittle hairs remain within the scarred expanse. Patients complain of mild pruritus or tenderness in the affected areas. Pustules and crusting may be found as well, and folliculitis decalvans may overlap. The disease generally progresses slowly, but long-standing or severe disease can result in scarring of the entire crown (Figure 14-12).

DIFFERENTIAL DIAGNOSIS	Central centrifugal cicatricial alopecia

- Female pattern hair loss
- Alopecia areata
- Lichen planopilaris (LPP)
- Telogen effluvium

Diagnostics

Skin biopsy of the scalp is required for definitive diagnosis and demonstrates specific findings of hyalinization of dermal collagen and broad tree trunk-like fibrous tracts.

Management

Early intervention may minimize the scarring process. Cessation of all heat treatments and relaxers as well as avoiding hair styles that require traction must be initiated.

If patients present with pustules, oral antibiotics such as doxycycline or minocycline may be used in addition to TCS. Hair transplantation is difficult. Because of the existing scarring, the transplanted hairs do not survive.

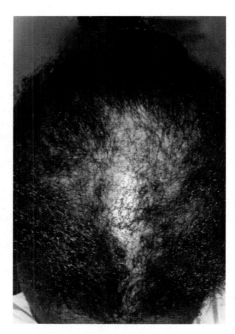

FIG. 14-12. Central centrifugal cicatricial alopecia. This condition occurs most commonly in African Americans and affects the crown and vertex scalp. Hair loss is permanent.

Patient education and follow-up

Thorough understanding of the etiology is essential to the discontinuation of these hair care practices. The Cicatricial Alopecia Research Foundation (CARF) has abundant literature and resources for these patients. Certain communities especially near large teaching hospitals have chapters of CARF and hold regular educational meetings for the patients.

Referral and consultation

Any scarring process on the scalp should be referred to a dermatology specialist as soon as possible. Early treatment may minimize additional scarring.

Lichen Planopilaris

LPP is a follicular form of lichen planus and is sometimes accompanied by characteristic lesions of lichen planus on the skin of the extremities and mucous membranes.

Pathophysiology

Although the etiology is unknown, LPP is an inflammatory reaction involving lymphocytes that attack the hair follicle. It is more common in women than in men and in Caucasians rather than in dark-skinned individuals.

Clinical presentation

The classic presentation of LPP is a centrifugal pattern on the frontal and vertex scalp. There are hyperkeratotic follicular papules with characteristic perifollicular scale.

In addition, there may be smooth, atrophic patches of alopecia. The lesions tend to spread outward, leaving the scarred areas in the center (Figure 14-13).

A variant of LPP is frontal fibrosing alopecia. This presents in postmenopausal women with bitemporal and frontal recession accompanied by eyebrow loss and erythema.

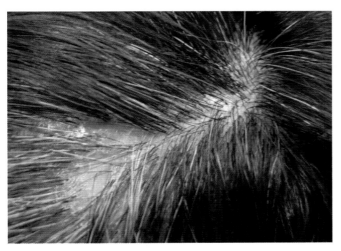

FIG. 14-13. Lichen planopilaris has a characteristic perifollicular erythema and scale.

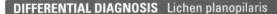
DIFFERENTIAL DIAGNOSIS Lichen planopilaris

- Lupus erythematosis
- Pseudopelade
- Folliculitis decalvans

Diagnostics

Biopsy is performed for confirmation of the diagnosis and should show a lichenoid dermatitis at the dermal–epidermal junction just as in lichen planus. There may be fibrosis around the hair follicles in advanced disease. Direct immunofluorescence is positive 50% of the time.

Management

LPP is very difficult to treat and may take years for the disease to burn out. No studies have shown truly effective treatment, and improvement may be due to the normal fluctuation in disease rather than treatment success. The first line of treatment would likely be a potent TCS solution such as clobetasol 0.05% b.i.d. for several weeks. Intralesional triamcinolone 5 to 10 mg per mL can also be tried if the areas are small. Widespread and worsening disease may require systemic agents such as doxycycline or minocycline 100 mg b.i.d. for their anti-inflammatory effect. Hydroxychloroquine, azathioprine, and cyclosporine have all been tried with varying success. Trials with biologic agents are also being attempted.

Referral and consultation

LPP is a cutaneous inflammatory process and is best treated by a dermatology specialist. An early intervention may be helpful to minimize scarring.

Dissecting Cellulitis

Dissecting cellulitis is an uncommon scarring alopecia which occurs most frequently in African American men between 20 and 40 years of age but can occur in any age, race, or sex. The etiology is unknown.

Clinical presentation

The active process is usually seen at the crown, vertex, or occiput. It presents with inflammatory nodules which evolve into fluctuant

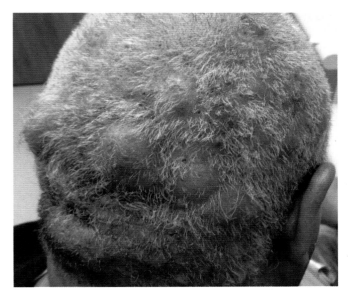

FIG. 14-14. Dissecting cellulitis.

boggy, oval, and linear ridges that progress to form extensive interconnected sinus tracts. Fibrosis and permanent hair loss ensue. Painful draining nodules may be present, and the scarring is extensive (Figure 14-14).

DIFFERENTIAL DIAGNOSIS Dissecting cellulitis

- Folliculitis decalvans
- Acne keloidalis
- Fungal kerion

Diagnostics

Physical examination by an experienced dermatology practitioner will generally result in a diagnosis. Skin biopsy can be helpful to confirm the diagnosis as the long-term prognosis is poor.

Management

Patients with this condition should not be managed in primary care until their condition is stable. Oral antibiotics are used extensively to minimize the inflammatory process and must be continued for the long term. A course of systemic antibiotics should be initiated by the primary care clinician, with immediate referral to a dermatology specialist. Drugs of choice are minocycline 100 mg b.i.d., doxycycline 100 mg b.i.d., and erythromycin 500 mg b.i.d. Other antibiotics such as clindamycin and rifampin may be initiated by a specialist.

Referral and consultation

In addition to the antibiotics, dermatology specialists may utilize intralesional triamcinolone 5 mg per mL to a few affected areas. Oral corticosteroids are sometimes used for a short time to decrease inflammation. Oral retinoids such as isotretinoin have been used to decrease the follicular keratinization as is seen in cystic acne. Dapsone, as well as the newer biologic agents which inhibit TNF-α, may be considered for long-term use. Surgical intervention may also be helpful to drain any large, painful nodules. Laser hair removal may be helpful, with resultant patches of alopecia. As a last resort, the patient should be informed about the use of wigs and hair pieces.

Patient education and follow-up

Patients must understand that the prognosis for this condition is poor and that treatment of new lesions should be done promptly. Good skin care regimen with antibacterial cleansers may help discourage secondary infection. Loss of weight has been shown to be helpful if the patient is overweight.

HAIR EXCESS

Hirsutism

Hirsutism in females is defined as the presence of dark, coarse terminal hairs on the face, chest, lower abdomen, and areola. In general, hair occurs in women where men usually have it and where women do not want it.

Pathophysiology

Hirsutism is usually the result of hyperandrogenism or an increased sensitivity of the hair follicle to the androgens. These high androgen levels convert the normal vellus hairs on the body to terminal hairs. Hirsutism may be seen with or without virilization (development of male sex characteristics). Hirsutism without virilization may simply be the result of genetic, racial, or familial differences. It may represent endocrine dysfunction such as hypothyroidism or be related to drug use, particularly glucocorticoids, minoxidil, oral contraceptives, and phenytoin. When hirsutism is associated with virilization, high androgen levels may be caused by polycystic ovary syndrome (PCOS), Cushing syndrome, adrenal hyperplasia, or androgen-secreting tumors. Idiopathic hirsutism can be seen in women with normal ovarian function and normal circulating androgen levels.

Clinical presentation

Hirsutism by definition is excessive hair growth in nine specific areas: face, chest, low back, upper back, buttocks, inner thighs, external genitalia, linea alba, and areola. Virilization may be manifest as acne, deepening of the voice, reduction in breast size, clitoral hypertrophy, frontal–temporal balding, increased muscle mass, infrequent or absent menses, heightened libido, and malodorous perspiration.

DIFFERENTIAL DIAGNOSIS Hirsutism

- Idiopathic hirsutism
- Polycystic ovary syndrome
- Congenital adrenal hyperplasia
- Androgen-secreting tumors (adrenal and ovarian)
- Anabolic corticosteroid use
- Porphyria
- Drugs
- Anorexia nervosa
- Hypothyroidism

Diagnostics

A detailed history should include a timeline of hair growth, the presence or absence of other signs of virilization, family history of hirsutism, and medication use (including anabolic corticosteroids). The physical examination should include the presence or absence of skin changes such as acne, androgenetic alopecia, and acanthosis nigricans.

Laboratory studies include 17-hydroxysteroid, thyroid stimulating hormone (THS) and prolactin if menses are irregular or absent, total testosterone, and DHEAS. If PCOS is suspected, then a complete work-up is required, including ultrasound, fasting glucose tolerance test (GTT), and lipid panel.

Management

Oral contraceptives and antiandrogens such as spironolactone or finasteride are helpful, and patients are usually followed up by an endocrinologist or gynecologist for treatment. Oral glucocorticoids may also be used.

If the hirsutism is idiopathic, then discussion with the patient regarding laser therapy or other hair removal methods may be helpful. Eflornithine, (Vaniqa™) in combination with hair removal, may slow the rate of regrowth. It is prescribed to be applied b.i.d. and must be continued long term.

Referral and consultation

If PCOS or other androgen-related disorders are suspected, referral to an endocrinologist is required.

Special considerations

Pediatrics. Hirsutism in children may occur as a result of familial or ethnic traits and usually begins during puberty. Hirsutism that occurs before puberty (precocious puberty) may be a sign of an underlying disease such as congenital adrenal hyperplasia (CAH) and usually occurs in early childhood. Late-onset CAH may occur with hirsutism after puberty.

Hypertrichosis

Hypertrichosis is the overgrowth of hair on the scalp and body. Unlike hirsutism, hypertrichosis affects both men and women and is in a nonsexual pattern. The cause is often heredity. Medications have also been implicated and include oral corticosteroids, minoxidil, phenytoin, and cyclosporine.

The porphyrias are also associated with hypertrichosis. These are a group of inherited disorders in which an enzymatic defect causes a disruption in the body's production of heme. The most common of the porphyrias is porphyria cutanea tarda and is discussed further in chapter 18.

HYPERHIDROSIS

Hyperhidrosis, by definition, is the production of increased amounts of sweat beyond what is necessary for thermoregulation. It is a common condition but can cause significant social and emotional consequences. It affects 1% to 3% of the population and affects males more than females. Family history is very common. Generally, it is a primary, idiopathic condition but can be secondary to other medical conditions or medications. When hyperhidrosis is limited to certain areas of the body, it is referred as primary focal hyperhidrosis, and most commonly affects the palms, soles, axilla, and face. When the sweating is generalized, it suggests a secondary cause.

Pathophysiology

The sweat glands, primarily the eccrine glands are responsible for creating sweat when it is needed to control the body's temperature by evaporation. The eccrine glands are most abundant in the palms and soles and less so in the axillae. The eccrine glands are innervated by the sympathetic nervous system. Sweating on the palms and soles is usually due to emotional stress, while sweating on the face, chest, and back is associated with heat stimuli. Histologically and functionally, the eccrine glands are normal; however, in primary focal hyperhidrosis, there may be an abnormal sympathetic response to the stress stimulus.

Clinical presentation

Patients with primary focal hyperhidrosis develop symptoms in childhood or adolescence, and it generally persists throughout life. It is usually bilateral and symmetrical, may be episodic or continuous and is rarely associated with bromhidrosis. Primary focal hyperhidrosis is usually associated with emotional stress that is not present during sleep. Generalized secondary hyperhidrosis usually presents in adults and is said to be present during sleep as well as waking hours.

Primary focal hyperhidrosis will affect the palms and soles, while secondary hyperhidrosis will be associated with an underlying disease or medication.

DIFFERENTIAL DIAGNOSIS Hyperhidrosis

- Thyroid disease
- Diabetes
- Infection

Diagnostics

The criteria for diagnosis include focal, visible excessive sweating for at least 6 months, with no apparent cause and at least two of the following:

- Bilateral and relatively symmetrical sweating
- Impairment of daily activities
- At least one episode per week
- Age of onset less than 25 years
- Positive family history
- Lack of sweating during sleep

A thermoregulatory sweat test is available but seldom used; refer to a dermatology specialist if desired.

Management

Ordinary, over-the-counter antiperspirants are usually about a 6% solution of aluminum chloride and are useful for mild sweating. Prescription strength 20% aluminum chloride is more effective. Patients should be informed to wash the area or shower first (usually at bedtime). Apply the solution to the entire area and cover with plastic wrap or gloves. Place each foot in a baggie or put on a T-shirt if the axillae are involved. Patients are directed to apply nightly until the sweating has ceased and then as often as needed to maintain control. The most common side effect is skin irritation which can be minimized by washing the solution off in the morning. Hydrocortisone 1% can be used if needed.

Iontophoresis is a method of delivering ionized substances through the skin by application of direct current. The exact mechanism is not clear, but it is thought to temporarily block the sweat glands. Equipment is available for home use and is marketed under the name Drionic and is available for hands, feet, and axillae.

Botulinum toxin is the most promising treatment to date but carries with it some disadvantages. It can be used successfully for hands, feet, and axillae but is a painful procedure. Temporary weakness in the muscles of the thenar eminence has been reported with injections into the palm.

Microwave energy is the newest treatment modality used for hyperhidrosis. This system focuses energy to selectively heat the interface between the skin and the fat where the sweat glands are present. It creates thermolysis and destroys the sweat glands. It is an in-office procedure.

Systemic agents have been used with some success. β-*Blockers* are used for episodic symptoms related to stress-induced perspiration.

Anticholinergics such as glycopyrrolate (Robinul) have been used successfully by some but are not FDA approved for this purpose. Dry mouth and dehydration are the most common side effects.

Surgical intervention has been tried by removing sweat glands primarily in the axilla. Transthoracic sympathectomy is a last resort.

Referral and consultation

Simple measures such as antiperspirants can certainly be initiated by the primary care clinician. Referral to a dermatology specialist may be useful if this initial treatment attempt is unsuccessful. Some dermatology or plastic surgery practices in the area may have the microwave device. Botox injections are administered by many different specialists, including dermatologists and plastic surgeons.

DISORDERS OF NAILS

Although the primary function of the nail is protection and the enhancement of sensation, changes in the nails can also be useful as a diagnostic sign. Nail changes occur normally as a process of aging. They often accompany cutaneous disease but may also provide clues to the diagnosis of certain systemic disease. Understanding the structure and function of the nail will allow you to identify and explain abnormalities (Figure 14-15).

The normal growth of the nail plate is very slow, but fingernails grow faster than toenails. The rate of growth is slowest at birth, increases through childhood, peaks in the teens and 20s, and sharply decreases after the age of 50. A fingernail takes approximately 5 to 6 months to completely regenerate from the matrix to the hyponychium, while toenails can take 12 to 18 months to achieve complete

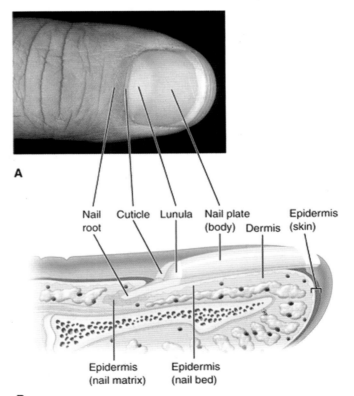

FIG. 14-15. Fingernail. **A:** External view. **B:** Anatomy of a nail.

growth. Because of this slow process, nails can provide information about conditions and changes that occurred months prior. They can also store information such as toxicology exposure and DNA.

Common Nail Changes

Variations seen in the nail apparatus can be the result of normal aging or can be related to infection, trauma, and cutaneous disorders or may reflect systemic disease such as liver, and pulmonary disorders (Table 14-3). Longitudinal ridging and beading are a normal finding in the geriatric population and is the result of the slowing down of the growth process. Median nail dystrophy and habit tic deformity are similar entities due to mechanical irritation to the cuticle at the proximal nail fold. This pressure results in longitudinal ridging and discoloration often in a fir tree pattern in the central nail and extending from proximal to distal

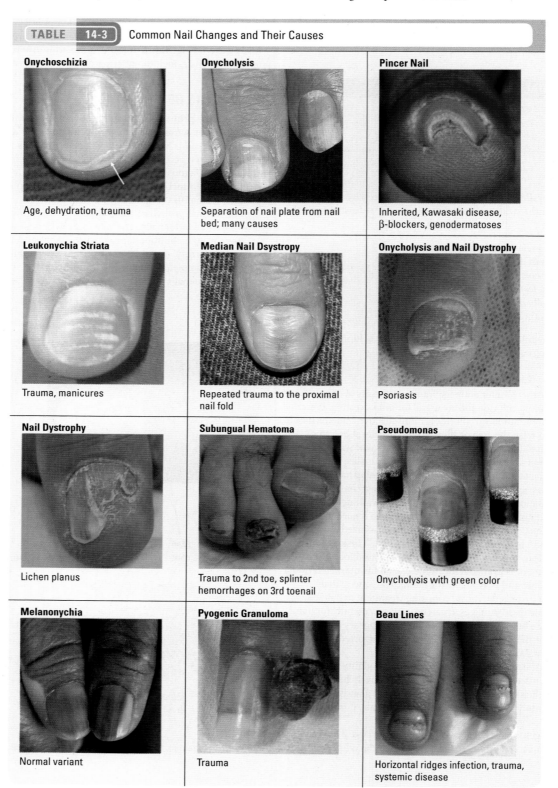

| TABLE 14-3 | Common Nail Changes and Their Causes |

Onychoschizia
Age, dehydration, trauma

Onycholysis
Separation of nail plate from nail bed; many causes

Pincer Nail
Inherited, Kawasaki disease, β-blockers, genodermatoses

Leukonychia Striata
Trauma, manicures

Median Nail Dsystropy
Repeated trauma to the proximal nail fold

Onycholysis and Nail Dystrophy
Psoriasis

Nail Dystrophy
Lichen planus

Subungual Hematoma
Trauma to 2nd toe, splinter hemorrhages on 3rd toenail

Pseudomonas
Onycholysis with green color

Melanonychia
Normal variant

Pyogenic Granuloma
Trauma

Beau Lines
Horizontal ridges infection, trauma, systemic disease

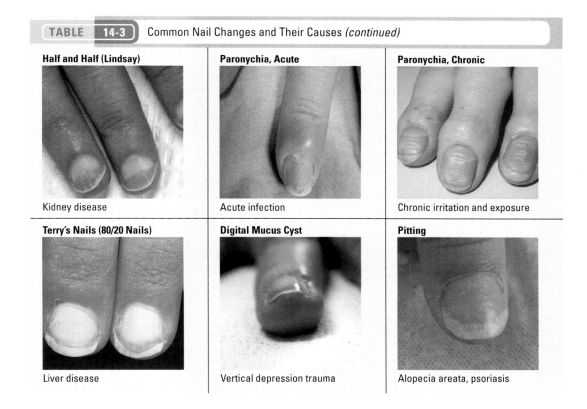

TABLE 14-3 Common Nail Changes and Their Causes *(continued)*

Half and Half (Lindsay) — Kidney disease

Paronychia, Acute — Acute infection

Paronychia, Chronic — Chronic irritation and exposure

Terry's Nails (80/20 Nails) — Liver disease

Digital Mucus Cyst — Vertical depression trauma

Pitting — Alopecia areata, psoriasis

Nail changes caused by infection
Onychomycosis
The most common cause of a nail infection is fungus and is caused by dermatophytes, yeast, or nondermatophyte molds. See chapter 12 for a detailed discussion of fungal nail infections and treatment.

Paronychia
Acute paronychia is an infection in the nail fold, causing erythema, pain, and swelling. Purulent material may be trapped behind the cuticle and should be relieved by gently separating the cuticle from the nail plate to release the purulent drainage and pressure, which is usually adequate treatment. If the patient is not responding, oral antibiotics and deeper incision may be indicated (see Table 14-3).

Chronic paronychia evolves slowly over time and is not a result of acute paronychia but is caused by repeated contact or irritant exposure (see chapter 12).

Pseudomonas
Appearing as a green/black discoloration of the nail bed, *Pseudomonas aeruginosa* ("green nail syndrome") infection of the nail bed is sometimes mistaken for hemorrhage from trauma but lacks a history of injury. *Pseudomonas*, gram-negative bacteria, is caused by repeated exposure to water and with resultant softening of the hyponychium, allowing the microorganism to enter beneath the nail plate. The greenish-black coloration is the result of the pigments secreted by the bacteria. This can be seen in women who wear artificial nails, where moisture becomes trapped under the cosmetic aid. *Pseudomonas* is treated with a white vinegar or bleach solution of 1:4 parts water. Distal fingers are submerged to soak where the separation has occurred. Trimming the nail or removing the artificial nail helps to remove the reservoir of moisture and hasten resolution of the infection (see Table 14-3).

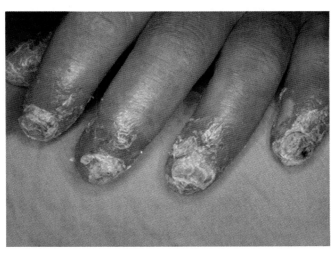

FIG. 14-16. Pustular psoriasis with destruction of the nail.

Nail abnormalities associated with skin disorders
Psoriasis
Nail changes are a common manifestation in patients diagnosed with psoriasis and are rarely the only symptom of psoriasis. Common changes are pitting, oil-staining, and nail dystrophy (see chapter 5). A severe form of pustular psoriasis may occur, and produces significant destruction of the nails and periungual skin (Figure 14-16).

Alopecia areata
AA is associated with nail changes less than 50% of the time, usually in the fingernails and with extensive disease. Pitting is the most predominant feature but is more geometric than the pitting of psoriasis. In AA, the pits are generally arranged in longitudinal rows. In psoriasis, they are more haphazard. A characteristic red lunula is also seen.

Lichen planus

The nail changes of lichen planus are seen about 10% of the time and are usually in association with other skin symptoms. The most common changes are longitudinal grooves, ridging, and hyperpigmentation, and onycholysis may also occur. In more extensive disease, a pterygium may occur when the proximal nail fold adheres to the matrix, resulting in destruction of the cuticle and a permanent scar. This is also known as "angel wing deformity" for its characteristic shape (Figure 14-17). Treatment is with intralesional corticosteroids by an experienced clinician. Further evaluation and treatment are done at the dermatology office.

Tumors of the nail

Benign tumors. Digital mucous cysts arise on the dorsum or lateral aspect of the distal digit adjacent to the DIP joint. They appear as translucent bluish cysts and may be tender when pressure is applied. To confirm the diagnosis, the cyst can be incised, and a clear gelatinous substance will emerge. The area should be prepped with alcohol and a no. 11 surgical blade or a medium-gauge needle (25G) is used to pierce the cyst approximately 1 to 2 mm. The cyst is then drained by manual pressure. As a result of pressure on the nail matrix at the site of the cyst, a vertical depression will appear in the nail and may be present even if the cyst is not visible. Mucous digital cysts do tend to reoccur but will become smaller or asymptomatic with repeated drainage. Cryosurgery can be performed by anesthetizing the area, removing the surface, and freezing for 20 to 30 seconds. A hemorrhagic bulla will result but should heal in 4 to 6 weeks.

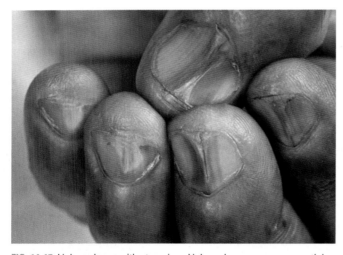

FIG. 14-17. Lichen planus with pterygium. Lichen planus can cause partial or complete destruction of the nail matrix, producing pterygium with the posterior nail fold overgrowing and connecting with the nail bed.

Pyogenic granulomas can appear near the lateral nail fold. These vascular lesions are removed by anesthetizing the lesion and performing a curettage and desiccation. The entire lesion should be removed to prevent reoccurrence. The lesion is sent for histologic examination by the dermatopathologist as these tumors may mimic an amelanotic melanoma.

Malignan t Processes. Melanomas of the nails are classified as acral lentiginous melanomas. They grow slowly and painlessly (see chapter 7). Squamous cell carcinoma of the nail bed is rare (see chapter 8).

BILLING CODES ICD-10

Androgenetic alopecia unspecified	L64.9
Alopecia areata	L63.8
Alopecia areata totalis	L 63
Alopecia areata universalis	L63.1
Central centrifugal scarring alopecia	L66.3
Chronic cutaneous lupus erythematosus	L93
Dissecting cellulitis	L03.90
Hirsutism	L68.0
Hyperhidrosis	R61
Hypertrichosis, localized	L62.2
Hypertrichosis, unspecified	L68.9
Lichen planopilaris	L66.1
Ophiasis pattern	L63.2
Other androgenetic alopecia	L64.8
Telogen effluvium	L65
Traction alopecia	L65.9
Trichotillomania	F63.3

READINGS

Blattner, C., Polley, D. C., Feritto, F., & Elston, D. M. (2013). Central centrifugal cicatricial alopecia. *Indian Dermatology Online Journal, 4*(1), 50–51.

Bolognia, J. L., Jorizzo, J. L., Rapini, R. P. (2008). *Dermatology* (2nd ed., pp. 965–1035). St. Louis, MO: Mosby Elsevier.

Freedberg, I. M., Eisen, A. Z. Wolff, K., Austen, K. F., Goldsmith, L. A., & Katz, S. I. (Eds.). (2003). *Fitzpatrick's dermatology in general medicine* (6th ed., pp. 148–163, 633–671). New York, NY: McGraw Hill.

Habif, T. P. (2004). *Clinical dermatology: A color guide to diagnosis and therapy* (4th ed., pp. 834–891). Edinburgh: Mosby.

Hoss, D. M., (2011). *Alopecia.* Retrieved from www.dermnet.com/videos/alopecia/

Linton, C. P. (2012). Describing nail abnormalities. *Journal of the Dermatology Nurses' Association, 4*(2), 149–150.

Linton, C. P. (2012). Describing the hair and related abnormalities. *Journal of the Dermatology Nurses' Association, 4*(3), 207–208.

Omori, M. S., (2012). *Herpetic whitlow.* Retrieved from http://emedicine.medscape.com/article/788056-overview

Tosti, A. (2013). *Onychomycosis.* Retrieved from http://emedicine.medscape.com/article/1105828-overview

Cutaneous Manifestations of Connective Tissue Diseases and Immune-Mediated Blistering Diseases

Margaret A. Bobonich

Connective tissue diseases (CTD) are autoimmune diseases which cause chronic inflammation, leading to the injury and destruction of tissue. Autoantibodies target collagen and elastin, which are found in almost every organ of the body. These proteins are essential for support and stretching, especially in connective tissue and skin. Hence, skin findings on physical examination can provide critical clues for the diagnosis of many CTD discussed in this chapter, including lupus erythematosus (LE), dermatomyositis (DM) and polymyositis (PM), cutaneous scleroderma (morphea), and Raynaud phenomenon and CREST syndrome.

CUTANEOUS LUPUS ERYTHEMATOSUS

LE is a multisystem autoimmune disease in which most patients manifest mucocutaneous symptoms. The American College of Rheumatology criteria require 4 of 11 symptoms for the diagnosis of systemic lupus erythematosus (SLE)—which could be met in patients who present with four cutaneous symptoms (Tan et al., 1982). Yet caution should be taken to understand that individuals can develop cutaneous lupus erythematosus (CLE), SLE, or both.

There are several subtypes of CLE, and they vary in their pathophysiology, clinical presentation, treatment, and prognoses. Genetic, environmental, and hormonal factors such as ultraviolet radiation exposure, smoking, family history, medications, infection, and specific HLA phenotypes have been identified as triggers. The strongest risk factor for CLE is gender, with women almost 10-fold higher than men and African Americans at greater risk than Caucasians. The age of onset is variable among the subtypes and is relative to an association with underlying SLE.

Patients suspected of having LE of any type should be referred to a rheumatologist for evaluation and management. A dermatologist may be involved for the management of cutaneous disease. Regardless of the type of LE diagnosis, the goals of care are control of the disease, early recognition of systemic involvement, and minimization morbidity and mortality. This section will focus on the recognition of CLE and not the diagnosis and management of SLE.

Pathophysiology

In a normal immune system, antibodies identify foreign proteins or organisms and trigger a cascade of inflammatory responses that attack the potential danger. Conversely, CTD can be characterized as a disease where the body's immune system does not recognize "self" and attacks it. Serum autoantibodies (antibodies directed at one of the body's own cellular components or target antigens) are directed at the body's normal tissue. Autoantibodies that develop are unique

for each CTD entity. Autoimmune diseases with systemic involvement are suspected when autoantibodies target nuclear antigens (antinuclear antibodies or ANA).

CLE can be classified into three groups: acute (ACLE), subacute (SCLE), and chronic (CCLE). Each disease is based on a continuum of systemic and cutaneous involvement (Figure 15-1).

Acute Cutaneous Lupus Erythematosus

ACLE is characterized as a transient skin eruption lasting for days or weeks in patients who usually have an underlying diagnosis of SLE with multisystem involvement. Lesions can be localized violaceous plaques or diffuse patches, papules, or plaques often exacerbated by sun exposure on the face, neck, chest, back, and arms. There is a wide range of cutaneous symptoms that should alert the clinician to a possible diagnosis of SLE (Box 15-1). The central face, in particular, often develops erythematous plaques and induration involving the malar prominences and commonly referred to as the *butterfly rash* (Figure 15-2). It can be confused with rosacea and seborrheic dermatitis except that ACLE does not involve the nasal labial fold or have an acneiform features. The plaques do not appear discoid, but the patient may develop discoid LE (DLE). Other cutaneous findings may include palmar telangiectasias, erythema of the dorsal fingers (between IP joints), periungual erythema, abnormal capillary loops of the nail folds, alopecia, and urticaria (Figures 15-3 and 15-4). ACLE

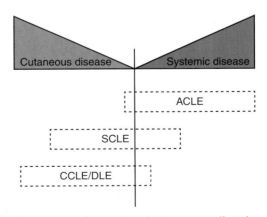

FIG. 15-1. The spectrum of systemic and cutaneous manifestations related to the three subtypes chronic cutaneous lupus erythematosus (CCLE) most commonly including DLE; subacute cutaneous lupus erythematosus (SCLE); and acute cutaneous lupus erythematosus (ACLE).

BOX 15-1	Cutaneous Symptoms of Lupus Erythematosus

Oral or mucosal ulcers
Periungual telangiectasias
Malar "butterfly" rash
Nonscarring alopecia
"Lupus hairs"
Discoid lesions
Nail fold capillary abnormalities
Urticaria
Livedo reticularis
Photosensitivity
Raynaud phenomenon

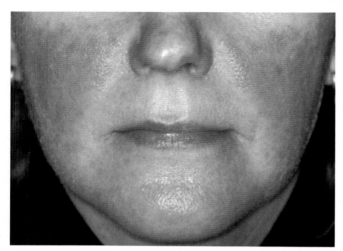

FIG. 15-2. The "butterfly" rash of SLE is erythema over the malar prominences and nose but usually spares the nasolabial folds.

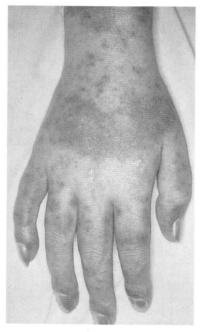

FIG. 15-3. Erythema on the dorsum of the hands and fingers is distributed *between* the intraphalangeal joints and not over them, as seen in dermatomyositis (Gottron papules).

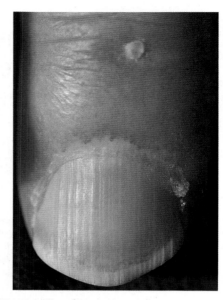

FIG. 15-4. Dilated capillary loops in the proximal nail folds, and periungual erythema can be an indicator of possible connective tissue disease.

lesions do not leave depigmentation or scarring. Patients commonly report arthralgia, photosensitivity, fever, and oral ulcerations. ACLE can accompany the systemic flares of SLE.

Subacute Cutaneous Lupus Erythematosus

The cutaneous eruptions of SCLE, on the other hand, lasts for weeks or months and may not be associated with underlying systemic disease. Involved areas are often photodistributed, favoring the upper trunk, extensor arms, and lateral aspects of the face and neck (sparing the central area). The morphology of SCLE is much more papulosquamous and less indurated than ACLE, sometimes resembling psoriasis or eczema. Patches and plaques can be annular or coalescing polycyclic plaques (Figure 15-5). As lesions resolve, hypopigmentation and telangiectasias may be permanent, but scarring is not typical. The course of SCLE is chronic and recurrent.

Chronic Cutaneous Lupus Erythematosus

There are several types of CCLE which are not typically associated with underlying SLE. Patients with SLE, however, may develop CCLE lesions.

Discoid lupus erythematosus

DLE is present in about one quarter of patients with SLE and may be the only presenting symptom of systemic involvement. While most DLE patients have a negative ANA, it is estimated that about 5% to 10% will go on to develop SLE. Lesions are usually distributed above the shoulders and favor the scalp, face, and conchal bowls of the ears. Because lesions develop deeper in the papillary and reticular dermis (compared to ACLE and SCLE), the result is erythematous, scaly, thick, atrophic, and hyperpigmented plaques that leave scarring and abnormal pigmentation (Figure 15-6). Adherent scale near hair follicles causes follicular plugging that can be seen on the underside of the scale ("carpet tack" effect).

Lupus profundus

Also referred to as lupus panniculitis, LP are painful, erythematous nodules caused by subcuticular inflammation and destruction. Lesions can occur anywhere but often distributed on the face, breasts,

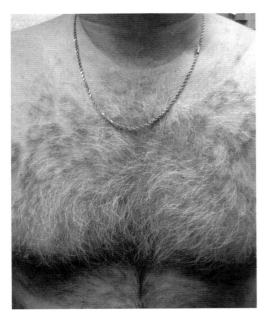

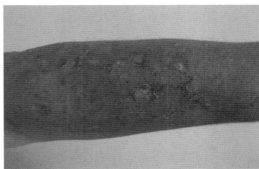

FIG. 15-5. Subacute lupus erythematosus are usually annular, scaly plaques. UVR often exacerbates cutaneous symptoms and results in papulosquamous eruptions in photodistributed areas.

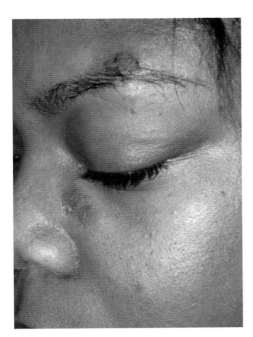

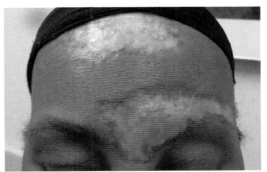

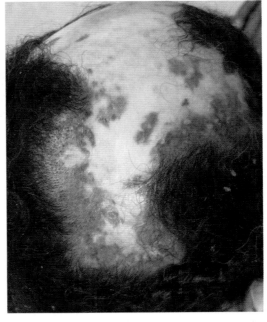

FIG. 15-6. Discoid lupus is highest in African American young women. It commonly occurs on the face, ears, and scalp, sometimes resulting in disfiguring scars and abnormal pigmentation.

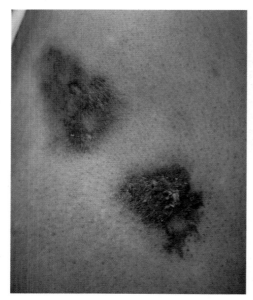

FIG. 15-7. Lupus profundus or lupus panniculitis are firm tender nodules often noted with a black crust with surrounding erythema.

buttocks, arms, and thighs. The tender plaques and nodules may ulcerate and then heal with a black hemorrhagic crust, leaving "dents" or atrophic scars (Figure 15-7). To diagnosis LP, an excisional biopsy (or deep punch) should be done to ensure subcutaneous fat in the specimen. LP may occur concomitantly with DLE.

Drug-induced lupus erythematosus

Drugs can be responsible for inducing a DILE which can mimic SLE (see chapter 17).

Neonatal lupus erythematosus

NLE is caused by vertical transmission of maternal autoantibodies (IgG anti-Ro, anti-La, or anti-RNP) to the fetus, resulting in cutaneous and systemic manifestations (see chapter 6).

Chilblain lupus (Lupus Pernio)

Chilblains present as small, erythematous (reddish-blue) papules that can be painful or itchy and occur on acral sites like the ears, nose, fingers, and toes (Figure 15-8). Lesions are a localized form of vasculitis induced by cold exposure and may ulcerate, swell, or bleed. One quarter of patients with chilblains meet the classification ACR criteria for

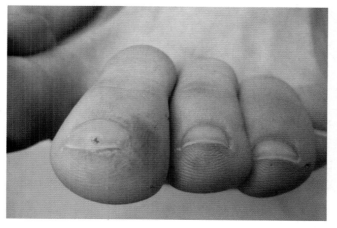

FIG. 15-8. Chilblains or lupus pernio presenting as a small tender, red, or bruise-like papules developing on the tip of the patient's toes.

SLE. Treatment should be focused on the avoidance of cold exposure, including gloves, socks, and shoes. Topical and oral corticosteroids, calcium channel blockers, and smoking cessation can be efficacious.

Diagnostics

Antinuclear antibodies

Serologic testing for a patient suspected of any CTD should start with an ANA screening. A negative result makes a CTD unlikely, whereas a false-positive finding can be caused by medications, disease, infections, and sometimes healthy individuals. Thus, a positive test does not infer disease but should prompt the clinician to make a clinicopathologic correlation. Serologies should include a complete blood count with differential, urinalysis, comprehensive metabolic panel, and sedimentation rate (ESR).

DIFFERENTIAL DIAGNOSIS	Subacute lupus erythematosus and acute cutaneous lupus erythematosus
• Sarcoidosis	
• Psoriasis	
• Lichen planus	
• Dermatomyositis	
• Syphilis	
• Drug eruption	
• Photodermatitis	
• Seborrheic dermatosis	
• Tinea corporis	
• Mycosis fungoides	

Autoantibodies

When the ANA is positive, the clinician should order additional autoantibodies to support or eliminate possible diseases from the differential diagnoses list. Specific types of autoantibodies develop and target antigens relative to the CTD. These specific tests may be ordered by the primary care provider or referred to a rheumatologist and dermatologist for more extensive testing.

Histopathologic analysis

Routine histologic analysis includes use of hematoxylin and eosin (H&E) staining from a punch biopsy. This, along with clinical correlation, is the preferred diagnostic test to establish a diagnosis of CLE.

Immunofluourescence

A direct immunofluorescence (DIF) for suspected diagnosis of CLE should be performed on *lesional* skin, which differs from the technique used to diagnose autoimmune blistering disease (AIBD). A positive DIF with deposition of IgG and/or IgM supports the diagnosis, while a negative DIF cannot exclude CLE. A DIF can also be performed on *normal* skin for evidence of strong, continuous antibody deposition (referred to as a "lupus band") at the basement membrane zone (BMZ).

Management

Treatment for CLE can be complex requiring systemic, topical, and intralesional drug therapy or a combination. Referral to dermatology for management is recommended.

Referral and Consultation

For patients with positive clinicopathologic findings of CLE, the importance of referral to a dermatologist or rheumatologist cannot be overstated. While the primary clinicians may be confident in their diagnosis of cutaneous disease, ensuring that SLE and concomitant autoimmune diseases are diagnosed can be challenging.

> **DIFFERENTIAL DIAGNOSIS** Discoid lupus erythematosus
> * Same as for subacute lupus erythematosus and acute cutaneous lupus erythematosus
> * Rosacea
> * Granuloma annulare and faciale

Patient Education and Follow-up

CLE can be photo-exacerbated; therefore, the importance of UVR protection should be discussed. Lifelong management and monitoring are paramount.

DERMATOMYOSITIS AND POLYMYOSITIS

DM is a rare autoimmune disease involving idiopathic inflammation of the skin, muscles, joints, and other organs. There is a wide variation in presentation and severity of both cutaneous and systemic manifestations. DM has a bimodal incidence, with peak onset in children between 5 and 10 years and adults after the age of 40 years. Women are twice as likely to be affected as men and without racial predilection. It has been suggested that there may be a genetic predisposition for some individuals with HLA phenotypes. Infections and drug-induced cases have also been reported. The most important disease association for DM is the high risk for underlying malignancies. Less common variants are PM, which is absent of cutaneous symptoms, and amyopathic DM (ADM), which does not have any muscle symptoms.

Pathophysiology

DM is idiopathic, and it is difficult to predict the course of the disease or the severity of symptoms. The complex pathogenesis includes both immune and nonimmune mechanisms responsible for the inflammation of muscles and capillaries, leading to muscle weakness and atrophy.

Clinical Presentation

Cutaneous symptoms are usually the first sign of DM but often go unrecognized. Musculoskeletal symptoms may also be overlooked as their onset is insidious. There is a variety of skin findings that are characteristic for DM and are not present in PM (Figure 15-9). Scaly or psoriasiform plaques commonly occur on the forehead and scalp. Extremely pruritic and erythematous patches/plaques that erupt on the body may have some fine scale but are usually diffuse and can become violaceous. Photo-exposed areas may develop pigmentary changes and telangiectasias. It is referred to as the "shawl sign" when located on the shoulders and "V" sign on the chest. Cutaneous

> **DIFFERENTIAL DIAGNOSIS** Dermatomyositis and polymyositis
> * Contact dermatitis
> * Atopic dermatitis
> * Drug eruptions
> * Psoriasis
> * Polymorphic light eruption
> * Lupus erythematosus
> * Cutaneous T-cell lymphoma
> * Tinea corporis
> * Lichen planus

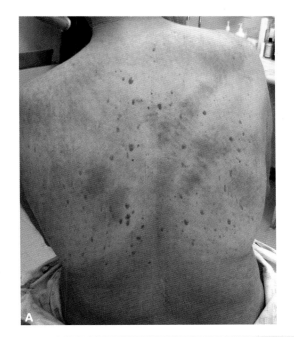

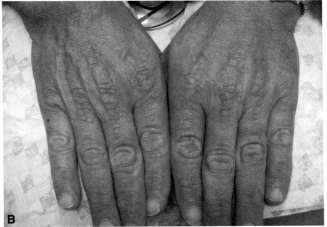

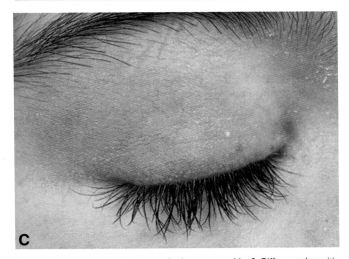

FIG. 15-9. Cutaneous symptoms seen in dermatomyositis. **A:** Diffuse and pruritic scaly eruptions on the trunk which is often misdiagnosed. **B:** *Gottron papules* erupt over the metacarpophalangeal and interphalangeal joints of extensor surfaces on the hands and fingers. Periungual erythema and dilated capillary loops may be noted, along with cuticular overgrowth. **C:** The hallmark *heliotrope* rash presents as erythema occurring around the eyes, especially the upper lids.

TABLE 15-1	Comparative Features of Dermatomyositis and Lupus Erythematosus Skin Involvement		
		DM	**LE**
Distribution of skin involvement			
Face			
	Malar eminences	+	+ +
	Eyelids, periorbital areas	+ +	+
Scalp		+ +	+ +
Oral mucosa		+	+ +
Extensor arms, forearms		+ +	+ +
Hands			
	Dorsal apsect	+ +	+ +
	Palmar aspect	+	+ +
Dorsal fingers		+	+ +
Knuckles		+ +	+
Periungual telangiectasia		+ +	+
Color of skin lesions			
	Violaceous	+ +	+
	Red, pink	+	+ +
Alopecia		+	+ +
Hyperkeratosis		+	+ +
Gottron papules		+ +	0
Pruritus		+ +	+
Pathology			
	Dermal mucinosis	+ +	+ +
	Intense mononuclear cell infiltrate	+	+ +
Immunopathology			
	D-E juncton band	+	+ +
Laboratory findings			
	ANA	+ +	+ +
	Anti-Ro/SS-A	+	+ +
	Anti-native DNA	0	+ +
	Anti-Sm	0	+ +
	Elevated ESR	+	+ +
Malignancy association		+ +	0

ANA, antinuclear antibody; DM, dermatomyositis; ESR, erythrocyte sedimentation rate; LE, lupus erythematosus; + +, frequently seen; +, occasionally seen; 0, absent.

Reprinted with permission from Sontheimer, R. D. & Provost, T. T. (2004). *Cutaneous manifestations of rheumatic diseases* (2nd ed.). Philadelphia, PA: Lippincott Williams & Wilkins.

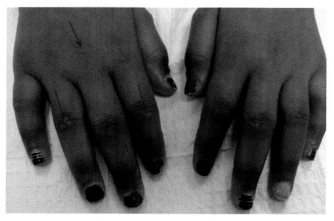

FIG. 15-10. Very subtle Gottron papules (*arrows*) starting in a 6-year-old African American girl diagnosed with dermatomyositis. Her initial complaint was swelling in her hands and fingers and hard papules on her elbows (calcinosis cutis).

evaluation and diagnostics such as radiographs, electromyography, and muscle biopsy (usually MRI guided).

Management

Patients with the presumed diagnosis of DM should be referred to a rheumatologist or dermatologist for collaborative care in the management and monitoring of their disease. Specialists may be consulted depending on systemic involvement and severity of disease.

Special Considerations

Juvenile DM can present with symptoms similar to adults (Figure 15-10). Calcinosis cutis is more commonly reported in childhood DM, and the association for underlying malignancy is much lower. Pediatric rheumatologists should be consulted for care of children with DM.

Prognosis and Complications

The severity of myopathy and presence of an underlying malignancy are the greatest prognostic factors for DM. If symptoms are limited to the skin, patients may achieve complete resolution in a few years. Flares can occur, especially with triggering events such as UVR exposure.

Patient Education and Follow-up

Initially, patients should be followed closely for disease control, drug therapy, and side effects. Once in remission, patients will not need as frequent office visits but should be monitored as medication is tapered off. Patients must be instructed that photo exposure can exacerbate the disease and that careful measures should be taken to avoid it. Most importantly, patients with DM should be carefully evaluated during the first 5 years after the onset for disease when the risk for malignancy is highest. Routine cancer screenings and other diagnostics should be performed as indicated. Patients must understand the importance of reporting the onset of any new symptoms.

SCLERODERMA

Scleroderma is a rare autoimmune disease affecting connective tissues, skin, and internal organs. The disease can be categorized into systemic scleroderma (SSc) and localized scleroderma. The incidence of scleroderma varies depending on the type, but there is an overall female predominance.

Systemic Scleroderma

SSc is usually diagnosed in between the ages of 30 and 50 years. It affects African Americans more than Caucasians or those from

symptoms of DM can appear very similar to those seen with CLE, which mandates an experienced rheumatology and/or dermatology specialist to provide further evaluation and diagnosis (Table 15-1).

Myopathies associated with DM can be significant and usually develop as proximal muscle weakness that slowly progresses. Initially, patients may have difficulty raising their hand to brush their hair or lifting their legs to walk and climb steps. Esophageal involvement may result in dysphagia, as well as cardiac symptoms including conduction abnormalities. Interstitial lung disease has been reported in up to 10% cases of DM. Furthermore, DM may present concomitantly with other autoimmune or CTD, making the clinical diagnosis challenging.

Diagnostics

Serologic testing for suspected DM should include an ANA, anti-Jo, anti-La, and anti-RNP to differentiate it from other CTDs. Serum levels of creatine kinase, glutamic oxaloacetic transaminase (SGOT), alanine aminotransferase (ALT), lactic dehydrogenase (LDH), aldolase, and AST may be elevated. A 24-hour urine for creatine is more sensitive than serum markers for DM. A punch biopsy of lesional skin for histology and nonlesional skin for DIF are helpful in supporting a suspected diagnosis of DM. Patients with positive findings suggestive of DM should be referred to a rheumatologist for further

European descent. Often, pitting edema of the fingers and other skin changes are the initial presenting symptoms. Most patients with SSc have internal organ involvement, which will not be addressed here.

Pathophysiology

SSc is a disruption in the immune system that results in complex extracellular changes in the matrix, including collagen deposition that leads to fibrotic changes and hardening of the tissue. Small blood vessels, like capillaries in the fingers, narrow or develop vasospasms especially with exposure to cold. Large vessels, such as the renal or pulmonary arteries, vasoconstrict and harden, causing disease (i.e., pulmonary hypertension). There may be some genetic predisposition for SSc, but it is not inheritable. Studies suggest that it may be triggered by environmental exposures, infections, and hormonal influences—but are not pathogenic.

Clinical presentation

SSc always has organ involvement but is divided into two subtypes that are differentiated based on cutaneous involvement. *Limited* SSc has cutaneous manifestations involving the distal extremities and face, whereas *diffuse* SSc also includes the proximal extremities and trunk. Box 15-2 identifies skin findings that are commonly seen in SSc.

Raynaud phenomenon is a syndrome that occurs in almost all patients with SSc, often preceding the diagnosis, and in association with other autoimmune diseases. In contrast, *Raynaud disease* is the presence of the syndrome without an underlying disease process. Raynaud phenomenon can be triggered by exposure to cold temperatures or from stress, causing vasoconstriction and/or vasospasms in the arteries and arterioles in the fingers. Patients complain of painful, cold, and numb fingers and toes (Figure 15-11). Their digits become white, cyanotic or bluish, and then red after reactive vasodilation. A close examination of the proximal nail folds may reveal changes in the capillaries (drop out) which would favor Raynaud *phenomenon* and indication for further evaluation for systemic disease.

CREST, the acronym for calcinosis cutis, Raynaud phenomenon, esophageal involvement (usually Barrett esophagitis), sclerodactyly, and telangiectasias, is a syndrome of localized SSc with specific disease characteristics (Figure 15-12). Calcinosis cutis, which erupts as firm nodules on the fingertips and pads, may harden, rupture, and persist as chronic ulcerations.

Localized Scleroderma/Morphea

Localized scleroderma, more commonly called *morphea*, affects a younger population, with an onset occurring between 20 and 40 years of age. Yet 20% of cases occur in children and adolescents. There is a higher incidence of localized scleroderma in individuals of European descent and Caucasians rather than in African Americans. Morphea

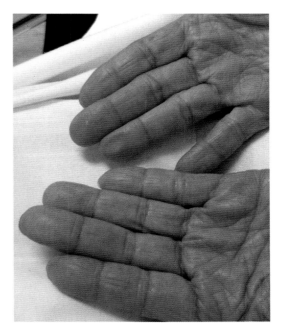

FIG. 15-11. Raynaud phenomenon.

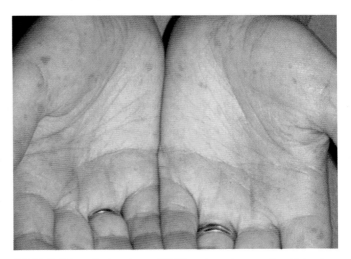

FIG. 15-12. A form of scleroderma, CREST syndrome has prominent telangiectasias on the hands, face, and mucosal surfaces.

is *not* associated with SSc or underlying autoimmune disease, which means patients will not have Raynaud phenomenon or CREST. Morphea is often misdiagnosed as lichen sclerosus et atrophicus.

Pathophysiology

Inflammation and collagen deposition in the dermis and subcutaneous layer cause a thickening and hardening of the skin, leaving atrophic plaques. It was once suspected that *Borrelia burgdorferi,* the same spirochete that causes Lyme disease, played a role in the etiology of morphea. However, studies do not support the theory.

Clinical presentation

New lesions erupt as solitary or multiple plaques with a sometimes violaceous hue. Active lesions retain a bluish-purple appearance on the periphery. As plaques age, they expand centrifugally, with a central white, shiny, scar-like (sclerosed) appearance without hair follicles.

There are several variants:

Plaque-type morphea is the most common type and develops on the trunk. Patients are often unaware of the asymptomatic lesions

BOX 15-2	Cutaneous Symptoms of Scleroderma

Raynaud phenomenon
Sclerodactyly
Pitting edema of the fingers/toes
Changes in skin texture
Calcinosis (tips of digits and near joints)
Matted telangiectasis (face, lips, palms)
Nail folds—tortuous capillaries or drop out
Atrophic or thickened patches of skin
Abnormal pigmentation
Leukoderma ("salt & pepper skin")
Pitted scars on fingertips
Ulcerations or contractures fingers/toes

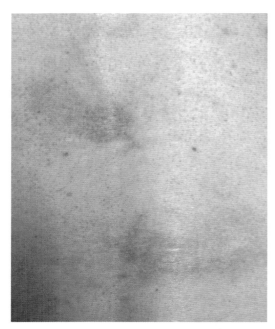

FIG. 15-13. Plaque-type morphea showing atrophic plaque with a shiny surface.

(Figure 15-13). *Linear* morphea initially presents as a plaque on the arms and legs that begins to extend longitudinally (Figure 15-14). This can be a problem as the thickened, scar-like skin can limit mobility, causing weakness, and shorten limb development. *En coup de sabre* or Parry–Romberg syndrome is morphea involving the face (Figure 15-15). Loss of subcutaneous tissue can lead to significant hemifacial atrophy or abnormal development of the underlying facial nerves and vessels.

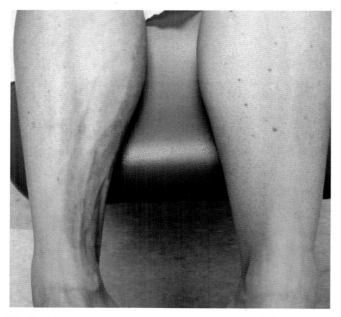

FIG. 15-14. Linear morphea in the lower leg of a woman with a notable loss of fat and muscle. This patient does not have a loss of function or mobility that can occur with linear morphea, especially near the joints.

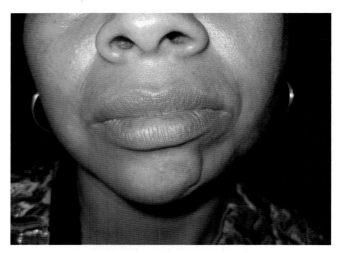

FIG. 15-15. *En coup de sabre,* a variant of linear morphea, describes lesions that appear like a sword striking the head.

Diagnosis
Patients suspected of SSc or localized should be referred to a rheumatologist and dermatologist for evaluation and diagnostics.

Management
Similarly, patients with SSc or complicated localized morphea will require lifelong management with a rheumatologist.

Prognosis and complications
SSc can have a high mortality and morbidity relative to the type and severity of organ involvement. Patients diagnosed with SSc require chronic disease management by a multidisciplinary team led by a rheumatologist. The psychosocial impact of SSc can be devastating for patients and their families and should not be overlooked. Cutaneous lesions can be disfiguring, especially on the face, and should be considered when caring for these patients.

Morphea, on the other hand, is a strictly cutaneous disease and usually has mild symptoms. There are no systemic complications and can resolve spontaneously. Complications may include hyperpigmentation or "hard" skin, which can rarely cause disability. Patients with morphea should be referred to a dermatologist and may require collaboration with a rheumatologist when there is an impaired muscle function.

IMMUNE-MEDIATED BULLOUS DISEASES

Clinicians often evaluate patients who present with vesicles and bullae that may be attributed to injury, infection, genetic disorders, eczematous dermatitis, or hypersensitivity reaction. However, there is a subgroup of patients who may go undiagnosed and be mismanaged if the clinician does not consider AIBD. Although not common, these chronic dermatoses can be associated with high mortality and morbidity. Prompt diagnosis, consideration of therapeutic options, and referral to experienced clinicians are requisite to optimize patient outcomes. Content will focus on pemphigus, bullous pemphigoid, linear immunoglobulin A (IgA) disease (LAD), and dermatitis herpetiformis (DH). There will be a brief overview of some of the other variants.

Pathophysiology

Vesicles and bullae (blisters) are the collection of fluid in the epidermis or basement membrane. Blisters may contain clear fluid or

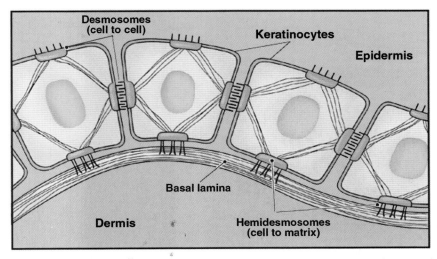

FIG. 15-16. Basement membrane zone. Keratinocytes in the epidermis attach to each other (cell-to-cell) with specialized cell junctions called *desmosomes*. Impaired function can result in an intraepidermal blister. *Hemidesmosomes* attach the basal keratinocytes to the dermis (cell-to-matrix) at basal lamina. Disruption of the hemidesmosomes can lead to subepidermal (below the basal keratinocyte) blisters, separating the epidermis from the dermis.

TABLE 15-2	Types of Autoimmune Bullous Diseases and Location of Blisters in the Skin

TYPE OF ADHESION	LOCATION OF BLISTERS

Cell-to-cell	Epidermal
	    Pemphigus vulgaris
	    Pemphigus foliaceous
	    Paraneoplastic pemphigus

Cell-to-matrix	Subepidermal
	    Bullous pemphigoid
	    Mucous membrane pemphigoid
	    Linear IgA
	    Epidermolysis bullosa acquisita
	    Bullous systemic lupus erythematosus
	    Dermatitis herpetiformis

blood-tinged (hemorrhagic) fluid from a disruption in blood vessels. This is compared to a pustule, which has yellow or cloudy fluid. An accurate diagnosis can be achieved more promptly if the clinician understands the pathophysiology of AIBD and has knowledge of the depth and other characteristics of the blister.

In general, AIBDs are separated into two categories: intraepidermal and subepidermal blistering diseases (Table 15-2). Individuals with AIBDs develop autoantibodies that target specific molecules in the epidermis called *desmosomes*, which are responsible for cell-to-cell adhesion. Impaired desmosomes result in *intraepidermal* (within the epidermis) blisters. Similarly, *hemidesmosomes* are responsible for basal keratinocyte adhesion to the epidermis or cell-to-matrix adhesion in the BMZ. Autoantibodies that target the hemidesmosomes, anchoring fibrils and filaments, and fibrin can result in subepidermal (below the basement membrane of the epidermis) blisters (Figure 15-16). AIBDs can involve the skin and/or mucous membranes and vary in clinical presentation relative to the level of involvement in the epidermis.

Diagnostics

Primary care clinicians should always consider AIBD as a differential diagnosis whenever patients present with blisters or erosions secondary to blisters. The morphology, distribution and location, severity of blisters, and comorbidities are critical for clinical correlation. The diagnosis of an AIBD requires both clinical and immunohistological correlation. Autoantibodies can be detected in the skin and the blood with the aid of immunofluorescent testing.

Histopathologic analysis

Two punch biopsy specimens are usually obtained. A biopsy for routine H&E staining can be helpful, but is not essential for the diagnosis of an AIBD. This biopsy sample should be performed near the edge of a new blister to allow for a full thickness histologic examination. Specimens are transported to the lab in formalin. Routine histopathology identifies the location/level of the blister in the skin (Figure 15-17).

The second punch biopsy performed on nonlesional skin (preferably 2–3 mm away from the blister's edge) is sent for DIF. This is the gold standard for detecting the presence and location of *tissue-bound* autoantibodies, complements, and fibrin deposits in skin or mucous membrane. Specimens for DIF should be transported in Michel's media and NOT in formaldehyde. DIF is important for the specificity and location of autoantibodies. Additionally, a DIF performed using "salt-split skin" technique (salt-split skin) allows further differentiation. Skin soaked in hyperosmolar saline causes separation of the BMZ. Antibodies tagged with immunofluorescence will bind to either the roof (epidermal side) or the floor (dermal side) of the BMZ. This enables the clinician to further distinguish between subepidermal blistering diseases.

Serologic testing

Indirect immunofluorescence (IIF) identifies *circulating* antibodies from the patient's serum and incubated on various substrates. IIF detects the specific antibody, patterns, and location, and should be

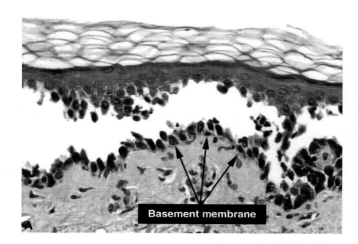

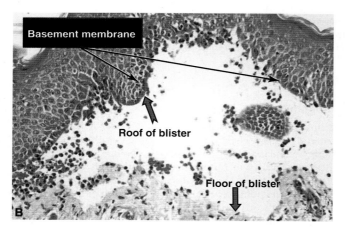

FIG. 15-17. **A:** Histopathologic analysis shows intraepidermal separation (blister) that occurs above the basal membrane zone in a patient with PV. **B:** Subepidermal blister below the basal layer (subepidermal) in a patient with pemphigoid.

ordered by dermatologists with experience. Enzyme-linked immunosorbent assays (ELISA) are available. ELISAs can detect the level of circulating autoantibodies against the hemidesmosomes (bullous pemphigoid [BP] 180 and 230 for pemphigoid) and desmosomes (desmoglein 1 and 3 for pemphigus). These levels can also be used to monitor disease activity and response to therapy. These diagnostic tests can be confusing to understand and expensive to analyze, and are best left to be ordered and interpreted by experienced dermatology specialists.

INTRAEPIDERMAL (CELL-TO-CELL) BLISTERING DISEASE

Pemphigus

Pemphigus is a family of rare skin disorders with immune-mediated, intraepidermal blisters. Pemphigus vulgaris (PV), the most common of the group, has been reported in all ages but is considered a disease of middle age (mean age 40–60 years), with increased incidence in Jewish and Mediterranean population. Subtypes include PV, pemphigus foliaceous (PF), and paraneoplastic pemphigus (PNP). Thymoma and myasthenia gravis have been associated with PV.

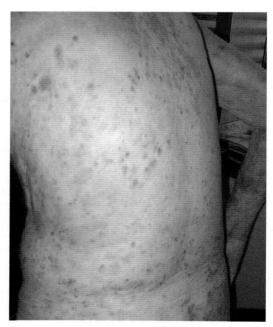

FIG. 15-18. Vesicles and bullae in PV are fragile and rupture easily with scratching.

Pathophysiology

The blistering that occurs in pemphigus is caused by a disruption or impaired cell-to-cell adhesion (*acantholysis*) within the epidermis. It is unclear why IgG autoantibodies target desmogleins 1 and 3, the antigens responsible for keratinocyte adhesion. In PNP, glycoproteins from the plakin family are also targeted.

Clinical presentation

Since the defect in pemphigus occurs within the epidermis, vesicles and bullae are flaccid and rupture easily. The physical examination may only reveal crusted erosions secondary to scratching (Figure 15-18). Blisters can be localized or generalized, with the majority of patients having mucosal involvement which typically precedes the skin eruption. When mucous membranes are involved, erosions and ulcerations can be seen on the conjunctiva, oral mucosa, nasopharynx, esophagus, urogenital mucosa, and anus (Figure 15-19). Mucosal lesions can cause dysphagia, hoarseness, and dehydration because of pain with eating and drinking. Severe burning, pain, and pruritus are commonly reported.

There are several variants of pemphigus which have distinct characteristics that aid in developing the diagnosis. More importantly, there are vast differences in treatment approaches depending on the subtype.

Subtypes

PV is the most common subtype of the pemphigus. Vesicles/bullae can be any size, often coalescing to become generalized erosions. Blisters often favor the head, upper body, and intertriginous areas. When mucous membranes are involved, the oral mucosa is the most common site. The pruritus of PV is variable.

Pemphigus vegetans is considered a variant of PV and has unique mucocutaneous lesions presenting initially as bullae that then develop into hypertrophic granulation or verruciform plaques (Figure 15-20). Lesions are malodorous and favor the extensor surfaces, oral mucosa, and intertriginous areas like the axilla, inguinal folds, and umbilicus.

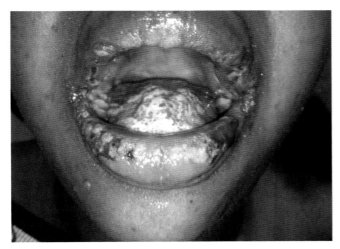

FIG. 15-19. Oral erosions and ulcerations in a patient with PV.

PF presents as crusted erosions that favor a seborrheic distribution of the scalp, face, upper chest, and back (Figure 15-21). Clinically, PF tends to have more shallow lesions, rarely involves mucous membranes, and has a milder disease course than PV.

PNP is a rare form of pemphigus characterized by a rapid and extensive stomatitis involving the lips, oral mucosa, throat, and conjunctiva. The oral mucosal lesions of PNP are extremely painful, leading to dehydration and poor nutrition. Dusky targetoid plaques, similar to those in erythema multiforme, may appear on the trunk and extremities. PNP patients have a very ill appearance. Unlike the other pemphigus types, the onset of PNP occurs in patients over 60 years and is usually associated with an underlying malignancy.

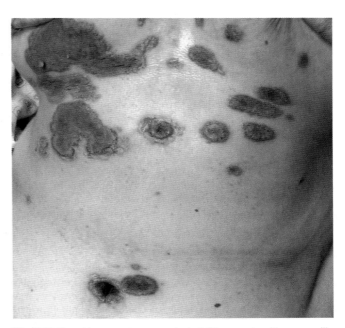

FIG. 15-20. Pemphigus vegetans, a variant of PV, presents with verruca-like plaques and pustules favoring intertriginous areas.

DIFFERENTIAL DIAGNOSIS Pemphigus

- Toxic epidermal necrolysis (positive Nikolsky sign)
- Other autoimmune blistering disorders
- Erythema multiforme
- Bullous impetigo
- Herpes simplex or zoster
- Drug eruption
- Lupus erythematosus

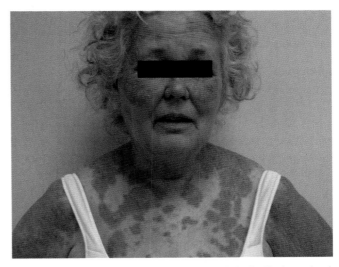

FIG. 15-21. Pemphigus foliaceous favors the seborrheic distribution and typically has a milder disease course than PV.

Diagnostics

It is not uncommon for there to be a delay in the diagnosis of pemphigus because erosions, not fluid-filled lesions, are typical on presentation. Thus, AIBDs may not initially be considered in the differential. A lesional biopsy for histopathology will show an intraepidermal blister with acantholysis. IgG and C3 staining will be evident on the DIF and ELISA testing for desmoglein 1 and 3 is highly sensitive for differentiating PV and PF. Patients with pemphigus can have a positive *Nikolsky sign* where the area surrounding the blister shears away when lateral pressure is applied. A positive Nikolsky is also seen in toxic epidermal necrolysis and staph scalded skin syndrome.

Management

Patients with pemphigus require management by a dermatologist experienced in AIBDs due to the high risk for morbidity and mortality.

Management of the disease depends on the type of pemphigus, severity of disease, patient age, and comorbidities. The initial first-line treatment for most every pemphigus patient includes systemic corticosteroids to halt the eruption of new vesicles or bullae. Prednisone is usually initiated at 1 to 2 mg/kg/day but may cautiously be titrated upward. As with any patient requiring systemic corticosteroids for more than 12 weeks, osteoporosis and peptic ulcer prevention and treatment should be considered along with monitoring for severe side effects (see chapter 2). The goal is to gain control of the disease with the lowest amount of corticosteroid.

Steroid-sparing agents such as mycophenolate mofetil (CellCept), azathioprine (Imuran), and dapsone are often started at the same time with the goal of tapering off the prednisone as soon as possible. However, the process is done very slowly to avoid flaring of the disease and may take months to years. In severe or recalcitrant cases, there are limited data for off-label use with alternative agents, including cyclophosphamide (Cytoxan), IVIG, and plasmapheresis. A few studies have examined the use of rituximab, with reported complete remission in patients with severe pemphigus; however, more controlled studies are needed. These therapies have higher risks for side effects and significant complications to consider.

The treatment approach for PNP differs in that clinicians should immediately perform screening for an underlying malignancy or benign neoplasm. If the initial search does not reveal the underlying etiology, one should maintain a high index of suspicion for an evolving neoplasm. When a malignancy or tumor is identified, treatment or excision must be instituted without delay. Immunosuppressive agents have not been efficacious and actually may contribute to complications.

Prognosis and complications
Achieving "complete" remission usually takes years for most pemphigus patients. Pemphigus has a higher morbidity and mortality than other AIBDs because of the compromised epidermal barrier in a large BSA, increased risk for infections, and fluid/electrolyte imbalance. The use of systemic corticosteroids in pemphigus has significantly reduced the mortality and morbidity of patients, yet the risk of immunosuppression can result in diabetes, hypertension, kidney and liver dysfunction, and hematologic complications. Cutaneous complications include secondary infections, hyperpigmentation, scaring, impaired function, and psychosocial sequelae. The prognosis for PNP is very poor even with prompt recognition and treatment.

Special considerations
The autoantibodies of PV can cross the placenta in pregnant women and affect the epidermis of the fetus. PV in children is rare but can occur.

Referral and consultation
Collaboration between the primary care clinician and the dermatologist is essential to promote optimal outcomes and minimize complications. Appropriate specialists should be consulted when there is involvement of mucous membranes.

Patient education and follow-up
Primary care clinicians and dermatologists should collaborate to screen annually for tuberculosis, as well as age-appropriate health screenings. Monitoring and prevention of corticosteroid-associated side effects and complications are essential (see chapter 2). Continuous disease monitoring and treatment may require changes in therapy, and the patient must be well educated regarding risks, side effects, and complications. Laboratory monitoring is usually frequent depending on the agent and level of immunosuppression. Patients with PV should be educated about recurrence and development of associated diseases (thyroid dysfunction, thymoma, and myasthenia gravis). Exposure to sun light should be limited to avoid a flare.

SUBEPIDERMAL (CELL-TO-MATRIX) BLISTERING DISEASES
Patients with subepidermal blistering have autoantibodies that target adhesion proteins in the BMZ that are responsible for anchoring keratinocytes to the matrix (cell-to-matrix). The specific type of subepidermal disease depends on the specific antigen targeted by autoantibodies.

Bullous Pemphigoid
BP is the most common AIBD and typically presents in patients 60 years and older, with an equal incidence in men and women. It is a chronic disease characterized by exacerbations and remission. There is an increased risk to develop BP in individuals with specific HLA alleles. New studies are examining an association between BP and neurologic diseases such as Parkinson's and cerebral vascular accident. Drug-induced BP has been linked to diuretics, antibiotics, captopril, and neuroleptic agents, contributing to the trigger of an already genetically susceptible individual. Infections have also been identified as an inciting event.

Pathophysiology
Blister formation occurs in BP when autoantibodies target the hemidesmosomes (BP 180 and 230), triggering complement activation and inflammatory mediators. The result is deposition of IgG and C3 in the BMZ. The recruitment of neutrophils and eosinophils results in destruction of the BMZ.

Clinical presentation
The symptoms of BP are highly variable, often presenting as urticarial plaques (nonbullous phase) that may last from weeks to months, then gradually evolve into tense vesicles/bullae (Figure 15-22). This stage may delay the diagnosis since clinicians may not recognize urticaria and pruritus as a key symptom in the early clinical presentation of BP. The fluid-filled blisters are located deeper in the skin (compared to pemphigus) and therefore form tense bullae that are more difficult to rupture. There is a negative Nikolsky sign in BP.

Vesicles/bullae are usually polymorphic and may be filled with either clear or hemorrhagic fluid. Bullae may be solitary lesions but can become very large and extensive involving the trunk (Figure 15-23). Lesions tend to favor the flexural areas on the arms and legs (Figure 15-24). Once bullae rupture, erosions take days or weeks to heal and may leave abnormal pigmentation. Oral lesions may be present in BP but are less common (24%) than in pemphigus.

Variants
Mucous membrane pemphigoid (MMP), which has also been referred to as "cicatricial (scarring) pemphigoid," is a rare but severe type of localized BP occurring in patients aged 60 to 80 years, with a higher incidence in women. The most common sites affected in MMP are the oral mucosa and conjunctiva, but may develop in the nasopharynx, esophagus, genitals, and anus. Painful erosions and desquamative gingivitis from the disease can be disabling. Ocular involvement

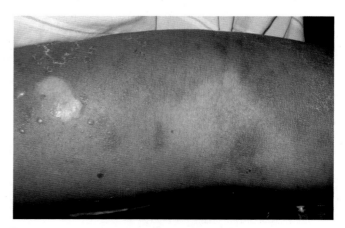

FIG. 15-22. The urticarial phase of BP is very pruritic and can precede the development of vesicles/bullae by weeks and months.

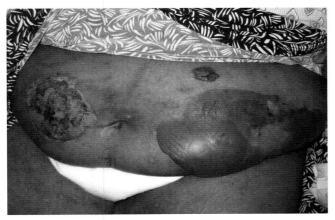

FIG. 15-23. Large hemorrhagic bullae in a BP patient who continues to develop new lesions.

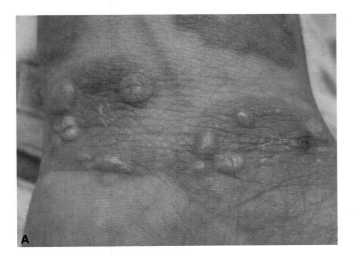

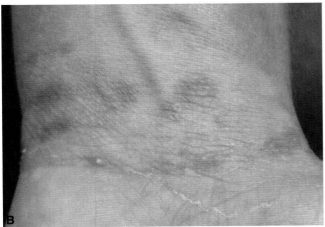

FIG. 15-24. **A:** The urticarial phase of BP starts as papules and plaques, then develops into vesicles and bullae. **B:** Three weeks after treatment with systemic prednisone and mycophenolate mofetil.

is usually severe and painful, and often progressive from erosions to fibrous conjunctival lesions or symblepharon (Figure 15-25). Patients suffer from reduced ability to tear, corneal opacities and ulcerations, ingrown eyelashes, and ultimately blindness. The skin is involved in about one quarter of the cases of MMP and usually affects the head, neck, and chest.

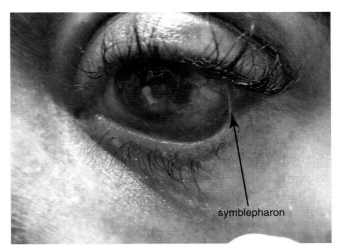

FIG. 15-25. Erosions in ocular mucous membrane pemphigoid heal with scarring or symblepharon.

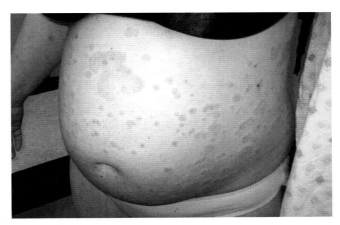

FIG. 15-26. Herpes gestationis (gestational pemphigoid) looks similar to PUPPP but is not concentrated in the striae and usually involves the umbilicus.

Herpes gestationis (HG), also known as gestational pemphigoid, presents during the 2nd and 3rd trimester of pregnancy and can flare after delivery. The name is a misnomer as HG is not related to the herpes virus. Pruritus, urticarial papules and plaques erupt on the trunk, and the umbilicus is commonly involved. (Figure 15-26). Lesions expand and can develop vesicles.

DIFFERENTIAL DIAGNOSIS   Bullous pemphigoid

- Other autoimmune blistering diseases
- Bullous drug eruption
- Bullous impetigo
- Erythema multiforme
- Contact dermatitis
- Stevens–Johnson syndrome/toxic epidermal necrolysis
- Urticaria or urticarial vasculitis
- Pruritic urticarial papules and plaques of pregnancy

Diagnostics

A subepidermal blister is noted on histopathology (lesional skin) in BP and will have an abundant infiltration of eosinophils and some neutrophils. Most importantly, DIF performed on nonlesional skin will show a linear deposition of IgG and C3 at the BMZ. Yet epidermal bullosa acquisita (EBA) and MMP have similar characteristics. A DIF on salt-split skin can help differentiate BP with immune deposits on the roof (epidermal side) in comparison to EBA, which binds to the floor (dermal side) of the BMZ. IIF of the patient's sera is positive for circulating IgG deposited in the epidermal side of salt-split skin. ELISA for BP 180 and 230 can be used for diagnostic purposes as well as a prognostic indicator in cessation of therapy and possible relapse.

Diagnostics for MMP should be ordered and evaluated by an experienced dermatologist. A DIF on salt-split skin may be limited as IgG may bind to both sides, but an ELISA for BP 180 and laminin 5 is much more sensitive.

Management
Careful consideration must be given to the treatment of patients with BP since it occurs more often in the elderly who are more likely to have comorbid conditions. Additional challenges to managing these patients may be due to their limited resources, ability to monitor for side effects or complications, and adherence to recommendations which can impact outcomes.

Treatment approach is based on severity, diffuse versus localized, and location of the blisters. Mild and localized BP may be effectively treated with potent topical corticosteroids and immunomodulators. Systemic therapies that may be added include nicotinamide, tetracycline class drugs, dapsone, and sulfonamides. In severe cases or those involving mucous membranes, dermatologists may initiate systemic corticosteroids starting at low doses. Steroid-sparing agents, often started at the same time, include mycophenolate mofetil, azathioprine, methotrexate, and sulfones, and help control disease while tapering off prednisone. Recalcitrant BP or severe oral involvement may require rituximab or IVIG.

The management approach for MMP must be initiated *immediately* by an experienced dermatology clinician if the patient is to avoid permanent impaired function. Aggressive immunosuppression often requires more than systemic corticosteroids. A combination of drug therapy and surgical modalities are often necessary. Women with HG can be treated effectively with mid- to high-potency topical corticosteroids and antihistamines.

Prognosis and complications
Although considered a more benign disease than PV, BP can result in significant morbidity and death. Close monitoring of the patient cannot be stressed enough as both corticosteroids and steroid-sparing agents can have severe or lethal side effects, especially in the elderly. Response to therapy can be monitored with serum BP 180 (ELISA) levels to identify disease remission for discontinuation of drug therapy. Women with HG have an increased risk for recurrence with subsequent pregnancies along with risk for Grave disease. The fetus has 10% risk to have skin lesions present.

The prognosis for MMP is very poor as impaired function of the eyes resulting in blindness is not uncommon. Other mucous membrane involvement of the mouth, nasopharynx, esophagus and trachea, and urogenital tract can also develop scarring and strictures. Patients with BP are at increased risk for adenocarcinoma and solid organ tumors. Additionally, high-risk immunosuppressive agents and long-term therapy increase the risk of complications and secondary infections.

Referral and consultation
Women with HG require collaboration between an obstetrician and a dermatologist for management. MMP patients require a multidisciplinary approach dependent of the mucous membrane involved.

An ophthalmologist, ENT specialist, dentist, and gastroenterologist are commonly consulted.

Patient education and follow-up
Routine and symptomatic follow-up with the primary care clinician is vital to any pemphigoid patient. Both patients and providers should have a heightened awareness for signs and symptom of infection. Age-appropriate and symptomatic cancer screenings are highly advised. Most of all, patients should understand and monitor for risks and complications of immunosuppressive therapy used to treat their disease. UVR protection and avoidance of trauma to the skin can help reduce exacerbations.

Linear IgA Disease
A rare blistering disorder, LAD is a subepidermal disorder presenting in adults over 60 years. It also occurs during childhood with a presentation typically before the age of 5 years and is referred to as chronic bullous disease of childhood (CBDC). Once thought to be related to DH, LAD is now considered a distinct entity.

Like many AIBDs, LAD has been associated with patients who have underlying lymphoproliferative or solid organ malignancy, infections, or inflammatory bowel diseases. LAD can be drug-induced by medications such as vancomycin, captopril, lithium, NSAIDs (especially diclofenac), penicillin, furosemide, cephalosporin, and others. There has also been some suggestion of a genetic association with specific HLA alleles.

Pathophysiology
The pathogenesis of LAD is not well understood. IgA autoantibodies target BP 180 antigen along the BMZ which has a major role in epidermal–dermal adhesion.

Clinical presentation
LAD can have a variable presentation and disease course. In adults, an abrupt onset of vesicles and bullae may develop centrally on an erythematous plaque or as annular lesions. LAD is symmetrical and favors the trunk, extensor surfaces of extremities (compared to flexor surfaces of BP), and perineum. Blisters quickly erode because of intense pruritus and scratching. The face and perioral mucosa are involved in the majority of adults with LAD.

The unique feature of LAD is the small clusters of vesicles or papules that appear on the periphery of erythematous round plaques and are often described as *rosettes*, *crown of jewels*, or *string of pearls*. The clinical presentation and symptoms of CBDC in children are different than in adults. The distribution of blisters is more generalized and commonly affects the extremities, including hands/feet, genitals, and oral mucosa in about half the cases (Figure 15-27).

> **DIFFERENTIAL DIAGNOSIS** Linear IgA disease
> - Dermatitis herpetiformis
> - Other autoimmune blistering diseases
> - Bullous impetigo
> - Erythema multiforme
> - Stevens–Johnson syndrome/toxic epidermal necrolysis
> - Drug eruption

Diagnostics
A lesional punch biopsy shows a subepidermal blister with an abundance of neutrophils with collections in the dermal papillae. A DIF

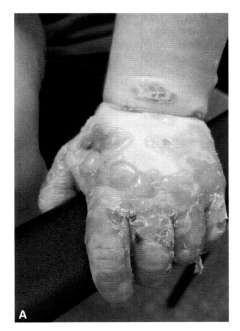

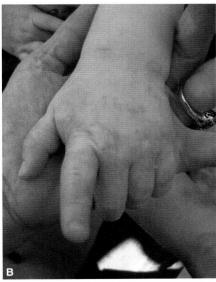

FIG. 15-27. **A:** Chronic bullous disease of childhood in a 16-month-old boy. **B:** After 2 weeks of oral prednisone and dapsone.

reveals a linear deposition of IgA along the BMZ (compared to the granular deposition in DH). An IIF on sera shows circulating IgA bound to the epidermal side (or roof) of salt-split skin.

Management

Most adults and children with LAD are managed successfully with dapsone. Patients usually have a rapid improvement within days and the drug is well tolerated. However, the dosing and administration of dapsone should be done by an experienced dermatology clinician. Adverse effects include hemolytic anemia, methemoglobinemia, leukopenia, agranulocytosis, hypersensitivity reaction, and gastrointestinal and hepatic events. A baseline CBC with differential, comprehensive chemistry (including LFTs), urinalysis, and G6PD should be evaluated before starting therapy. Initially,

weekly monitoring is advised for the response to therapy and side effects.

Severe LAD, disease not responding to dapsone, or patients with a G6PD deficiency may require systemic prednisone or other second-line agents such as sulfapyridine, mycophenolate mofetil, and colchicine. Potent topical corticosteroids can be effective when applied to lesions on the trunk and extremities. Low-potency corticosteroids or calcineurin inhibitors (off-label) are recommended for the face, genitals, or intertriginous regions. If drug-induced LAD is suspected, the drug should be discontinued immediately.

Prognosis and complications

The disease course of LAD in adults is unpredictable and can spontaneously resolve or last for years with episodes of remission. Clinicians should intermittently attempt to slowly taper off the patient's medications while monitoring for flares. Again, the prognosis of CBDC differs from that of adults. In most cases, spontaneously resolution occurs within 2 years.

Complications from LAD and CBDC are usually minimal since the lesions do not scar or result in abnormal pigmentation. However, disease involving the mucous membrane can cause scarring and disability. Secondary infections as well as conditions inherent with the use of both systemic and topical corticosteroid therapy may occur.

Referral and consultation

Patients with LAD or CBDC should be referred immediately to a dermatologist. Evaluation by an ophthalmologist should be done on any patient with ocular involvement. Other consultations may include the gynecologist, gastroenterologist, and otolaryngologist, depending on the severity and type of mucous membrane involvement.

Patient education and follow-up

Patients treated with dapsone or other steroid-sparing agents must have regular follow-up and monitoring. Initially, weekly visits and laboratory monitoring are recommended until the disease is stabilized and risk of complications from drug therapy is lowered. Education regarding side effects and risk of secondary infections are important. Patients are counseled to avoid direct sun and to use sunscreen.

Dermatitis Herpetiformis

DH is a rare (11 per 100,000 in the United States), lifelong subepidermal blistering disease associated with gluten sensitivity. Systemic symptoms of gluten-sensitive enteropathy are celiac disease (CD), which can range from mild to severe or no intestinal symptoms. DH predominantly affects Caucasians, with a higher incidence in individuals with northern European ancestry. It is rarely seen in African Americans and Asians. The onset of DH occurs during the third and fourth decades of life, with a 2:1 predominance in males to females. Several autoimmune disorders have been associated with DH, most common being Hoshimoto thyroiditis and insulin-dependent diabetes melitis. Individuals with the immunogenic HLA-DQ2 genotype are at higher risk for both DH and CD.

Pathophysiology

There are suggested environmental and genetic influences that play a role in the development of CD and DH. The pathogenesis of DH begins with the ingestion of grains (wheat, barley, and rye) which contain the protein gliadin. Tissue transglutaminase (TG), an enzyme necessary for metabolism, is the target of IgA antiendomysial antibodies (IgA-EmA) resulting in damage to the mucosa in CD.

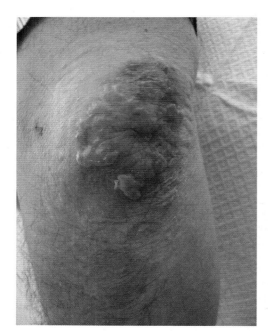

FIG. 15-28. Vesicles erupting on the extensor aspect of the elbow in a patient with DH.

Later, antibodies to epidermal transglutaminase (ET) develop and are more specific to DH. IgA antibodies to ET in the dermis lead to neutrophilic chemotaxis and blister formation in the BMZ at the lamina lucida.

Clinical presentation

The cutaneous eruption of DH is symmetrical and favors the extensor aspects of the arms and legs as well as the back and buttocks (Figure 15-28). It usually spares the face and genitals but sometimes involves the scalp. Erythematous papules, vesicles, and bullae on an urticarial base are clustered in groups (herpetiform arrangement). DH can be localized or diffuse involving the trunk and extremities. There is such severe pruritus associated with the lesions that the clinician often sees only erosions, ulcers, and crusts secondary to scratching.

Since most patients with DH also have CD, a gastrointestinal evaluation is vitally important. Almost all patients with DH have evidence of CD on intestinal biopsy; however, they may not have any signs or symptoms of intestinal disease. Subclinical symptoms are easily overlooked by patients and clinicians.

DIFFERENTIAL DIAGNOSIS Dermatitis herpetiformis

- Bullous pemphigoid
- Linear IgA disease
- Lupus erythematosus
- Scabies
- Erythema multiforme
- Atopic dermatitis

Diagnostics

Histopathologic analysis will show a subepidermal blister (at the level of the lamina lucida), with neutrophilic microabscesses in the dermal papillae and perivascular lymphocytic infiltrates. DIF from skin just outside the blister will have *granular* deposition at the BMZ compared to the linear deposition of LAD. Furthermore, a definitive

characteristic of DH is granular IgA in the dermal papillae on the DIF. Additional diagnostics such as IIF, ELISAs, or serum IgA may be indicated and should be directed by a dermatologist.

Other laboratory tests that aid in the diagnosis and management of DH include serum IgA-EmA titers, indicative of jejunal involvement and will indicate adherence to a gluten-free diet. Screening diagnostics for Hashimoto thyroiditis and diabetes are recommended. Baseline labs, including complete blood count, comprehensive metabolic panel, and G6PD, should be ordered in anticipation for treatment with dapsone.

Management

First-line treatment and maintenance of DH is a gluten-free diet, which is extremely challenging. Patients must exclude all grains from their diet but are allowed corn, rice, and oat products. A growing public interest in the relationship between gluten and many other conditions has sparked an industry surge of "gluten-free" products now available to consumers. Most, but not all, DH patients respond well to the cessation of gluten. Yet it may take months to years to achieve resolution. Patients who knowingly or unknowingly consume gluten can anticipate and prepare for a flare of their cutaneous symptoms. Serum titers of IgA-EmA are indicative of dietary adherence and will eventually fall to zero if gluten is completely omitted from the diet.

Many patients with DH also require pharmacologic therapy in addition to dietary modification. Dapsone is considered a first-line drug effective in neutrophilic dermatoses such as DH. Improvement or resolution typically occurs quickly or may take months. A combination of dietary and drug therapy often allows for a quicker tapering off of the dapsone. Patients unable to tolerate or who are unresponsive to dapsone may be treated with sulfasalazine. Successful treatment with tetracycline and nicotinamide has been reported. Topical corticosteroids can be effective for small, localized outbreaks.

Prognosis and complications

DH is a lifelong skin condition that can go into remission or flares that last weeks to months to years. The pruritic lesions of DH eventually heal but leave hyperpigmentation. Secondary infections from erosions and ulcerations are a complication when cutaneous symptoms are not controlled. CD is also a chronic condition and should be addressed with the patient even if they are asymptomatic. Malabsorption can be a chronic problem leading to other systemic disease and illness. Patients with DH are at higher risk of developing autoimmune disorders, anemia, and lymphoma (gastrointestinal and nongastrointestinal). Although cutaneous symptoms of DH are responsive to gluten-free diet, it is uncertain whether it lowers their risk of intestinal lymphoma.

Referral and consultation

Patients with DH are managed by a dermatologist for cutaneous symptoms and a gastroenterologist for the evaluation, diagnosis, and monitoring of CD. Perhaps the most valuable referral for patients with DH is to a nutritionist to teach and support the patient about a gluten-free lifestyle.

Patient education and follow-up

The role of primary care cannot be overstated in patients with DH and CD. Routine screening examinations and symptomatic evaluation are essential. An increased risk for the development of associated diseases (thyroiditis, anemia, diabetes, and lymphoma) should always be at the forefront of the clinician's thoughts. Age appropriate and symptomatic screening should be current. Patients on dapsone should be instructed about the risk of side effects and complications, along with the importance of frequent laboratory monitoring. Clinicians should routinely evaluate and reaffirm the importance of lifelong compliance to a gluten-free diet and avoidance of iodide and NSAIDs.

MISCELLANEOUS AUTOIMMUNE BLISTERING DISEASES

Epidermal Bullosa Acquisita

A very rare subepidermal AIBD, epidermal bullosa acquisita (EBA) is an acquired disorder in adults and occasionally in childhood. It should be noted that EBA is different from the inherited blistering disorder epidermal bullosa (EB). Some case studies have suggested an association between EBA and inflammatory bowel diseases that may predate the blistering disease. IgG autoantibodies targeting type VII collagen in the BMZ, in addition to chronic trauma and friction, are pathogenic for EBA.

Characteristic blisters erupt on trauma-prone areas like the extensor surfaces of the knees, elbows, dorsal hands, and fingers. Chronic inflammation and erosions result in scarring and milia. EBA can be difficult to differentiate from BP, porphyria cutanea tarda, and EB. DIF on salt-split skin shows linear deposits of IgG on the floor (dermal side) of the BMZ compared to BP or base side of the DIF on salt-split skin.

The primary focus for treatment of EBA is avoidance of trauma or friction. EBA is resistant to treatment, and chronic inflammation results in destruction of the hair, skin, nails, and mucous membranes. Systemic and topical corticosteroids, colchicine, azathioprine, dapsone, and methotrexate have had reported success but lack data to make recommendations. EBA has a low mortality rate but high morbidity. Complications associated with immunosuppressive therapies (secondary infections, osteoporosis, diabetes, etc.) and malignancies from chronic inflammation should be monitored.

Patients must be educated about protecting their skin from friction and injury. Wound care and healing is paramount to limiting morbidity. During flares, patients should be followed up monthly; otherwise annual follow-up with primary care and age-appropriate cancer screenings will be enough.

Bullous Eruption of Systemic Lupus Erythematosus

A subepidermal AIBD, bullous systemic lupus erythematosus (BSLE) is a rare subtype of SLE. Patients must meet the American College of Rheumatology diagnostic criteria for SLE. Hence, the incidence is highest in 20- to 40-year olds, African Americans, and women. BSLE is caused by IgG autoantibodies targeting type VII collagen and anchoring fibrils in BMZ. The DIF shows a continuous granular band along the BMZ and often shows a lupus band.

Clinical presentation of BSLE can vary from small grouped vesicles to bullae symmetrically involving the upper trunk, face, neck, and upper extremities. Blisters can last for days or months and is exacerbated by photo exposure. Unlike many other AIBDs, BSLE responds well to first-line treatment with dapsone. The disease does not usually result in scarring but may leave hyperpigmentation. Diagnosis and management of BSLE should be done through collaboration between a dermatologist and a rheumatologist.

BILLING CODES ICD 10

Acquired epidermolysis bullosa	L12.3
Bullous disorder, unspecified	L13.9
Bullous pemphigoid	L12.0
Calcinosis cutis	L94.2
Cicatricial pemphigoid	L12.1
Chronic bullous disease of childhood	L12.2
Dermatitis herpetiformis	L13.0
Linear scleroderma	L94.1
Localized scleroderma (morphea)	L94.0
Lupus erythematosus	L93
Discoid lupus erythematosus	L93.0
Subacute cutaneous lupus erythematosus	L93.1
Other local lupus erythematosus	L93.2
Other localized connective tissue disorders	L94
Pemphigus	L10
Pemphigus foliaceous	L10.2
Pemphigus vegetans	L10.1
Pemphigus vulgaris	L10.0

CLINICAL PEARLS

- Erosions on the skin may have developed secondary to blisters.
- DIF is the gold standard for diagnosing an AIBD. A biopsy for histopathology alone is not sufficient to make the diagnosis.
- Once identified as a blistering condition, it is critical to diagnose the SPECIFIC AIBD which guides treatment and prognosis.
- HG can be differentiated from papular urticarial papules and plaques of pregnancy (PUPPP) that develops in the striae and spares the umbilicus.
- All blisters are not indicative of an AIBD. Consider infection, injury, hypersensitivity, drugs, and genetic disorders.
- H&E staining should be performed on an intact vesicle, if possible.
- Biopsy for DIF should be performed on perilesional skin and must be transported in Michel's media, not formaldehyde.
- Systemic corticosteroids may be necessary for patients with AIBD. However, steroid-sparing agents should be started as soon as possible to allow for the tapering off of corticosteroids.
- Always consider osteoporosis and peptic ulcer prevention for patients treated with systemic corticosteroids for more than 3 months.

READINGS

Bernard, P., & Borradori, L. (2012). In J. L. Bolognia, J. L. Jorizzo, & J. V. Schaffer, (Eds.), *Dermatology* (3rd ed.). Philadelphia, PA: Saunders Elsevier.

Chan, L. S. (2014). *Bullous pemphigoid.* Retrieved from http://emedicine.medscape.com/article/1062391-overview on May 1, 2014.

Connolly, M. K. (2012). Systemic sclerosis (scleroderma) and related disorders. In J. L. Bolognia, J. L. Jorizzo, & J. V. Schaffer, (Eds.), *Dermatology* (3rd ed.). Philadelphia, PA: Saunders Elsevier.

Habif, T. P. (2010). *Clinical dermatology: A color guide to diagnosis and therapy* (5th ed). St. Louis, MO: Mosby.

Herti, M., & Sitaru, C. (n.d.). Pathogenesis, clinical manifestations, and diagnosis of pemphigus. In J. J. Zone, (Ed.), *UpToDate*. Waltham, MA.

Hull, C. M., & Zone, J. J. (2012). Dermatitis herpetifomis and linear EgA bullous dermatosis. In J. L. Bolognia, J. L. Jorizzo, & J. V. Schaffer (Eds.), *Dermatology* (3rd ed.). Philadelphia, PA: Saunders Elsevier.

Lee, L. A., & Werth, V. P. (2012). Lupus erythematosus. In J. L. Bolognia, J. L. Jorizzo, & J. V. Schaffer, (Eds.), *Dermatology* (3rd ed.). Philadelphia, PA: Saunders Elsevier.

Leiferman, K. M. (n.d.). Epidemiology and pathogenesis of bullous pemphigoid and mucous membrane pemphigoid. In J. J. Zone, (Ed.), *UpToDate*. Waltham: MA.

Ljubojevic, S., & Lipozencic, J. (2012) Autoimmune bullous diseases associations. *Clinics in Dermatology, 30*(1), 17–33.

Miller, M. L., & Vleugels, R. A. (n.d.). Clinical manifestations of dermatomyositis and polymyositis in adults. In I. N. Targoff, J. M. Shefner, & J. Callen, (Eds.), *UpToDate*. Waltham, MA.

Pomeranz, M. K. (n.d.). Dermatoses of pregnancy. In C. J. Lockwoeed, & R. P. Dellavalle (Eds.), *UpToDate*. Waltham, MA.

Rheumatology. 1997 Update of the 1982 American College of Rheumatology revised criteria for classification of systemic lupus erythematosus. Available at http://tinyurl.com/1997SLEcriteria. Accessed July 6, 2014.

Rocken, M., & Ghoreschi, K. (2012). Morphea and lichen sclerosus. In J. L. Bolognia, J. L. Jorizzo, & J. V. Schaffer (Eds.), *Dermatology* (3rd ed.). Philadelphia, PA: Saunders Elsevier.

Schmidt, E., della Torre, R., & Borradori, L. (2011). Clinical features and practical diagnosis of bullous pemphigoid. *Dermatology Clinics, 29,* 427–438.

Schur, P. H., & Moschella, S. L. Mucocutaneous manifestations of systemic lupus erythematosus. In Pisetsky, D. S., and Callen, J. (Eds.), *UpToDate*, Waltham, MA.

Schur, P. H. (n.d.). Measurement and clinical significance of antinuclear antibodies. In R. H. Shmerling (Ed.). *UpToDate*. Waltham, MA.

Schur, P. H. (n.d.). In R. H. Shmerling (Ed.). *UpToDate*. Waltham, MA.

Sontheimer, R. D. (2004). Skin manifestations of systemic autoimmune connective tissue disease: Diagnostics and therapeutics. *Best Practice & Research. Clinical Rheumatology, 18*(3), 429–462.

Sontheimer, R. D., & Provost, T. T. (2003). *Cutaneous manifestations of rheumatic diseases.* Philadelphia, PA: Lippincott Wilkins & Williams.

Tan, E. M., Cohen, A. S., Fries, J. F., Masi, A. T., McShane, D. J., Rothfield, N. F., . . . Winchester, R. J. (1982). The 1982 revised criteria for the classification of systemic lupus erythematosus. *Arthritis and Rheumatism, 25*, 1271–1277.

Wjoodley, D. T., Che, M., & Kim, G. (n.d.). Epidermolysis bullosa acquisita. In J. J. Zone, (Ed.), *UpToDate*. Waltham, MA.

Wolveron, S. E. (2013). *Comprehensive dermatologic drug therapy.* Philadelphia, PA: Saunders Elsevier.

Yancy, K. B. (2012). The biology of the basement membrane zone. In J. L. Bolognia, J. L. Jorizzo, & J. V. Schaffer (Eds.), *Dermatology* (3rd ed.). Philadelphia, PA: Saunders Elsevier.

16 Vasculitis and Hypersensitivity

Cathleen Case

A hypersensitivity reaction is an exaggerated and pathologic response by the immune system to a self- or foreign antigen. Hypersensitivity reactions differ in the mediators involved, mechanisms, timing, and clinical manifestations; however, there may be similar morphologic appearances making clinical diagnosis a challenge. There are four types of hypersensitivity reactions: Type I is immediate, anaphylactic; mediated by IgE, histamine, leukotrienes; and includes urticaria and angioedema. Type II is cytotoxic; mediated by IgM or IgG, complement; and includes some drug reactions and transfusion reaction. Type III is mediated by IgG or IgM antibodies in immune complexes; includes serum sickness, arthus reaction, vasculitis, or systemic lupus erythematosus. Type IV is delayed/cell mediated; activates reactions with antigen-specific T cells, such as poison ivy, allergic contact dermatitis, tuberculin reaction.

The hypersensitivity reactions addressed in this chapter include vasculitis, urticaria and angioedema, erythema multiforme (EM), and erythema nodosum (EN). These reactions range in severity from mild to life-threatening and can be triggered by drugs, infectious agents, foods, environmental allergens, malignancies, autoimmune disorders, other systemic illness, or unknown etiologies.

VASCULITIS

Vasculitis is an inflammatory process which involves the walls of any size or type of vessel causing damage that results in tissue necrosis. Cutaneous vasculitis may be limited to the skin only, may be a primary cutaneous vasculitis with secondary systemic involvement; or a cutaneous manifestation of a systemic vasculitis. All categories of vessels can be affected, including small, medium-sized, and large vessels of the arterial and/or venous systems. *Small vessels* include arterioles, capillaries, and postcapillary venules that are found in the superficial and mid-dermis of the skin (Table 16-1). Medium-sized vessels refer to the main visceral arteries and veins, and the small arteries and veins within the deep dermis or subcutaneous tissue (Table 16-2). *Large vessels* are the aorta, its major branches and corresponding veins, and other named arteries such as pulmonary or temporal artery. Cutaneous involvement occurs almost always with vasculitis of small and medium-size vessels and therefore the large-vessel vasculitides will only be briefly mentioned in this chapter.

The clinical spectrum of vasculitis presents a diagnostic challenge even for the experienced dermatology or rheumatology provider. In an attempt to classify the vasculitides, several schemes have been proposed; historically the classification was based on vessel size. Other criteria have been developed based on clinical signs and symptoms, histopathology, historical data, and the presence or absence of internal organ involvement. Most recently, The International Chapel Hill Consensus Conference on the Nomenclature of Systemic Vasculitides (CHCC2012) updated their original work of 1994. This is neither a classification system nor a diagnostic system, but rather it defines the nomenclature that should be used for a specifically defined disease process (Figure 16-1). For example, if a vasculitis is caused by direct invasion of pathogens, then the vasculitis should be specified

as such (i.e., rickettsial vasculitis or syphilitic aortitis) rather than "infectious vasculitis." Although there are differences among these criteria, a shared defining feature of vasculitis is an inflammation of blood vessel walls at some time during the course of the disease.

Furthermore, CCHC has renamed the vasculitis previously known as cutaneous leukocytoclastic vasculitis and is now referred to as *cutaneous small-vessel vasculitis* (CSVV). By definition, CSVV has the histologic findings associated with leukocytoclastic vasculitis but the involvement is limited to the small blood vessels of the skin, and no other organ system is involved. This may also be referred to as *single-organ vasculitis*. The following section will focus on the CSVV that is more commonly seen in the primary care setting, the importance of screening for systemic organ involvement, differential diagnoses, diagnostics, and prompt management.

Pathophysiology

The etiology of vasculitis can be broadly labeled as infectious or noninfectious, while the pathogenesis is poorly understood. Possible mechanisms of vascular damage include the deposition of immune complexes (i.e., Henoch–Schönlein purpura), presence of autoantibodies, or cell-mediated granuloma formation (T-cell response). Each pathway results in endothelial cell activation, leading to vessel obstruction and ischemia of dependent tissue.

Immune complex vasculitis. When vasculitis is caused by a hypersensitivity to an antigen, immune complexes form and are deposited in the vessel walls, which in turn activate complement that attracts neutrophils. The classic histologic features demonstrate transmural infiltration in and around small blood vessels (postcapillary venules) by neutrophils showing fragmentation of nuclei (karyorrhexis or leukocytoclasia), fibrinoid necrosis of the vessel walls, extravasation of erythrocytes, and swelling, shrinkage, or sloughing of endothelial cells. The late phase of the disease will show thrombosis of the affected postcapillary venules. Occlusion and necrosis in arteries and veins also occur secondary to aberrant coagulation caused by a hypercoagulable state or *vasculopathy*.

The difference between vasculitis and vasculopathy is subtle but needs to be considered throughout the diagnostic process since there may be similar clinical features and divergent diagnoses and treatments. The primary process in *vasculitis* is an inflammatory cell infiltrate triggering the clotting cascade and thrombosis, and may be seen in the late stages of healing vasculitic lesions. In *vasculopathy*, the primary process is thrombosis, usually due to a hypercoagulable state. Inflammatory cells enter the vessel and vessel wall in order to reestablish the local circulation. Thus, vascular inflammation is seen late in this *primarily* thrombotic process and can be misinterpreted as vasculitis on biopsy. The presence of livedo reticularis on clinical examination is usually, but not always, more consistent with vasculopathy.

Antineutrophil cytoplasmic antibodies-associated vasculitis. Antineutrophil cytoplasmic antibodies (ANCAs) are autoantibodies directed against an antigen in the cytoplasm of neutrophils. ANCAs are often associated with some system vasculitides, referred

TABLE 16-1 Small-Vessel Vasculidities

NOMENCLATURE	DESCRIPTION
ANCA – Associated Vasculitides Necrotizing vasculitis, few or no immune deposits. Associated with pANCA or cANCA. Involves small arteries, arterioles, capillaries, and venules, but may also affect medium arteries and veins.	
Microscopic polyangiitis*	Necrotizing vasculitis, few or no immune deposits. Necrotizing arteritis in small and medium-sized arteries may be present, necrotizing glomerulonephritis very common, and pulmonary capillaritis often occurs
Granulomatosis with polyangiitis* (Wegener's)	Necrotizing granulomatous inflammation involving upper and lower respiratory tract; necrotizing vasculitis in small-to-medium-sized vessels. Necrotizing glomerulonephritis is common.
Eosinophilic granulomatosis with polyangiitis* (Churg–Strauss syndrome)	Necrotizing vasculitis of small and medium-sized vessels, associated with asthma and eosinophilia. Necrotizing granulomatous inflammation involves the respiratory tract. If glomerulonephritis is present, then usually ANCA is positive.
Immune Complex Vasculitides* Notable deposits of immunoglobulin and/or complement of the vessel walls. Frequent glomerulonephritis. Involves small arteries, arterioles, capillaries, and venules.	
Antiglomerular basement membrane disease	Involving glomerular and/or pulmonary capillaries with deposition of anti-GBM autoantibodies Inflammation can result in necrotizing glomerulonephritis or pulmonary hemorrhage.
Cryoglobulinemic vasculitis	Cryoglobulin immune deposits associated with serum cryoglobulins Cutaneous, glomeruli, peripheral nerves often involved.
IgA vasculitis	IgA1-dominant immune deposits Involve skin and gastrointestinal tract, frequently causing arthritis Glomerulonephritis indistinguishable from IgA nephropathy Onset often associated with URI or GI infection. Example: HSP
Hypocomplementemic urticarial vasculitis	Presents with urticaria and hypocomplementemia. Associated with anti-C1q antibodies, glomerulonephritis, arthritis, COPD, and ocular inflammation
Cutaneous leukocytoclastic vasculitis† (LCV)	Isolated cutaneous small-vessel vasculitis/leukocytoclastic vasculitis without systemic vasculitis or glomerulonephritis Usually limited to one organ

*Some may also be categorized as vasculitis associated with systemic or unknown etiologies.

†LCV, traditionally classified as a single-organ vasculitis according to CHCC.

Adapted from Jennett, J. C., Falk, R.J., Bacon, P.A., Basu, N., Cid, M.C., Ferrario, F.... Watts, R. A. (2013). 2012 Revised International Chapel Hill Consensus Conference Nomenclature of Vasculitides. *Arthritis & Rheumatism, 65*(1), 1–11.

to as ANCA-associated vasculitis affecting mixed small- and medium-sized vessels. Indirect immunofluorescence (IIF) produces two major staining *patterns*: cytoplasmic ANCA (cANCA) and perinuclear ANCA (pANCA), while ELISA will identify antibodies to *specific* antigens.

Many small-vessel vasculitides, particularly CSVV, have little or no vascular immune deposits and are idiopathic. There are many precipitating agents associated with vasculitis, such as chronic disease, malignancy, infections, or drugs (Table 16-3). It is worthwhile mentioning the occurrence of *cocaine-associated* vasculitis. Dermatologists, urgent care providers, emergency physicians, and primary care providers should be able to recognize the vasculitic lesions associated with the intravenous or intranasal use of cocaine. Characteristically, there is purpura and necrosis of the ears (Figure 16-2), nose, cheeks, and various other locations including the trunk. Levamisole, a drug contaminate in cocaine, is the suspected culprit, although a direct causal relationship has not been established.

Clinical Presentation

The importance of a detailed physical examination that accurately identifies the morphology of the presenting lesions cannot be over-emphasized. Clinical presentation is critical in developing a differential diagnoses for vasculitis. It is absolutely essential that clinicians evaluate the patient for systemic involvement, which may present as fever, cough, myalgia, hemoptysis, abdominal pain, melena, weight loss, nausea/vomiting, diarrhea, hypertension, headache, visual disturbances, and renal insufficiency (urine sediment with protein and red and white cells).

The morphology of the cutaneous findings in any vasculitis will depend on the size of the vessels primarily affected and will provide clues to the type of vasculitis. Clinicians should understand the terminology frequently used in discussing these dermatoses (Table 16-4). Small-vessel vasculitis (SVV) results in petechia, purpura, erythematous macules, papules, and pustules (Figure 16-3). *Palpable purpura* occurs when vasculitis is present

TABLE 16-2	Medium- and Large-Vessel Vasculitides (Other Than Small Vessel)
NOMENCLATURE	**DESCRIPTION**
Large-Vessel Vasculitis Large arteries and aorta	
Takayasu arteritis	Arteritis, often granulomatous, usually patients <50 years
Giant cell arteritis	Arteritis, often granulomatous, usually patients >50 years. Predominantly the carotid and vertebral arteries; most commonly the temporal artery
Medium-Vessel Vasculitis Any size artery, especially medium-sized artery like main visceral arteries & branches	
Polyarteritis nodosa	Necrotizing arteritis without glomerulonephritis (of medium-sized or small arteries), or vasculitis not associated with ANCAs (arterioles, capillaries, or venules)
Kawasaki disease	Arteritis associated with mucocutaneous lymph node syndrome (small, medium-sized, large arteries, and aorta) Coronary artery involvement usually seen in young children and infants
Variable Vessel Vasculitis No predominant size or type of vessel	
Behçet disease, Cogan syndrome	Primary categories of vasculitis because of the frequency of vasculitis in these conditions
Single-Organ Vasculitis Any size artery and in a single organ	
Named according to the affected organ or vessel	Distribution may be unifocal or diffuse within an organ/system Examples: cutaneous small-vessel vasculitis; testicular vasculitis; or central nervous system vasculitis
Vasculitis Associated with Systemic Disease Caused by or associated with a systemic disease	
Named according to disease-related etiology	Sometimes considered secondary vasculitis Examples: rheumatoid vasculitis; lupus vasculitis; or sarcoidosis vasculitis
Vasculitis Associated with Probable Etiology Based on specific etiology	
Named according to etiology	Sometimes considered a secondary vasculitis Examples: Hydralazine-associated microscopic polyangiitis; hepatitis B virus-associated vasculitis; syphilis-associated aortitis; or cancer-associated vasculitis

in postcapillary venules and is the hallmark of cutaneous vasculitis (Figures 16-4 to 16-6). Lesions typically evolve within 7 to 10 days of a causative exposure, and erupt in crops lasting about 1 to 4 weeks. The size of SVV lesions can range from 1 mm to several centimeters and may be asymptomatic, itchy, or painful. Edema may develop if nephritis is present. Painful nodules, pustules, and necrotic ulcers can present in specific types of SVV like granulomatosis with polyangiitis (GPA). The unusual distribution of lesions in GPA found in the oral and nasal mucosa should heighten the clinician's index of suspicion. Yet most SVV lesions favor dependent sites such as legs and feet, or areas affected by trauma and tight-fitting clothing. The buttocks or back of a bedridden patient may be involved and reflects the influence of venous pressure due to gravity.

Medium-vessel vasculitis occurs predominately in medium-size and small arteries (i.e., visceral arteries and branches). Polyarteritis nodosa (PAN) is a necrotizing medium-vessel vasculitis presenting as nodules (similar to EN), palpable purpura, and vesicles/bullae. Livedo reticularis may progress to ulcerations usually located on the lower extremities. The lesions are painful and may be accompanied by edema. Patients with PAN often have systemic symptoms.

Kawasaki disease (KD) is also a vasculitis of medium-size arteries, including coronary arteries and aorta. Although it is rare and self-limiting, recognition of the clinical presentation is important to avoid cardiac sequelae. It is more common in childhood and is discussed under Childhood Vasculitis.

Large-vessel vasculitis involving the aorta and large arteries means that affected patients have systemic involvement and appear much sicker. Ulcerations and sometimes gangrenous digits are seen with large-vessel involvement. Giant cell arteritis (GCA) occurs in patients over 50 years, who report constitutional symptoms along with temporal artery tenderness, visual loss, polymyalgia rheumatica, headache, jaw claudication, and temporal enlargement with absent pulse is common. Clinicians should assess the patient for aortic involvement, including signs and symptoms of aneurysm. In contrast, Takayasu arteritis is more prevalent in females younger than 50 years and affects the aorta and major branches. Granulomatous inflammation affects any or all of the organs, resulting in significant morbidity and mortality.

DIFFERENTIAL DIAGNOSIS Vasculitis	
MORPHOLOGIC PRESENTATION	**DIFFERENTIAL DIAGNOSIS**
Palpable purpuric papules/ plaques (raised)	Arthropod bite
	Erythema multiforme
	Morbilliform drug eruption with hemorrhage
	Infectious emboli
	Cellulitis
Purpuric macules/patches (flat)	Hemorrhage
	Trauma, solar/actinic purpura, medication-related (e.g., aspirin), thrombocytopenia, viral exanthem, scurvy
	Thrombosis
	Hypercoagulable state, purpura fulminans (e.g., DIC or sepsis), heparin or warfarin necrosis, livedoid vasculopathy
	Emboli
	Cholesterol, cardiac, fat, air
	Inflammation
	Pigmented purpura/capillaritis
Urticarial lesions	Urticaria
	Arthropod bites
	Papular urticaria
	Serum sickness–like reaction
	Erythema multiforme
	Viral exanthem
	Sweet syndrome
	Urticarial phase of bullous pemphigoid
Ulcers	Venous or arterial disease
	Pyoderma gangrenosum
	Livedoid vasculopathy
	Hypercoagulable state
	Calciphylaxis
	Infections (e.g., bacterial, mycobacterial, fungal)
Nodules	Panniculitis
	Superficial migratory thrombophlebitis
	Dermal neoplasms
	Infections (e.g., bacterial, mycobacterial, fungal)
	Systemic vasculitides

Diagnostics

The general approach for any patient with vasculitis should be to rule out other diseases that may mimic vasculitis; look for any underlying or secondary cause (disease, infection, drug, or malignancy); perform diagnostics to confirm the presence of a vasculitis; and conduct additional tests to identify the type and severity of the vasculitis.

A detailed history, review of systems, and clinical presentation will be invaluable in guiding the clinician's development of a differential diagnosis or suspicion for secondary causes (Table 16-5). The initial diagnostic test should be a punch or excisional biopsy, the gold standard for evaluation of vasculitis, which should be taken from the center of a new lesion (preferably 24–48 hours old), making sure to collect some of the subcutaneous tissue if evaluating deeper, larger vessels. The histopathologic features of the biopsy can aid in identifying the type of vasculitis as well as other features which may indicate other systemic disease (i.e., interface dermatitis suggestive of connective tissue disease). Additional punch biopsy for direct immunofluorescence (preserved in Michel's medium) may be helpful in identifying the deposition of immunoglobulins and complements in the blood vessels (i.e., Henoch–Schönlein purpura [HSP]).

A complete blood count with differential should be part of the initial workup. Patients with a primary vasculitis rarely have leukocytosis or thrombocytopenia, which, if present, should prompt further evaluation for an underlying disease, malignancy, or infection. Eosinophilia is seen in Churg–Strauss syndrome. Anemia could signify underlying lupus erythematosus or malignancy. A C-reactive protein (CRP) and erythrocyte sedimentation rate (ESR) are usually elevated but are nonspecific markers of systemic inflammation. Blood urea nitrogen, creatinine, and electrolyte abnormalities may reflect kidney involvement. Abnormal liver function tests may be associated with underlying liver disease or malignancy. A stool guaiac will help assess for vasculitis of the bowel in patients with abdominal pain. Urinalysis with microscopy that is positive for red blood cell casts is suggestive of glomerulonephritis, while proteinuria is common in lupus nephritis. A chest x-ray may be recommended if the patient's review of symptoms or clinical presentation suggests pulmonary involvement and may reveal pulmonary infiltrates, nodules, patchy consolidation, pleural effusion, and cardiomegaly.

Management

Treatment of vasculitis should be based on type and severity, as well as the presence of organ involvement. Management of primary CSVV seen in primary care will be the focus of this section. Medium- and large-vessel vasculitis are beyond the scope of this text and should be managed by dermatologists or appropriate specialists.

Most primary CSVV is mild and self-limiting. If an offending antigen like a drug is identified, then removing the source is the obvious first step. Underlying infection or disease should be treated at the outset. Treatment of CSVV (without systemic involvement) should proceed with supportive care, including leg elevation, rest, and gentle compression of legs for comfort. However, tight restrictive clothing may aggravate susceptible skin regions and should be avoided. Pain and inflammation can be treated with nonsteroidal anti-inflammatory drugs (NSAIDs), and pruritus may be attenuated with antihistamines such as hydroxyzine or diphenhydramine. Class I topical corticosteroid (TCS) ointment may also be helpful for adult patients, most of whom will not require systemic measures.

Short-term oral corticosteroids (prednisone) may be considered in patients with chronic (active disease that persists for more than 4 weeks) or recurring CSVV if hemorrhagic blisters and ulcerations are present. The dose and duration of treatment are dependent on the severity. A dosage of 0.5 mg/kg/day can be prescribed for 1 to 2 weeks or until new lesions cease to erupt. A taper over 2 to 4 weeks may be necessary and usually meets with complete resolution. Chronic forms of CSVV, or those with more severe cutaneous

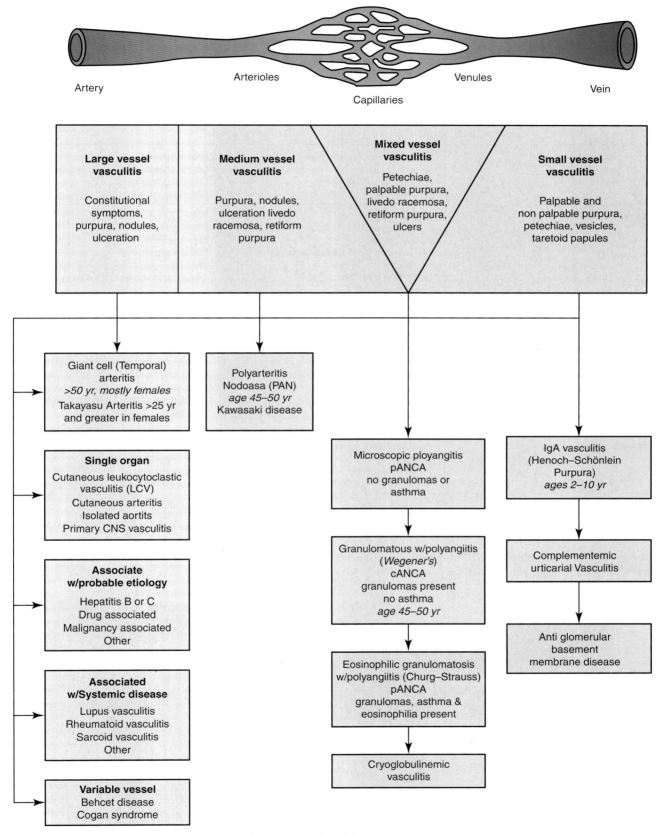

FIG. 16-1. Diagram of vasculitis showing vessel size, morphology, and related conditions.

TABLE 16-3 Cutaneous Vasculitis: Causes and Precipitating Agents

CAUSE	AGENT	
Infection	Bacterial	Parvovirus B19
	β-hemolytic *Streptococcus* group A	Fungal
	Staphylococcus aureus	*Candida albicans*
	Mycobacterium leprae	Protozoan
	Mycobacterium tuberculosis	*Plasmodium malariae*
	Viral	Helminthic infections
	Hepatitis A, B, C (including vaccines)	*Schistosoma haematobium*
	HSV	*Schistosoma mansoni*
	HIV	
Chronic disease state	Systemic lupus erythematosis	Behcet disease
	Sjogren syndrome	Cystic fibrosis
	Rheumatoid arthritis	Cryoglobulinemia
	Inflammatory bowel disease	Bowel bypass syndrome
Drug exposure	Common	Macrolide antibiotics
	Anti-TNF agents	Phenytoin
	COX-2 inhibitors	Retinoids
	Granulocyte colony-stimulating factor	Sulfonylureas
	Hydralazine	Thiazides
	Leukotriene inhibitors	Trimethoprim–sulfamethoxazole
	Minocycline	Vancomycin
	NSAIDs	Rare
	Penicillins	Aspirin
	Quinolones	Atypical antipsychotics
	Streptokinase	Cocaine/levamisole contaminated
	Occasional	Gabapentin
	ACE inhibitors	Insulin
	Allopurinol	Metformin
	β-blockers	Rituximab
	Coumarins	Selective serotonin-reuptake inhibitors
	Furosemide	Vitamins
	Interferons	
Neoplasm	Lymphoproliferative disorders	Lymphosarcoma
	Hodgkin disease	Multiple myeloma
	Mycosis fungoides	Solid organ tumors
	Myeloproliferative disorders	Adult T-cell leukemia
Other	Chemicals	Food stuff allergens
	Insecticides	Milk proteins
	Petroleum products	Gluten

HSV, herpes simplex virus; COX, cyclooxygenase; NSAIDs, nonsteroidal anti-inflammatory drugs; TNF, tumor necrosis factor.

Adapted from Chung, L., Kea, B., & Fiorentino, D. F. (2008). Cutaneous vasculitis. In J. L. Bolognia, J. L. Jorizzo, & R. P. Rapini (Eds.), Dermatology (2nd ed., pp. 347–367). Spain: Mosby Elsevier.

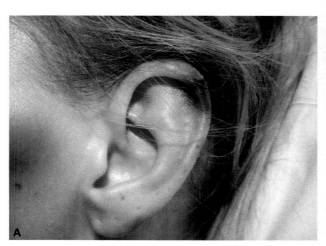 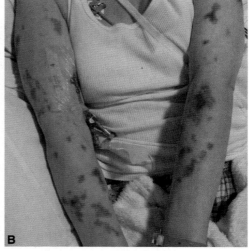

FIG. 16-2. Characteristic purpura associated with levamisole (common contaminate in cocaine) induced small-vessel vasculitis on the ear (**A**) and arms (**B**).

TABLE 16-4	Terminology
Purpura	Lesions caused by extravasated red blood cells into skin, appearing red-brown or purple, flat (macule or patch)
Palpable purpura	Papules or plaques (raised) which are blanchable erythema or nonblanchable component of visible hemorrhage. Diascopy can help distinguish between the two (below).
Petechiae	Small pinpoint (<4 mm) purpuric macules, initially bright red that turn brown or rust-colored, and can be seen in thrombocytopenic states, as shown in Figure 16-3
Livedo	Macular violaceous netlike patterned erythema of the skin; may indicate vasculopathy
Retiform purpura	Angulated or branched configuration of purpura reflecting the vascular architecture in the skin; vasculopathy diagnosis should be favored
Ecchymosis	Large (>1 cm) blue-purple areas of interstitial hemorrhage
Infarct	Areas of cutaneous necrosis secondary to occlusion of blood vessels. Lesions are dusky red and gray irregular macules surrounded by pink hyperemia and eventually turning black. It can be present in vasculitis, vasculopathy, or embolic disorders.
Diascopy	Application of pressure using a glass slide on a red lesion to distinguish vascular dilatation (erythema) which blanches compared to redness due to extravasated red blood cells (purpura), which does not blanch.

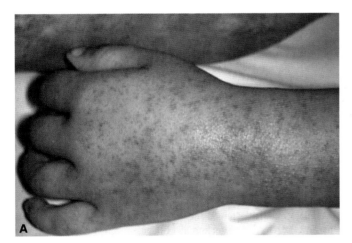
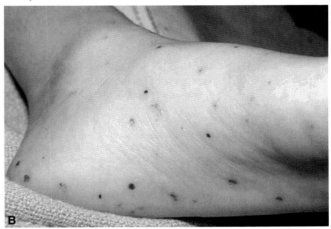

FIG. 16-3. **A:** Tiny skin hemorrhages (petechiae) in a child with thrombocytopenia. **B:** Petechiae on the foot and sole of a child with HSP with palpable purpura.

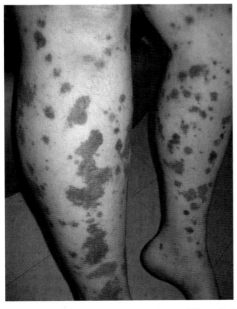
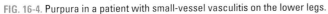
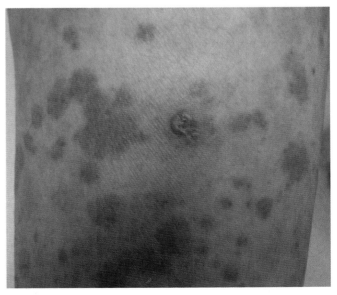

FIG. 16-4. Purpura in a patient with small-vessel vasculitis on the lower legs.

FIG. 16-5. Purpura with a bulla on the lower leg.

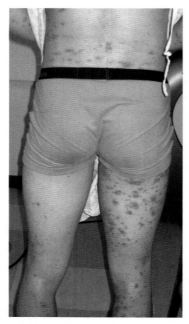

FIG. 16-6. Nonpalpable purpura of leukocytoclastic vasculitis, also called single-organ vasculitis, on man with an allergy to shellfish.

TABLE 16-5	Assessment of the Patient with Cutaneous Vasculitis
History	Timing, lesions develop 7–10 days after inciting agent. Special focus on history of malignancy, infections, connective tissue disorder, and recent drug administration or ingestion, including illicit drug use
Review of systems	Critical for assessment of systemic involvement: cardiovascular, pulmonary, abdominal, and neurologic symptoms
Physical examination	Detailed: For the initial evaluation, assess patient for signs of systemic involvement. Special attention should be paid to dependent areas, body areas affected by trauma or tight clothing Constitutional: fever, weight loss, chills, night sweats, and fatigue Weight loss, myalgia, arthralgia Positive findings: diplopia, headache, eye or ear pain, cough, shortness of breath, hemoptysis, nausea, vomiting, diarrhea, abdominal pain, blood in stool, weakness, neuropathy, myalgia, arthralgia, hair loss, sicca symptoms, sinus tenderness, oral or nasal inflammation, otitis media, keratitis, hepatosplenomegaly, and lymphadenopathy

disease, may require higher doses of prednisone dosed 1 mg/kg/day to control symptoms. Since long-term use of corticosteroids has the risk of significant side effects, transitioning the patient to a steroid-sparing agent (i.e., colchicine, dapsone) is important. Patients on dapsone need G6PD testing prior to initiating therapy and careful monitoring for hemolytic anemia during therapy. Pentoxifylline

has been effective when the CSVV is resistant. Recalcitrant CSVV or SVV with systemic involvement often requires management by dermatology specialists with azathioprine, methotrexate, cyclophosphamide, intravenous immunoglobulin, mycophenolate mofetil, rituximab, or plasmapheresis.

Referral and Consultation

The initial presentation and evaluation of vasculitis may begin in the primary care office, and patients with localized or early vasculitis can be managed symptomatically with removal of an offending antigen. Most patients are referred to a dermatology provider when there is extensive cutaneous involvement, threatened organ involvement, and relapse or disease progression despite treatment. A number of specialists should be consulted based on findings, including a nephrologist, pulmonologist, cardiologist, and otolaryngologist. Surgical consult may be necessary if necrotizing or ulcerative lesions are present.

Prognosis and Complications

If a drug or infection is the cause, there may only be one episode with spontaneous resolution; however, if SVV is associated with a systemic disease, such as hepatitis C infection or rheumatoid arthritis, treatment considerations will be different. Ultimately, the best indicator of prognosis in any vasculitis with systemic involvement depends on the size of the vessel and organ involved. Long-term implications include the possibility of multiple episodes with recurrent crops of vasculitic lesions appearing for months or years.

Patient Education and Follow-up

Patients receiving short-term corticosteroids should be advised of possible adverse effects, including hypertension, glucose intolerance, sleep disturbance, hirsutism, weight gain, and avascular necrosis of the hip. Patients on prednisone for extended periods of time should have baseline bone mineral density testing and receive education about corticosteroid-induced osteoporosis, including weight-bearing exercise, smoking and alcohol cessation, and fall prevention in the elderly. Consider calcium with vitamin D supplementation and bisphosphonates for high-risk individuals. Blood pressure and serum glucose should be monitored. Patients of childbearing age should always be counseled regarding adequate birth control measures, especially if treated with teratogenic medications. Close follow-up of patients with systemic vasculitis by multiple providers may be required to halt disease progression, evaluate response to therapy, and prevention of complications.

Special Considerations

Childhood vasculitis

Henoch–Schönlein purpura. IgA vasculitis or HSP is the most common vasculitis in childhood, usually occurring in children aged 2 to 10 years. It is rare but can affect adults. HSP is an SVV typically preceded by a respiratory tract infection or sometimes an allergy, drug therapy, or vaccination. The features of HSP can be attributed to IgA-containing immune complexes entrapped in small-vessel walls of skin and target organ. Although it may be limited to the skin, 80% of HSP have systemic involvement, most often the intestines, kidneys, and joints.

HSP presents with a classic tetrad of purpura, abdominal pain, arthralgias, and hematuria, if it has progressed to nephritis. Erythematous macules or urticarial papules develop in crops, progressing into palpable purpura with a dusky or necrotic center (Figure 16-7). Presenting lesions can include vesicles, bullae, and pustules. Lesions

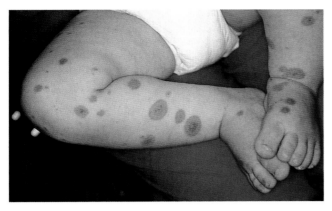

FIG. 16-7. Henoch–Schonlein purpura. Lesions are macular and papular, purpuric, varying shades of purple and blue, and necrotizing centers are noted.

favor the extensor aspect of the lower extremities and buttocks, but can include arms, face, and ears. It is not commonly seen on the trunk (Figure 16-8A). Joint symptoms including arthralgia of ankles, knees, and dorsum of hands and feet are common and disabling—children don't want to walk.

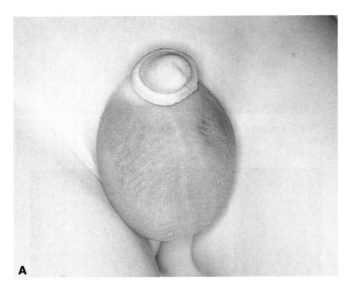

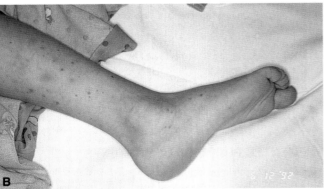

FIG. 16-8. Henoch–Schonlein purpura. **A:** Edema and possible purpura seen in the scrotum of a 6-year-old patient referred for possible torsion. **B:** Typical purpura of the legs noted on further examination, providing a great clue to the diagnosis of Henoch–Schonlein purpura.

GI manifestations of HSP include abdominal pain, nausea, vomiting, diarrhea, GI bleeding, and bloody stool. Scrotal involvement is common in affected males (Figure 16-8B), and intussusception can be a major complication. Renal involvement detected with a urinalysis shows hematuria and minimal proteinuria, which is usually mild and self-limiting. The onset of renal disease, however, may be delayed for weeks or months. Nephrotic syndrome or renal failure can develop.

The priority is the identification and treatment of the precedent infection or removal of the offending agent. Diagnosis can be made on clinical presentation when classic signs and symptoms are present. All children should have a urinalysis with microscopy to rule out renal involvement. Biopsy and laboratory diagnostics are not usually necessary unless the diagnosis is questionable or an abnormal urinalysis is noted. HSP is usually self-limiting and resolves spontaneously in 6 to 8 weeks. Care of children with HSP is mostly supportive with NSAIDs for the arthralgias, painful skin lesions, and edema. Oral corticosteroids are reserved for cases with severe systemic symptoms and may hasten recovery.

Patients with severe or prolonged disease should be referred to dermatology or other specialists (nephrology or gastroenterology) as appropriate. HSP can recur and may leave postinflammatory hyperpigmentation. Follow-up with periodic urinalysis for at least 6 months is recommended since renal involvement can be delayed. Long-term follow-up is warranted for adults or children with associated nephritis.

Acute hemorrhagic edema of infancy (AHEI) is a rare, self-limiting SVV with mostly cutaneous manifestations and rarely systemic involvement. AHEI affects children aged 2 months to 3 years and is considered the leukocytoclastic vasculitis (LCV) of childhood with an unknown etiology. It has been associated with infections (upper respiratory, GI, or urinary tract), drug exposure, and immunizations.

AHEI presents abruptly with large and erythematous plaques (medallion-like appearance) that are purpuric, favoring the face, ears, and distal extremities. They may progress to a targetoid, annular, or rosette-like appearance and become painful and edematous. Joint pain, abdominal pain, or scrotal pain may occur, but unlike HSP these findings are rare. The unique characteristics of AHEI are the sudden onset and impressive lesions, but the patient does not appear ill. Diagnostics are not necessary, but a skin biopsy for histopathology would reveal LCV. The course of the disease is usually 1 to 3 weeks and only requires supportive care. Recurrence is rare.

Kawasaki disease, also called mucocutaneous lymph node syndrome, is an important childhood febrile vasculitis that clinicians should recognize as it is the leading cause of acquired heart disease. Classified as a medium- and small-vessel disease, KD can affect the aorta and main coronary arteries, leading to aneurysm and death. The etiology is unknown, but there is a higher incidence in Japanese and Asian Americans, usually in children under the age of 5 years and peaking at 2 years old. KD also appears to be seasonal, with a higher incidence in winter and early spring. The diagnosis can be very easy to miss, but the consequences of an untreated occurrence carry high morbidity and mortality.

Children with KD appear very ill (toxic) and have high fevers (>38.5 °C) lasting for days or weeks and is unresponsive to antipyretics. The fever may precede other clinical symptoms. The guidelines for diagnosing KD are based on presenting symptoms in children with high fever lasting 5 days or more and without an unknown cause. Yet about 10% of children who develop coronary artery aneurysms do not meet the outlined criteria for KD. The American Heart Association set forth clinical criteria for the diagnosis of KD (Table 16-6).

In addition to the diagnostic features, the child may have diarrhea, nausea and vomiting, abdominal pain, inconsolable irritability,

TABLE 16-6	Clinial Criteria for the Diagnosis of Kawasaki Disease

Persistent fever ≥5 days *and* the presence of at least 4 of the following features*:

Bilateral injection of the bulbar conjunctiva (nonexudative)
Mucositis or changes in oral mucosal membranes and lips (strawberry tongue, hyperemic and fissured lips, injected pharynx)
Polymorphous eruption
Cervical lymphadenopathy >1.5 cm (usually obvious)
Peripheral changes in extremities (erythema of soles, palms, and feet); periungual desquamation of the fingers and toes (usually after 2 wk)

*Experienced clinicians can make the diagnoses before 5 days or before day 4 if all five clinical features are present. See also Differential Diagnosis: Kawasaki Disease.

Adapted from Newberger, J. W., Takahashi, M., Gerber, M. A., Gewitz, M. H., Tani, L. Y., Burns, J. C.,.... American Academy of Pediatrics. (2004). Diagnosis, treatment, and long-term management of Kawasaki Disease: A Statement for Health Professionals from the Committee on Rheumatic Fever, Endocarditis and Kawasaki Disease, Council on Cardiovascular Disease in the Young, American Heart Association. *Circulation, 110,* 2747–2771.

cough, rhinorrhea, erythema, and nonpitting edema of the extremities (especially the hands and feet). Mucositis including the classic "strawberry tongue," along with fissured lips, can lead to a decreased fluid intake and dehydration (Figure 16-9). Laboratory studies are not diagnostic of KD but are important in supporting the diagnosis. Ideally, diagnosis should be made within the first 10 days of symptoms to reduce the risk of coronary artery aneurysm. Treatment includes high-dose aspirin and intravenous immunoglobulins. Late diagnosis may be accompanied by cardiac abnormalities (pericardial effusion, tachycardia, murmur, arrhythmias, etc.), CNS involvement, lethargy, gastrointestinal symptoms (including hepatic involvement), and long-term cardiac sequelae.

CLINICAL PEARLS Vasculitis

- *Always* evaluate patients for systemic involvement.
- Purpura above the waist has been reported to be an indicator of renal complication.
- HSP rarely occurs in adults but has been associated with an underlying malignancy.
- Age can be an important diagnostic clue for identifying the type of vasculitis.

DIFFERENTIAL DIAGNOSIS Kawasaki disease

- Viral exanthems
- Exudative conjunctivitis or pharyngitis
- Scarlet fever
- Toxic shock syndrome
- Rocky Mountain spotted fever
- Stephens–Johnson syndrome
- Serum sickness
- Mercury hypersensitivity
- Staph scaled skin syndrome
- Juvenile arthritis
- Leptospirosis

CLINICAL PEARLS Kawasaki Disease

- Clinicians should have a high index of suspicion for KD in children with high fevers for more than 5 days that have little or no response to antipyretics.
- Infants with KD may have intermittent high fevers without a known cause and can be extremely irritable, even inconsolable at times.
- Desquamation of the periungal skin occurs later in the disease (Figure 16-10).
- Perineal erythema (and subsequent desquamation) is an *early* and common symptom.

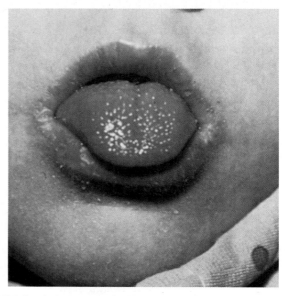

FIG. 16-9. Cracked, erythematous lips and "strawberry" tongue in Kawasaki disease.

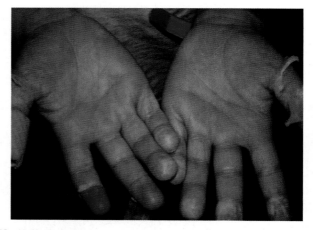

FIG. 16-10. Periungual desquamation during the convalescent phase of Kawasaki disease.

PIGMENTED PURPURIC DERMATOSES

Pigmented purpuric eruptions are characterized by clustered petechial hemorrhages secondary to capillaritis, on a background of yellow-brown discoloration that is due to hemosiderin deposits (Figure 16-11).

These conditions have no systemic findings, and are not associated with venous insufficiency, and hematologic or coagulation

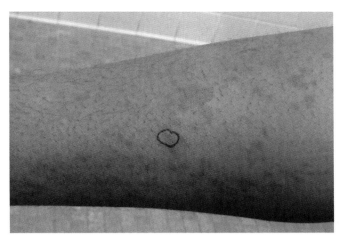

FIG. 16-11. Schamberg purpura; cayenne pepper spots on lower leg.

disorders. Synonyms include capillaritis, pigmented purpuric dermatitis, purpura simplex, and purpura pigmentosa chronica. This brief discussion will focus on *Schamberg disease*, the most common variant of pigmented purpura. Schamberg disease is a progressive dermatosis usually seen in middle-aged and older men but can be seen in women and children.

Pathophysiology

Histology shows minimal inflammation and hemorrhage of superficial papillary dermal vessels usually capillaries without fibrinoid necrosis of vessels.

Clinical Presentation

The primary lesion is red-brown pinpoint, "cayenne pepper" macules that are superimposed over irregular but discrete yellow-pink or yellow-brown patches. Pigmented purpura develops slowly on the lower extremities; however, upper body and oral mucosa may be involved. The lesions are usually symmetric and asymptomatic. The petechiae are nonblanchable purpura (diascopy). Lesions may become violaceous with age and palpable as blood leaks out of damaged capillaries, leaving brown dotting.

DIFFERENTIAL DIAGNOSIS Pigmented purpuric
dermatoses

- Drug-induced purpura
- Contact dermatitis
- Postinflammatory hyperpigmentation (hemosiderin staining)
- Leukocytoclastic vasculitis
- Nummular eczema
- Purpuric mycosis fungoides

Diagnostics

Clinical presentation is usually diagnostic, but a skin biopsy may be done to rule out vasculitis, especially when the lesions are palpable or lichenoid, making the diagnosis less obvious (Figure 16-12).

Management

TCS can be effective for pruritus and extensive erythema. Compression stockings should be considered when venous stasis coexists.

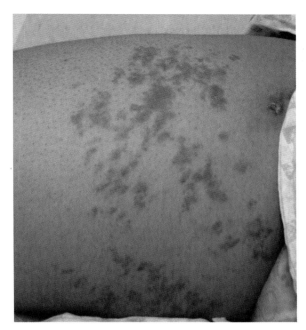

FIG. 16-12. Pigmented purpuric dermatosis may have lichenoid or palpable lesions.

Prognosis and Complications

Schamberg disease is usually chronic, with hyperpigmentation persisting for years.

URTICARIA

Urticaria is a common vascular reaction of the skin characterized by rapidly fluctuating, transient skin and/or mucosal edema due to plasma leakage. Wheals (also known as hives) result from edema in the superficial dermis compared to angioedema occurring in the deep dermis and subcutaneous tissue. Urticaria is wheals, with or without angioedema.

Pathophysiology

The mast cell is the primary effector cell in urticarial reactions. There are several types of stimuli that can cause urticaria, which include immunologic, nonimmunologic, physical, and chemical etiologies (Table 16-7). Release of mast cell mediators causes inflammation and mast cell degranulation, resulting in the release of histamine and inflammatory mediators, as well as an accumulation and activation of other cells, including eosinophils, neutrophils, and possibly basophils. Histamine causes endothelial cell contraction, which allows vascular fluid to leak between the cells through vessel walls, causing tissue edema and wheal formation. When histamine is injected into the skin, there is vasodilation, causing *local erythema*, a *peripheral flare* characterized by erythema beyond the border of local erythema (axon reflex), and a *wheal* produced by leakage of fluid from the postcapillary venules. It is difficult to know the exact pathogenesis of individual cases of urticaria. The majority of urticaria is not allergic, and many cases remain idiopathic after evaluation.

Clinical Presentation

Characteristic hives are pink or pale raised, well-circumscribed, edematous papules or plaques that change in size and shape (regression or peripheral extension) (Figure 16-13). Lesions may

TABLE 16-7	Identifiable Causes of Urticaria
CAUSE	**AGENT**
Infection	Bacterial (sinus, dental, pulmonary, urinary tract) Viral (preicteric phase of hepatitis B or C, mononucleosis, coxsackie) Fungal infections Protozoan and helminthic (intestinal worms, malaria)
IgE mediated	Medications (penicillin, sulfonamides, aspirin) Insects (stinging or biting) Latex Foods (children: milk, egg, peanuts, tree nuts, wheat, seafood; adults: seafood, tree nuts, peanuts) Food additives (benzoates, salicylates, sulfites) Contact allergens (chemicals, textiles, wood, saliva, cosmetics, perfumes, bacitracin)
Direct mast cell activation	Narcotics/opiates Muscle relaxants (succinylcholine, curare) Radiocontrast medium Stinging nettle plant
Physical stimuli	Pressure urticarias Exercise-induced anaphylactic syndrome
Internal disease	Serum sickness Systemic lupus erythematosus Rheumatoid arthritis Sjogren syndrome Autoimmune thyroid disease Hyperthyroidism Carcinomas, lymphomas Rheumatic fever Juvenile rheumatoid arthritis Polycythemia vera
Hormones	Pregnancy Premenstrual flare (progesterone)

Adapted from Habif, T. P. (2010). Clinical dermatology: A color guide to diagnosis and therapy (5th ed.). Philadelphia, PA: Mosby.

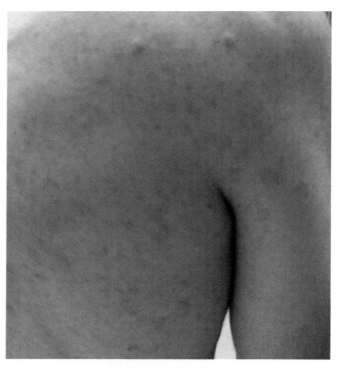

FIG. 16-13. Urticaria on a back and arm. Note the pale wheal and erythematous ring.

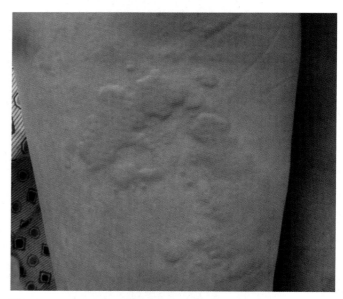

FIG. 16-14. Large urticarial plaques with dermal vasodilation and coalescing into polycyclic plaques.

range from a few millimeters to more than 5 cm in size and can coalesce and form annular or polycyclic plaques (Figure 16-14). Generally, there is a central edematous area (wheal) that will be pale compared to the surrounding erythema (flare) (Figures 16-15 and 16-16). Patients report pruritus and sometimes burning. Hives continually evolve and resolve but usually do not last more than 24 hours. Subcutaneous or submucosal edema (angioedema) may also be present.

Ordinary urticaria

There are two types of ordinary urticaria, acute and chronic. Hives erupt spontaneously and without specific stimulus, physical trigger, or evidence of vasculitis. The overall distribution of ordinary urticaria is usually haphazard, and the fluctuating wheals may be accompanied by angioedema.

Acute urticaria

All urticarias are initially acute. The term *episodic or recurrent* urticaria may be used for hives that occur less frequently over a long period of time since this presentation may have an environmental trigger that can be identified. Acute urticaria lasts up to 6 weeks and is usually an IgE-mediated, type I hypersensitivity reaction. It can be triggered by foods, drugs, inhalants, or insect bites; however, most cases are idiopathic. Food allergies are important in infantile urticaria, often to cow's milk; the frequency of acute urticaria resulting from foods is higher in children and decreases with age. Latex allergy is an IgE-mediated urticaria; yellow jackets are the most common cause of insect-induced urticaria and anaphylaxis in the United States. Acute urticaria is common in children and young adults,

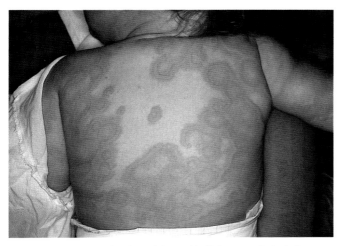

FIG. 16-15. Dramatic urticaria on infant with distinct morphologic features: wheal, flare, and central clearing of larger plaques.

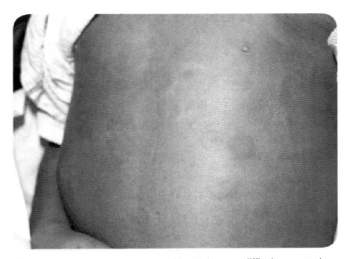

FIG. 16-16. Hives or urticaria on dark skin can be more difficult to appreciate.

compared to chronic urticaria accounting for about 1% of cases and mainly affects adults. It is usually managed by primary practitioners and is often seen in the emergency room setting.

Chronic urticaria

Lasting more than 6 weeks, chronic urticaria presents with signs and symptoms recurring at least 2 days out of the week-off treatment. Many cases are associated with autoimmune conditions, including Hashimoto disease, vitiligo, insulin dependent diabetes, rheumatoid arthritis, and pernicious anemia. The diagnosis, etiology, and management of chronic urticaria can be challenging and may be accompanied by physical urticaria. It is often a diagnosis of exclusion requiring a detailed history and physical examination. Patients are referred to a dermatology or allergy specialist if hives persist.

Physical urticarias

The physical urticarias are listed separately since their presence depends on an eliciting nonimmunologic external (exogenous) physical factor. They are classified by the predominant stimulus, and

provocative testing can usually confirm the diagnosis. The attacks are often brief, resolving within hours except for delayed pressure urticaria and delayed dermatographism; both of these may present after a delay of several hours and last for 72 hours or more. Angioedema can be seen with any of the physical urticarias except with symptomatic dermatographism.

Dermatographism. Simple dermatographism occurs in response to moderate stroking of the skin and is considered an exaggerated physiologic response. To test for dermatographism, draw a tongue blade across the arm or back of a patient and monitor for the wheal to present within several minutes (Figure 16-17). Symptomatic dermatographism will occur on sites of friction from clothing or gentle stroking of the skin, and pruritus may be present before the wheals. The general course is unpredictable, but the tendency to remain dermatographic may last for years. Symptomatic dermatographism may follow scabies infestation or penicillin allergy. There is no association with systemic disease, atopy, food allergy, or autoimmunity. Delayed dermatographism will appear 30 to 60 minutes after the stroking stimulus.

Delayed pressure urticaria. Lesions of delayed pressure urticaria are induced by standing, walking, manual use of hands, prolonged sitting, wearing tight garments, or sexual intercourse. Systemic features may include malaise, fatigue, fever, headache, or arthralgias. The mean duration for the condition is 6 to 9 years, and many patients have moderate-to-severe disease that is disabling. Pressure urticaria, chronic urticaria, and angioedema will often occur in the same patient.

Cholinergic urticaria. The attack starts with itching, burning, tingling, warmth, or irritation of the skin precipitated by overheating the body particularly with exercise. Concurrent systemic symptoms are rare but may include angioedema, hypotension, wheezing, and abdominal pain. Lesions are papules and pruritic wheals. An episode may last for an hour, and the condition may last for years (Figure 16-18).

Adrenergic urticaria. This is distinguishable from cholinergic urticaria by the presence of blanched vasoconstricted skin surrounding pink wheals that is provoked by sudden stress.

Exercise-induced anaphylaxis (EIA). EIA presents with pruritus, urticaria, respiratory distress, and hypotension after exercise. Attacks of food- and exercise-induced angioedema and anaphylaxis occur when the patient exercises within 30 minutes of ingesting the food (wheat, celery, shellfish, fruit, and fish). EIA is elicited by

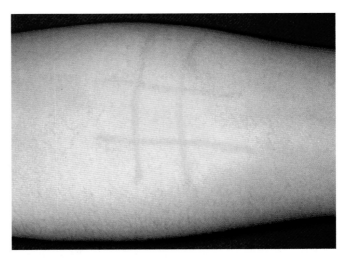

FIG. 16-17. Dermatographism or skin writing is an exaggerated response to pressure.

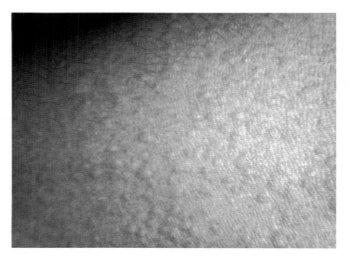

FIG. 16-18. Cholinergic urticaria.

exercise and not by an increase in core body temperature, differentiating EIA from cholinergic urticaria.

Cold urticaria. Cold urticaria syndromes are a group of conditions in which urticaria, angioedema, or anaphylaxis can occur within minutes of cold exposure, and can occur within minutes of rewarming. Primary acquired/essential cold urticaria most frequently occurs in young adults, and may follow a recent respiratory infection, arthropod bite or sting, drug therapy, or stress. Local whealing, burning, and itching occur within a few minutes of applying a solid or liquid cold stimulus to the skin. Wheals last for approximately an hour, and the condition may last for several years (Figure 16-19). Systemic symptoms of flushing, headache, syncope, and abdominal pain can develop if large skin areas are involved. Hives can occur with a sudden drop in air temperature or with exposure to cold water; swimming in cold water can cause a severe reaction with hypotension, shock, and possibly death. Secondary acquired cold urticaria is a rare presentation of cold urticaria associated with the presence of cryoglobulin, cryofibrinogen, or cold agglutinin.

Solar urticaria. It occurs within minutes of sun exposure on sun-exposed areas; the wheals of solar urticaria disappear in less than an hour. Severe reactions can include headache and syncope. Solar urticaria can be caused by natural or artificial UVR. Patients should be reminded that solar radiation can penetrate light clothing.

Aquagenic urticaria. It develops after contact with water of any temperature and the eruption will resemble a mild cholinergic urticaria.

Localized heat urticaria. This reaction is very rare; itching and whealing occur at the site of contact with heat within minutes of contact. Sources can include warm water, radiant heat, or warm sunlight.

Contact urticaria. Triggered by a biologic or chemical agent, contact urticaria is characterized by development of wheal and flare at the site of contact with skin or mucosa, or a generalized urticarial attack. Some patients only complain of localized itching, burning, or tingling; this should be contrasted with the eczematous reaction seen with allergic contact dermatitis, which is a cell-mediated immunity. The wheal and flare response will typically develop 30 to 60 minutes after exposure; there are immunologic and nonimmunologic forms. *Allergic contact urticaria* is associated with atopic disease, and these young patients become sensitized to environmental allergens like grass, animals, foods, and in some cases latex. The nonimmunologic type of contact urticaria is most common and most benign, does not require prior sensitization, is due to effects of urticants on blood vessels, and may take 30 to 50 minutes to appear. This includes exposure to histamine-releasing substances such as plants (nettles), animals (caterpillars, jellyfish), medications (dimethyl sulfoxide [DMSO]), bacitracin, cobalt chloride, cinnamic aldehyde, benzoic acid, and sorbic acid.

DIFFERENTIAL DIAGNOSIS   Urticaria

Acute
- Drug eruption
- Acute facial contact dermatitis
- Urticarial phase of bullous pemphigoid
- Dermatitis herpetiformis
- Insect bite reactions
- Other types of urticaria
- Erythema marginatum
- Erythema multiforme
- Urticaria pigmentosa

Chronic: includes all of the above, plus
- Systemic lupus eurythermous
- Sweet syndrome
- Fixed drug eruption

Urticaria must be differentiated from *urticarial vasculitis*, also known as hypocomplementemic urticarial vasculitis (HUV) or *anti-C1q vasculitis*, which is a rare immune complex SVV. Although most cases are idiopathic, it has been associated with connective tissue diseases, infections, medications, malignancies, and serum sickness. In addition to the urticarial plaques, systemic involvement often may include glomerulonephritis, pulmonary disease, arthritis, and ocular inflammation. Although similar in appearance, urticarial plaques of HUV, which may be painful, exist in the same location, persist for 1 to 7 days, and often leave a residual scaling and hyperpigmentation. Urticaria, on the other hand, is more pruritic, has migrating lesions that do not last for more than 24 hour, and does not leave any signs of the lesions. Histologically, HUV has a pattern similar to LCV.

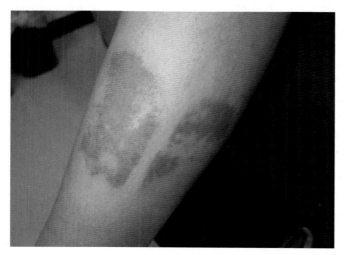

FIG. 16-19. Cold urticaria on a lower leg after the use of an ice pack.

Diagnostics

A detailed history is essential for the evaluation and diagnosis of urticaria and may identify the underlying etiology, saving the patient the pain and expense of an extensive diagnostic workup. In addition to the patient's medical history, a history as it relates to the urticaria should be the clinician's focus, especially in cases that do not respond to initial therapy or in chronic urticaria. Box 16-1 provides a list of important questions to ask. Particular attention should also be given to known causes of urticaria, which may be identified during the patient interview. The reported duration of the urticaria will immediately categorize the urticaria as acute or chronic.

Physical examination of the skin, noting the size, thickness, distribution, and duration of the lesions, can be crucial for a differential diagnoses. Localized distribution should indicate physical or contact urticaria; generalized distribution is more indicative of internal disease, ingestants, or inhalants. Most urticaria will be superficial plaques; however, papules might indicate insect bites or cholinergic urticaria; deep urticarial lesions indicate angioedema. Stroking the patient's arm with a dull object may illicit a red, raised hive-like plaque indicating dermatographism ("skin writing"), which may indicate a physical urticaria. Provocation tests, exposing the patient to the suspected causative stimulus, can be diagnostic of most physical urticarias. It is important to remember that for many patients the urticaria will be idiopathic.

A punch biopsy of the skin is indicated when urticarial lesions are painful or last for more than 24 hours, to rule out urticarial vasculitis. If the histologic features are consistent with leukocytoclastic vasculitis, further evaluation is necessary. Angioedema will show similar infiltrates to urticaria but has more edema in the interstitial tissues. Laboratory studies and imaging are not usually indicated but may be considered for suspicion of underlying etiologies (autoimmune disease, infections, and allergies). An initial screening would include a complete blood count with differential, ESR, TSH, T_3, T_4, and thyroid autoantibodies.

Management

Primary care providers are well placed to evaluate and treat acute spontaneous urticaria. Many patients will have a good idea of the cause for their acute urticaria and may not require intervention beyond removal or avoidance of the offending agent. Treatment of the underlying infection or disease by the primary care provider may result in complete resolution of the urticaria. Yet patients with chronic urticaria may be more challenging and should focus on possible triggers such as ingestants, inhalants, injectants (including stings and bites), infections, and internal diseases. Patients diagnosed with a physical urticaria will be managed according to the type or stimulus.

Whether or not the underlying cause of the urticaria has been identified, the goal of pharmacologic therapy for urticaria is to provide symptom relief (Figure 16-20). Control of pruritus is critical. Avoiding exacerbation of urticaria may include the use of cooling lotions (calamine, menthol, and/or pramoxine); tepid showers or baths with colloidal oatmeal; and avoidance of overheating or warm/humid environment. Patients should avoid aspirin, NSAIDs, opiates, alcohol, and any potential foods (and food additives) that may be suspected as an allergen.

Special Considerations

Pediatric. The most common cause of acute urticaria in children is infection, followed by drug hypersensitivity and food allergy. If the urticaria is chronic, autoimmune and thyroid diseases must also be considered. Physical urticarias are most often diagnosed in childhood, with dermatographic and cold urticaria being most common and potentially most severe. Pite, Wedi, Bornego, Kaap, & Raap (2013) reported that up to 50% of children with cold urticaria will have anaphylaxis due to cold exposure. Management is similar to that in adults (with appropriate dosage adjustments) except for the use of first-generation H_1 antihistamines. Systemic corticosteroids should be avoided whenever possible.

Geriatric. The most important consideration for the geriatric patient is the sedative effects of antihistamines, even the second-generation "nonsedating" ones.

Pregnancy. Treatment of urticaria in pregnancy can be problematic. Antihistamines should be avoided, especially in the first trimester. Chlorpheniramine is often recommended when necessary since it has a long safety record, although it is not approved for this indication. Additional information regarding pruritic urticarial papules and plaques of pregnancy (PUPPP) will be discussed later.

Prognosis and Complications

Most patients with chronic urticaria will benefit from treatment and at least 50% will clear within 1 year; however, patients with urticaria

---

| BOX 16-1 | **Questions to Elicit History of Urticaria** |

1. Time of onset
2. Time of appearance
3. Time of day
4. Time of year (seasonal may indicate inhalant allergy, constant may indicate internal disease)
5. Relation to menstrual cycle
6. Frequency of wheals
7. Duration of wheals (acute—days to a few weeks; chronic—more than 6 wk)
8. Duration of individual lesions
   <1 hour physical urticaria, typical hives
   <24 hours typical hives
   >25 hours urticarial vasculitis
9. Size, shape, and distribution of wheals
10. Environment, including home, work, vacation
11. Exposure to pollen, chemicals, travel
12. Associated angioedema
13. Symptoms of lesions: itch or pain
14. Constitutional symptoms of arthralgia, fever, gastrointestinal
15. Appearance with physical stimuli (physical urticarias, scratch, pressure, exercise, sun exposure, cold)
16. Prior allergy, infections, internal disease (juvenile rheumatoid arthritis, serum sickness, systemic lupus, urticarial vasculitis, viral hepatitis, chronic sinus infections)
17. Personal or family history of urticaria or atopy
18. Psychiatric or psychosomatic conditions
19. Surgical implants or events during surgery
20. Exercise induced
21. Drugs, injections, immunizations, hormones, laxatives, suppositories, eye or ear drops, supplements, and vitamins
22. Food or drink correlation
23. Smoking history
24. Hobbies
25. Stress
26. Quality of life and emotional impact
27. Previous therapy and response

Adapted from Zuberbier (2012).

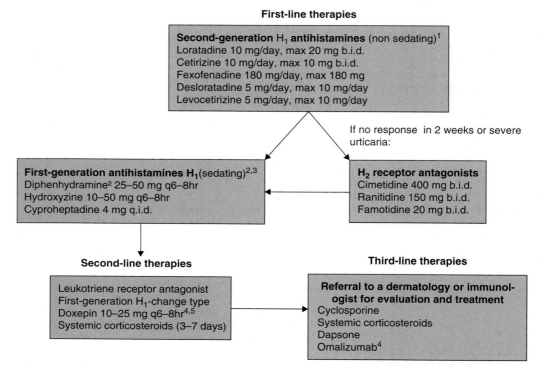

First-line therapies

Second-generation H$_1$ antihistamines (non sedating)[1]
Loratadine 10 mg/day, max 20 mg b.i.d.
Cetirizine 10 mg/day, max 10 mg b.i.d.
Fexofenadine 180 mg/day, max 180 mg
Desloratadine 5 mg/day, max 10 mg/day
Levocetirizine 5 mg/day, max 10 mg/day

If no response in 2 weeks or severe urticaria:

First-generation antihistamines H$_1$ (sedating)[2,3]
Diphenhydramine[2] 25–50 mg q6–8hr
Hydroxyzine 10–50 mg q6–8hr
Cyproheptadine 4 mg q.i.d.

H$_2$ receptor antagonists
Cimetidine 400 mg b.i.d.
Ranitidine 150 mg b.i.d.
Famotidine 20 mg b.i.d.

Second-line therapies

Leukotriene receptor antagonist
First-generation H$_1$-change type
Doxepin 10–25 mg q6–8hr[4,5]
Systemic corticosteroids (3–7 days)

Third-line therapies

Referral to a dermatology or immunologist for evaluation and treatment
Cyclosporine
Systemic corticosteroids
Dapsone
Omalizumab[4]

FIG. 16-20. Algorithm for pharmacologic treatment of urticaria. [1]Adjust doses for pediatric use. [2]Caution patient about sedative effects, given at bedtime. [3]More effective for patients with angioedema. [4]FDA off-label use for urticaria. [5]Use precautions with TCA drug class. Modified from Zuberbier T. (2012).

and angioedema are more likely to continue to have symptoms 20 years from the time of onset. Identifying and avoiding triggers can help prevent recurrence of symptoms. Often, even if the trigger source is not identified, there can be spontaneous remission. Rare complication of severe anaphylaxis or severe respiratory tract angioedema can develop, and these patients are seen and treated in urgent care or emergency departments. Emergency pharmacotherapy includes intramuscular (IM) epinephrine, IM diphenhydramine, and intravenous hydrocortisone or methylprednisolone.

Patient Education and Follow-up

In addition to patient education around treatment modalities and skin care, it may be important to help patients understand the unpredictable nature of chronic urticaria. It may last for months or years, and often a lengthy workup may be unrewarding. Urticaria can occur at any time, and may be worse at night, interfering with sleep, which will compound the distress for patients. Other quality-of-life issues include self-image, effect on sexual relationships, and other social and professional interactions. When there has been no specific cause identified for chronic hives, patients should be taught to avoid the following:

- Heat, hot showers, humidity
- Tight clothing, especially straps and waistline
- NSAIDs
- Aspirin
- Alcohol
- Spicy foods
- Stress
- Upper respiratory tract infections
- Poor sleep or lack of sleep

Patients need to be reassured that treatments, especially antihistamines, will decrease symptoms and discomfort, and in most cases, the urticaria will resolve spontaneously.

Patients should be counseled on the sedation, diplopia, blurred vision, urinary retention, dry mouth, vaginal dryness, and constipation that can occur with antihistamines. Education on the use of systemic corticosteroids should include the dangers of long-term use, and the clinical rebound that can occur with short-term use. Known allergens or triggers of urticaria should be avoided and recurrent infections addressed promptly. Patient education should include the signs and symptoms of dangerous reactions or anaphylaxis. If the patient experiences trouble breathing, tightness in their chest or throat, nausea, vomiting, fainting, and swelling of their eyes, mouth, or tongue, they should call local emergency services. Epi-pens prescribed for patients with severe reactions or anaphylaxis should also be accompanied with the instructions to proceed to the nearest emergency department as the effects of the epi-pen may be ineffective or only last a few minutes.

Referral and Consultation

Referral to dermatology specialists is recommended for evaluation and management of urticaria and angioedema that does not respond to first-line treatment or if symptoms of urticaria persist for more than 6 weeks in spite of treatment with antihistamines. If an allergy is suspected, referral to an allergist is indicated. Patients with chronic urticaria, especially if it is difficult to manage, or those who have had life-threatening symptoms should be referred to an allergist or urticaria specialist.

Patient Education and Follow-up

When possible, identifying and eliminating the eliciting factors of all forms of urticaria is important for control. Most cases of acute urticaria and angioedema are self-limited and will disappear within a few days. Individualized evaluation and treatment approach is necessary because of the large number of potential causes, as well as the high variability of symptoms and patient response. A suspected allergy to food or a medication should be adequately substantiated and documented. Many medication allergies are incorrectly blamed for an urticarial reaction, and this has significant implications for patients regarding their care in the future.

ANGIOEDEMA

Angioedema (angioneurotic edema) is a hive-like swelling in the subcutaneous tissue of skin, mucosa, and submucosal layers of the respiratory and GI tracts. The reaction is similar to that of hives in the upper dermis; hives and angioedema often occur simultaneously and may have the same etiology. Angioedema will occur with or without urticaria.

Clinical Presentation

Angioedema consists of thicker/deeper plaques that result from interstitial fluid in the dermis and subcutaneous tissues; the deeper reaction compared to hives produces more diffuse swelling. Angioedema can result from trauma, and like typical hives these large, thick, and firm plaques may form on any skin surface but typically involve the lips, eyes, larynx, and mucosa of the GI tract, palms, soles, limbs, trunk, and genitalia (Figures 16-21 and 16-22). Lesions of angioedema are typically skin colored, painful, larger, and longer lasting than wheals. Itching is usually absent; however, burning and painful swelling are common. Symptoms of gastrointestinal (abdominal pain, vomiting, diarrhea) involvement could indicate hereditary angioedema (HAE) or acquired angioedema (AAE). Angioedema without wheals can be recurrent and idiopathic; however, drug reaction needs to be excluded and C1 esterase inhibitor (C1 INH) deficiency should be investigated.

Angioedema with wheals

Idiopathic angioedema sometimes occurs with urticaria, can occur at any age, with an unpredictable pattern of recurrence. There may be GI and respiratory involvement but no asphyxiation danger. Allergic or IgE-mediated angioedema results from severe allergic type I immediate hypersensitivity reaction causing acute angioedema and urticaria that can occur with or without other symptoms of anaphylaxis. Common triggers include food, drugs, venom, latex, or environmental allergen. Medication- and chemical-induced angioedema is usually a nonimmunologic response. Common examples include contrast dye used in radiology

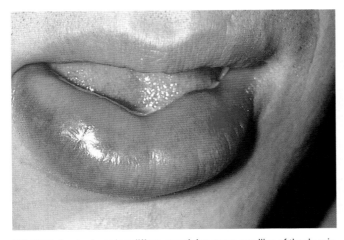

FIG. 16-21. Angioedema is a diffuse, nonpitting, tense swelling of the dermis, and subcutaneous tissue that can develop rapidly. Although usually allergic in nature and sometimes associated with hives, angioedema does not itch.

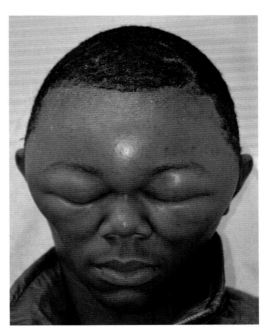

FIG. 16-22. Periorbital angioedema from contact allergy to a shampoo.

and NSAIDs. Angiotensin-converting enzyme (ACE) inhibitors are a frequent cause of acute angioedema and are potentially life-threatening. There is a higher incidence in black Americans and smokers, and a propensity for the face and tongue; the reaction can occur within hours, weeks, months, or years of taking the drug. Longer-acting ACE inhibitors may present with more severe symptoms than the short-acting form.

Angioedema without wheals

HAE is an inherited C1 INH deficiency, and patients present solely with angioedema. Most commonly affected areas include the face, tongue, throat, hands, arms, legs, abdomen, genitalia, or buttocks. HAE is characterized by an insufficient production of C1 INH or normal concentrations of a functionally deficient protein. Minor trauma, surgery, sudden emotional stress, and other unknown triggers can lead to release of vasoactive peptides that produce swelling of the airway and GI tract that can result in death. Any patient who experiences recurrent angioedema or abdominal pain in the absence of urticaria should be evaluated for HAE. Acquired angioedema is an autoimmune response resulting from the formation of inhibitory autoantibodies against C1 INH or associated with lymphoproliferative diseases and high-grade lymphomas. Clinical presentation of patients with AAE is similar to HAE.

DIFFERENTIAL DIAGNOSIS Angioedema
- See urticaria

Diagnostics

Same as for urticaria. History needs to include inquiry for C1 inhibitor deficiency. Testing should include a C4 level to determine the need for quantitative and functional levels of C1 INH and C1q levels.

Management

Angioedema is treated with antihistamines or corticosteroids with epinephrine for laryngeal edema, removal of the offending drug if indicated with supportive therapy of acute symptoms. Prophylactic therapy for angioedema is similar to that for urticaria with daily antihistamine, although angioedema may not respond as well as urticaria. Treatment of C1 inhibitor deficiency is guided by the severity of disease and individual needs, and managed by specialist in dermatology or immunology. Acute treatment for severe attacks may include infusion of C1 inhibitor concentrate, and attenuated androgens and/or tranexamic acid may be used for minor attacks or prophylaxis.

PRURITIC URTICARIAL PAPULES AND PLAQUES OF PREGNANCY

PUPPP, also called polymorphic eruption of pregnancy, is the most common dermatosis affecting pregnant women. It is seen most frequently in primigravidas, and usually begins in the late third trimester or very early in the postpartum period. The incidence is unknown but is estimated to occur in about 1 in 150 pregnancies. PUPPP may be associated with rapid and excessive weight gain, multiple gestation, labor induction, and hypertensive disorders.

The eruption usually begins within the striae on the abdomen, pink or red papules surrounded by a narrow pale halo that will coalesce to large urticaria-like plaques. The eruption may be broadly erythematous with discrete papules; papulovesicles may develop, but blisters are not seen. Distribution includes the abdomen, upper thighs, umbilicus, face, and palms, but the soles are generally spared (Figure 16-23). Unlike urticaria, the lesions are fixed. PUPPP generally spreads over a few days, with a mean duration of 6 weeks.

DIFFERENTIAL DIAGNOSIS	Pruritic urticarial papules and plaques of pregnancy

- Contact dermatitis
- Drug eruption
- Urticaria
- Viral exanthema
- Urticarial pemphigoid gestationis

Diagnostics

Diagnosis is generally made on clinical presentation; however, biopsy may be indicated if there is suspicion for pemphigoid gestationis.

Management

Treatment is supportive with cool baths or compresses for pruritus, Class V topical corticosteroids, antipruritic topical lotions with menthol, and antihistamines (usually diphenhydramine) as needed.

Prognosis and Complications

Most cases of PUPPP clear within 1 week of delivery. Lesions do not leave any residual scars or hyperpigmentation.

Referral and Consultation

Women with PUPPP are usually diagnosed and managed by their obstetrician.

ERYTHEMA MULTIFORME

EM is generally an acute, self-limited, inflammatory skin disease associated with infectious agents in approximately 90% of cases. EM is most commonly linked to a preceding herpes simplex virus (HSV) infection and less commonly to Epstein–Barr virus, bacteria (i.e., *Mycoplasma pneumoniae*), or dermatophyte infections. Drugs have also been implicated and include nonsteroidal anti-inflammatory drugs, sulfonamides, antiepileptics, and antibiotics.

For the purposes of this chapter, this author suggests that *EM major* is a disease with mucosal involvement and systemic symptoms, while *EM minor* does not have mucosal involvement. EM major is now considered a disorder distinct from Stevens–Johnson syndrome (SJS) with similar mucosal erosions but different lesion morphology and distribution. Table 16-8 outlines the EM and SJS/toxic epidermal necrosis (TEN) spectrum. SJS and TEN are discussed in chapter 17; this chapter will focus primarily on EM minor.

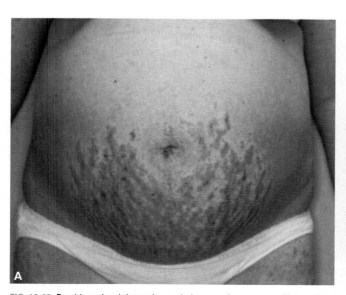
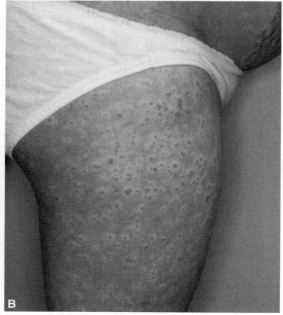

FIG. 16-23. Pruritic urticarial papules and plaques of pregnancy. Note urticaria within striae on the abdomen **(A)** and on the thighs **(B)**.

TABLE 16-8	Spectrum Comparison for Erythema Multiforme Minor, Erythema Multiforme Major, and Stevens–Johnson Syndrome		
	ERYTHEMA MULTIFORME MINOR	**ERYTHEMA MULTIFORME MAJOR**	**STEVENS–JOHNSON SYNDROME**
Morphology	Targetoid Atypical papular targetoid	Targetoid Atypical papular targetoid	Purpuric macules Atypical macular targetoid Bullous lesions
Distribution	Elbows, knees, wrists, hands, face	Extremities and face	Trunk and face
Mucosal involvement	None or mild	Severe	Severe
Precipitating factors	HSV, other infections	HSV, *Mycoplasma pneumoniae* Other infections Drugs (rare)	Drugs
Prognosis	Often recurrent Low morbidity	Increased morbidity	High morbidity

HSV, herpes simplex virus.

The overall incidence of EM is unknown, but there is a preponderance for young adults. Prodromal symptoms of malaise, fever, and myalgia are not common in EM minor, but occur in about half of the patients with EM major, especially if there is mucosal involvement. Recurrences are very likely to occur in individuals with a history of EM.

Pathophysiology

EM is a type IV hypersensitivity reaction in response to a stimulus, most often HSV. A cell-mediated immune reaction results in destruction of keratinocytes expressing HSV antigen, triggering an inflammatory cascade and causing cell death of HSV-infected keratinocytes and the recruitment of autoreactive T cells. This leads to the epidermal damage and the inflammatory infiltrate that creates classic EM lesions. EM associated with a drug is due to abnormal metabolism resulting in toxic metabolites binding to the surface of keratinocytes and triggering an immune reaction.

Clinical Presentation

The term *multiforme* implies the varied clinical manifestations that can be observed with EM. The primary and characteristic lesion of EM is a typical *target* or *iris* lesion (Figure 16-24). The typical target size is usually under 3 cm in diameter, round, erythematous, and edematous papule that spreads outward, and the center can become cyanotic, purpuric, or vesicular (Figure 16-25). Lesions will evolve during the course of the illness and may develop polycyclic and annular configurations. However, atypical papular target lesions are round, edematous, and palpable but may have only two zones and poorly demarcated edges (Figure 16-26). Partially formed targets with annular borders, or target lesions on the palms and soles, may resemble urticaria on clinical examination. A complete skin examination is essential since some patients will have target lesions that are not yet typical and only a few completely developed typical target lesions.

A classic eruption of EM begins symmetrically on extremities; particularly target lesions favoring the extensor surfaces of the upper extremities and dorsal hands (palms may be involved). Lesions then spread centripetally to the trunk, neck, and face. Early lesions may burn or be asymptomatic but generally not pruritic. Mucosal lesions are usually absent in EM minor and if present are mildly symptomatic and few in number. Severe mucosal involvement is characteristic for EM major, with erosions and hemorrhagic crusting on the lips, as well as ulcerations on the buccal mucosa and gingiva, conjunctiva, and genital mucosa.

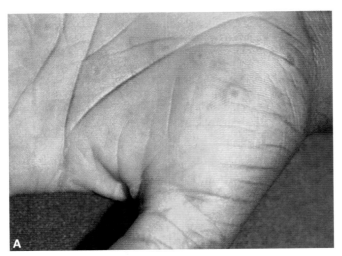
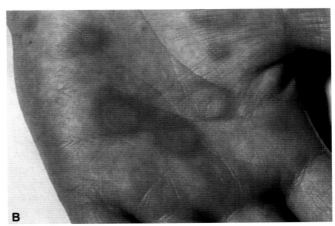

FIG. 16-24. **A,** Erythema multiforme minor with small target or iris lesions on the palm. **B,** Larger target papules with central bullae surrounding erythema appearing after antibiotic therapy.

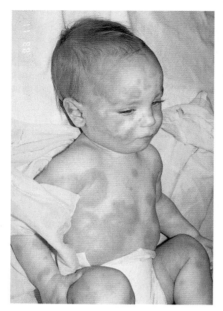

FIG. 16-25. Target lesions of EM characterized by a distinct red ring around central clearing (sometimes with a central bull's eye) that can coalesce into larger polycyclic plaques.

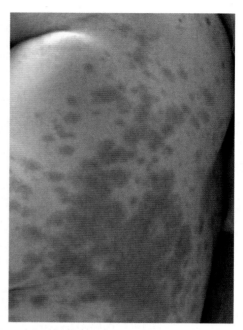

FIG. 16-26. Atypical EM secondary to hydroxychloroquine.

The onset of EM lesions is sudden and occurs over about 2 to 3 days. The initial papules and plaques that expand to form targetoid lesions with vesicles are typically monomorphic, fixed, and last at least 7 days. These can be differentiated from urticaria, which present as edematousplaques with normal skin in the central portion. Urticaria is a polymorphic eruption which migrates around the body, and lasts less than 24 hours.

DIFFERENTIAL DIAGNOSIS Erythema multiforme

- Stevens–Johnson syndrome
- Toxic epidermal necrosis
- Fixed drug eruption
- Subacute cutaneous lupus erythematosus
- Bullous pemphigoid
- Pityriasis rosea
- Polymorphous light eruption
- Urticaria, giant urticaria
- Viral exanthem
- Urticarial vasculitis

Diagnostics

The diagnosis of EM is usually based on clinical presentations with classic morphology of the primary lesion, distribution, presence of mucosal lesions, and signs or symptoms of systemic illness. History of the illness will further support the diagnosis since EM is commonly associated with a preceding upper respiratory tract infection, HSV, or *M. pneumoniae*. Atypical presentations or severe disease may necessitate a punch skin biopsy to rule out other skin diseases like vasculitis or lupus erythematosus. An additional punch biopsy should be performed for direct immunofluorescence if a blistering disease is suspected. More severe cases may have an elevated ESR and mild leukocytosis. Clinical criteria separate the EM spectrum

from the SJS/TEN spectrum. SJS/TEN is usually a severe drug-induced reaction characterized by widespread blisters/epidermal detachment and purpuric macules.

Management

The initial treatment of EM always includes the identification of the precipitating factor and appropriate treatment or discontinuation of the offending medication. The precipitating factor and treat appropriate infection or stop the offending medication. Further disease management will depend on the severity of the disease. In most cases of EM minor, symptomatic treatment is all that is necessary. Oral antihistamines may reduce swelling, burning, and pruritus of the skin. If needed, soothing mouthwashes (e.g., warm saline rinse, or solution of equal parts diphenhydramine, viscous xylocaine, and aluminum/magnesium antacid) may be used. Consider class II TCS for localized skin relief.

Patients with EM major or severe symptoms can be treated with a short course of oral corticosteroid (prednisone 40–80 mg/day) until cleared, then followed by a 1-week taper. In patients with more than five attacks a year of herpes-associated EM, oral acyclovir 400 mg prescribed twice daily has been used for suppressive therapy. Antiviral suppressive therapy can also be used for idiopathic recurrent EM. Valacyclovir and famciclovir are better absorbed and may be used if there is no response to acyclovir. In recalcitrant cases, dapsone, azathioprine, and cyclosporine may be considered. Suppressive antiviral therapy can prevent HSV-associated EM, but antiviral therapy started after the EM outbreak has no effect on the course of that outbreak.

Special Considerations

EM is uncommon in children. When it occurs, it can mimic polymorphous light eruption.

Prognosis and Complications

EM is generally self-limited and uncomplicated, usually resolving in about 1 month without major sequelae. Individual lesions may leave postinflammatory hyper- or hypopigmentation. In general, recurrences are common, especially in HSV-associated disease. EM major may require hospitalization, and patients with mucosal involvement need specialized care to avoid complications such as infection and sepsis; eye complications, including purulent conjunctivitis with scarring, anterior uveitis, or corneal scarring; pneumoniae; dehydration; gastrointestinal hemorrhage; renal failure.

Referral and Consultation

Referral to a dermatology specialist is recommended unless the case of EM is mild with no mucosal involvement, and a correlation with HSV is clear. Infectious disease specialists may be recommended for intercurrent infections and treatment recommendations. Referral to an ophthalmologist is recommended for topical ophthalmic therapy recommendations.

Patient Education and Follow-up

Patients should be educated about appropriate symptomatic treatment, and reassurance that EM minor is self-limited. It is also important for patients to be made aware of the risk of recurrent EM, and reminded to avoid any specific etiologic agent.

Follow-up will depend on individual response to treatment. A patient with recurrent HSV and EM will be followed up long term by a dermatology specialist.

ERYTHEMA NODOSUM

Panniculitis is the term used for a group of inflammatory disorders primarily located in the subcutaneous fat. Clinically, lesions of all panniculitides present as subcutaneous nodules. EN is the most common of these panniculitides. EN is a hypersensitivity reaction to a variety of antigenic stimuli, several diseases, and/or certain drug therapy. Pregnancy and oral contraceptive use can also cause EN. Approximately 55% of cases of EN are idiopathic. It is more frequently observed between second and fourth decades of life, and the female to male ratio is approximately 5:1 (Habif, 2010). Choice of biopsy is crucial for pathologic evaluation and must include a generous portion of subcutaneous fat.

Pathophysiology

EN is generally considered a delayed hypersensitivity response to a wide variety of disorders; the most common causes are listed in Table 16-9. More rare causes include rheumatologic diseases, autoimmune disorders, and malignancies. There are a variety of adhesion molecules and inflammatory mediators associated with the disease.

Subcutaneous fat is homogenous tissue that responds to insult in a limited number of ways, and thus histologically, there is an overlap of different forms of panniculitis. EN is considered the prototypic septal panniculitis; the biopsy specimens show inflammatory infiltrate involving the connective tissue septa between fat lobules. Neutrophils, lymphocytes, and/or other mononuclear cells will be present depending on the stage of the lesion. Histiocytes and multinucleate giant cells may predominate older lesions. Leukocytoclastic vasculitis is not a histologic feature of EN; however, a "secondary" vasculitis may be present in lesions with heavy mixed or neutrophil-rich inflammatory infiltrate (Patterson, 2008).

Clinical Presentation

The onset of EN is usually acute and often associated with malaise, leg edema, arthritis or arthralgia, and fever; these systemic symptoms do not necessarily relate to an underlying systemic disorder. Initially,

TABLE 16-9	Causes of Erythema Nodosum
Common causes	Idiopathic: ⅓ to ½ of cases
	Streptococcal infection, especially upper respiratory tract
	Other infections: bacterial gastroenteritis (*Yersinia, Salmonella,* or *Shigella*); viral upper respiratory tract infection; coccidioidomycosis.
	Drugs: estrogens and oral contraceptive pills; sulfonamides, penicillin, bromides
	Sarcoidosis
	Inflammatory bowel disease: Crohn disease with a stronger association with ulcerative colitis
Uncommon causes	Infectious: Brucellosis; *Chlamydia pneumoniae* or *trachomatis, Mycoplasma pneumoniae*; tuberculosis; hepatitis B; histoplasmosis
	Neutrophilic dermatoses (Behcet and Sweet syndromes)
	Pregnancy

Adapted from Patterson, J. W. (2008). Panniculitis. In J. L. Bolognia, J. L. Jorizzo, & R. P. Rapini (Eds.), Dermatology (2nd ed., pp. 1511–1535). Spain: Mosby Elsevier.

EN may appear like tests bruising to the patient (Figure 16-27). Then, painful, erythematous, shiny, and tender nodules present on the bilateral pretibial regions and lateral shins (Figure 16-28). Although there can be solitary nodules, EN usually typically presents as multiple lesions that range in size from 1 to 10 cm in diameter that arise in crops. Forearms and thighs may be involved; however, nodules on the trunk, neck, and face should prompt consideration of other

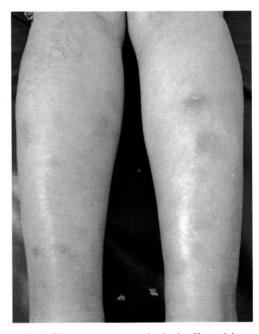

FIG. 16-27. Initially, EN can present as tender, bruise-like nodules on the legs.

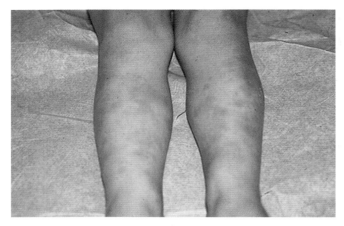

FIG. 16-28. Bilateral and tender nodules of EN on the pretibial aspects of lower legs.

diagnoses. Ulceration is not a feature of EN; however, it may be seen in other forms of panniculitis.

EN nodules change over days or weeks and become more fluctuant and change color from red to more yellow and bruise-like. They will generally disappear after 2 weeks with desquamation of the overlying skin, but new lesions continue to erupt for 3 to 6 weeks. Ankle swelling and leg aching may persist for weeks, and the condition may recur for months or years.

DIFFERENTIAL DIAGNOSIS Erythema nodosum
• Erythema induratum
• Nodular vasculitis
• Cellulitis
• Superficial and deep thrombophlebitis
• Erysipelas

Diagnostics

Other forms of panniculitis must be considered in the differential diagnosis and physical assessment of EN, although an acute eruption of tender subcutaneous nodules over both shins in a young person is highly suggestive of EN. When lesions are located in areas other than the lower legs, few in number, or of longer duration (>6 weeks), it may be difficult to differentiate EN from other forms of panniculitis. Atypical lesions or distribution, or chronic lesions should suggest an alternative diagnosis such as erythema induratum or pancreatic panniculitis.

In most cases, the clinical picture of EN is characteristic and biopsy is not needed. However, if the presentation is atypical or the case does not evolve typically, it is critical that an incisional biopsy be performed. The biopsy technique ensures that the specimen includes a generous sample of subcutaneous fat. Inadequate sampling can lead to misinterpretation and misdiagnosis. An evaluation for an infectious cause should include throat culture and ASO titer, ESR, and CBC. A chest x-ray will provide initial screening for evidence of pulmonary sarcoidosis; hilar adenopathy may indicate coccidioidomycosis, histoplasmosis, tuberculosis, or lymphoma.

Patients with gastrointestinal symptoms should have stool culture for *Yersinia enterocolitica*, *Salmonella*, and *Campylobacter pylori*. Test for infectious agents prevalent in local area are based on travel and exposure history.

Management

The initial treatment of EN includes rest and elevation of the affected extremities, salicylates, and nonsteroidal anti-inflammatory drugs. Gentle support hose and limiting physical activities can also be helpful and may prevent exacerbations and recurrences. Identifying the underlying trigger is of primary importance, although treating an infectious cause may not necessarily shorten the course of EN.

Saturated solution of potassium iodide (SSKI) has been used with response within 2 weeks. The adult dose dose ranges from 300 to 1,500 mg per day, starting 150 to 300 mg three times daily. Dosing should be adjusted for younger children, 150 mg three times daily. Side effects include nausea, bitter taste, urticaria, and headache. Long-term use can lead to hypo- or hyperthyroidism; SSKI should be avoided in pregnancy. Oral corticosteroids are effective but should not be needed for limited disease.

Prognosis and Complications

Uncomplicated EN is usually self-limited. The prognosis for acute EN is generally good, with resolution of symptoms in 2 to 6 weeks. If the underlying condition or infection persists, or if physical activity has been resumed too quickly, there may be recurrence.

Referral and Consultation

EN that is prolonged, unusually painful, or recurrent will require referral to a dermatology specialist for confirmation of diagnosis with appropriate biopsy technique and more aggressive treatment.

Patient Education and Follow-up

The most important recommendation for patients is rest and limitation of physical activity, especially during the acute phase of EN, to hasten recovery and prevent exacerbation.

BILLING CODES ICD-10	
Angioedema, hereditary	D84.1
Angioedema with hives	T78.3
Dermatographism	L50.3
Erythema multiforme	L51
Erythema nodosum	L52
Henoch–Schönlein purpura	D69.0
Kawasaki disease	M30.3
Pruritic urticarial papules and plaques of pregnancy	026.86
Progressive pigmentary purpura	L81.7
Urticaria, acute	L50
Urticaria, cold	L50.2
Urticaria, cholinergic	L50.9
Urticaria, chronic	L50.8
Urticaria, idiopathic	L50.1
Urticaria, solar	L50.9
Vasculitis	L95.0
Vasculitis, skin only	177.6

READINGS

Aurelian, L., Ono, F., & Burnett, J. (2003). Herpes simplex virus (HSV)-associated erythema multiforme (HAEM): A viral disease with an autoimmune component. *Dermatology Online Journal*, *9*(1), 1.

Chung, L., Kea, B., & Fiorentino, D. F. (2008). Cutaneous vasculitis. In J. L. Bolognia, J. L. Jorizzo, & R. P. Rapini (Eds.), *Dermatology* (2nd ed., pp. 347–367). Spain: Mosby Elsevier.

Fiorentino, D. F. (2003). Cutaneous vasculitis. *Journal of the American Academy of Dermatology, 48*(3), 311–340.

French, L. E., & Prius, C. (2008). Erythema multiforme, Stevens-Johnson syndrome, and toxic epidermal necrolysis. In J. L. Bolognia, J. L. Jorizzo, & R. P. Rapini (Eds.), *Dermatology* (2nd ed., pp. 287–291). Spain: Mosby Elsevier.

Fritsch, P. O., & Ruiz-Maldonado, R. (2003). Erythema multiforme, Stevens-Johnson syndrome, and toxic epidermal necrolysis. In I. M. Freedman, A. Z. Eisen, K. Wolff, L. A. Goldsmith, & S. I. Katz (Eds.), *Fitzpatrick's dermatology in general medicine* (6th ed., pp. 543–557). New York, NY: McGraw Hill.

Grattan, C. E. H., & Black, A. K. (2008). Urticaria and angioedema. In J. L. Bolognia, J. L. Jorizzo, & R. P. Rapini (Eds.), *Dermatology* (2nd ed., pp. 261–276). Spain: Mosby Elsevier.

Grattan, C. E. H., Sabroe, R. A., & Greaves, M. W. (2002). Chronic urticaria. *Journal of the Academy of Dermatology, 46*(5), 645–647.

Habif, T. P. (2010). *Clinical dermatology: A color guide to diagnosis and therapy* (5th ed.). Philadelphia, PA: Mosby.

Habif, T. P., Campbell, J. L., Chapman, M. S., Dinulos, J. G., Sug, K. A. (2011). *Skin disease: Diagnosis & treatment* (3rd ed.). Philadelphia, PA: Elsevier Saunders.

Jennette, J. C., Falk, R. J., Bacon, P. A., Basu, N., Cid, M. C., Ferrario, F. . . . Watts, R. A. (2013). 2012 Revised International Chapel Hill Consensus Conference Nomenclature of Vasculitides. *Arthritis & Rheumatism, 65*(1), 1–11.

Lotti, T., Ghersetick, I., Comacci, G., & Jorizzo, J. (1998). Cutaneous small vessel vasculitis. *Journal of the Academy of Dermatology, 39*(5), 667–687.

Newberger, J. W., Takahashi, M., Gerber, M. A., Gewitz, M. H., Tani, L. Y., Burns, J. C.,. . . American Academy of Pediatrics. (2004). Diagnosis, treatment, and long-term management of Kawasaki Disease: A Statement for Health Professionals from the Committee on Rheumatic Fever, Endocarditis and Kawasaki Disease, Council on Cardiovascular Disease in the Young, American Heart Association. *Circulation, 110*, 2747–2771.

Patterson, J. W. (2008). Panniculitis. In J. L. Bolognia, J. L. Jorizzo, & R. P. Rapini (Eds.), *Dermatology* (2nd ed., pp. 1511–1535). Spain: Mosby Elsevier.

Pite, H., Wedi, B., Bornego, L. M., Kapp, A., & Raap, U. (2013). Management of childhood urticaria: Current knowledge and practical recommendations. *Acta Dermato-Vereneologica, 93*. http://www.medicaljournals.se/acta/content/?doi=10.2340/00015555-1573&html=1

Scharma, P., Sharma, S., Baltaro, R., & Hurley, J. (2011). Systemic vasculitis. *American Family Physicians, 83*(5), 556–565.

Sokumbi, O., & Wetter, D.A. (2012). Clinical features, diagnosis, and treatment of erythema multiforme: A review for the practicing dermatologist. *International Journal of Dermatology, 51*, 889–902.

Waller, J. M., Feramisco, J. D., Alberta-Wzolek, L., McCalmont, T. H., & Fox, L. P. (2010). Cocaine-associated retiform purpura and neutropenia: is levamisole the culprit? *Journal of the American Academy of Dermatology, 63*, 530–535.

Zuberbier, T. (2012). A summary of the New International EAACI/GA²LEN/EDF/WAO Guidelines in urticaria. *World Allergy Organization Journal, 5*, S1–S5.

Zuberbier, T., Asero, R., Bindslev-Jensen, C., Walter, C. G., Church, M. K., Giménez-Arnau, A. M.,. . . World Allery Organization. (2009). EAACI/GA²LEN/EDF/WAO guideline: Management of urticaria. *Allergy, 64*, 1427–1443. doi:10.1111/j.1398-9995.2009.02178.x

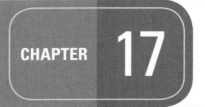

CHAPTER 17

Cutaneous Drug Eruptions

Glen Blair, Victoria Griffin, Margaret A. Bobonich, and Mary E. Nolen

Medications are commonly prescribed by health care providers as part of the management of patient illness and wellness. Many individuals, especially the elderly, have multiple chronic diseases accompanied by a long list of drugs prescribed by various clinicians. Adverse drug reactions (ADRs) are common and can range from a mild exanthematous eruption to a potentially life-threatening condition. Nearly 100,000 deaths are attributed to ADRs each year in the United States. Cutaneous manifestations are frequently associated with an ADR and can provide clinical clues for early diagnosis and prompt management. Hence, clinicians must be mindful to consider the possibility of an ADR or side effect in patients presenting with skin eruptions.

This chapter will review the most common and important cutaneous eruptions associated with drug use and guide clinicians in the evaluation and treatment of these conditions. Urticarial drug eruptions and angioedema are discussed in chapter 16.

ADVERSE DRUG REACTIONS

An ADR is an unintended and toxic response to a drug given for the purposes of prevention, diagnosis, or therapeutics (WHO, 2008). The reaction cannot be explained by another disease state or drugs and does not include drug abuse, overdose, withdrawal, or errors in administration. A *serious* ADR is considered one that results in death, disability, birth defect, or requires medical or surgical intervention (FDA, 2014). In contrast, *side effects* (SEs) are predictable and less toxic adverse effects that occur more frequently. SEs are usually dose related.

Risk Factors

Multiple factors place an individual at increased risk for developing an ADR including the drug itself. Clinicians should maintain a heightened awareness when their patients are receiving medications that are known to be high risk for ADR. Overall, aminopenicillins, sulfonamides, and nonsteroidal anti-inflammatory drugs (NSAIDs) account for the largest number of drug-related cutaneous eruptions. Other risk factors include the following:

- *Host.* The elderly are at greater risk for ADRs that may be attributed to polypharmacy and changes in drug metabolism and/or excretion with aging. Children are also at higher risk due to their smaller body size. Females are affected more than males, and individuals with a history of an ADR have an increased risk of developing one to another medication.
- *Immune status.* Patients who are immunosuppressed, have HIV, or have malignancies such as lymphoma have an increased risk for ADRs, the degree of which may correlate with the severity of their disease state.
- *Genetics.* There is an association with HLA types present in identified races that predispose them to an ADR induced by a specific drug like phenytoin, carbamazepine, allopurinol,

sulfamethoxazole, and abacavir. Patients with a history of an ADR may have family members who may not be able to metabolize that drug or tolerate its metabolite.
- *Medications.* The drug itself may have factors that increase the risk for an ADR, including the class of drug, dose, route of administration, and drug–drug interactions.
- *Infection.* Patients are at greater risk of developing a hypersensitivity reaction during viral illnesses. The most well-known example is an ampicillin-induced rash in patients with Epstein–Barr virus (EBV) or a trimethoprim-sulfamethoxazole-induced rash in patients with HIV. Drugs can also trigger latent viral infections.

Pathophysiology

ADRs are classified as immunologic, nonimmunologic, or idiosyncratic. It is helpful to recognize the type so that appropriate treatment may be initiated and future reactions avoided.

Immune-mediated reactions

Most ADRs are an immunologic response to a drug and considered a hypersensitivity reaction (see chapter 16). Cutaneous ADRs can be classified as type I to IV reaction patterns:

- *Type I* (immediate): IgE mediated, occurs within minutes of ingesting medication. ADRs include urticaria, angioedema, and anaphylaxis.
- *Type II*: IgG mediated and cytotoxic. Examples would include drug-induced hemolytic anemia or pemphigus.
- *Type III*: antigen–antibody complexes deposited in skin and vessels. The onset is minutes to days after ingestion. ADRs include serum sickness, urticarial vasculitis.
- *Type IV* (delayed): sensitized T cells with four subtypes. This is the most common type of ADR and typically occurs 1 to 3 weeks after initiation of the suspected culprit drug. Type IV hypersensitivity ADRs include Stevens–Johnson syndrome/toxic epidermal necrolysis (SJS/TEN), drug reaction with eosinophilia and systemic symptoms (DRESS), contact dermatitis, and acute generalized exanthematous pustulosis (AGEP).

Nonimmunologic reactions

High drug doses or overdosage, as well as undesirable drug SEs (i.e., chemotherapy), can illicit non-immune-mediated cutaneous reactions. Extended therapy on a medication may result in cumulative toxicity to the drug or its metabolites which may be an immediate (i.e., amiodarone) or delayed (i.e., arsenic) reaction. Drug–drug interactions can also occur via numerous mechanisms including the displacement of medication from binding proteins or receptor sites (i.e., tetracycline and calcium). As mentioned, drugs can alter the metabolism of other drugs or metabolic changes within the body. And lastly, drugs can exacerbate a disease or trigger a latent disease process (i.e., lithium and psoriasis).

Idiosyncratic reactions

When an ADR cannot be attributed as an immunologic or nonimmunologic reaction, it is considered idiosyncratic.

History

The diagnosis of a cutaneous ADR is based on clinical suspicion, presentation, chronology, and probability. The most important factor in the diagnosis of an ADR is the history and timing of the intake of the suspected drug. A *detailed* history of all prescription, nonprescription, and recreational drugs taken by the patient must be collected; however, it can be a lengthy process especially in the elderly where polypharmacy is common. It can be helpful to inquire about all routes of administration when accounting for their medications (Box 17-1). The chronology is critical to identifying the causative agent of an ADR, including date of initiation, dosage, and first sign of the reaction. And a family history of ADRs should be noted, given the genetic associations that have been observed.

Clinical Presentation

Physical examination findings often mimic other skin disorders and may occur days or even years after beginning drug therapy, making the diagnosis challenging. An important variable that impacts the quality of the physical assessment is a complete body examination. Often, patients perceived their "rash" to be independent of any other symptoms or lesions occurring on other parts of their body (see chapter 1).

A detailed physical examination should be performed carefully, making note of the primary morphology and distribution of the cutaneous symptoms. Close examination of the oral cavity and other mucous membranes is extremely important. Vital signs should be taken to assess for fever, hypotension, tachycardia, and other systemic symptoms signaling a possible life-threatening ADR.

Diagnosis of a cutaneous ADR eruption is based on clinical suspicion, chronology, and probability. Clinicians should always consider drug eruption in the differential diagnosis in patients presenting with pruritic, symmetrical, and generalized skin rashes. There are several valuable resources and online databases available, such as *Litt's Drug Eruption Manual* (2009), which can enable clinicians to view specific drug information, reaction, and incidence. It also provides content regarding the most common drug eruptions and patterns that can aid in predicting, diagnosing, and managing the patients with suspected ADRs.

Diagnostics

Most ADRs are diagnosed based on history and physical findings and do not require any diagnostics. In severe or persistent cases, further testing may be necessary. Skin biopsy may be indicated to

---

| BOX 17-1 | **The Seven "I"s for History of Patient Medications** |

Instill (eye, ear drops, contact lens solution)
Ingest (capsules, tabs, gels, liquids)
Inhale (cortico steroids)
Inject (IM, IV, SC)
Insert (suppositories)
In secret (sharing among elders or teens)
Intermittent (not taken every day)

| BOX 17-2 | **Approach to Identifying Cause of Adverse Drug Reaction** |

1. Identify the morphology, distribution, and location for a clinical pattern
2. Assess for signs and symptoms of systemic organ involvement
3. Determine any/all medications that have been ingested
4. Establish an accurate chronology of medication intake; create a timeline
5. Inquire about a personal and family history of prior ADRs
6. Determine the probability of ADR
7. Consider a nondrug etiology
8. Discontinue the suspected offending drug
9. Consider additional labs or biopsy, if indicated
10. Educate the patient that the ADR will not resolve immediately
11. Ensure the patient understands importance of documenting the allergy
12. Consider rechallenge at a later date, if appropriate

---

support the clinician's suspicion and to rule out other disease processes. Histologic findings typically show spongiosis with perivascular infiltrates of lymphocytes and eosinophils, and require clinicopathologic correlation. Patients and clinicians must understand that even if histology supports the diagnosis of an ADR, it cannot identify the offending agent. This is a patient expectation that should be discussed and managed before a biopsy is performed. Immunofluorescence is performed when a connective tissue disease or autoimmune blistering disease is suspected.

Other diagnostics including laboratory studies are indicated in patients with systemic symptoms. In addition to a complete blood count with differential and chemistry panel, antinuclear antibodies (ANA) screening can be helpful. Antihistone antibodies may support a diagnosis of drug-induced lupus. Blood cultures, urinalysis, and stool guaiac will help to rule out infection and vasculitis. Provocation testing is only considered in specific circumstances and is generally performed in carefully controlled settings.

Management

Management of an ADR is relative to the specific drug and reaction type which will be discussed in this chapter. However, the first and universal approach to all ADRs is discontinuation of the offending drug (Box 17-2).

Patient Education and Follow-up

Regardless of the type of drug eruption, any patient diagnosed with an ADR must be educated about lifelong avoidance of the offending drug, medications in the same drug class, or other classes that may have potential cross-reactivity. Good communication between the patient and health care team should ensure that all personal health records and medic-alert identifiers reflect the patient's history of serious ADRs. Most importantly, patients with an ADR should be instructed to notify their health care provider should the rash recur or worsen, indicating a severe hypersensitivity reaction. Clinicians should be alerted if the patient develops fever, redness that starts to expand over the body, blisters, ulcerations, or sores on any mucous membrane, or the patient experiences a new onset of pain. In the event that the provider is unavailable, the patient should be referred to the emergency department (Box 17-3).

CUTANEOUS DRUG REACTION PATTERNS

ADRs are often described by the pattern of symptoms, morphology, distribution, and/or underlying etiology. The spectrum of clinical presentations can be categorized into one of the following patterns: exanthematous, fixed drug, bullous, neutrophilic, acneiform, drug-induced lupus, photosensitivity, and pigmentary eruptions. The reaction pattern can aid in the diagnosis as many drugs are known for specific reaction patterns.

BOX 17-3	Red-Flag Symptoms for Systemic Involvement in Adverse Drug Reaction

Fever
Purpura
Erosions/blisters of mucosal membranes
Angioedema
Erythroderma
Blisters (especially positive Nikolsky sign) or necrosis
Facial edema
Lymphadenopathy
Chest pain or dyspnea
Meningism
Arthralgia

EXANTHEMATOUS DRUG REACTIONS

Exanthematous drug eruptions account for about 95% of all drug reactions. As the name implies, exanthematous eruptions are maculopapular or morbilliform (measle-like in appearance) and are often difficult to distinguish from viral exanthems such as EBV, enterovirus, adenovirus, acute HIV, HHV-6, parvovirus (Box 17-4).

Pathophysiology

The exact mechanism of these reactions is unknown, but it is believed to represent a type IV hypersensitivity reaction characterized by a T-cell-mediated response, causing direct cellular damage.

BOX 17-4	Drugs Frequently Implicated in Exanthematous Drug Reactions

Allopurinol	Isoniazid
Amoxicillin	Lithium
Ampicillin	Naproxen
Cephalosporins	Penicillin
Barbiturates	Phenothiazines
Captopril	Phenylbutazone
Enalapril	Phenytoin
Carbamazepine	Piroxicam
Chlorpromazine	Quinidine
Diflunisal	Sulfonamides
Gentamycin	Thiazides
Gold salts	Thiouracil
Glipizide	TMP/SMX
Glyburide	

Adapted from Habif, *Clinical Dermatology (2010).*

Clinical Presentation

The onset of exanthematous ADRs usually occurs within hours to weeks after initiation of the drug. They generally develop as bright red, pruritic macules and papules that symmetrically appear on the trunk but may coalesce and spread to the extremities (Figure 17-1A). In adults, it usually spares the face, whereas in children, it may be limited to the face and extremities. Confluent lesions may develop bilaterally (Figure 17-1B) and in the intertriginous areas. Palms, soles, and mucous membranes can be involved. The associated pruritus often disturbs sleep. A low-grade fever and/or chills may be present compared to the high-grade fever associated with a hypersensitivity syndrome reaction. The onset of exanthematous eruptions usually occurs within hours to weeks after initiation of the drug.

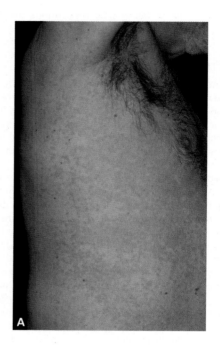

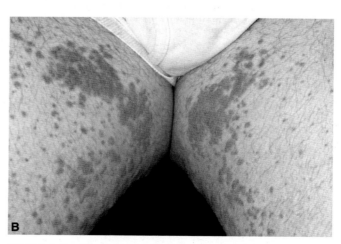

FIG. 17-1. **A:** Exanthematous eruption. **B:** Exanthematous eruption coalescing plaques.

Diagnostics

An exanthematous drug eruption is usually a clinical diagnosis that correlates with a history of drug administration. In most cases, it is not necessary to perform a skin biopsy except when the diagnosis is in question or to rule out other causes. Histopathology typically shows eosinophilia, perivascular lymphocytes, and vacuolar if the patient interface dermatitis. If the patient's morbilliform rash progresses or if the patient develops fever, chills, lymphadenopathy, or angioedema, additional diagnostics would be indicated for evaluation of systemic involvement.

Management

In addition to discontinuing the suspected drug, symptomatic treatment is all that is needed for a mild or moderate exanthematous drug eruption. Antihistamines, both H_1 and H_2 blockers, may be used to reduce pruritus. Mid-potency topical corticosteroids may be used during the acute phase, if necessary. Since this eruption is often widespread, triamcinolone 0.1% cream or ointment, prescribed in a large quantity (1-lb jar), is usually sufficient but should be avoided on the face, skin folds, and genital areas (see chapter 2). Application of cool compresses, fragrance-free moisturizing creams, and anti-itch lotions can be helpful in controlling discomfort. In a rare instance that the offending drug cannot be discontinued or the patient has a severe eruption, a short course of oral prednisone may be prescribed at a dose of 1.0 to 2.0 mg/kg/day for 7 to 10 days to provide symptomatic relief and induce rapid remission.

Prognosis and Complications

An exanthematous drug rash lasts for 1 to 2 weeks and then fades. Resolving lesions have hues of tan and purple, scaling, or desquamation. Clinicians should use great caution when patients with a morbilliform rash progress to develop fever, mucositis, erythroderma, facial edema, or blisters. They should be seen and evaluated immediately.

FIXED DRUG ERUPTION

A fixed drug eruption (FDE) is a localized adverse skin reaction to an ingested drug. The hallmark of FDE is the appearance of the same type of lesion(s) on the same location of the body with subsequent exposure. The specific location may be a clue as to the drug. Tetracyclines, for example, often produce lesions on the glans penis. Other drugs that are known to cause FDEs include NSAIDs, sulfonamides, barbiturates, allopurinol, propranolol, and laxatives.

Pathophysiology

FDE is a cell-mediated process involving $CD8^+$ T cells. These T cells are increased in the lesions of FDE and apparently play a dual role in the skin. Normally, these intraepidermal T cells have a protective function. However, when there is overactivation by an antigen as in FDE, they may actually be responsible for tissue injury.

Clinical Presentation

FDE takes a few days to appear after initiation of the culprit drug. Yet if the patient has been previously sensitized to the drug, lesions could develop within minutes of taking a single dose. A classic feature of FDE is the reappearance of lesions with subsequent exposures to the drug. Lesions usually recur in the same localized areas as the initial eruptions. New lesions can develop in new areas as well. FDE can occur anywhere on the body but favors the dorsal hands, glans penis and groin area, periorbital, perioral, and occasionally the oral mucosa (Figure 17-2A). In males presenting with penile lesions, FDE should always be at the top of the differential diagnosis (Figure 17-2B).

FDE has a distinct appearance as sharply demarcated, round/oval, dusky-red patches or plaques that may be solitary or multiple. Plaques sometimes become edematous and form central vesicle/

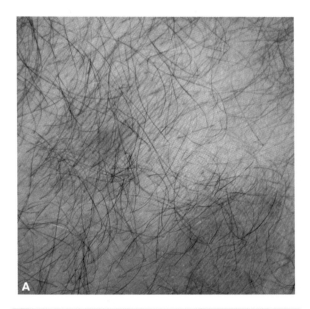

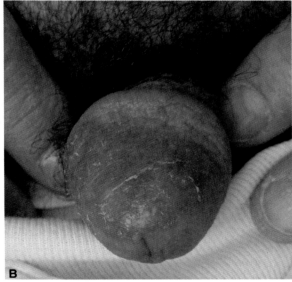

FIG. 17-2. Fixed drug eruption. **A:** An early lesion will present with an erythematous border and dusky center. **B:** The glans penis is a common location, especially with reaction to tetracyclines.

bulla, giving it a target-like appearance and then eroding. There may be no other associated symptoms or there may be some mild itching or burning.

> **DIFFERENTIAL DIAGNOSIS** Fixed drug eruption
>
> - Spider or arthropod bite (single lesion)
> - Cellulitis
> - Erythema annulare centrifugum
> - Acute urticaria
> - Herpes simplex (genital lesion)
> - Erythema multiforme/Stevens–Johnson syndrome
> - Autoimmune blistering disease
> - Lichen planus
> - Aphthous stomatitis

Diagnostics

FDR is generally a clinical diagnosis. History is the most helpful diagnostic tool as patients often do not correlate the offending medication with the eruption. Sometimes, a biopsy is performed and shows basal cell destruction and pigment incontinence.

Prognosis and Complications

Skin lesions typically persist for as long as the medication is taken and may take weeks to resolve after the drug is discontinued. The initially erythematous lesions fade to a dark brown-purple area of hyperpigmentation, especially in skin of color.

ACUTE GENERALIZED EXANTHEMATOUS PUSTULOSIS

AGEP is a rare cutaneous pustular eruption that occurs at a rate of one to five cases per million per year. AGEP generally develops after taking certain medications, especially calcium channel blockers, NSAIDs, anticonvulsants, enalapril, griseofulvin, itraconazole, aminopenicillins, macrolides, and quinolones. Viral infections have been known to also trigger AGEP.

Pathophysiology

While the pathophysiological mechanism is not yet understood, a genetic hypersensitivity or a type IV allergic reaction is suggested.

Clinical Presentation

AGEP has an acute onset and typically takes 1 to 3 weeks to develop in nonsensitized individuals. It is characterized by numerous pinpoint sterile pustules surrounded by bright-red erythema and edema. They are not perifollicular and can be either grouped or irregularly dispersed. Initially, lesions erupt on the face (Figure 17-3A) and intertriginous areas, especially the neck, axillae, and inguinal folds (Figure 17-3B). Pustules rapidly expand to cover the entire trunk. High fever and leukocytosis are common from the outset. Facial edema and nonviral hepatitis may develop (Figure 17-3C).

> **DIFFERENTIAL DIAGNOSIS** Acute generalized exanthematous pustulosis
>
> - Pustular psoriasis
> - Sweet syndrome
> - Stevens–Johnson syndrome/toxic epidermal necrolysis
> - Drug reaction with eosinophilia and systemic symptoms
> - Subcorneal pustulosis (Sneddon–Wilkinson syndrome)
> - Bullous impetigo

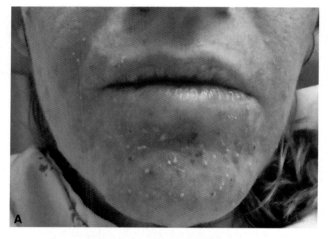

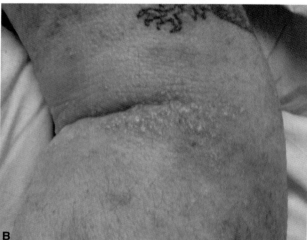

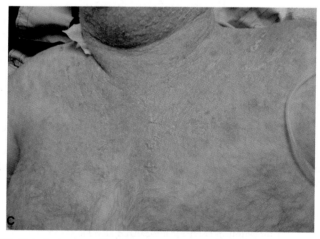

FIG. 17-3. Acute generalized exanthematous pustulosis. **A:** Eruption beginning on the face. **B:** Sheets of pustules in an intertriginous area. **C:** The entire trunk is involved and beginning to desquamate.

Diagnostics

A CBC with differential typically reveals a marked leukocytosis with very elevated neutrophils and mild eosinophilia. Serum BUN, creatinine, and 24-hour urine may reflect a transient reduction in creatinine clearance, whereas liver function studies are usually normal. AGEP histology has spongiform subcorneal and/or intraepidermal pustules, vasculitis, and marked edema of the papillary dermis.

It differs from pustular psoriasis which has acanthosis (epidermal thickening) and neutrophils in the epidermis.

Management

Resolution of this condition is spontaneous; however, patients may require hospitalization depending on the extent and severity of pustulosis or organ dysfunction. Treatment modalities include systemic corticosteroids, intravenous hydration, moisturizing creams and emollients, oral antihistamines and analgesics. The patient should be monitored closely until fever and pustules have resolved.

Referral and Consultation

Consultation with dermatology can be helpful for the reassurance that this will likely resolve with just supportive measures when the offending drug is discontinued. A referral to other specialists may be indicated if there are complications.

Prognosis and Complications

Hospitalization for supportive care and monitoring is not uncommon for patients with AGEP. The prognosis for full recovery is excellent once the drug has been identified and discontinued. The pustules spontaneously resolve in about 2 weeks, and a generalized desquamation occurs. Complications are rare but may include hepatitis; so careful monitoring of liver function tests is important until all symptoms and adverse reactions have resolved (Table 17-1).

URTICARIA AND ANGIOEDEMA

Urticarial drug eruptions are the second most common pattern of ADRs. See chapter 16 for additional information.

DRUG REACTION WITH EOSINOPHILIA AND SYSTEMIC SYMPTOMS

Formerly known as drug-induced hypersensitivity syndrome, DRESS is an uncommon but potentially life-threatening drug-induced reaction with cutaneous, hematologic, and systemic organ involvement. Anticonvulsants, including phenytoin, carbamazepine, lamotrigine, phenobarbital, as well as allopurinol, are the most commonly associated drugs with DRESS. Other drugs implicated less commonly are vancomycin, sulfonamide antibiotics, dapsone, and minocycline. DRESS is rare in children and does not have predilection for gender, but there is some evidence to support the association with HLA phenotypes.

Pathophysiology

DRESS is thought to be a drug-specific immune response; however, in approximately 20% of cases, no drug is identified. One theory of pathogenesis is a hypersensitivity reaction to a drug which triggers a reactivation of human herpes virus (HHV-6, -7), cytomegalovirus, or EBV by unknown mechanisms. Certain individuals may also be genetically predisposed because of their inability to metabolize certain drugs quickly enough (slow acetylators), causing a higher concentration of drug to remain in the system, which produces toxic metabolites. Activation of cytotoxic T cells is responsible for tissue damage.

Clinical Presentation

The onset of cutaneous symptoms in DRESS occurs around 3 to 4 weeks after intake of the drug. An erythematous, morbilliform eruption occurs on the face, upper trunk, and extremities but may encompass the entire skin surface and may become exfoliative. This eruption may occur up to 3 weeks after beginning the drug and may occur with the primary exposure to the drug. Facial edema is a hallmark sign but is not present in all cases. Cutaneous manifestation is accompanied by a high fever (>38°C), leukocytosis, atypical lymphocytosis, lymphadenopathy, and malaise, which should send a red flag to the clinician and prompt immediate hospitalization for evaluation and management of possible DRESS. Symptoms may persist for more than 2 weeks after the drug is discontinued.

The liver is the organ most commonly affected in DRESS but is not always discernable. Typically the patient does not have liver tenderness or hepatosplenomegaly, but has elevated liver function. If not recognized and managed in the early stages, it can progress to fulminant hepatitis. Other symptoms from organ dysfunction may include intestinal bleeding, encephalitis, aseptic meningitis, parotid sialadenitis, interstitial pneumonitis, respiratory distress syndrome, and myocarditis.

DIFFERENTIAL DIAGNOSIS Drug reaction with eosinophilia and systemic symptoms
• Acute generalized exanthematous pustulosis
• Acute viral infection
• Hypereosinophilic syndromes
• Exfoliative dermatitis
• Lymphoma/pseudolymphoma
• Stevens–Johnson syndrome/toxic epidermal necrolysis
• Acute cutaneous lupus erythematosus

Diagnostics

Because the onset of DRESS is slower than all of the other ADRs and can occur up to 8 weeks following administration of the drug, the importance of a detailed drug history cannot be overemphasized. A complete blood count with peripheral eosinophilia (>700 μL) is suggestive of DRESS. Elevated serum ALT and AST on two separate occasions and negative screening for hepatitis B and C are suggestive of liver involvement secondary to DRESS.

A punch biopsy of a lesion would show perivascular lymphocytic infiltrates in the superficial dermis with some eosinophils and dermal edema. Other imaging, liver biopsy, and serologies may be necessary based on the severity of systemic involvement. Overall, the drug history, morbilliform rash, systemic symptoms, including peripheral eosinophilia, lymphadenopathy, and elevated liver enzymes should distinguish DRESS from other ADRs.

Management

When DRESS is suspected, the patient should be immediately referred to the emergency department, where hospitalization, often in intensive care, is necessary to stabilize and monitor the patient. The priority for any patient with DRESS is to identify and withdraw the offending drug. In mild cases, high-potency topical (class I or II) corticosteroids or a short course of systemic corticosteroids can provide relief from the pruritus and inflammation.

Prognosis and Complications

Most cases of DRESS resolve in weeks to months after discontinuation of the drug. Complications occur secondary to organ involvement with up to 90% of patients with DRESS having at least one internal organ affected (liver, kidneys, lungs, and heart). Patients

TABLE 17-1 Comparison of Common Adverse Drug Reaction Patterns

	EXANTHEMATOUS (95% OF ADRs)	FIXED DRUG ERUPTION	ACUTE GENERALIZED EXANTHEMATOUS PUSTULOSIS
Onset	Insidious, 1–4 wk after initiation of drug	Rapid, hours to days	1–4 wk after initiation of drug
Etiology *	Drugs—sulfonamides, aminopenicillins, anticonvulsants, cephalosporins, antiretrovirals (see Box 17-4 for full list) IM or CMV + PCN HIV + sulfonamides Allopurinol + PCNs	Drugs—ASA, NSAIDs, sulfonamides, aminopenicillins, tetracyclines, TMP/SMX, phenolphthalein, barbiturates	Drugs: β-lactam and macrolide antibiotics, tetracyclines, calcium channel blockers, antifungals, NSAIDs, anticonvulsants Enterovirus, Epstein–Barr virus
Systemic	If present, including fever, consider *hypersensitivity syndrome reaction*	Typically none	Fever and leukocytosis, rare liver involvement (hepatitis) Watch LFTs
Morphology and Distribution	Morbilliform (papules and macules) *No blisters or pustules* Symmetrical, starts on trunk, then to extremities Favors pressure bearing areas Children: face & extremities Very similar presentation to viral exanthem	Discrete, solitary or multiple, red/dusky macules, papules, or plaques Edematous, ± *bullae* Lips, extremities, glans penis, lesions often recur in same location if offending agent reintroduced	Nonfollicular *pustules* with erythematous base Face & intertriginous areas, spreading quickly to trunk
Distribution			
Prognosis	Lesions fade with discontinuation, ± desquamation 1–2 wk	Lesions resolve with discontinuation, ± hyperpigmentation	Lesions resolve with discontinuation, desquamation 1–2 wk

* Most common cause or groups, not inclusive.

↓ Direction of spread.

CMV, cytomegalovirus; IM, infectious mononucleosis; PCN, aminopenicillins; TMP/SMX, trimethoprim/sulfamethoxazole; NSAID, nonsteroidal anti-inflammatory drug.

with hepatitis alone account for 10% of the mortality. There have been reports of patients developing autoimmune disorders after recovery from DRESS.

Referral and Consultation

Hospitalization is required, and consultations with a hepatologist, cardiologist, oncologist, and pulmonologist are often necessary.

Patient Education and Follow-up

Patients diagnosed with DRESS should maintain regular follow-up care with both primary care and specialists as indicated. Aggressive treatment with systemic corticosteroids require ongoing monitoring of glucose, blood pressure, symptoms of GERD, and other sequelae associated with corticosteroid therapy (see chapter 2). Patients should also be monitored for signs and symptoms of autoimmune disorders that have been reported in DRESS patients during the postrecovery period. Lastly, patients with DRESS and their families should avoid any exposure to the offending drug or similar drugs in its class.

PHOTOSENSITIVITY DRUG REACTIONS

See chapter 18 for a discussion of photosensitive reactions.

STEVENS–JOHNSON SYNDROME AND TOXIC EPIDERMAL NECROLYSIS

SJS and TEN are acute, systemic, and true medical emergencies. These potentially life-threatening ADRs are characterized by full-thickness denudation of the cutaneous and mucosal surfaces. Although their occurrence is rare, primary care clinicians need to recognize and emergently manage these patients because of the high mortality and morbidity with the disease. It is important to understand that SJS and TEN are the same skin disease on a continuum. They have the same pathologic process and are only differentiated by the percentage of body surface area (BSA) involved. For clarity, SJS involves less than 10% BSA, while TEN means that 30% or more BSA is involved. There is a gray area in the diagnosis when 10% to 30% of BSA is involved and is commonly referred to as "SJS/TEN overlap" (Figure 17-4).

The incidence of SJS/TEN is estimated to range from two to eight persons per million per year depending on geographic location and the offending drug or agent. In the United States, sulfonamides, anti-epileptics, and NSAIDs are implicated in the majority of cases. Less common causative drugs are cephalosporins, macrolides, benzodiazepines, H_1 antihistamines, and mucolytic agents.

The peak occurrence of SJS/TEN is during summer and early spring season. Infections, immunizations, and other disorders have also been implicated but are much less common. Data support a strong association between genetic susceptibility associated with HLA subtypes and the lack of ability to process specific drug metabolites. Patient populations from East Asian and European descent should be tested for the specific HLA subtypes before starting on oxicam, sulfamethoxazole, carbamazepine, lamotrigine, oxcarbazepine, phenytoin, abacavir, and allopurinol. The elderly, HIV-infected individuals, and those with autoimmune diseases (i.e., inflammatory bowel disease or systemic lupus erythematosus [SLE]) are at higher risk (Table 17-1).

Pathophysiology

Most experts consider SJS/TEN to be a delayed hypersensitivity reaction to a drug for unknown reasons. Cytotoxic T lymphocytes (drug-specific $CD8^+$ cells), along with natural killer T cells, trigger keratinocyte destruction (programed cell death), resulting in a separation of the epidermis from the dermis.

Clinical Presentation

SJS occurs more often in children and young adults and is often preceded by a prodrome of symptoms that includes high fever, sore throat, cough, malaise, arthralgia, stinging eyes, and upper respiratory tract infection. These symptoms can occur 1 to 3 days prior to

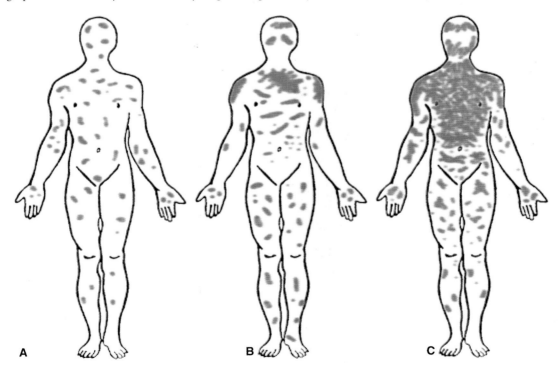

FIG. 17-4. Body surface area involvement of SJS/TEN. **A:** SJS: <10%. **B:** SJS/TEN: 10% to 30%. **C:** TEN: >30%.

the mucocutaneous lesions. In SJS, group erythematous targetoid (2 zones) or atypical (3 zones) lesions erupt, some with a central vesicle (Figure 17-5A). Palms and soles can be the first site of cutaneous eruption. Purpuric macules develop on the trunk and can spread to the face, neck, and extremities, developing into flaccid blisters, erosions, and detachment of the epidermis. The oral mucosa is almost always involved, often developing hemorrhagic crusts on the lips. Other mucous membranes like the conjunctiva, oral and nasal mucosa, and anogenital and vulvovaginal areas can be involved (Figure 17-5B).

TEN can present initially as SJS that rapidly progresses to involve more than 30% BSA with full-thickness desquamation of the epidermis. Yet clinicians should be cautioned that all TEN does not occur in this "linear" progression (Table 17-2). About half the cases of TEN develop rapidly from diffuse erythema to necrosis and epidermal detachment. The slightest pressure or friction on the skin near the bullae can result in a shearing off (positive Nikolsky sign) of sheets of the epidermis, exposing an erythematous, oozing dermis (Figure 17-6). Patients with TEN have a toxic appearance with high fever, cardiovascular compromise, metabolic imbalances, and severe pain. Organ involvement ensues rapidly with associated ocular, pulmonary, cardiovascular, neurologic, gastrointestinal, hematologic, and renal symptoms.

DIFFERENTIAL DIAGNOSIS Stevens–Johnson syndrome/toxic epidermal necrolysis

- Exanthematous drug eruption
- Other drug eruptions (acute generalized exanthematous pustulosis, drug reaction with eosinophilia and systemic symptoms, fixed drug eruption)
- Erythema multiforme major
- Scarlet fever
- Phototoxic eruptions
- Toxic shock syndrome
- Acute graft-versus-host disease
- Staphylococcal scalded skin syndrome
- Thermal burns
- Exfoliative dermatitis
- Generalized morbilliform eruption
- Drug-induced linear IgA bullous dermatosis
- Erythroderma

Diagnostics

The diagnosis of SJS/TEN is a clinical one supported by histologic findings. Patients with SJS/TEN will have a positive Nikolsky sign that can be elicited when lateral pressure applied near the bullae results in a shearing away of the surrounding epidermis. However, this can also be positive in pemphigus and staphylococcal scalded skin syndrome. Likewise, a positive Asboe–Hansen sign can be elicited when pressure is applied to the top of a bulla, causing lateral extension of the blister to adjacent skin.

The primary diagnostic test is a punch biopsy taken from an early lesion which histologically shows epidermal necrosis and detachment with apoptosis of the keratinocytes. There is usually inflammatory infiltrates in the dermis. A punch biopsy for direct immunofluorescence will differentiate SJS/TEN from other autoimmune blistering diseases. Laboratory testing is not diagnostic for SJS/TEN but is critical in assessing and monitoring systemic involvement and complications from the ADR. When it is unclear which drug is the offending agent in a patient with SJS/TEN, a carefully monitored provocation test or patch testing may be considered at a later time.

Management

It is imperative to immediately discontinue the suspected drug and admit any patient with suspected SJS/TEN to the hospital, preferably one with a burn unit. Aggressive management of fluid and electrolytes and wound care are a priority. Due to significant epidermal loss, patients are at high risk for secondary infections and need intensive monitoring and supportive therapy. *This is a true dermatologic emergency.* Treatment with high-dose parenteral corticosteroids, intravenously administered immunoglobulin, biologics, and cyclosporine have been used, but there are no proven therapies to be recommended.

The primary goal of treatment is to protect the dermis and promote reepithelialization while minimizing the risk of infection. Skin care during the acute phases is similar to the treatment for burn patients, using moist, nonadhering dressings. Surgical debridement is not recommended. Sometimes bullae are gently ruptured by piercing them with a sterile needle and allowing the roof to act as a biologic dressing. The effectiveness of adjuvant therapies including systemic corticosteroids, intravenous immunoglobulins,

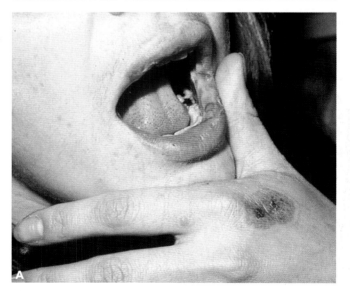

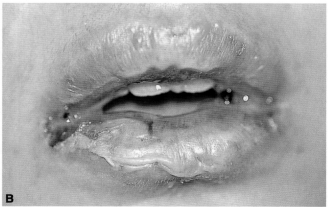

FIG. 17-5. Stevens–Johnson syndrome. **A:** Bullae and crusts are noted on the lips, and targetoid lesions are seen on the hand. **B:** Mucous membrane involvement.

TABLE 17-2	Comparison of Erythema Multiforme, Stevens–Johnson Syndrome, and Toxic Epidermal Necrolysis		
	ERYTHEMA MULTIFORME* (EM)	**STEVENS–JOHNSON SYNDROME (SJS) (%BSA)**	**TOXIC EPIDERMAL NECROLYSIS (%BSA)**
Onset	Acute onset, spring and fall Adolescents	Children & young adults Slightly higher F > M	
Etiology†	Common: HSV infection Sometimes: *Mycoplasma pneumoniae*, drugs, other infections	Common: Drugs—antibiotics (sulfonamides, quinolones, aminopenicillins, etc.), anticonvulsants, NSAIDs Uncommon: *M. pneumoniae*, viruses, immunizations, CMV	
Systemic	*Mild*, if any	*Sick* appearance	*Toxic* appearance
Prodrome	Abrupt onset Usually no illness	High fever, malaise, ST, influenza-like symptoms, starts as macular rash aphthous ulcers	Same as SJS Increasing systemic symptoms, pulmonary involvement 25%
Morphology & Distribution	*Targetoid* (3 zones) Red with darker center *Raised* Expanding then erosions Symmetric, acral extremities favors the extensors, palms, & soles	*Atypical* targetoid (2 zones) or typical targetoid, red *Flat* Central *vesicle* Starts on trunk, usually involves palms & soles Pruritic Negative Nikolsky sign	Papules/plaques, dusky, diffuse/increasing BSA Flaccid *bullae* *Full-thickness* desquamation >30% BSA and increasing Extracutaneous symptoms Painful Positive Nikolsky sign
Distribution			
Mucus Membranes	*Few* or no oral lesions	*Usually* oral Conjunctivitis is uncommon Hemorrhagic crusts	*Always* (before the rash) Usually more than one area *Conjunctival edema*
Prognosis	Self-limiting Lesions resolve 1 mo Usually no sequelae	5%–15% Mortality Heals without scarring Usually dyspigmentation	30%–40% Mortality Late withdrawal of drug leads to increased mortality

*Erythema multiforme is discussed in chapter 16.
†High-risk causes or groups, not inclusive.
HSV, herpes simplex virus; CMV, cytomegalovirus; BSA, body surface area.
Adapted from James, W. D. (2011). Drug reactions. In *Andrews' diseases of the skin: clinical dermatology* (11th ed., pp. 111). China: Elsevier.

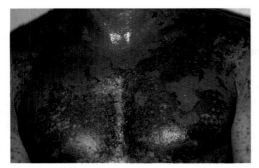

FIG. 17-6. Toxic epidermal necrolysis from treatment with nevirapine.

plasmapheresis, cyclosporine, and biologics has not been convincing and has shown varied rates of efficacy. Pain management is critical and similar to that of a burn patient but also includes extremely painful lesions in the mouth, nose, and eyes. Parenteral therapy is often needed for hydration and nutritional support. These lesions can last for weeks or months.

Prognosis and Complications

The overall mortality for SJS/TEN is estimated to be 10% to 30%. Ocular sequelae are the most common complication and can occur with either SJS or TEN. Ocular complications can range from severe corneal ulcerations, symblepharon, and blindness to dry eyes or trichiasis (eyelashes growing inward toward the eye). Long-term cutaneous sequela also includes scarring, dyspigmentation, strictures, or adhesions. Systemic complications include sepsis and organ failure that can be fatal or result in extensive morbidity. Long-term sequelae can include genitourinary, pulmonary, and cardiovascular disease, along with kidney failure requiring dialysis.

Referral and Consultation

Upon admission to the hospital, patients suspected with SJS/TEN should have immediate consultation with a dermatologist, burn care or wound specialist, and infectious disease specialist. Critical care intensivists often coordinate their care in ICU. After the acute phase has passed, ongoing medical care and support is paramount and often requires a multidisciplinary team to provide tertiary care. Early involvement of an ophthalmologist is recommended during the acute illness and continued throughout recovery.

Patient Education and Follow-up

Patients with a personal history or family history of SJS/TEN must avoid the potential causative agent and any cross-reacting agents in the drug class. The FDA recommends that patients who have Asian or South Asian ancestry and are being considered for treatment with the antiepileptic carbamazepine be screened for HLA-B*1502 as this population is at increased risk for SJS/TEN.

DRUG-INDUCED LUPUS

Drug-induced lupus (DIL) is an ADR associated with several drugs that trigger a lupus-like illness in patients who have not been previously diagnosed with lupus erythematosus. It is estimated that there are about 20,000 cases of DIL each year; however, it is a condition that is underrecognized and probably underreported. The highest

risk of DIL is associated with hydralazine and procainamide and somewhat less with quinidine. A low-risk association has been noted with carbamazepine, phenytoin, minocycline, terbinafine, griseofulvin, isoniazid, sulfasalazine, penicillamine, anti-TNF alphas, interferons, and propylthiouracil. There is some predilection for gender, race, and age in the incidence of DIL but it may be in relation to the underlying medical condition and socioeconomics associated with the drug therapy.

Pathophysiology

The etiology of DIL is uncertain but is proposed to be related to inhibition of DNA methylation, genetic predisposition (HLA and C_4 alleles), hormonal influences (estrogen), TNF-α inhibition, and reactive drug metabolites.

Clinical Presentation

The onset of DIL can occur weeks to years after the initiation of the drug therapy. DIL can mimic the signs and symptoms of SLE but typically has a milder clinical presentation. This is a syndrome characterized by fever, arthritis, myalgia, and myositis—all of which can be present in SLE. DIL typically presents as psoriasiform plaques and annular lesions, especially in photoexposed areas (Figure 17-7). They may be clinically and histologically indistinguishable from subacute cutaneous lupus erythematosus (see chapter 15). There are some subtle variations in the clinical findings that may help differentiate SLE and DIL. Alopecia, malar and discoid rash, and mucosal ulcers are not as prevalent in DIL. Lymphadenopathy, pleuritis, Raynaud syndrome, renal and neurologic symptoms, and myalgias are more common in SLE.

DIFFERENTIAL DIAGNOSIS Drug-induced lupus
• Discoid lupus erythematosus
• Subacute cutaneous lupus erythematosus
• Systemic lupus erythematosus
• Psoriasis

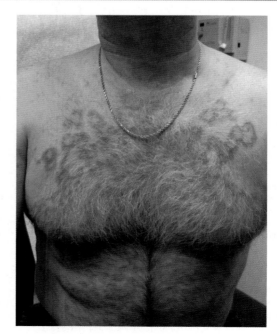

FIG. 17-7. Drug-induced cutaneous lupus.

Diagnostics

The history should seek to determine whether the patient has any signs, symptoms, or diagnosis of SLE or other autoimmune conditions prior to the skin eruption. Serology for ANA is usually positive with a homogenous pattern. Positive antihistones are seen in 95% of cases and positive anti-SSA/Ro, especially if the causative agent is a thiazide diuretic. Anti-dsDNA is usually negative and anti-ssDNA is positive in DIL. Punch biopsy histology and direct immunofluorescence offer very little diagnostic value.

The recommendation for a diagnosis of DIL is made when the patient has no history of LE; positive ANA; at least one clinical symptom of SLE after the initiation of drug therapy; and symptom resolution after discontinuance of the suspected causative drug.

Management

Prompt diagnosis and discontinuation of the drug are the priority for patients suspected of DIL. Symptomatic treatment may be needed to relieve arthritis and myalgias. The eruption may not resolve immediately after the drug's withdrawal and requires treatment with topical or intralesional corticosteroids and occasionally a short course of systemic corticosteroids. Emollients and antihistamines can be used for symptomatic relief of the pruritus.

Prognosis and Complications

Clinical symptoms usually resolve within 4 to 6 weeks after the drug is discontinued. Repeat antibody titers may be slow to return to normal. Most patients do not have any further problems or development of SLE. Rechallenge can be performed at a later date if there is a question about the causative agent.

Patient Education and Follow-up

Patients should follow up in about 2 weeks after the drug has been discontinued to ensure the rash and systemic symptoms have resolved. Repeat ANA usually returns to normal but can remain elevated. Patients should be vigilant in avoiding ingestion of the drug (or drug class) in the future.

RED MAN SYNDROME

Red man syndrome (RMS) is a hypersensitivity reaction associated with the administration of intravenous vancomycin. It was originally thought to be related to impurities in the product itself; however, these reactions continued despite improvements in the vancomycin preparations. The reaction occurs between 5% and 10% of the time, especially if the infusion is administered in less than a 60-minute period. Patients at greater risk for RMS are individuals 40 years and older or 2 years old and younger. Concurrent use of vancomycin and other antibiotics, opioid analgesics, muscle relaxants, or contrast dyes, increases the risk of RMS attributed to their histamine-releasing effects.

Pathophysiology

RMS is not a true allergic reaction and does not involve drug-specific antibodies. This anaphylactoid reaction is the result of mast cell degranulation and the release of histamine relative to the amount and rate of vancomycin infused.

Clinical Presentation

Signs of RMS can appear within minutes of initiating a vancomycin infusion or after completion of the treatment. It usually occurs with the first dose but may be delayed and react after several doses. Patients complain of diffuse burning and itching, with a rapid onset of dizziness and agitation. Flushing, rash, or redness of face, back of neck, upper body, and arms are common. Muscle spasms in the back or neck, fever, chills, nausea, vomiting, dyspnea, and hypotension may occur. In some patients, there is very subtle pruritus at the completion of the treatment and the reaction may go unnoticed.

Management

As soon as the clinician recognizes RMS, the vancomycin infusion should be stopped and diphenhydramine 50 mg given intravenously. The patient should be assessed for developing signs of anaphylaxis, which can sometimes occur. Vitals signs should be monitored. Most cases are mild and result in immediate resolution of symptoms.

Once symptoms have subsided, consideration can be given to reattempt the infusion of vancomycin. RMS does not prohibit subsequent doses; however, infusion of smaller doses over a longer period of time (at least 60 minutes) is recommended. Pretreatment with hydroxyzine is recommended for patients with known RMS in the past.

CORTICOSTEROID-INDUCED ACNE

Pustular eruptions resembling acne can occur acutely on the face and upper trunk 1 to 3 weeks after initiation of systemic corticosteroids. True acne is characterized by *comedones* (plugged follicular units); however, the lesions associated with drug-related acne are monomorphous and not comedonal in nature (see chapter 4). Although ideal treatment is the discontinuation of the causative agent, it may not always be possible. Use of topical acne medications such as benzoyl peroxide wash and topical retinoids can be effective until clearance is achieved.

DRUG-INDUCED DYSPIGMENTATION

The drugs most commonly associated with pigmentary changes are amiodarone, minocycline, and bleomycin. NSAIDs, heavy metals, antimalarials, and psychotropic drugs have also been implicated as causative drugs.

Pathophysiology

There are several mechanisms that can be responsible for drug-induced pigment abnormalities. Pathogenesis includes an accumulation of melanin caused by the drug itself, especially with sun exposure; postinflammatory changes secondary to drug therapy (hemosiderin staining); and actual deposits of the drug or drug metabolites along the basement membrane.

Clinical Presentation

There is a variable range of color, patterns, and locations of drug-induced pigmentation that is often specific to the offending agent. *Amiodarone dyspigmentation* is characterized by a violaceous coloration on sun-exposed skin surfaces, especially the face. Cutaneous changes usually develop with long-term, continuous therapy. The discoloration may fade after discontinuation of the drug but sometimes remains as a permanent dyspigmentation. *Minocycline* can induce a blue-black coloration that affects the skin, nails, sclerae, oral mucosa, and teeth (Figure 17-8A). Scar tissue, such as acne scars, and anterior

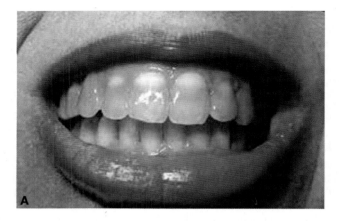

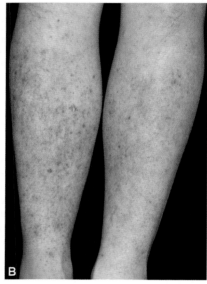

FIG. 17-8. Minocycline hyperpigmentation. **A:** Oral mucosa and teeth. **B:** Bluish-black minocycline pigmentation is often on the legs, related to trauma.

shins are commonly affected and often confused with bruising. Three patterns of minocycline hyperpigmentation have been described:

- *Type I*: blue-black color that appears in sites of previous inflammation or scarring, typically within facial acne scars. Histology shows iron deposition in the dermis.
- *Type II*: blue-gray discoloration that affects otherwise normal skin, often on lower extremities. Histologic analysis exhibits melanin and iron deposits in the deeper dermis and fat (Figure 17-8B).
- *Type III*: muddy brown discoloration accentuated in sun-exposed areas. Histology shows superficial melanin deposition in epidermis or dermis.

Bleomycin causes changes in pigmentation that are characterized as "flagellate pigmentation" which appears as a brown-gray linear hyperpigmentation. The lesions can be diffuse, often developing on the chest, back, and extremities, and can be photo-exacerbated. It develops anywhere from 1 day to 9 weeks after systemic treatment with bleomycin. The discoloration will fade about 3 to 4 months after the bleomycin has been discontinued. Mild pruritus can be managed with low- to mid-potency topical corticosteroids or oral antihistamines (Figure 17-9).

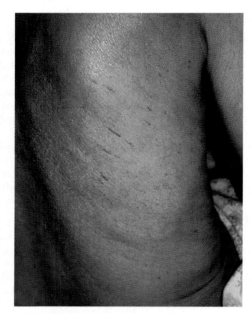

FIG. 17-9. Bleomycin flagellate pigmentation.

Management

Photoprotection and drug avoidance, if possible, are the recommended treatment for drug-induced hyperpigmentation. Many times the pigmentation will fade, while others become a permanent residual from drug therapy. There are some reports of success using laser therapy.

VASCULITIS

Cutaneous small vessel vasculitis has been associated with drugs from almost every drug class and is thought to develop when drug antigen immune complexes deposit in postcapillary venules. Vasculitis typically occurs within 1 to 3 weeks of drug administration. Rechallenge results in symptoms within 3 days. Clinically, the patient presents with palpable purpura, but can also present with urticarial lesions, ulcers, nodules, and digital necrosis (Figure 17-10). Constitutional

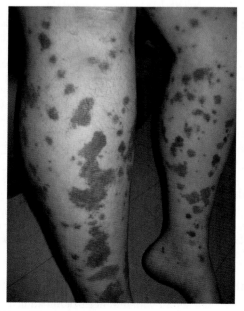

FIG. 17-10. Vasculitis.

signs and symptoms such as fever, headache, myalgia and arthralgia, arthritis, peripheral edema, and tachypnea warrant an investigation into additional organ system involvement. Medications associated with drug-induced vasculitis include penicillins, NSAIDs, sulfonamides, and cephalosporins among others. See chapter 16 for a complete discussion of vasculitis.

CLINICAL PEARLS

- The three most common types of drugs that cause ADRs are antibiotics, NSAIDs, and anticonvulsants.

- Skin eruptions in patients taking *high-risk* drugs with mucosal involvement, blisters, or targetoid lesions should be suspected of SJS/TEN.

- Fixed drug eruption should always be considered for any erythematous macules or plaques on the glans penis.

- Patients with mucocutaneous blistering should be referred to dermatology immediately.

- Clinicians should be cautious with ADRs accompanied by fever.

- Most ADRs are morbilliform and caused by drugs, infections, or immunizations.

BILLING CODES ICD-10

Acute generalized exanthematous pustulosis	L27.0
Adverse cutaneous drug eruption	T88.7
Drug-induced photosensitivity	L56.0
Drug-induced lupus erythematosus	L93.2
Drug reaction with eosinophilia and systemic symptoms	L27.0
Fixed drug eruption	L27.1
Stevens–Johnson syndrome	L51.1
Stevens–Johnson syndrome/toxic epidermal necrolysis overlap	L51.3
Toxic epidermal necrolysis	L51.2
Vasculitis	L95.9

READINGS

American Society of Health-System Pharmacists. (1995). ASHP guidelines on adverse drug reaction monitoring and reporting. *American Journal of Health-System Pharmacy, 52*, 417–419.

Cacoub, P., Musette, P., Descamps, V., Meyer, O., Speirs, C., Finzi, L., & Roujeau, J. C. (2011). The DRESS syndrome: A literature review. *The American Journal of Medicine, 124*, 588–597.

FDA US.S. and Food Drug Administration. *MedWatch: The FDA Safety Information and Adverse Event Reporting Program.* http://www.fda.gov/Safety/MedWatch/default. Accessed on May 10, 2014

Habif, T. P. (2010). *Clinical dermatology: A color guide to diagnosis and therapy* (5th ed.). St. Louis, MO: Mosby Elsevier.

Husain, Z., Reddy, B. Y., & Schwart, R. A. (2013). DRESS syndrome: Part I. Clinical perspectives. *Journal of the American Academy of Dermatology, 68*(5), 693–703.

Heinzerlin, L., Tomsitz, D., & Anliker, M. D. (2011). Is drug allergy less prevalent than previously assumed? A 5-year analysis. *British Journal of Dermatology, 166*(1), 107–114.

Hutson, C., & Carlson, T. (2013). Wound management. In T. M. Buttaro, J. Trybulski, P. Polgar Bailey, J. Sandberg-Cook. (Eds.), *Primary care: A collaborative practice* (4th ed., pp. 302–312). St. Louis, MO: Mosby Elsevier.

James, W. D. (2011). *Andrews' diseases of the skin: Clinical dermatology* (11th ed., pp. 1086). St. Louis, MO: Elsevier.

Litt, J. Z. (2009). *Litt's drug eruptions & reactions manual* (15th ed.). New York, NY: Informa Healthcare.

Noguera-Morel, L., Hernandez-Marin, A., & Torrelo, A. (2014). Cutaneous drug reactions in the pediatric population. *Pediatric Clinics of North America, 61*(2), 403–426.

Revuz, J., & Valeyrie-Allanore, L. (2012). Drug reactions. In J. L. Bolognia, J. L. Jorizzo, & J. V. Schaffer (Eds.), *Dermatology* (3rd ed., pp. 335–356). Philadelphia, PA: Elsevier Saunders.

Schwartz, R. A., McDonough, P. H., & Lee, B. (2013). Toxic epidermal necrosis: Part I. Introduction, history, classification, clinical features, systemic manifestations, etiology, and immunopathogenesis. *Journal of the American Academy of Dermatology, 69*(2), 173.e1–173.e13.

Schwartz, R. A., McDonough, P. H., & Lee, B. (2013). Toxic epidermal necrosis: Part II. Prognosis, sequelae, diagnosis, differential diagnosis, prevention, and treatment. *Journal of the American Academy of Dermatology, 69*(2), 187.e1–187.e16.

Speekaert, M. M., Speekaert, R., Lambert, J., & Brochez, L. (2010). Acute generalized exanthematous pustulosis: an overview of the clinical, immunological and diagnostic concepts. *European Journal of Dermatology, 20*, 425–433.

US Food and Drug Administration. (2014). *MedWatch: The FDA Safety Information and Adverse Event Reporting Program.* Retrieved from http://www.fda.gov/Safety/MedWatch/default

Wolverton, S. E. (2012) *Comprehensive dermatologic drug therapy* (2nd ed.). China: Elsevier.

Wolff, K., & Johnson, R. A. (2013). *Fitzpatrick's color atlas & synopsis of clinical dermatology* (7th ed., pp. 173–177). New York, NY: McGraw-Hill.

World Health Organization, Media Centre. (2008). *Medicines: Adverse drug reactions. Fact sheet.* Retrieved from http://www.who.int/mediacentre/factsheets/en/Query Log

CHAPTER 18

Pigmentation and Light-Related Dermatoses

Katie B. O'Brien

The presence of pigmentation in skin is largely determined by genetic makeup. Skin type is related to the amount of melanin that is produced by an individual. A general understanding of the process of melanin synthesis is essential to understanding the conditions of dyspigmentation. Disturbances in the process of pigment production can yield significant alterations in one's appearance. Cosmetic and physiologic changes may occur as a result of genetic, environmental, and even pharmacologic influences. The sun alone can play a major role, not only in the overproduction of pigmentation which is seen in normal tanning but as a predisposing factor in the development of skin cancer. In this chapter, we review the biology and function of melanocytes, the role of melanosomes in the production of melanin, and the common types of dyspigmentation which can result when this normal process is interrupted.

BIOLOGY OF PIGMENTATION

Melanocytes are derived from the neural crest and migrate to the epidermis, hair follicles, uveal tract of the eye (choroid, ciliary body, and iris), the leptomeninges, and the inner ear (cochlea). They contain the melanin-producing cells called melanosomes, where, under genetic influence, and with the aid of the enzyme tyrosinase, melanin is synthesized. There are two types of melanin: eumelanin (brown/black) and pheomelanin (yellow-red). The melanocyte resides in the basal layer of the epidermis and via its dendritic processes attaches to the keratinocytes and deposits the melanin-containing melanosome. A person's skin color is determined by the size and number of these melanosomes, the amount of melanin they produce, and their distribution within the epidermis.

DISORDERS OF PIGMENT LOSS

Hypopigmentation and depigmentation can occur if there is a loss of melanocytes, an inability of melanocytes to produce melanin, or an inability to transport melanin correctly. The term *hypopigmentation* refers to a partial loss of melanocytes, while *depigmentation* refers to a total loss of melanocytes. Patients with large body surface areas (BSAs) of pigment abnormality may be challenging for the clinician to identify a patient's normal skin color.

Vitiligo

Vitiligo is an unpredictable disease of depigmentation. The exact cause of melanocyte destruction is unknown. It affects males and females equally, and is present in all ethnicities. The prevalence of vitiligo is estimated to be 1% of the world's population, with 50% of all cases occurring before the age of 20 years. Thirty percent of patients with vitiligo have other family members who also have the disease. Some people attribute the initial onset to emotional stress, illness, or skin trauma such as sunburn.

Risk factors for developing vitiligo include heredity, autoimmune disease, especially Hashimoto thyroiditis, and a variety of systemic diseases such as diabetes, pernicious anemia, Addison disease, and hypoparathyroidism. Interestingly, patients who have received bone marrow transplants, or lymphocyte infusions from a donor with vitiligo, have developed vitiligo themselves.

Pathophysiology

The mechanism of depigmentation in vitiligo is not well understood. It is thought that there is an absence of functional melanocytes caused by both genetic and nongenetic factors. In addition to the belief that vitiligo is hereditary, it is theorized that specific autoantibodies are directed against tyrosinase, the enzyme that converts tyrosine into melanin, resulting in pigment loss. Others suggest that vitiligo is caused by an intrinsic defect in the structure and function of melanocytes or that there is a defective free-radical defense, which results in the destruction of melanocytes, leading to depigmentation.

Clinical presentation

A patient with vitiligo typically presents with well-demarcated, depigmented white macules or patches surrounded by normal skin. The onset of the lesions is insidious with expanding, irregularly shaped patches that rarely have inflamed borders. Hair follicles present in the depigmented patch are usually white. When the scalp area is involved, it usually presents as a solitary patch called *poliosis* or *white forelock* (Figure 18-1). The eyebrows and eyelashes may also be affected. There may also be focal blue-gray hyperpigmented macules on the skin representing melanin incontinence.

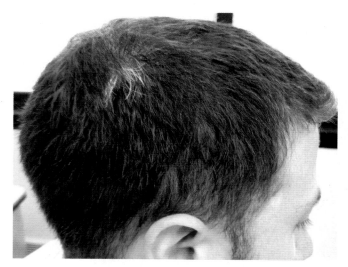

FIG. 18-1. Poliosis or white forelock is the localized loss of pigment in the hair and skin on the scalp and can occur in the eyebrow and eyelashes.

There are six different types of vitiligo: localized, segmental, generalized, universal, acrofacial, and mucosal.

Generalized vitiligo is the most common type, accounting for 90% of all cases. It is usually symmetrically distributed on the face, upper chest, dorsal hands, axillae, and groin (Figure 18-2A). It has a predilection for orifices, including the eyes (Figure 18-2B), nostrils, mouth, nipples, umbilicus, and anogenital areas. Sites of trauma are commonly affected.

Localized vitiligo may affect one nondermatomal site, or asymmetrically affect one region (e.g., an extremity).

Segmental vitiligo has a distribution similar to localized vitiligo, but is often dermatomally distributed. It is more often seen in younger patients, and is less likely to be related to autoimmune disease.

Acrofacial vitiligo affects facial orifices and/or distal fingers and toes (think "lips and tips").

Mucosal vitiligo, as its name clearly states, affects the mucous membranes alone, and is commonly seen on the lips and genital and perianal areas (Figure 18-2C).

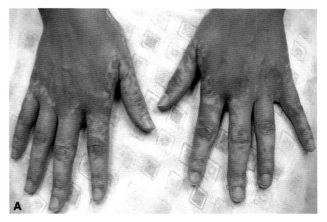

DIFFERENTIAL DIAGNOSIS Vitiligo

- Chemical leukoderma
- Leukoderma associated with melanoma
- Postinflammatory depigmentation
- Tinea versicolor
- Morphea
- Lichen sclerosis
- Pityriasis alba

Diagnostics

The diagnosis of vitiligo is usually made based on clinical findings. A skin biopsy will show an absence of melanocytes and sometimes inflammation. Vitiligo macules/patches may not be obvious upon a general examination, especially around the eyes, nose, axilla, hands/fingers, and groin. Wood's lamp examination is a low-cost and convenient diagnostic tool that can help differentiate depigmented lesions from hypopigmented lesions. Lesions become markedly enhanced on wood's lamp examination and help to define specific areas of depigmentation (Figure 18-3A, B).

Because vitiligo is often associated with systemic disease, it is important to screen for underlying thyroid disease, pernicious anemia, and diabetes. If indicated, laboratory studies should include CBC, TSH, T_3, T_4, glycosylated hemoglobin, thyroid antibodies (antithyroglobulin and antithyroid peroxidase antibodies), and antinuclear antibody (ANA) screening.

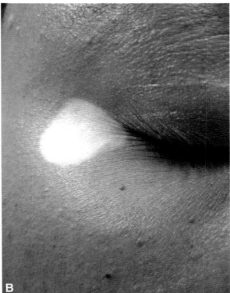

Management

In patients with fair skin, nontreatment may be an option as the disfigurement from vitiligo may not be severe. However, these patients must adhere to strict sun-protective practices. Camouflage makeup can be used as well. Some brand-name products available for patients with dyspigmentation are Dermablend, Dermacolor, Keromask, Veil Cover, Perfect Cover, and Covermark. Aestheticians can be helpful in assisting patients with application and matching their skin tone.

Topical corticosteroids (TCS). TCS are the treatment of choice for vitiligo when small areas of skin are involved (<20% BSA) and for children. High-potency TCS should be initiated with these

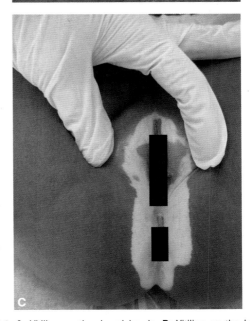

FIG. 18-2. **A:** Vitiligo on the dorsal hands. **B:** Vitiligo on the lateral eye. **C:** Vitiligo at the anogenital area.

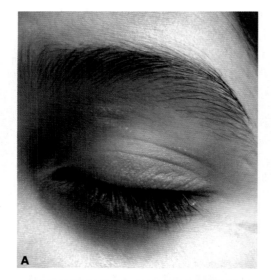

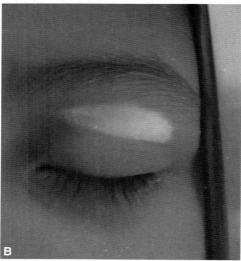

FIG. 18-3. **A:** Vitiligo can have a subtle presentation that is difficult to discern, especially in patients with fair skin. **B:** Wood's light examination can be used to accentuate areas of pigment loss and help to diagnose vitiligo.

patients and continued for 2 months. If there is no response, then the treatment should be discontinued. If the lesions are repigmenting, a slow taper to lower-potency TCS should be continued for 4 to 6 months. An exception to this general approach is lesions located around the eyes due to concern for increased intraocular pressure. Clinicians should regularly monitor patients for side effects and response to treatment.

It is important to educate the patient on the risks of using TCS, especially on the face, including, but not limited to acne, atrophy, and telangiectasias. Occlusion of any form of topical therapy may enhance efficacy and side effects. Pulse dosing can be used to minimize these side effects by alternating days of application with several days off. A common example is to apply Monday to Friday and omit the weekend.

Phototherapy. Narrow-band UVB (NBUVB) and psoralen with UVA (PUVA) have been shown to be effective treatment for vitiligo; however, the exact mechanism of action is unknown. The primary objective is to stimulate the few remaining melanocytes which

reside in the hair follicle. Ultraviolet light (UVL) activates the melanocytes, which migrate up the hair follicle and then spread to the surrounding area. Initially, repigmentation occurs at the hair follicle and presents as small hyperpigmented dots within the area of depigmentation.

Phototherapy can be inconvenient for the patient, however, as it is an in-office therapy usually recommended two to three times per week.

Excimer laser treatment may also be used for localized lesions twice weekly for 24 to 48 sessions.

Topical immunomodulators (TIMS). Off-label use of pimecrolimus (Elidel) and tacrolimus 0.3% to 0.1% (Protopic) is an alternative to TCS and has been effective in treating facial vitiligo. Some studies have shown that these drugs are more efficacious when used in combination with NBUVB phototherapy (Bolognia, Jorizzo, & Rapini, 2008). However, TIMS should not be on the skin while the patient is receiving a phototherapy treatment. The FDA has issued a "black-box" warning for pimecrolimus and tacrolimus, stating that they may increase the risk of lymphoma and skin cancers. Please see chapter 3 for details.

Calcipotriol. Topical calcipotriol has also proven to be effective in producing repigmentation of vitiligo when used in combination with corticosteroids. This has been observed in patients who have previously failed topical corticosteroid treatment as a monotherapy.

In general, Cochrane review states that most of the trials assessed combination therapies using phototherapy to enhance repigmentation.

Total depigmentation. Depigmentation is usually reserved for vitiligo patients with a 40% or greater BSA involvement. The treatment approach considers that it is easier to remove the remaining normal pigment to match the large depigmented areas. This is permanent and requires lifelong sun protection. A 20% cream of monobenzylether of hydroquinone may be applied b.i.d. for 6 to 18 months.

Systemic therapy. Systemic corticosteroids and immunosuppressants are not commonly used in the treatment of vitiligo. They should only be used to arrest rapidly spreading disease.

Micropigmentation. Medical tattooing or micropigmentation may be useful for sites that have a poor response to treatment such as the lips and distal fingers.

Surgical therapies. Punch grafting may be successful for carefully chosen individuals who fail to respond to other therapies. Small punch grafts (1–2 mm) are taken from uninvolved skin and implanted 5 to 8 mm apart into the depigmented areas. Criteria for punch grafting include stable vitiligo for at least 6 months, no Koebner phenomenon, no tendency to develop keloid scars, a positive mini-grafting test, and at least 12 years of age (Bolognia et al., 2008).

Special considerations
Pediatrics. Pigment loss in children is either congenital or acquired; therefore, the onset of the disease can provide important diagnostic clues. Congenital depigmentation is an uncommon occurrence that presents at birth or during infancy and is usually associated with a genetic disorder. A white forelock on an infant would be concerning for autosomal dominant piebaldism in comparison to patients with vitiligo that may develop a forelock later in life. Children have a higher propensity for autoimmune disease than adults.

Pregnancy. Corticosteroids, pimecrolimus, tacrolimus, calcipotriol, monobenzone, and psoralens are pregnancy category C. It is best to postpone topical vitiligo treatment until after pregnancy. NBUVB treatment is safe during pregnancy.

Prognosis and complications

Treatment of vitiligo is challenging, unpredictable, and often very frustrating. Any therapy used in the treatment of vitiligo should be accompanied by the warning that lesions may not resolve and can recur. If the patient does respond to treatment, it is usually very slowly and improvement may depend on anatomic location. Facial lesions achieve greater than 90% improvement in pigmentation with TCS, whereas lesions located on the trunk only achieve a 40% response to treatment.

Repigmentation of facial lesions occurs diffusely, but it occurs perifollicularly in lesions on the trunk. Darker skin tones are more responsive to TCS than lighter skin. Cochrane review also states that none of the studies reported long-term benefit, that is, sustained repigmentation for at least 2 years.

Referral and consultation

Referral to dermatology should be made if vitiligo fails to respond to topical treatment or expands to involve large BSA as the patient may require advanced therapies. Newly diagnosed patients should be advised to have an ophthalmologic examination as there has been some association with uveitis and vitiligo. Newborns and infants with depigmented skin should be referred immediately to a pediatric dermatologist, if available. Lastly, vitiligo can have a significant impact on a patient's quality of life and social development due to disfigurement. A referral to a mental health professional may be helpful.

Patient education and follow-up

Patients should be counseled on their increased risk for skin cancer and the importance of UVR protection. A broad-spectrum sunscreen containing zinc oxide or titanium dioxide should be worn and sun-protective clothing encouraged (see chapter 2). As many patients will be using TCS at some point during the treatment of their disease, the potential side effects should always be explained to the patient.

Patients should be closely monitored for efficacy and side effects of treatment. As the risk of skin cancer is increased in fair-skinned individuals with vitiligo, a thorough skin examination should be performed annually. Treated areas should be checked for pigmented macules at the site of hair follicles at each visit. Lack of improvement may be discouraging to the patient. It is important to be empathetic and understand the psychological impact that this disease has on the patient. Vitiligo can be especially disfiguring for dark-skinned individuals and children.

Pityriasis Alba

Pityriasis alba is a common dermatosis in which patients present with ill-defined patches of hypopigmentation. It is most commonly seen in children and adolescents who have a history of atopy. Males and females are affected equally. Like vitiligo, it is more cosmetically distressing for those with darkly pigmented skin.

Pathophysiology

The exact etiology of pityriasis alba is unknown, but the cause of hypopigmentation has been classified as postinflammatory. It seems to appear after a flare of eczema or atopic dermatitis. The hypopigmentation resolves spontaneously, usually before young adulthood. Histopathology reveals a reduction in the number of melanocytes.

Clinical presentation

Patients with pityriasis alba are asymptomatic. Small, slightly elevated, hypopigmented, ill-defined patches are most commonly distributed on the cheeks but may also appear on the proximal upper and lower extremities. In the early stage of pityriasis alba, lesions may be mildly erythematous, then become hypopigmented and scaly. The lesions are more apparent on unaffected skin that has been tanned, creating an even greater contrast next to the hypopigmentation patches (Figure 18-4).

DIFFERENTIAL DIAGNOSIS Pityriasis alba
• Vitiligo
• Chemical leukoderma
• Tinea versicolor
• Eczematous dermatitis

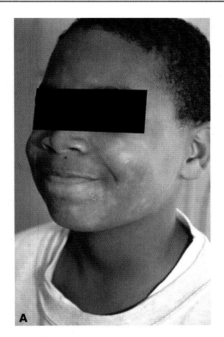

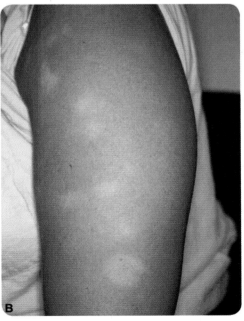

FIG. 18-4. **A:** Pityriasis alba on the face. **B:** Pityriasis alba on the arm.

Diagnostics

A negative KOH prep can differentiate pityriasis alba from tinea versicolor. In pityriasis alba, nondiscrete lesions can be visualized with wood's lamp examination. Some melanin is present, so there is no accentuation of the color as is seen in the markedly depigmented lesions observed in vitiligo.

Management

Emollients are effective at reducing scale. Mild TCS or TIMS may be helpful, as they can reduce subtle inflammation allowing repigmentation to occur. Phototherapy has not shown an improvement in pigmentation.

Prognosis and complications

Pityriasis alba is a benign hypopigmented skin condition that resolves spontaneously. It can have psychosocial impact on darkly skinned individuals, as lesions are more noticeable.

Referral and consultation

Refer to dermatology if the pityriasis alba fails to resolve spontaneously or spreads. A referral is also warranted if the patient's atopic dermatitis is poorly controlled.

Patient education and follow-up

It is important to listen to patients' concerns, be empathetic, and reassure them that the hypopigmentation will resolve. Sun protection should be encouraged, as tanning may make hypopigmentation more noticeable. Patients should be educated on the proper use of emollients. If they are being treated with TCS, the side effects and risks should be discussed.

Idiopathic Guttate Hypomelanosis

Idiopathic guttate hypomelanosis (IGH) is a common dermatosis of unknown etiology. It consists of photo-distributed, hypopigmented macules on the upper and lower extremities. It affects 50% to 70% of people over the age of 50, and 80% of patients over the age of 70. It seems to be more common in females, perhaps because females seek medical attention more frequently than men.

Pathophysiology

Histopathology shows a loss of melanocytes in the skin, but not a complete absence. Some melanocytes function normally, while others do not. This is thought to be a result of actinic damage, as patients exhibit signs of photoaging in the same locations. Others propose that it is a degenerative sign of aging.

Clinical presentation

Patients usually present with IGH out of cosmetic concern. There are well-circumscribed, 2- to 5-mm, hypopigmented macules distributed on the sun-exposed (extensor) surfaces of the upper and lower extremities. Lentigines and xerosis are typically present. Once these hypopigmented macules present, they do not usually become larger and are permanent (Figure 18-5).

DIFFERENTIAL DIAGNOSIS Idiopathic guttate hypomelanosis
• Pityriasis alba
• Vitiligo
• Tinea versicolor
• Flat warts

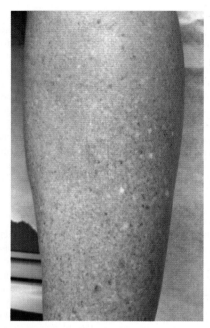

FIG. 18-5. Idiopathic guttate hypomelanosis.

Diagnostics

IGH is usually a clinical diagnosis. A skin biopsy is not usually needed, but may confirm an incomplete loss of melanocytes and melanin. A KOH prep may be done if tinea versicolor is suspected.

Management

The patient should be reassured that this is a benign skin finding. There have been some reports that liquid nitrogen has caused repigmentation. Cryotherapy may cause leukoderma or postinflammatory hyperpigmentation, so patients should be well aware of this risk. Tinted makeup, such as Dermablend or Covermark, can be used to cover hypopigmented macules. Self-tanners are not helpful as the macules do not absorb the topical.

Prognosis and complications

Patients tend to develop more lesions as they age; however, the size of the lesions should remain stable. Future sun exposure or tanning may darken the surrounding area and accentuate the appearance of the hypopigmented macules.

Patient education and follow-up

Patients should be reassured that treatment is not medically necessary as it is a benign condition. They should be counseled on sun protection.

Follow-up is generally not needed; however, these patients often have significant actinic damage, so careful skin cancer screening should be performed.

DISORDERS OF PIGMENT EXCESS

Melasma

Melasma, also known as chloasma or the mask of pregnancy, is a common disorder of hyperpigmentation. Melasma is more common in females of childbearing age, and those with darker skin phenotypes. Genetics is suspected to play a role in melasma in Asian and Hispanic ethnicities. Sun exposure is the greatest risk factor for the development of melasma, and hormones have also been implicated. Therefore, pregnant women and those taking oral contraceptives or hormone replacement therapy are at higher risk.

Pathophysiology

The exact cause of melasma is unknown. The theory is that the melanocytes in the affected skin produce greater amounts of melanin than they do in the uninvolved skin. This hyperfunctioning of the melanocytes is thought to be triggered by UV exposure, hormonal or other systemic conditions such as thyroid disease. These stimuli can cause increased levels of nitric oxide, which stimulates tyrosinase activity, causing increased localized melanin production.

Clinical presentation

Tan to dark brown irregularly bordered, symmetric patches are most commonly distributed on the face and sometimes forearms (Figure 18-6). Three patterns of hypermelanosis are observed and are described as centrofacial, malar, and mandibular. The central facial pattern is the most common, affecting the forehead, cheeks, nose, upper lip, and chin. The malar and mandibular patterns exclusively affect the cheeks, nose, and the mandible.

> **DIFFERENTIAL DIAGNOSIS** Melasma
> - Drug-induced hyperpigmentation
> - Postinflammatory hyperpigmentation
> - Solar lentigines
> - Nevus of Ota
> - Discoid Lupus

Management

Melasma can be stubborn to treat and frustrating for both the patient and clinician. There are many prescribed, over-the-counter products and procedures that are reported to be effective. Yet despite advanced and expensive therapies, melasma is often recalcitrant and recurrent. Selection of treatment modalities should be based on the location, size, and severity of hyperpigmentation. Caution should be used as over treatment or aggressive therapies that cause inflammation, may in turn cause more hyperpigmentation.

Topical therapies. Treatment of melasma is generally managed with topical lightening agents such as hydroquinone either alone or in combination with a topical retinoid (tretinoin or adapalene) and at times a mild TCS to counteract the irritation from the retinoid. Hydroquinone blocks the production of tyrosinase and selectively damages melanosomes and melanocytes. Hydroquinone 2% to 4% cream may be applied twice daily to the affected areas. Hydroquinone 2% can still be purchased without prescription. Tretinoin cream 0.025%, 0.05%, and 0.1% is effective as a monotherapy, but has greater efficacy if used in combination with the hydroquinone. Treatment results are slow and may take 6 months to achieve desired results. Caution should be used with higher strengths of topical retinoids (tretinoin 0.1%) as they can cause significant inflammation. Triluma Cream which is a combination of hydroquinone, tretinoin, and fluocinolone, is often prescribed for efficacy and ease of administration. The hyperpigmentation should be reassessed after 2 months of treatment and is more likely to improve and less likely to recur if patients avoid the sun and any causative agents.

Recently, a number of skin-lightening agents without hydroquinone have become available. They contain numerous agents that claim to be more natural and nontoxic, such as vitamin C. Most cosmetic companies have a skin-lightening product on the shelf. Chemical peels including glycolic acid and salicylic acid may be effective when used in low concentrations and in combination with

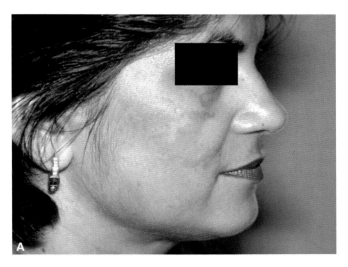

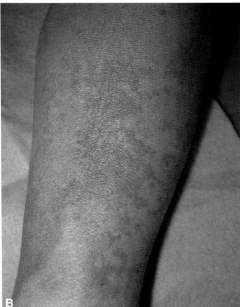

FIG. 18-6. **A:** Melasma on the cheek. **B:** Melasma on the forearm.

hydroquinone cream. High-concentration chemical peels should be avoided as the inflammation may cause hyperpigmentation.

Laser therapy. Laser treatment has not been consistently effective, and the side effects may be greater than the benefits. As this condition exists primarily in patients with darker skin, a resulting hypopigmentation from the laser is a definite concern.

Special considerations

Pregnancy. The state of pregnancy is often the cause of melasma; so care must be taken to avoid most of the usual treatments. Hydroquinone is pregnancy category C and tretinoin is pregnancy category D, and should absolutely be avoided during pregnancy. Azaleic acid is pregnancy category B. It has not shown any adverse fetal effects, and is probably safe to use during pregnancy and or breastfeeding. Pregnant patients should be reassured that melasma usually fades postpartum.

Prognosis and complications

Epidermal melasma typically has a better response to treatment than dermal melasma. Melasma usually improves or resolves slowly over a few months postpartum or after discontinuing oral contraceptives. Patients using high-strength hydroquinone for long periods may be at risk for worsening pigmentation which can be a sign of ochronosis, a known side effect of long-term use.

Referral and consultation

If a patient's melasma is not responding to topical therapy, referral to a cosmetic dermatology provider may be necessary.

Patient education and follow-up

Strict sun protection with broad-spectrum sunscreens, hats, and sun avoidance is imperative for patients with melasma. Patients should be advised that their daily moisturizer with a sunscreen is not adequate and their treatment will fail if they do not adhere to these sun-protection practices. Patients taking oral contraceptives should decide if discontinuation or change to a low-estrogen oral contraceptive is necessary. Patients should also be advised to watch for any worsening pigmentation during treatment , and if it occurs, discontinue use of hydroquinone.

Café au Lait Macules

Café au lait macules (CALMs) are well-demarcated light brown patches, which measure approximately 2 to 5 cm. CALMs are usually noted during early childhood and may persist into adulthood. The term "café au lait" refers to the lesion's color, which resembles coffee with milk, which can be light tan to brown. Multiple lesions (>5) are sometimes an indicator for various syndromes. Single CALMs are found in 10% to 20% of the population. African Americans are affected more often than Caucasians.

Pathophysiology

The hyperpigmentation seen in CALMs is due to increased amounts of melanin within the keratinocytes. The underlying cause of this is not known.

Clinical presentation

CALMs are typically oval-shaped, completely macular patches, which may be located anywhere on the body, except the mucous membranes. Their usual size ranges from 2 to 5 cm, but may sometimes be smaller or larger. CALMs tend to grow as the body grows and are not associated with malignancy (Figure 18-7). Rarely, CALMs are associated with an underlying systemic disorder such as neurofibromatosis (see chapter 6 for details).

DIFFERENTIAL DIAGNOSIS Café au lait macules

- Linear nevoid hyperpigmentation
- Early nevus spilus (before nevi appear within the tan patch)
- Postinflammatory hyperpigmentation (PIH)
- Phytophotodermatitis

Management

It is not medically necessary to treat CALMs, as malignant transformation has not been reported. Hydroquinone is not effective, and laser treatment has had variable results. The risks of laser surgery include scarring, dyspigmentation, incomplete clearance, and recurrence.

Prognosis and complications

CALMs sometimes fade after childhood. Most CALMs are not associated with systemic disease; however, the provider should examine patients who present with multiple CALMs closely for additional features that may indicate an associated syndrome.

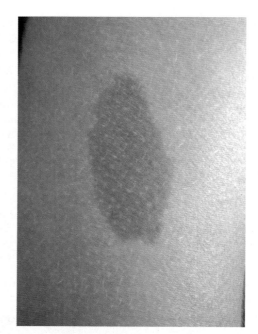

FIG. 18-7. Café au lait macule.

Referral and consultation

If there is clinical suspicion for any associated syndromes with CALMs, referral to the appropriate specialists for evaluation and management should be done promptly. Genetic counseling and testing may be indicated. If neurofibromatosis is suspected, multidisciplinary evaluation and management are essential (see chapter 6).

Patient education and follow-up

Patients and their parents should be reassured that CALMs are typically benign lesions. They should notify their provider if any change develops within the lesion(s).

A full skin examination should be performed on patients with CALMs to look for other signs of associated syndromes.

Erythema Ab Igne

Erythema Ab Igne (EAI), also known as *toasted skin syndrome* or *fire stains*, describes a local area of erythema and reticulated hyperpigmentation. It is caused by chronic exposure of the skin to heat sources such as heating pads or open fire. The incidence of this condition had dramatically declined with the invention of central heating; however, the introduction of the laptop computer has brought a resurgence in the condition. Other heat sources include hot water bottles, electric heaters, radiators, car heaters, heated reclining chairs, and electric blankets.

Pathophysiology

EAI develops from long-term exposure to heat below 113° F. The exposure is not hot enough to cause a thermal burn, but does cause injury to the epidermis and superficial vasculature. Reticulated erythema develops, followed by reticulated hyperpigmentation. The exact pathogenesis is unknown.

Clinical presentation

Early EAI presents with reticular, net-like erythema that blanches easily. It is most commonly seen in the lumbosacral region, abdomen,

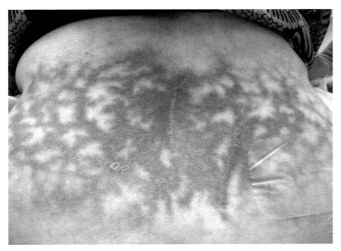

FIG. 18-8. Erythema Ab Igne on the lower back with a Fentanyl patch providing a clue about the underlying chronic back pain.

and anterior legs (Figure 18-8). Over time, the erythema evolves into hyperpigmentation and does not blanch. Lesions are typically asymptomatic. Patients will usually have a history of chronic local heat exposure. There may be a history of chronic back pain where the patient often uses a heating pad. The developing abnormal pigmentation may go undetected as the patient has difficulty viewing their back. Children and adults who lived in undeveloped countries may have EAI from lying close to a fire for warmth. If the heat source is not obvious, the provider should inquire about occupation and hobbies.

DIFFERENTIAL DIAGNOSIS Erythema Ab Igne

- Livedo reticularis
- Cutis mammorata telanciectasia congenita
- Poikiloderma
- Vasculitis

Diagnostics
EAI is usually a clinical diagnosis when the source of heat exposure has been identified. A punch biopsy may be done if EAI is uncertain.

Management
Discontinuation of offending heat source is most important. If caught early, EAI may sometimes be responsive to topical therapies including off-label use of tretinoin, Tri Luma, and corticosteroids. Chronic changes of EAI are very stubborn and not usually responsive. If a patient presents with EAI from heating pad use, the source of pain must be managed.

Prognosis and complications
After removal of the chronic heat source, early EAI sometimes resolves spontaneously. Pigmentation from chronic or severe EAI may be permanent. Epithelial atypia can develop from the chronic inflammation and potentially lead to squamous cell carcinoma (SCC) and Bowen disease.

Referral and consultation
If the patient is applying heat chronically, the source of pain and discomfort must be identified. A full review of systems must be performed to uncover any unknown systemic disease.

Patient education and follow-up
Patients should be instructed to avoid the source of heat exposure, if possible. Skin cancer education and prevention should be provided and the increased risk of developing SCC in the affected area must be explained. Patients should be advised to follow up for any changes in the skin.

Confluent and Reticulated Papillomatosis of Gougerot and Carteaud

Confluent and reticulated papillomatosis of Gougerot and Carteaud (CARP) is a disorder of reticulated or net-like hyperpigmentation that typically occurs on the chest and upper back. Young adult females are affected more often than males, and individuals with dark skin are affected more often than those with light skin. There have been some familial cases reported.

Pathophysiology
The exact etiology of CARP is unknown. A genetic defect in keratinization, overproduction of yeast (*Malassezia* or *Pityrosporum*) and bacteria, endocrine abnormalities, and response to UVR exposure are among the suspected causes.

Clinical presentation
Scaly hyperpigmented macules and papules begin on the midsternal chest or the midline of the back. Lesions coalesce to form larger plaques with reticular or net-like borders (Figure 18-9). Lesions may be itchy or asymptomatic. Sometimes lesions appear to be hypopigmented with fine white scale and are often mistaken for tinea versicolor.

DIFFERENTIAL DIAGNOSIS Confluent and reticulated papillomatosis of Gougerot and Carteaud

- Tinea versicolor
- Postinflammatory hyperpigmentation
- Acanthosis nigricans

Diagnostics
KOH preparation should eliminate the diagnosis of tinea versicolor. However, if KOH prep is equivocal, a tissue sample should be sent for periodic acid–Schiff (PAS) fungal staining to help detect the presence of a fungal organism. CARP associated with metabolic and hormonal disturbances should include patient screening for diabetes, thyroid disease, and polycystic ovary syndrome.

Management
Although the cause of CARP is unclear, several therapies have been effective in treating it. Minocycline 100 mg twice daily for 6 weeks is effective in most cases. Amoxicillin, azithromycin, and topical mupirocin have also been successful. Topical tretinoin and/or oral retinoids (isotretinoin or acitretin) have been used successfully, as they reduce abnormal cell turnover and reduce the hyperkeratotic surface of the papules/plaques. CARP has responded to oral contraceptives when occurring along with polycystic ovary syndrome. Systemic or topical antifungal agents have also been effective, if fungal elements are present.

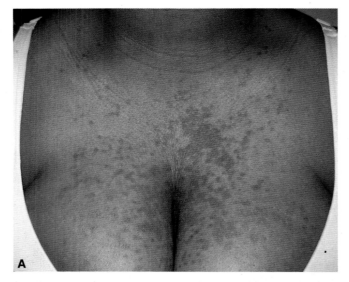

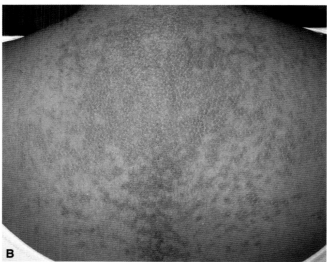

FIG. 18-9. CARP. **A:** The chest and back are the most commonly affected areas. **B:** Note the raised, hyperkeratotic coalesced papules on upper back that are sometimes misdiagnosed as acanthosis nigricans.

Prognosis and complications

CARP is a chronic condition with periods of exacerbation and remission. It is responsive to treatment but often recurs when treatment is discontinued.

Patient education and follow-up

Patients should have the expectation that this is a chronic condition with exacerbations and remissions, and there is no cure.

Postinflammatory Hyperpigmentation

Postinflammatory hyperpigmentation (PIH) can occur commonly as a result of inflammatory dermatoses and as a complication of many therapeutic interventions and mechanical injuries. PIH is more common in those with darker skin tones, but it also affects Caucasians. Many patients confuse PIH with scarring.

Pathophysiology

PIH occurs when epidermal and/or dermal melanocytes are stimulated by inflammation, causing an increase in melanogenesis, as well as an increase in pigment deposition in surrounding keratinocytes. The inflammation may have an endogenous cause from systemic disease or cutaneous skin conditions such as acne or cystic lesions. Exogenous inflammation can be induced by many mechanisms such as chronic friction/scratching or manipulation of acne lesions.

Clinical presentation

Patients who have PIH have a history of a preceding inflammation or injury to the skin. Lesions can range from light brown color occurring in the epidermis to a deeper dermal melanosis appearing dark brown, gray, or bluish. PIH will appear differently on various skin types. It will appear darker in those with darker skin tones and pink or light purple in individuals with skin type I to III (Figure 18-10).

PIH commonly results from acne, lichen planus, systemic lupus erythematosus, and chronic eczematous dermatitis. Some lesions may fade significantly, while others may be permanently disfiguring. PIH can worsen with sun exposure.

DIFFERENTIAL DIAGNOSIS Postinflammatory hyperpigmentation

- Melasma
- Acanthosis nigricans
- Drug-induced hyperpigmentation
- Systemic lupus
- Discoid lupus
- Sarcoidosis

Diagnostics

The diagnosis of PIH is typically made clinically by history and physical examination. Epidermal lesions have accentuated borders under wood lamp examination, while dermal lesions are not accentuated and are poorly demarcated. A skin biopsy may be performed if definitive diagnosis cannot be made.

Management

Treatment of PIH requires time and patience, as it may take 6 to 12 months. Acne should be treated early and efficiently to prevent PIH, especially in darkly pigmented skin. Topical preparations, such as tretinoin and azelaic acid, are used to treat acne and may

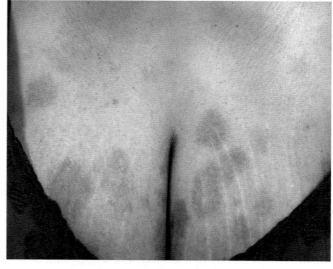

FIG. 18-10. Postinflammatory hyperpigmentation in a patient after acute eczematous dermatitis.

also be effective at minimizing hyperpigmentation. Patients should also be advised to wear sunscreen daily to avoid worsening of the symptoms. Other topical therapies may be used for PIH with variable responses (see management of Melasma above). Caution must be used in darkly-skinned individuals because of the increased risk of hypopigmentation.

Prognosis and complications

PIH can be emotionally difficult for adolescents and those with darker skin types. PIH usually fades within 6 to 12 months, but may not resolve completely in severely inflammatory conditions such as lichen planus or lupus. Sun protection and the topical treatments stated above are usually effective.

Referral and consultation

If PIH is refractory to treatment or severe, then refer to a cosmetic dermatology provider who has experience in laser treatment and specifically one who has experience using lasers on darkly pigmented skin.

Patient education and follow-up

Patients often think that PIH is the same as scarring and must be informed of the difference. Patients should be instructed to avoid manipulation of acne lesions, friction or irritation to their skin. Sun protection is important to minimize worsening of the condition.

PHOTODERMATOSES

Photodermatoses are a group of cutaneous disorders which occur only in the presence of ultraviolet light exposure. UVL causes acute and chronic changes in the skin which may necessitate a visit to a primary care clinician and/or dermatologist. In this section, we will review some of the most common light-related disorders.

In chapter 2, the spectrum of ultraviolet light was reviewed. UVA and UVB wavelengths were identified as major causes of skin disorders. UVA with its capacity for deeper penetration is the spectrum of light that causes photoallergic and phototoxic reactions, which will be discussed in this section.

Phototoxic Reaction

Phototoxic reactions are not immune-mediated skin reactions and occur when an individual is exposed to sunlight while using a sensitizing systemic or topical agent (Box 18-1).

Pathophysiology

The inflammatory reaction occurs when an appropriate concentration of a photosensitizer is absorbed into the skin and is subsequently exposed to UVA light. In theory, all exposed individuals should have the same reaction, but they do not. Photoactivation of the drug by UVA causes cellular damage, resulting in the inflammatory eruption.

Clinical presentation

A phototoxic reaction results in a sunburn-like appearance. The intensity of the reaction depends on the dose of the photosensitizer used. Typically, the "sunburn" begins within 2 to 6 hours after exposure and then worsens for 2 to 3 days before it subsides. The reaction only occurs on sun-exposed skin.

DIFFERENTIAL DIAGNOSIS Phototoxic reaction

- Photoallergic dermatitis
- Porphyria cutanea tarda
- Subacute cutaneous lupus erythematosis

BOX 18-1 | **Agents That Cause Phototoxic Reactions**

Topical agents
Coal tar derivatives
Perfume (Bergamot)

Systemic agents
5-Aminolevulinic acid
5-Fluouracil
Acitretin
Fluoroquinolones
Furosemide
Hydrochlorothiazide
Isotretinoin
Itraconazole
Methyl-5-aminolevulinic acid
Nonsteroidal anti-inflammatory drugs
PABA
PDT prophotosensitizers
Phenothiazines
Sulfonamide
Tetracyclines
Voriconazole

Adapted from Habif, T. P. (2010). *Clinical dermatology: A color guide to diagnosis and therapy* (5th ed.). Philadelphia, PA: Mosby.

Diagnostics

Laboratory testing should be considered based on the patient's history and review of symptoms. An ANA screening may be performed to check the patient for lupus erythematosus. A negative result means that acute cutaneous lupus erythematosus is unlikely, but subacute and discoid lupus may still be considered. ANA screening should be interpreted with clinicopathologic correlation. A 24-hour urine analysis can be done for uroporphyrin and corproporphyrin levels. This should be normal in a photoallergic reaction.

Photopatch testing is a great tool to aid in the diagnosis of photoallergic contact dermatitis. Suspected photoallergens are applied to the skin in two sets. After 24 hours, one set is irradiated with UVA. Both sets are evaluated for reaction after 48 hours. Erythema, edema, and/or blistering indicate a positive reaction. If the positive reaction is at the irradiated site only, then it is a photoallergic reaction. If a positive reaction occurs at both sites, it indicates allergic contact dermatitis. If a reaction is seen at both sites, but the reaction is stronger at the irradiated site, then the test result should be interpreted as both photoallergic contact dermatitis and allergic contact dermatitis.

Skin biopsy (preferably punch technique) can be helpful. Histologic changes show epidermal spongiosis with dermal lymphocytic infiltrates, which is very similar to the histologic findings seen in contact dermatitis, but the presence of necrotic keratinocytes is suggestive of phototoxicity. A skin biopsy may also differentiate cutaneous lupus or porphyria cutanea tarda from a phototoxic reaction.

Management

First, identification and avoidance of the photosensitizing agent must be done. Topical and systemic corticosteroids may provide relief to the erupted skin. Cool compresses are helpful in relieving discomfort. Nonsteroidal anti-inflammatory drugs (NSAIDs) are not recommended, as they may potentiate the phototoxic reaction. As phototoxic reactions are primarily triggered by UVA, patients should use sunscreens that contain UVA-protective ingredients such as avobenzone, titanium dioxide, and zinc oxide. A phototoxic reaction cannot occur in the absence of UVR exposure.

Prognosis and complications

Sun protection usually prevents reactions. If repeated phototoxic injury occurs, there may be chronic effects on the skin. These effects include premature aging of the skin and increased risk of skin cancer. Phototoxic reactions, especially those resulting from topical photosensitizers, may cause significant hyperpigmentation.

Generally, most patients' symptoms resolve once the offending agent is removed, although it may take weeks to months depending on the compound. TCS are often used to provide relief of symptoms. Systemic corticosteroids should only be used in severe cases.

Referral and consultation

Patients should be referred to dermatology for photopatch testing.

Patient education and follow-up

Patients with phototoxic reactions should avoid the causative agent, and protect themselves from the sun. Even normal UVR exposure that has not caused problems in the past may result in a severe reaction with these drugs. The patient must be educated on the potential for phototoxicity if they are being prescribed any new medication. Sunscreens should be broad-spectrum UVA/UVB protective, containing zinc oxide, titanium dioxide, or avobenzone.

Phytophotodermatitis

Phytophotodermatitis (PPD) is a phototoxic reaction that may occur at any time, without prior sensitization to the offending agent. It occurs when the skin comes in contact with a plant or fragrance containing *furocoumarin*. Furocoumarins are chemical compounds which occur naturally in a variety of plants and vegetables commonly ingested. In nature, they are used as a defense against predators and are responsible for the classic eruption known as PPD in humans. The average dose commonly ingested, however, is apparently too low to elicit this phototoxic reaction.

Pathophysiology

Skin is exposed to furocoumarins or other photosensitizing substances and is then exposed to UVA light, which is the spectrum responsible for PPD.

When UVL comes in contact with furocoumarin, the energy is absorbed, raising furocoumarin from its ground state to a triple excited state. When it returns to its ground state, energy is released and causes damage to the keratinocytes. Postinflammatory pigment alteration follows, and resolves spontaneously.

Clinical presentation

Symptoms start several hours after exposure. Patients initially experience burning and erythema of the affected area. Sometimes erythema, vesicles, and/or bullae follow. Residual brown hyperpigmentation persists for weeks to months.

Patients may have had an exposure to a furocoumarin-containing plant or have used a fragrance product containing oil of Bergamot (Box 18-2). The exposure to the latter usually causes the eruption to appear on the face and neck. Sometimes grocery workers or celery farmers are affected, as celery, as well as celery roots contains furocoumarin. Limes very commonly cause PPD (Figure 18-11). This is frequently seen in patients who have recently returned from vacation in a sunny climate where they may have squeezed lime into beverages while lounging on the beach. Sometimes people will rinse their hair in lime juice, and then expose themselves to the sun. This will result in the dermatitis being distributed on the neck and hairline.

BOX 18-2	**Plants Containing Psoralen Compounds**

Angelica
Carrot (wild)
Celery
Cow parsley
False bishop's weed
Fig (wild)
Hogweed
Meadow grass (agrimony)
Parsnip (wild parsnip)
Persian limes
Rue
Sweet orange
Wild angelica

DIFFERENTIAL DIAGNOSIS Phytophotodermatitis

- Allergic contact dermatitis
- Autoimmune bullous disorder
- Herpes simplex virus
- Porphyria cutanea tarda

Diagnostics

PPD is usually a clinical diagnosis. Laboratory tests are done to rule out other suspected diseases. If clinically indicated, porphyrin levels should be checked. If there is clinical suspicion of herpes simplex virus, then a viral culture may be helpful. Photopatch testing should be done if phototoxic and photo allergic dermatitis cannot be distinguished from each other clinically. If the clinical picture remains unclear, skin biopsy should be helpful, as PPD has distinct histopathologic features.

Management

Reassurance that PPD will resolve with discontinuation of offending agent is important once the diagnosis is made. Cool compresses, NSAIDs, and TCS may provide relief of acute inflammation. The

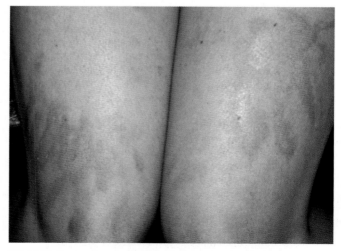

FIG. 18-11. Phototoxic reaction. Note the hyperpigmentation that follows the acute phase of phytophotodermatitis.

hyperpigmentation that follows will resolve spontaneously over time. Sun avoidance will help to speed that process.

Prognosis and complications

The prognosis of PPD is good once the patient is aware of and avoids the offending agent. If the patient cannot comply with removal of the offending agent, they should either avoid the sun completely or use a sunscreen that effectively blocks UVA.

Photoallergy

Photoallergic dermatoses are true allergic reactions (type IV hypersensitivity), which require the patient's immune system to be sensitized to a particular allergen when triggered by UVL. It can be related to a systemic medication or a topical agent (Box 18-3).

Pathophysiology

Photoallergic reactions are a cell-mediated immune response that occurs when a photosensitizing drug is activated by the sun and is transformed into a new molecule. This new molecule is then interpreted as foreign material by the body. Langerhans cells present the new material (antigen) to the T lymphocytes, which become activated and initiate an inflammatory response in the skin.

Clinical presentation

Photoallergic reactions typically begin on sensitized patients 24 to 48 hours after exposure. If the offending allergen is administered systemically, the reaction may be more widespread than an allergen exposed through contact. In the acute phase of this type IV hypersensitivity reaction, moderate-to-severe erythema and vesiculation are presenting signs. In later stages or with chronic exposure, the eruption evolves into a milder erythematous scaling or may present with lichenified papules or plaques.

Skin eruptions from photoallergic reactions are typically seen in areas of direct sun exposure (photodistribution) and spare the areas that are not exposed (e.g., axillae, bathing suit area, buttocks, inframammary folds; Figure 18-12). If a photo eruption is suspected, examine the unexposed areas for diagnostic clues as they should be uninvolved.

DIFFERENTIAL DIAGNOSIS Photoallergy

- Sunburn
- Subacute cutaneous lupus erythematosis
- Drug eruption
- Polymorphous light eruption
- Porphyria cutanea tarda

Diagnostics

See phototoxic reaction.

Management

Identification and avoidance of the allergen and sun protection are crucial. Unless sunscreens are the suspected cause of the photoallergy, they should be used. As photoallergic reactions are primarily triggered by UVA, patients should use sunscreens that contain UVA-protective ingredients such as avobenzone, titanium dioxide, and zinc oxide. TCS may provide relief to the erupted skin. Oral corticosteroids should only be used in severe cases.

Prognosis and complications

The prognosis for a photoallergic reaction is good once the offending agent is discovered and removed, although the photosensitivity

---

BOX 18-3 | **Agents That May Cause Photoallergic Dermatitis**

5-Fluorouracil
Celecoxib
Cinnamates
Dapsone
Hydrochlorothiazide
Itraconazole
Ketoprofen
Oral contraceptives
PABA
Phenothiazines
Quinidine
Salicylates
Sulfonylureas

Adapted from Habif, T. P. (2010.) *Clinical dermatology: A color guide to diagnosis and therapy* (5th ed.). Philadelphia, PA: Mosby.

---

and lesions may take weeks to months to resolve. If light reactivity persists, premature aging of the skin may occur, and the risk of developing skin cancer increases. Hyperpigmentation does not usually result from photoallergic reactions.

Referral and consultation

Patients with suspected photoallergic eruptions without an identifiable cause should be referred to dermatology for possible photopatch testing.

Patient education and follow-up

Patients should be reassured that once the offending allergen is identified and avoided, their symptoms will resolve. Patients must be counseled about the potential photosensitizing properties of medications they are taking.

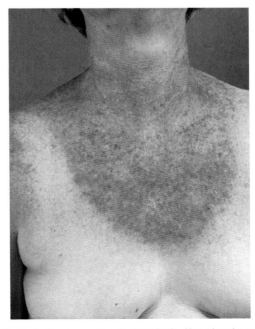

FIG. 18-12. Photoallergic reaction to griseofulvin. Note that the eruption is only occurring in the sun-exposed area. Upper chest involvement is common.

Polymorphous Light Eruption

Polymorphous light eruption (PMLE) is a common, idiopathic photodermatitis that typically occurs in springtime; following a person's first few sun exposures and often referred to as sun poisoning. It affects all races and age groups, and there is a hereditary form of PMLE seen in Native Americans. It is more common in northern climates where the sun is more intense in the spring and residents have more episodic exposure. It is less common in climates where the sun is intense all year presumably because of a type of desensitization.

Pathophysiology

PMLE is triggered by both wavelengths UVA and UVB. PMLE seems to be a delayed-type hypersensitivity reaction. Photo-provocation studies have shown perivascular infiltrates of $CD4^+$ T lymphocytes occurring within hours of UVL exposure, and $CD8^+$ cells within days of UVR exposure. The responsible antigens have yet to be defined. The susceptibility to PMLE is thought to be genetic.

Clinical presentation

Patients usually present after an early spring exposure or during a tropical vacation where the sun is more intense than usual. It may develop hours to days after sun exposure, and may last for days or weeks if exposure is continued. The eruption tends to improve as the summer continues, as the skin becomes "hardened" to UVR.

The early symptoms of PMLE are burning, itching, and erythema on sun-exposed skin. Areas that are commonly affected are the face, upper chest, dorsal hands, forearms, and the lower legs. Several different patterns of PMLE can be observed. The most common type is the *papular type,* in which small erythematous dermal papules appear on a patchy erythematous base (Figure 18-13). The second most common type is the *plaque type,* where superficial urticarial plaques are seen. The least common type is the *papulovesicular* type, where urticarial plaques develop into vesicles.

DIFFERENTIAL DIAGNOSIS Polymorphous light eruption
• Lupus erythematosis
• Photodrug eruption

Diagnostics

Diagnosis may be made clinically. Skin biopsy may be helpful in ruling out lupus erythematosis. In PMLE, the biopsy shows dermal edema, lymphocytic perivascular infiltrates, minimal epidermal damage, and no mucin. Mucin is generally seen histologically in lupus. An ANA screening should be performed if lupus is suspected; however, patients with PMLE may have a positive ANA as well. Review of systems should help to further differentiate between the two.

Management

High-potency TCS are usually effective at relieving the eruption. Brief courses of oral corticosteroids may be used in severe cases. Hydroxychloroquine 400 mg per day for the first month, then 200 mg per day throughout the summer is effective. Phototherapy with either NBUVB or PUVA may be used to increase the skin's tolerance to sun exposure by desensitizing the skin. Patients who have PMLE should minimize sun exposure, wear sun-protective clothing, and use broad-spectrum sunscreens.

Prognosis and complication

Lesions may last for 7 to 10 days, and patients will generally develop increased tolerance to UVR into the summer. The same type of

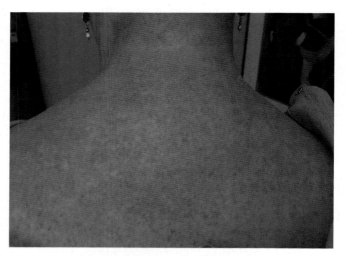

FIG. 18-13. Polymorphous light eruption on the upper back.

PMLE rash may recur the following spring or with the intense exposure and may develop for many years.

Referral and consultation

If TCS and sun protection are not working well, refer to a dermatology for consideration of phototherapy as the next desired modality of treatment.

Patient education and follow-up

Patients need to be counseled on sun protection. Extensive discussion about sun avoidance and proper sunscreen use is imperative. Dermaguard is a sun-protective film that may be applied to windows at home and in their car and needs to be replaced every 5 years. (See chapter 2 for a full discussion of sun protection.) Once the diagnosis of PMLE is made, a follow-up appointment can be made for the next early spring.

BILLING CODES ICD-10	
Chronic photodermatitis	L57.8
Café au lait macules	L81.3
Drug-induced pigmentation	L59.8
Erythema Ab Igne	L81.9
Hypopigmentation	L81.9
Lentigo	L81.4
Melasma	L81.1
Photodermatitis	L56.8
Phytophotodermatitis	L56.2
Pityriasis alba	L30.5
Vitiligo	L80

READINGS

Bolognia, J. L., Jorizzo, J. L., & Rapini, R. P. (2008). *Dermatology* (2nd ed.). Philadelphia, PA: Mosby.

Habif, T. P. (2010) *Clinical dermatology: A color guide to diagnosis and therapy* (5th ed.). Philadelphia, PA: Mosby.

Habif, T. P., Campbell, J. L., Chapman, M. S., Dinulos, J. G. H., & Zug, K. A. (2011). *Skin disease diagnosis and treatment* (3rd ed.). Edinburgh: Saunders Elsevier.

James, W. D., Berger, T. G., & Elston, D. M. (2011). *Andrews' diseases of the skin: Clinical dermatology* (11th ed.). Philadelphia, PA: Saunders.

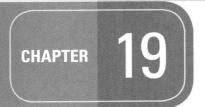

CHAPTER 19

Cutaneous Manifestations of Systemic Diseases

Susan Thompson Voss

Of all the organs of the human body, the skin is the largest. There are skin diseases which affect only the skin. However, there are many conditions of the skin that may signal to the clinician a potential internal disease or dysfunction. The patient will often seek advice from their primary care provider (PCP) when these skin symptoms arise. The ability to identify these cutaneous manifestations of internal or systemic conditions and malignancy is important.

PRURITUS

Pruritus is defined as an unpleasant sensation of the skin leading to the desire to scratch. It can be acute or chronic (>6 weeks in duration) and can arise from a variety of skin disorders and systemic diseases. Chronic itch has been reported in 10% to 50% of patients with a systemic disease or illness. It is estimated that less than 1% to 8% involve a malignancy. Systemic diseases associated with chronic pruritus include endocrine and metabolic disorders, infections, hematological and lymphoproliferative diseases, solid tumor neoplasms, and dermatologic conditions. Pruritus may be drug induced as well as have a neurogenic or psychogenic etiology (Table 19-1). Individuals of any age can be plagued by chronic itch, but it is more prevalent in the elderly, and females are more affected than males.

Pathophysiology

The skin does not contain dedicated receptors for pruritus. Pain and pruritus are both transmitted through unmyelinated C fibers of polymodal nociceptors, each of the sensations by a distinct subgroup of neurons which enter the dorsal cord of the spinal cord, synapse, cross the midline, and ascend to the spinothalamic tract. Keratinocytes release a variety of mediators in response to the pruritic stimuli, including histamines, cytokines, leukotrienes, opioids, kinins,

TABLE 19-1 Drugs Associated with Pruritus

DRUG CLASS/INDICATION	AGENT(S)
Antiarrhythmic	Amiodarone
Anticoagulant	Ticlopidine, fractionated heparin
Antidiabetic	Biguanide, sulfonylurea derivatives
Antiepileptic	Carbamazepine, oxcarbazepine, phenytoin, fosphenytoin, topiramate
Antihypertensive	Angiotensin-converting enzyme inhibitors*, angiotensin II antagonists, β-adrenergic blockers, calcium-channel blockers, methyldopa
Antimicrobial, chemotherapeutic	Penicillin*, cephalosporin, macrolides, carbapenem, monobactam, quinolone, tetracycline, lincosamide, streptogramin, metronidazole, rifampin, thiamphenicol, trimethoprim/ sulfamethoxazole, antimalarial (chloroquine*[†])
Cytokines, growth factors, monoclonal antibodies	Granulocyte macrophage colony-stimulating factor, interleukin 2*, mitumomab, lapatinib
Cytostatic	Chlorambucil, paclitaxel, tamoxifen
Erectile dysfunction	Sildenafil
Lipid lowering	Statins*
Plasma volume expander	Hydroxyethyl starch (HES)*
Psychotropic	Tricyclic antidepressants, selective serotonin reuptake inhibitors, neuroleptics
Other	Antithyroid agents, nonsteroidal anti-inflammatory drugs, corticosteroids, sex hormones, opioids*, inhibitors of xanthine oxidase, allopurinol

* Most common.

[†] Especially in 60% to 70% African Americans.

Adapted from Reich, A., Stander, S., & Szepietowski, J. C. (2009). Drug-induced pruritus: A review. *Acta Dermato Venereologica, 89,* 236–244. doi: 10.2340/00015555-0650.

prostaglandins, and many others. The pathophysiology of pruritus has been debated and studied by many. It is complex and multifactorial, thus complicating diagnosis and treatment.

Clinical Presentation

Itch is a symptom without a primary lesion. A rash can be misleading since scratching can create secondary lesions, which can confuse the clinical picture and underlying etiology. In the absence of primary lesions, clinicians should assess that patient for underlying disease. The characteristics of the patient's itch may give the clinician clues about the etiology.

Renal causes

Chronic kidney disease (CKD) is the most common systemic cause for chronic pruritus. Patients with chronic renal failure (20%–80%) often experience generalized, intractable, and severe pruritus. It may be paroxysmal and remit spontaneously, or it may persist day and night. Dialysis-associated pruritus varies, in that patients may have episodic and more localized pruritus.

Many factors may be involved in pruritus from CKD. Peripheral neuropathy, elevated levels of calcium, magnesium, and sulfate secondary hyperparathyroidism, increased histamine levels, hypervitaminosis A, and iron-deficiency anemia may contribute to pruritus with CKD. Uremic pruritus is reported in about half of the patients undergoing dialysis. The etiology is unknown but is thought to be immunologic. Classic xerosis (dry skin) in these patients can exacerbate the symptoms (Figure 19-1).

Treatment of pruritus associated with CKD includes capsaicin 0.025% or 0.05% cream applied topically, calcineurin inhibitors, phototherapy (UVB), and acupuncture. Severe disease may require oral gabapentin, thalidomide, cholestyramine, and activated charcoal.

Hepatic causes

Chronic liver disease with or without cholestasis (obstruction of bile flow) may cause itch. The cause of the pruritus is probably multifactorial and not because of deposits of bile salts in the skin as first thought. The symptoms may be intermittent, mild, localized, or generalized and often have an insidious onset. Pruritus is reported by 20% of patients with hepatitis C virus (HCV), making it the most common symptom with the infection. Accordingly, HCV screening is warranted for patients complaining of severe pruritus with no obvious cause.

The main goal of treatment for pruritus in patients with known liver disease is treatment of the disease itself. Additional treatments may include naltrexone (opioid antagonist), cholestyramine, rifampin, and phototherapy. Due to the potential side effects and the need for close monitoring, collaboration between a gastroenterologist, dermatologist, and PCP is important.

Neuropathic causes

Neuropathic pruritus refers to an itch that results from a disease or disorder of the central or peripheral nervous system. Neuronal damage can cause pruritus. Notalgia paresthetica (NP) is an example of a neuropathic pruritus that is a common yet often missed diagnosis. NP is thought to be due to compression of posterior rami of the spinal nerves at the T2-T6 level. It is characterized by pruritus, burning, increased sensitivity, or tenderness around the angle of the scapula (Figure 19-2). A pigmented patch may be localized to the area of pruritus. Multiple sclerosis, neoplasms, brachioradial pruritus, postherpetic neuralgia, and vulvodynia are other neuropathic conditions that can cause pruritus.

Psychodermatoses

Many psychogenic conditions have been associated with pruritus, making diagnosis and treatment challenging. Depression, anxiety, obsessive-compulsive disorder, somatoform disorder, mania, psychosis, fatigue, and substance abuse may all be associated with an intense itch. Secondary lesions, such as neurotic excoriations, result from scratching or picking and are limited to body areas where the patient can reach. The lateral areas of the back and shoulders may be involved, while the midline back is spared ("butterfly sign"). Scarring may be present in a linear pattern and is indicative of a chronic problem. Lesions are also commonly found on the lateral and extensor aspects of the patient's arms and legs (Figure 19-3). Characteristic erosions have an angular or punched-out appearance from the patient picking with their nails or implements like tweezers. Chronic lesions may appear like prurigo nodules.

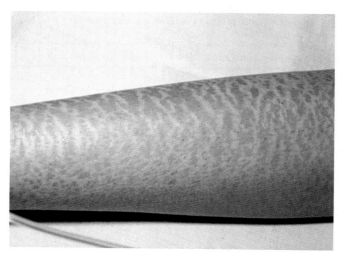

FIG. 19-1. Severe xerosis associated with renal failure.

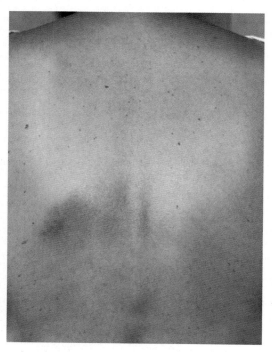

FIG. 19-2. Characteristics of NP include hyperpigmentation from severe pruritus near the angle of the scapula.

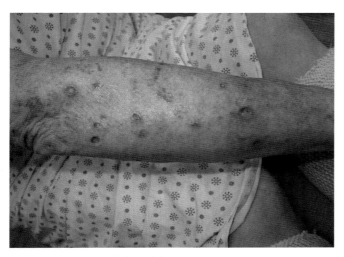

FIG. 19-3. Neurotic excoriations of the arm.

Patients with a psychodermatosis may not be aware of their scratching behavior, especially at night time, and may vehemently deny any scratching behavior. It can become a habit that is difficult to change and require behavioral therapy. Thus, identifying and treating the underlying psychological condition is extremely important.

Delusions of parasitosis are one example of a psychodermatitis. Patients suffering from this condition believe that they have "bugs" in their skin. Patients may bring in containers with pieces of skin or crusts that they have removed and are convinced that they are bugs. This can be an extremely difficult patient to manage but should begin with establishing the clinician–patient relationship. Clinicians must do a complete examination and carefully consider the possibility of a true infestation. Even when there is no identified cause, the clinician should acknowledge the strong physical and psychological stress that the patient is reporting. Offering good skin care education as well as low- to moderate-potency topical corticosteroids (TCS) can be helpful in alleviating the pruritus. On a follow-up visit, the clinician should introduce the idea of psychological counseling, not because the patient is "crazy," but because this condition is causing the patient so much anxiety and emotional upset.

Malignancy

For many PCPs, one of the most worrisome causes of pruritus is an underlying malignancy. This heightened concern occurs because pruritus is a reported symptom in virtually every form of carcinoma but varies in location and severity. For example, patients with leukemia usually have milder and generalized symptoms compared to pruritus associated with lymphoma which can be continuous and severe with burning characteristics. In Hodgkin lymphoma, pruritus is present in 10% to 30% of patients, with 7% reporting pruritus as their first symptom. Pruritus is reported in up to 15% of non-Hodgkin lymphoma patients.

Unfortunately, the symptom of itch associated with malignancies has resulted in unnecessary and extensive workups in pruritic patients without an obvious underlying cause. For this reason, it is important to evaluate the pruritic patient in a logical process. Clinicians should consider evaluation for an underlying malignancy when pruritus is generalized and persistent and without an identified cause. A workup is also warranted if the pruritus does not respond to conventional therapy. It should be noted that patients with idiopathic pruritus do not have a significant increased risk for malignant neoplasms when compared to the general population.

Human immunodeficiency virus/AIDS

Individuals with HIV often suffer from pruritus, and it may be the initial symptom in a few patients. A declining CD4 count seems to be associated with increased itch. For some patients with HIV, pruritus may be from a secondary infection or process such as Norwegian scabies, candidiasis, colonization of *Staphylococcus aureus*, an overgrowth of the Demodex mite, seborrheic dermatitis, acquired ichthyosis, Kaposi sarcoma, pruritic papular eruptions, and eosinophilic folliculitis.

DIFFERENTIAL DIAGNOSIS Pruritus

- Pruritus in the absence of a rash is a symptom
- Focus is on determining the underlying cause (Table 19-2)

TABLE 19-2	Diseases Associated with Pruritus
Dermatologic Diseases	
Inflammatory	Atopic dermatitis, psoriasis, contact dermatitis, dry skin, drug reactions, scars, "invisible dermatoses"
Infectious	Mycotic, bacterial and viral infections; folliculitis, scabies, pediculosis, arthropod reactions, insect bites
Autoimmune	Bullous dermatoses, especially dermatitis herpetiformis, bullous pemphigoid, dermatomyositis
Genodermatoses	Darier disease, Hailey–Hailey disease, ichthyoses, Sjögren–Larsson syndrome, epidermolysis bullosa pruriginosa
Dermatoses of pregnancy	Polymorphic eruption of pregnancy, pemphigoid gestationis, prurigo gestationis
Neoplasms	Cutaneous T-cell lymphoma, cutaneous B-cell lymphoma, leukemic infiltrates of the skin
Systemic Diseases	
Endocrine and metabolic	Chronic renal failure, liver diseases with or without cholestasis, hyperthyroid, hypothyroid, malabsorption, perimenopausal pruritus
Infectious	HIV infection, helminthiasis, parasitosis

TABLE 19-2 Diseases Associated with Pruritus *(continued)*	
Hematologic and lymphoproliferative	Iron deficiency, polycythemia vera, Hodgkin disease, Non-Hodgkin lymphoma, plasmocytoma
Visceral	Solid tumors of the cervix, prostate, or colon, carcinoid syndrome
Pregnancy	Pruritus gravidarum with and without cholestasis
Drug induced	Opioids, ACE inhibitors, amiodarone, hydrochlorothiazide, estrogens, simvastatin, hydroxyethyl starch, allopurinol
Neurologic and Psychiatric Diseases	
Neuropathic	Multiple sclerosis, neoplasms, abscesses, cerebral or spinal infarcts, brachioradial pruritus, nostalgia paresthetica, postherpetic neuralgia, vulvodynia, small fiber neuropathy
Somatoform	Psychiatric/psychosomatic diseases, depression, anxiety disorders, obsessive-compulsive disorders, schizophrenia, tactile hallucinosis, fatigue

ACE, angiotensin-converting enzyme.

Adapted from Stander, S., Weisshaar, E., Mettang, T., Szepietowski, J. C., Carstens, E., Ikoma, A., Bernhard, D. (2007). Clinical classification of itch: A position paper of the international forum for the study of itch. *Acta Dermato-Vernereologica, 87*, 291–294.

Diagnostics

Diagnosing the cause of chronic pruritus, on otherwise normal appearing skin, can be difficult and frustrating for the patient, their family, and the provider. The goal is to diagnose the etiology of the pruritus. The importance of a detailed review of symptoms, medical history, and physical examination cannot be overstated. Noting the start dates and duration of both over-the-counter and prescription medications is vital. A detailed history of the itch should note the following: when it started, aggravating factors, treatments that alleviate symptoms, and prior treatments. A review of symptoms may reveal other symptoms, not obvious to the patient, corresponding with the pruritus. Psychosocial symptoms should not be overlooked.

There is no consensus on the exact diagnostic workup for patients with severe pruritus without evidence of an underlying disease. Thus, an algorithmic approach to the initial diagnostics can be helpful (Figure 19-4). Be sure that the patient is current on their age-appropriate screening examinations. Diagnostic studies should also be considered based on the patient's family history or risk factors, even in the absence of symptoms. Positive findings should guide the clinician in ordering additional diagnostic tests. Caution should be used if prescribing systemic corticosteroids before the patient has been fully evaluated.

Management

To manage pruritus effectively, it is necessary to identify the underlying etiology. It is imperative that the provider first do a thorough history, including the patient's medical history, detailed history of the pruritus.

The initial treatment or first-line therapeutic approach for all patients should include good skin care as xerosis can contribute to severity of pruritus and should always be included in the management of pruritus (Box 19-1). This involves moisturizing the skin well and avoiding irritants (including fragrances, dyes, and other additives). Some moisturizers and emollients that contain menthol and/or camphor can be used intermittently to help alleviate the itch. However, good skin care provides only limited relief from the underlying disease causes.

Managing pruritus can be very challenging as there is no one treatment plan that suits every patient. If the underlying cause has not been identified, a stepwise approach should begin with first-line

therapies (Box 19-2). The plan of care for therapy should consider the patient's age, causative factors, comorbidities, expense, and psychological impact.

Topical therapy

Topical therapy is the treatment of choice for pruritus without a skin eruption. The goal is to decrease the itch sensation by directly applying the medication to the pruritic area. Topical anesthetics that can be utilized include capsaicin in concentrations up to 0.1%, pramoxine 1% or 2.5% cream, and a mixture of lidocaine and prilocaine 2.5% cream. Topical menthol provides a coolant effect. Doxepin 5% cream (a tricyclic antidepressant) may give some relief. Calcineurin inhibitors can be beneficial in facial and anogenital pruritus. TCS may be helpful but must be used with caution. Whenever TCS are used, patients should be educated about the signs and symptoms of secondary infections. The patient should be monitored closely to avoid skin atrophy from the corticosteroid. When topical therapy fails to control the itch or if the body surface area (BSA) involved is too extensive, then the clinician may need to add or change to systemic therapy.

Systemic therapy

Systemic therapies for pruritus should be utilized in combination with topical therapies when the topical therapies alone are unsuccessful. When possible, the systemic treatment should be targeted at the cause of the itch. Unfortunately, research has failed to reveal a singular effective drug for pruritus. An "add-on" approach is employed. Antihistamines at three to four times the usual recommended dosage are utilized initially. Antihistamines are often of limited efficacy. If ineffective, other medications may be added in a stepwise fashion.

Oral glucocorticoids should be limited to controlling acute severe forms of pruritus. In the literature, neuroactive medications—gabapentin and pregabalin—have been effective for treating pruritus caused by CKD as well as neuropathic pruritus. Selective serotonin reuptake inhibitors have also been reported to be beneficial for various forms of chronic pruritus. Mirtazapine, a noradrenergic and specific serotonergic antidepressant, may relieve nocturnal itch. Tricyclic antidepressants are sometimes utilized despite randomized trials for pruritus. Opiate agonists and antagonist may also aid in relief of resistant chronic pruritus.

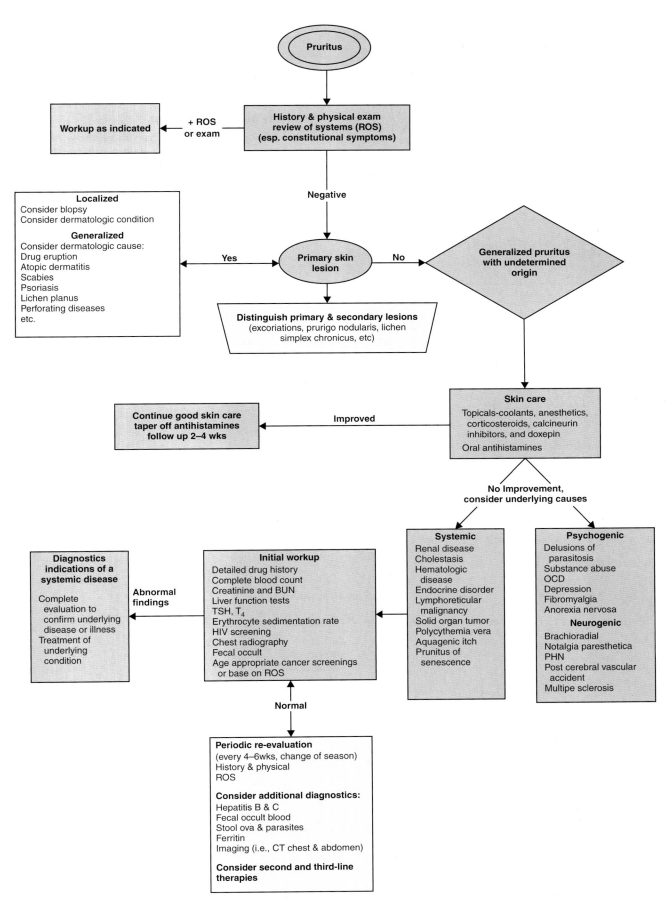

FIG. 19-4. Approach to assessing patients with chronic pruritus.

BOX 19-1 **Basic Care of Pruritic Skin**

Avoid hot water.

Bathe or shower in tepid/lukewarm water for 20 minutes.

Avoid washing with soap. When cleanser is needed, use a gentle, nondrying, fragrance-free one. Use mild soap only on the underarms, genitalia, and soles of the feet.

Apply topical emollients/moisturizers immediately after bathing to skin that has been gently patted dry.

Moisturizers with ceramides and lipids are preferred. If cost is an issue, petrolatum (petroleum jelly) may be used.

Moisturize an additional one to two times daily. Apply gently in the direction of hair growth. Caution: heavy emollients or occlusion can cause folliculitis.

Topicals with menthol and camphor may be utilized. Refrigeration may aid in the calming effect.

Avoid fragrance and dyes.

Other therapies

Occasionally, pruritus can be severe and recalcitrant to conventional therapies and require complex management. Primary care clinicians should refer these patients to dermatology for consideration of phototherapy with narrow-band phototherapy, intravenous immunoglobulin, and extracorporeal photophoresis. Consider behavioral-modification therapy that can complement other treatment modalities.

Prognosis and Complications

Chronic pruritus can have a significant physical as well as a psychological impact on the quality of life of the patients and their households. Symptomatic relief is often the focus of treatment unless there is an identified underlying cause. This can be frustrating for the patient and clinician. While treating the itch, it is important to monitor for signs and symptoms of secondary infection, such as impetigo, cellulitis, and herpes simplex virus, that may occur from scratching. A culture and sensitivity should be performed for diagnosis and treatment. Prognosis depends on the possible underlying disease associated with the pruritus.

Referral and Consultation

Referral to a dermatology provider should be considered when the cause of the pruritus is not apparent or when basic treatments have provided no relief. Other specialists may be consulted depending on the underlying disease. Collaboration with psychiatry can be helpful

BOX 19-2 | **Treatment for Pruritus**

First-Line Topical Therapies

Good skin care
Emollients—petrolatum, ceramide-based creams
Topical anti-inflammatory—corticosteroids, calcineurin inhibitors
Cooling agents—menthol, camphor, ice
Topical anesthetics—capsaicin, pramoxine, lidocaine/prilocaine
Predominantly nerve modulation—doxepin (topical amitriptyline)

 If little or no improvement, consider adding

Systemic: Antihistamines (AH)

Low dose—nonsedating AH daily
High dose—nonsedating AH b.i.d.–q.i.d., or combination with sedating AH at bedtime

First-Generation, Sedating	Second-Generation, Nonsedating
Hydroxyzine	Cetirizine
Diphenhydramine	Levocetirizine
	Fexofinidine
	Loratidine
	Desloratidine

 If little or no improvement, consider adding or changing

Other Systemic Agents*

1st choice	2nd choice	3rd choice
Gabapentin	SSRI	Naltrexone
Pregabalin	Mirtazapine	Lidocaine 5% patch
Selective serotonin reuptake inhibitors (SSRI), especially for paraneoplastic, polycythemia vera, or depression	Tricyclic and tetracyclic antidepressant	
Naltrexone, especially for renal or liver dysfunction	Phototherapy: narrow-band UVR	

*Off-label use.

Adapted from Steinhoff, M., Cevikbas, F., Ikoma, A., & Berger, T. G. (2011). Pruritus: Management algorithms and experimental therapies. *Seminars in Cutaneous Medicine and Surgery, 30,* 127–137. doi:10.1016/j.sder.2011.05.001

in patients with psychodermatoses. The introduction of this topic should be done carefully and after the clinician has developed a relationship with the patient.

Patient Education and Follow-up

It is prudent to monitor pruritic patients closely. Follow-up appointments made prior to the patient leaving the provider's office can help to facilitate compliance. Providers will often assume that lack of communication from the patient means that the treatment plan is working. Unfortunately, this is not always the case. Pruritic patients can become frustrated and depressed and lose hope that the itch will ever subside. To limit patient frustration, discussions about the challenging nature of pruritus treatment and the proposed treatment plan are appropriate. It is paramount that patients with pruritus be educated on good skin care.

DERMATITIS HERPETIFORMIS

Dermatitis herpetiformis (DH) is a chronic autoimmune blistering disease associated most commonly with celiac sprue disease or gluten sensitivity. Patients with DH have an increased incidence of other autoimmune diseases, including thyroid disease (40%), diabetes mellitus (DM), connective tissue disease, and small bowel lymphoma. DH has been reported internationally to be as high as 10 cases for a population of 100,000 and in the United States as high as 11.2 cases per population of 100,000 in one study. DH is rare in children. The typical age of onset is in the 20s to 40s, with males affected more than females (2:1). There is a higher incidence in individuals of Northern European descent and rare in those of Asian or African descent. See chapter 15 for additional information.

PEUTZ–JEGHERS SYNDROME

Peutz–Jeghers Syndrome (PJS) is an autosomal dominant inherited disorder characterized by extensive hamartomatous polyps and distinct hyperpigmented mucocutaneous lesions. The prevalence of PJS is estimated in the range of 1 in 8,300 to 280,000 individuals. The median age of diagnosis for PJS is 24.3 years. There is no increased prevalence based on sex, race, or ethnic group.

Polyps of PJS can cause intestinal obstruction, gastrointestinal bleeding, intussusception, and pain. Individuals with the disorder have a high risk of developing gastrointestinal cancers like stomach, pancreas, small intestines, and colorectal. Nongastrointestinal cancers include breasts, cervix, testicular, ovarian, and thyroid.

Pathophysiology

The cause of PJS in most cases appears to be a mutation of the *STK11/LKB1*, a tumor suppressor gene predisposing the individual to the formation of benign and malignant tumors. A parent with the gene has a 50% chance of passing it on to their child.

Clinical Presentation

Patients with PJS present with flat pigmented macules measuring 1 to 5 mm on the lips (often crossing the vermillion border), perioral area, nose, buccal mucosa, eyes, soles of the feet and palms, fingertips and under the nails, and anal area. They are typically blue-gray to brown and differ from freckles in that freckles never appear in the oral cavity (Figure 19-5). The pigmentation of PJS may occur at any age and most commonly during childhood but not at birth. Occasionally, the hyperpigmented macules of PJS can disappear during adolescence. Polyps found in the stomach and small intestines are likely diagnosed in childhood and young adults.

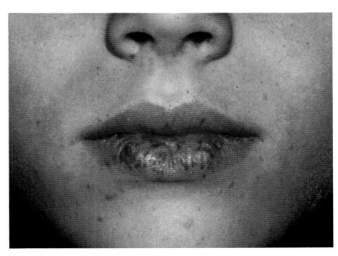

FIG. 19-5. Peutz–Jeghers syndrome: brown pigmented macules occurring in and around the oral mucosa and lips.

DIFFERENTIAL DIAGNOSIS Peutz–Jeghers syndrome
• Ephelides (freckles)
• Cowden syndrome
• Carney complex
• LEOPARD syndrome

Diagnostics

Diagnosis is defined by the presence of histopathologically confirmed hamartomatous polyps and at least two of the following clinical criteria: family history, characteristic hyperpigmentation, and polyps in the small bowel. Genetic testing is available for confirmation of PJS. The frequency of screening examinations is determined by family history, and gastrointestinal screening includes upper endoscopy, small intestine x-ray or capsule endoscopy, and colorectal examinations. Regular and frequent health screening includes pap and pelvic, breasts, prostate, testicles, and thyroid examinations.

Management

For the PCP, much of the management of the PJS patient involves prevention of symptoms and early detection of cancer. Coordinating and monitoring the appropriate cancer screenings at recommended intervals are paramount. Close surveillance should begin in childhood.

Prognosis and Complications

PJS is associated with significant morbidity, variable clinical course, and considerable predisposition to malignancies, especially gastrointestinal neoplasms. They also have increased risk of breast cancer, pancreatic cancer, and reproductive neoplasms when compared to the general population.

Referral and Consultation

Referral to a gastroenterology provider is important for appropriate screening, diagnosis, and management. PJS patients also benefit from genetic counseling.

Patient Education and Follow-up

Patient education should focus on signs and symptoms of gastrointestinal bleeding and obstruction. The importance of all cancer screenings and early recognition of disease should be reinforced. Close monitoring of the PJS patient is important. PCPs may assume that the patient is keeping all follow-up appointments with specialists, but this may not be true.

PORPHYRIA

Porphyria refers to a group of diseases caused by enzymatic defects in the heme biosynthetic pathway. Porphyrias may be classified by the primary site of enzymatic defect or clinically as acute and nonacute types (Figure 19-6). Acute types include variegate porphyria, hereditary coproporphyria, acute intermittent porphyria, and ALA dehydratase deficiency porphyria. Of the nonacute types, porphyria

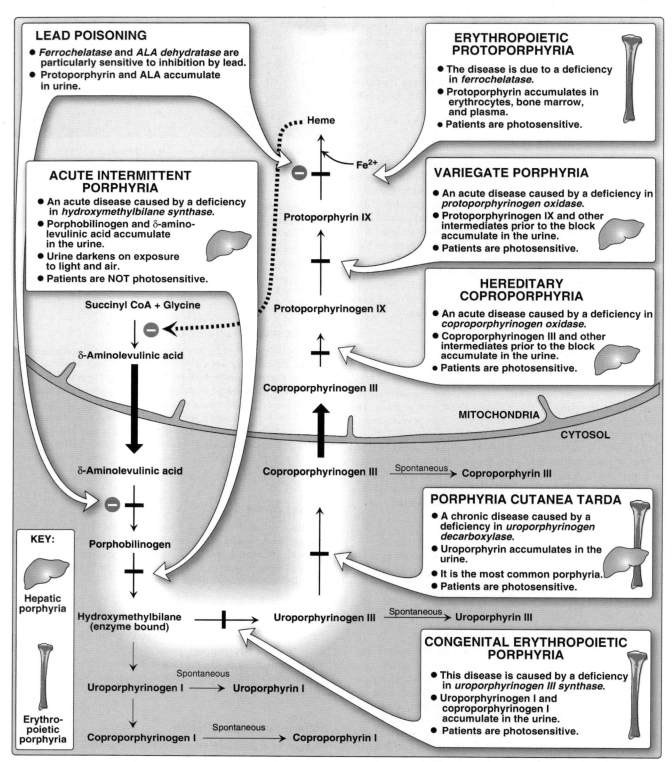

FIG. 19-6. Summary of heme synthesis in porphyrias.

cutanea tarda (PCT) is the most common and will be the focus of this section. Hepatoerythropoietic porphyria, congenital erythropoietic porphyria, and erythropoietic protoporphyria are also nonacute types that are uncommon.

Porphyria cutanea tarda is the most common and most readily treated type of porphyria. It is estimated that PCT rates are 1 case per 10,000 to 25,000 individuals. Both genders and all races are affected. The majority of PCT is acquired (80%) with a few familial cases (20%). The onset of PCT is usually in the third or fourth decade compared to the other nonacute porphyrias which begin during infancy or early childhood. It is associated with individuals who have hepatic iron overload and liver disease. There is a strong association between PCT and HCV and with mutations of the hemochromatosis gene.

Pathophysiology

In PCT, the activity of the heme synthetic enzyme uroporphyrinogen decarboxylase (UROD) is deficient, thus leading to increased uroporphyrin. UVR triggers the photoactivation of porphyrins, which causes oxidative damage to biomolecular targets and activation of the complement system. The result is the release (or activation) of dermal mast cells, leading to skin fragility, vesicles, and bullae.

The development of PCT can be influenced by both genetic and environmental factors. PCT can be precipitated by extrinsic factors such as alcohol abuse, medications (primarily estrogens and oral contraceptives), environmental pollutants, and viral infections (especially HCV), including HIV.

Clinical Presentation

Photosensitivity is the most common cutaneous manifestation of nonacute porphyrias. In a patient with PCT, the presenting features on sun-exposed areas include vesicles, bullae, erosions, burning, and edema (Figure 19-7). The dorsum of the hands is a common site and may reveal scars, milia, and hyper- or hypopigmentation from previous lesions (Figure 19-8). Increased skin fragility and scleroderma-like plaques (indurated and waxy) may be present on the neck, preauricular area, chest, and back. These classic findings should prompt the clinician to perform diagnostic testing for PCT.

Patients with PCT may report similar changes on their face and scalp in addition to violaceous coloration of the periorbital and malar areas. Facial hypertrichosis is a hallmark characteristic that occurs on the zygoma and malar prominences. This can be cosmetically

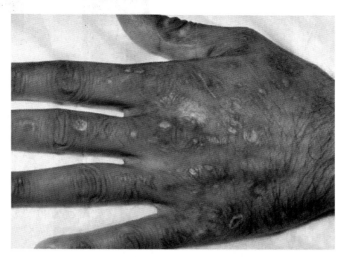
FIG. 19-8. Healing lesions of PCT with milia, scars, and abnormal pigmentation.

distressing in females and may be the impetus for their visit to a PCP or dermatologist. Males may complain about an increase in shaving. It has been suggested that the hypertrichosis of PCT led to the myth of werewolves. Alcohol ingestion can exacerbate porphyrias and flares of PCT.

DIFFERENTIAL DIAGNOSIS   Porphyria

- Epidermolysis bullosa (children)
- Epidermolysis bullosa acquisita (adults)
- Erythropoietic porphyria
- Pemphigus vulgaris
- Hydroa vacciniforme
- Bullous lupus erythematosus
- Pseudoporphyria

Diagnostics

Patients seeking treatment for cutaneous symptoms of PCT are likely to have a skin biopsy for histology, showing a subepidermal blister and festooning. However, skin biopsy is neither essential nor diagnostic. A perilesional biopsy for direct immunofluorescence can help differentiate PCT from an immunobullous disease.

A noninvasive analysis of the patient's fecal, plasma, urinary, and red blood cell porphyrins can be done. A 24-hour urine sample will have elevated levels of porphyrins, which confirms the diagnosis of PCT. Stool samples may only have trace amounts. If PCT is suspected, the clinician can perform a simple screening test and collect a random urine sample in the office. Using the Wood's light in a dark room, the urine specimen will fluoresce a bright red-pink (Figure 19-9). However, the absence of fluorescence does not exclude the diagnosis of PCT.

Serologic testing should include a complete blood count and serum ferritin levels which may be elevated in patients with PCT. A chemistry panel with special attention to liver function studies is important to evaluate the patient for liver disease. Patients should be screened for HCV and HIV.

Management

Treatment for PCT is threefold. It is imperative to identify and avoid triggers such as sun exposure, alcohol, and estrogen therapy.

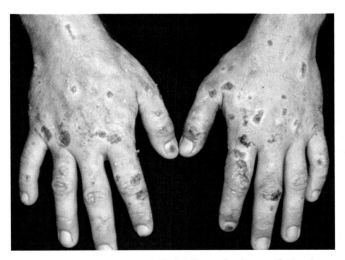
FIG. 19-7. Erosions, vesicles, and skin fragility on the dorsum of a hand suggest the need to test for PCT.

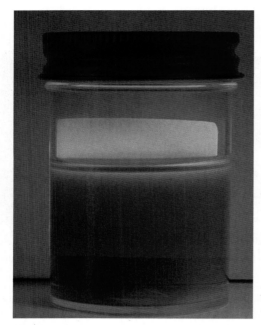

FIG. 19-9. Red fluorescence of urine with Wood light in PCT.

Removal of the offending agents can result in improving symptoms. Phlebotomy is the most common treatment used to reduce the iron overload and performed regularly until ferritin levels normalize. Low-dose antimalarials, iron chelators, and cholestyramine have been effective. Equally important, any associated HCV or HIV must be managed.

Prognosis and Complications

Given appropriate treatment, prognosis for PCT is very good. However, the skin fragility, blistering, and associated pain make performing certain jobs difficult, if not impossible. Mila, scarring, and pigment abnormalities are usually permanent. Secondary skin infections are common and should be treated appropriately. There may be an association between PCT and the development of hepatocellular carcinoma.

Referral and Consultation

Since PCT is a hepatic form of porphyria, consultation with a gastroenterologist or hepatologist is essential. Consultation with a dermatology provider for skin evaluation and biopsy may be considered. Phlebotomy and iron chelation therapies may best be managed by a referral to a hematologist. Females with PCT should be evaluated and counseled regarding birth control methods other than estrogen containing therapies. Patients with PCT who have alcohol dependency should be referred to counseling and support for avoidance.

Patient Education and Follow-up

Patients should be educated on the importance of following the prescribed treatment plan and follow-up. Knowledge regarding sun exposure and triggers for the disease is helpful. Physical blockers like titanium dioxide and zinc oxide, which reflect UVR, are the best type of sunscreens for these patients. However, sun avoidance and UV-protective clothing is the most important recommendation to help the patient achieve remission and avoid exacerbations.

PCT patients must be monitored closely for response to therapy. Hemoglobin, serum ferritin, and serum or plasma porphyrin levels must be monitored at least quarterly. Regular health maintenance and monitoring for complications including hepatic tumors should be emphasized.

PSEUDOPORPHYRIA

Pseudoporphyria is a bullous photosensitivity disorder that mimics PCT both clinically and histologically. Many think that it is not uncommon and is underreported in the literature. It affects males and females equally. No specific race is more impacted. Reported cases have ranged from 2 to 81 years of age.

Pathophysiology

The pathophysiology of pseudoporphyria is not fully understood but is attributed to medications, excessive sun exposure, UVA radiation from tanning beds, and chronic renal failure with hemodialysis. Naproxen is the most frequent offending agent in drug-induced pseudoporphyria. It has a higher incidence in children (fair-skinned) compared to adults, and women more than men. Other causative medications include antibiotics (tetracyclines and quinolones), furosemide, amiodarone, dapsone, voriconazole, nabumetone, and oxaprozin.

Clinical Presentation

Clinically, it is very difficult to distinguish pseudoporphyria from PCT as they both present with bullae, erosions, skin fragility, and milia on same sun-exposed areas of the head, face, and dorsal hands. Yet patients with pseudoporphyria do not have hypertrichosis, hyperpigmentation, or sclerodermoid changes—important diagnostic clues.

DIFFERENTIAL DIAGNOSIS Pseudoporphyria

- Bullous pemphigoid
- Epidermolysis bullosa
- Epidermolysis bullosa acquisita
- Erythropoietic protoporphyria
- Lupus erythematosus, bullous
- Porphyria cutanea tarda

Diagnostics

True porphyria must be ruled out in patients suspected of having pseudoporphyria. Unlike PCT, pseudoporphyria will have normal porphyrin levels in the urine, blood, and stools. Biopsy for histopathology will not differentiate pseudoporphyria from PCT.

Management

Elimination of the offending drug is usually adequate for cure. However, it can take several months for remission and skin lesions to heal.

Prognosis and Complications

The prognosis for pseudoporphyria is good except for possible permanent scarring and abnormal pigmentation from the lesions.

Referral and Consultation

Consultation with a dermatologist may be necessary for a skin evaluation and biopsy.

Patient Education and Follow-up

If pseudoporphyria was drug induced, it is important for the patient to avoid that drug and all others in the drug classification. The patient should be instructed to avoid excessive sun exposure and to avoid tanning beds. Periodic follow-up is helpful to make sure the patient is following the recommended plan of avoidance therapy.

LICHEN PLANUS

Lichen planus (LP) is a self-limiting pruritic inflammatory condition of unknown etiology. It is thought that cytotoxic T cells are activated in response to an antigen. LP may be idiopathic, or it may be associated with HCV infection. The cutaneous manifestation of LP may be the chief complaint of a patient who is unaware of their HCV infection (see chapter 5).

PERFORATING DERMATOSES

Perforating dermatoses (PDs) are most often associated with chronic renal failure and sometimes with DM. Eleven percent of patients on hemodialysis report a PD compared to its rare occurrence in the general population. It presents more frequently in African Americans and in women. PDs comprise Kyrle disease, perforating folliculitis, reactive perforating collagenosis, and elastosis perforans serpiginosa. Discriminating between the four types can be difficult; thus the term PD was proposed and is utilized to address and include all four forms.

Pathophysiology

The hallmark of PD is transepidermal elimination of material from the dermis with minimal damage to surrounding structures. The cause of this extrusion is unclear. The dermal theory of pathogenesis proposes that the metabolic derangement associated with chronic renal failure and diabetes induce superficial dermal connective tissue changes triggering the transepidermal elimination. Others suggest that it is a primary defect in the epidermis or an abnormal healing response to injury.

Clinical Presentation

Patients present with umbilicated dome-shaped papules on the arms and legs. Lesions less commonly occur on the trunk, neck, or scalp. The papules of PD are usually hyperkeratotic (crusted) and umbilicated, ranging in size from 2 to 10 mm (Figure 19-10). Varying degrees of pruritus are reported. A linear configuration suggests a koebnerization (lesions in the location of previous trauma or pressure). PD tends to be distributed on trauma-prone areas and often can be reproduced by scratching.

DIFFERENTIAL DIAGNOSIS Perforating dermatoses

- Folliculitis
- Hyperkeratosis lenticularis perstans (Flegel disease)
- Keratoacanthoma
- Keratosis follicularis (Darier disease)
- Keratosis pilaris
- Lichen planus
- Prurigo nodularis
- Squamous cell carcinoma

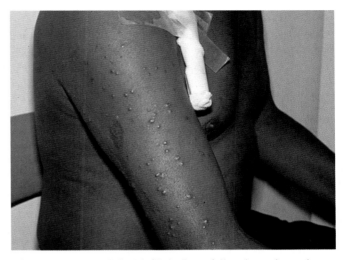

FIG. 19-10. Perforating folliculitis (Kyrle disease). Hyperkeratotic papules are present on extensor areas of the upper extremity in a diabetic patient with renal failure and undergoing dialysis.

Diagnostics

Skin biopsy for hematoxylin and eosin staining is usually diagnostic for the PDs. If confirmed, serology should include a basic metabolic panel to assess for diabetes and renal failure. Additional studies by a dermatologist may be indicated to help differentiate the type of PD.

Management

Recognition and treatment of any underlying disease is the first priority. The disorder may remit after patients receive kidney transplantation. Scratching, friction, and trauma should be avoided. Topical keratolytics such as salicylic acid, lactic acid, or urea may be initiated but should be used cautiously if there is broken skin or erosions. Topical retinoids used off label have been reported to be effective. Oral antihistamines and TCS may provide modest relief from pruritus (see Pruritus).

Dermatology clinicians may utilize phototherapy when a large BSA is involved or lesions are not responsive to topicals. Alternatively, intralesional corticosteroids, systemic retinoids, and cryotherapy have also been reported with mixed response.

Prognosis and Complications

The main complication from PDs is pruritus, which may contribute to secondary skin infections, scarring, and difficulty sleeping. Otherwise, the prognosis and complications are based on the underlying disease state.

Referral and Consultation

Most of the patients with PD associated with renal failure are already being cared for by nephrology and internal medicine. Referral to a dermatologist is usually for diagnosis and management of severe cutaneous symptoms.

Patient Education and Follow-up

Patients should be educated to avoid scratching, rubbing, and other trauma to the areas. Educating the patient on proper hydration of the skin and use of emollients is helpful.

CALCIPHYLAXIS

Calciphylaxis is a rare syndrome involving vascular calcification and skin necrosis. It is associated mainly with individuals with chronic renal failure and secondary hyperparathyroidism.

Pathophysiology

Accumulation of calcium deposits in the tunica media of the walls of small- and medium-sized vessels results in occlusion and ultimately tissue necrosis. The pathogenesis of calciphylaxis is poorly understood. It has been suggested that it may be due to a uremic-induced defect, chronic inflammation, or other processes that impact bone metabolism and calcification.

Clinical Presentation

Early presentation of calciphylaxis resembles livedo reticularis with the mottled pattern of cyanosis. There is rapid progression into the subcutaneous tissue, as purple nodules expand into large, stellate, and necrotic ulcers (Figure 19-11). There may be one or several lesions that are commonly located on the lower legs, thighs, buttocks, and lower abdomen. Patients with calciphylaxis experience excruciating and unremitting pain. Secondary infections may be present.

DIFFERENTIAL DIAGNOSIS Calciphylaxis

- Brown recluse spider bite
- Bullous pemphigoid
- Cellulitis
- Erythema nodosum
- Hypersensitivity vasculitis (leukocytoclastic vasculitis)
- Lupus erythematosus, bullous
- Necrotizing fasciitis
- Pyoderma gangrenosum
- Venous ulcer
- Vibrio vulnificus infection
- Wegener granulomatosis

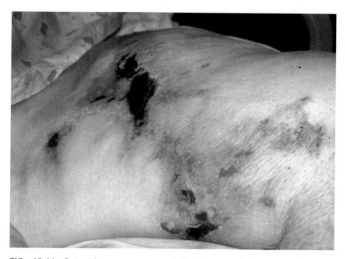

FIG. 19-11. Petechiae, purpura, and frank necrosis in a patient with calciphylaxis.

Diagnostics

Patients suspected of having calciphylaxis should be referred to a dermatologist immediately. Diagnosis of calciphylaxis requires a deep excisional biopsy to ensure that subcutaneous tissue is submitted for histological analysis. Patients should be screened for diabetes and hypercoagulability conditions. Serum calcium, phosphorus, parathyroid hormone, aluminum, urea nitrogen, creatinine, and albumin are critical. Imaging may be ordered to identify calcium deposits.

Management

A treatment plan for the calciphylaxis patient should begin with ongoing assessment and treatment of renal failure by nephrology. Hyperparathyroidism should be addressed to manage abnormal serum calcium and phosphorus levels. A parathyroidectomy is sometimes necessary. Surgical and wound care specialists may consider hyperbaric oxygen therapy or sodium thiosulfate infusions. Some novel treatments have been employed but require a multidisciplinary team approach from experienced specialists.

Prognosis and Complications

Calciphylaxis, especially when it has progressed to ulcerations, has a high mortality rate of 60% to 80%. The 1-year and 5-year survival rates have been reported at 45% and 35%, respectively. The most common cause of death is usually secondary sepsis.

Referral and Consultation

Patients presenting with lesions suspicious for calciphylaxis are typically diagnosed and managed by dermatology or wound care specialist in consultation with a PCP and nephrologist. Pain management may become involved due to the severe pain. Counseling can be important in helping patients and their families deal with this physically and psychologically devastating disease.

Patient Education and Follow-up

Weekly, and sometimes more often, follow-ups are usually necessary for these patients.

DIABETES MELITUS

With the current obesity epidemic in the United States, the incidence of DM is escalating. Individuals are being diagnosed in greater numbers and at younger ages. Early diagnosis of DM and initiation of treatment can decrease the long-term sequelae of the disease. DM impacts all systems of the body. There are distinct cutaneous features that indicate the potential for DM.

Acanthosis Nigricans

Acanthosis nigricans (AN) is a skin disorder that can easily be identified in primary care. AN can be benign or be a red flag for an existing or developing medical condition. Metabolic syndrome is a combination of obesity (especially truncal), elevated blood glucose, hyperlipidemia, and hypertension. It is believed that the obesity results in the insulin resistance. Other underlying endocrine diseases are associated with AN and include type II DM, hypothyroidism, Addison disease, polycystic ovarian syndrome, acromegaly, pituitary or adrenal adenomas, and Cushing syndrome. Individuals with lymphoma and GU/GI malignancies may present with AN. AN can begin at any age and has many speculating that it may be genetic. It impacts males and females equally. It is more common in dark skin tone races, including Native Americans, Hispanics, and African Americans.

Pathophysiology

The cause of AN is not fully known. Most individuals with AN have elevated insulin levels. AN is seen in situations of insulin resistance, including type II DM, obesity, and total lipodystrophy. In these situations, the cause may be related to insulin binding insulin-like growth factor receptors on keratinocytes and dermal fibroblast proliferation. In benign AN, there may be cases that are genetically inherited. The darkened skin appearance of AN is not due to increased melanin but from hyperkeratosis and papillomatosis. The stratum spinosum of the epidermis is thickened.

Clinical presentation

The typical presentation of AN involves hyperpigmentation and hyperkeratinization that results in velvety thickening of the skin folds and areas of friction. The onset is insidious as the lesions start out as flat patches that thicken and darken over time (Figure 19-12A). The most common site is around the neck. Initially, patients may attempt to wash or exfoliate it off but have no success. The axillae, groin, umbilicus, areolae, submammary regions, and hands can develop these characteristic lesions. The affected skin may be pruritic and have a foul odor. Children and adolescents with AN often experience ridicule and are called "dirty" (Figure 19-12B).

DIFFERENTIAL DIAGNOSIS Acanthosis nigricans

- Addison disease
- Hemochromatosis
- Pellagra
- Confluent and reticulated papillomatosis

Diagnostics

AN is easily identified by the experienced practitioner and rarely requires biopsy. A thorough history and physical may identify potential underlying disease. Screening for insulin resistance should include a glycosylated hemoglobin (hemoglobin A_{1c}) and fasting blood sugar, although a normal level does not rule out insulin resistance. Most importantly, a plasma insulin level is the best predictor. If AN onset is in an adult, a basic workup for underlying malignancy should be done.

Management

When obesity is a factor, weight loss can eliminate or improve the lesions. Low-carbohydrate diets and exercise can help to moderate the insulin resistance. If a malignancy is diagnosed, excision or treatment can resolve the lesions. Cutaneous symptoms may be very difficult. Cosmetic improvement may be achieved with application of topical retinoids, preparations with salicylic acid, ammonium lactate lotion or cream, 20% topical urea, or alpha hydroxyl acids. Oral retinoids, fish oil, and metformin have shown some promise but are not FDA approved. Laser and dermabrasion can help but are usually not covered by insurance.

Prognosis and complications

Benign AN has few complications. AN associated with underlying disease carries a prognosis directly related to the disease and treatment. Patients with AN are at higher risk to develop type II DM. An onset during adulthood has a higher association with internal malignancy, especially if the AN occurs suddenly, is extensive, or is pruritic in a patient with ideal BMI. Malignant AN is often associated with aggressive tumors and poor prognosis. The psychological complications from AN can have an impact on the patient's self-esteem, especially children and young adults.

Referral and consultation

Often patients with benign AN can be managed in the primary care setting. Referral to dermatology is only needed if the diagnosis is not obvious, the patient is not responding to treatment, or if they desire

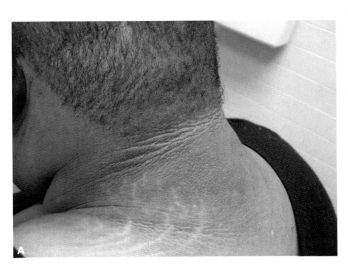
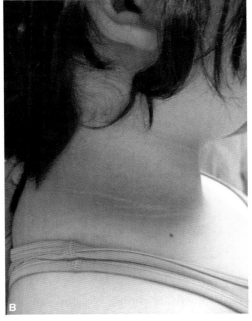

FIG. 19-12. **A:** Woman with classic ANs with a thick, hyperpigmented, velvety plaque. **B:** A 10-year-old girl with early ANs and the "dirty" appearance of an early plaque forming around her neck.

cosmetic treatment. Endocrinology may be consulted as needed to assist in the diagnosis and management of a possible metabolic disorder.

Patient education and follow-up

Patients should be empowered with the knowledge that control of AN (benign) is within their ability. Utilizing the topical therapies and following the lifestyle changes and medication when appropriate can greatly reduce, if not eliminate, AN. Patients need reassurance that AN is not related to hygiene. Follow-up should be done to evaluate the efficacy of therapy and to monitor the insulin resistance. Periodic screening for DM is advised.

Necrobiosis Lipoidica

Necrobiosis lipoidica (NL) is a chronic granulomatous dermatitis (see chapter 20). There is a strong relationship between NL and type I DM and, to a lesser extent, type II DM.

Granuloma Annulare

Granuloma annulare (GA) is a relatively common, self-limited, idiopathic dermatosis of the dermis and subcutaneous tissue. GA has been associated with type I DM, and less often with type II DM and thyroid dysfunction. Few patients with DM develop NL. In contrast, 75% of patients with NL have or will develop DM (see chapter 20). PCPs should be alert for signs and symptoms and screen the patient appropriately.

Diabetic Dermopathy

Diabetic dermopathy (DD) is commonly known as "shin spots" or "pigmented pretibial papules." It is the most common cutaneous manifestation of DM. It is more predominant in men over the age of 50 years.

Pathophysiology

The etiology of DD is unclear though trauma seems to be a modifying factor. It is speculated that microangiopathic changes associated with DM play a role in the development of DD. Research has failed to demonstrate a correlation between glucose control and DD.

Clinical presentation

DD presents as multiple, bilateral, asymmetrical, annular, or irregular red papules or plaques on the anterior aspect of the lower legs. The lesions gradually evolve into atrophic hyperpigmented finely scaled macules (Figure 19-13). While it is most common on the "shins," DD can present on the lateral malleoli, thighs, or forearms.

DIFFERENTIAL DIAGNOSIS Diabetic dermopathy
• Necrobiosis lipoidica
• Stasis dermatitis
• Pigmented purpura
• Posttraumatic scarring
• Postinflammatory hyperpigmentation
• Lymphedema

Diagnostics

DD is a clinical diagnosis and skin biopsy is usually not necessary. If considered, the benefit of biopsy must be weighed against the risk of slow healing, infection, and ulceration on the lower extremities of a diabetic patient.

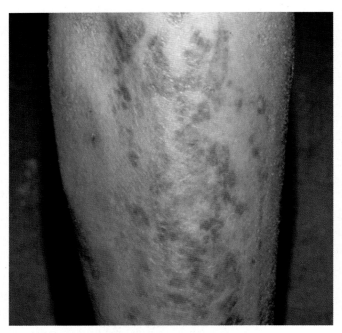

FIG. 19-13. Diabetic dermopathy.

Management

DD is largely asymptomatic and rarely progresses to ulceration. The lesions should be monitored, but there is no effective treatment. It is largely a cosmetic issue.

Referral and consultation

DD is a common problem managed by PCPs and rarely requiring referral to dermatology unless the diagnosis is uncertain.

Patient education and follow-up

Patients should be educated on importance of good glycemic control, proper skin care avoidance of trauma to the affected areas.

Diabetic Bullae

Diabetic bullae or bullosis diabeticorum develop in approximately 0.5% of individuals with DM. It has been reported only in adults and is most common in men. It is more common in long-term diabetics who suffer from neuropathy.

Pathophysiology

The pathogenesis of diabetic bullae is poorly understood and is likely multifactorial. Evidence also suggests an abnormality of anchoring fibrils that are essential for the integrity of the dermoepidermal junction. The prominence of bullae on acral surfaces is suggestive of trauma. The threshold for suction related blister formation is lower for diabetics than nondiabetics. UVR also seems to play a role. Recurrence is not uncommon.

Clinical presentation

These bullae appear suddenly and favor acral skin areas, especially the dorsal and lateral aspects of the lower legs and feet. Diabetic bullae are painless with clear fluid lesions ranging in size from a few millimeters to several centimeters (Figure 19-14). After they rupture, the bullae heal in 2 to 5 weeks without treatment.

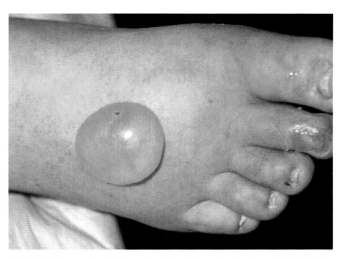

FIG. 19-14. Large clear bulla on the foot or lower leg is characteristic of diabetic bullae.

DIFFERENTIAL DIAGNOSIS Diabetic bullae

- Bullous pemphigoid
- Autoimmune blistering diseases
- Porphyria cutanea tarda
- Bullous impetigo
- Erythema multiforme
- Bullous tinea
- Arthropod assault

Diagnostics

A tissue biopsy for histology and direct immunofluorescence is indicated to exclude other blistering disorders of the skin. This will be best accomplished by a dermatologist since it would require a lesional biopsy for histology and a perilesional specimen for direct immunofluorescence (requires Michel's solution not formaldehyde). If PCT is in the differential (especially if bullae are located on the dorsal hands), porphyrin levels should be evaluated. Bacterial and fungal cultures may be necessary if an infection is suspected.

Management

Since the bullae heal spontaneously, treatment is focused on the avoidance and treatment of secondary infections. If there is discomfort, bullae can be aspirated with a sterile small-bore needle. Should the blister become unroofed, aggressive wound healing measures should be taken. Appropriate antibiotics should be utilized for secondary bacterial infections.

Referral and consultation

Refer diabetic bullae patients to dermatology for appropriate biopsy if needed to rule out other blistering skin disorders. If wounds from unroofed blisters are resistant to healing, refer to dermatology as soon as possible to avoid ulceration and necrosis. Once necrosis occurs the patient may require referral to a surgeon for debridement and skin grafting.

Patient education and follow-up

Patients with diabetic bullae should be monitored closely until the bullae have healed and resolved. Scarring is rare. Since the bullae are prone to recur, the patient should be evaluated with each episode. Good skin care and diabetic foot care should be taught and stressed. Patients should continue with appropriate diabetic care and monitoring.

HYPERTHYROIDISM AND HYPOTHYROIDISM

Thyroid hormones are primarily responsible for regulation of metabolism and can affect any organ in the body. There are a wide variety of skin changes and disorders that are associated or caused by dysregulation of the thyroid gland. Skin changes may be the patient's chief complaint and should prompt the clinician to consider evaluation of thyroid function. Correcting the thyroid hormone levels can lead to resolution of the skin conditions.

Low levels of circulating thyroid hormone or cell resistance to thyroid hormone action can result in hypothyroidism. The most common cause for hypothyroidism is the autoimmune disease Hashimoto thyroiditis, which results in glandular failure. Hypothyroidism can be genetic, or it may also be the result of surgical procedures and radiation to the head and neck. Treatment to correct hyperthyroidism can result in hypothyroidism. It can be drug induced with lithium being the common medication. Pregnancy and iron deficiency may cause hypothyroidism.

Hyperthyroidism results when there are excessive levels of circulating thyroid hormones usually due to an autoimmune disease called Graves disease. Hyperthyroidism can also develop due to thyroid adenomas, inflammation of the thyroid, excess iron intake, and in the postpartum period. It can be drug induced by amiodarone (Cordarone) and some IV contrasts.

Pathophysiology

Thyroid hormones appear to play a pivotal role in cellular metabolism, including the growth and formation of hair, nails, skin, and sebum production. The skin responds when there are inadequate or excessive amounts of circulating thyroid hormone. There can be a direct or indirect effect on the skin as thyroid dysfunction affects all organs and body systems, thus resulting in cutaneous systems. In a hyperthyroid state, many cutaneous manifestations are due to increased cutaneous blood flow and peripheral vasodilatation. In a hypothyroid state, symptoms may be associated with a reduced core body temperature and reflex cutaneous vasoconstriction.

Clinical Presentation

In addition to the skin changes noted in Table 19-3, other cutaneous manifestations may be present from disease or conditions associated with thyroid disease. For example, dyslipidemia resulting from hypothyroidism may manifest symptoms of AN.

Diagnostics

Screening for thyroid disease or dysfunction should begin with a thyrotropin or TSH. A free or total T_4 should be performed but may be affected by pregnancy, disease states, or genetic predisposition. Free T_3 levels are important when hyperthyroidism is suspected. In autoimmune thyroid disease, including Graves disease and Hashimoto thyroiditis, thyroid autoantibodies antithyroid peroxidase (anti-TPO) and antithyroglobulin (anti-Tg) are usually elevated, the latter being associated with infertility and spontaneous abortion. Additional studies may be ordered for further evaluation.

Management

Most of the cutaneous manifestations of thyroid dysfunction are managed by treating the specific thyroid problem. Thyroid

TABLE 19-3	Cutaneous Symptoms of Thyroid Dysfunction and Initial Workup	
	HYPERTHYROID (*GRAVES OR THYROTOXICOSIS*)	**HYPOTHYROID (*MYXEDEMA*)**
Skin	Vasodilatation Thin Warm Moist Smooth Excessive sweating Pruritus	Vasoconstriction Weight gain Cool Dry/xerosis Pale Decreased sweating Thickening of palms & soles Impaired wound healing
Hair	Soft & fine Diffuse, nonscarring alopecia	Dry, coarse, & brittle Diffuse or partial alopecia Loss of lateral ⅓ eyebrow "Queen Anne" sign (Figure 19-15)
Nails	"Plummer's nail" or separation from the nail bed Swelling and tenderness Soft, friable	"Plummer's nail" or separation from the nail bed Brittle nails
Pigmentation	Hyperpigmentation (palms and soles, gingival and buccal mucosa) Vitiligo	Yellowish hue on the skin (palms, soles, and nasolabial folds)
Myxedema changes	Scleromyxedema: firm, white, yellow, or pink papules scattered on the face, trunk, axillae, and extremities	Myxedema, facial and/or generalized: thickened, nonpitting edematous changes to the soft tissues
Diagnostics	Initial screening: serum TSH low/normal T_4*/free T_4 high or normal Free T_3 high or normal Thyroid autoantibodies elevated in Graves disease Radioactive iodine uptake and imaging	Initial screening: serum TSH-high/normal T_4*/free T_4 low to normal Free T_3 low to normal Thyroid autoantibodies elevated in Hoshimoto thyroiditis

*Results can be affected by disease, pregnancy, or genetic predisposition.

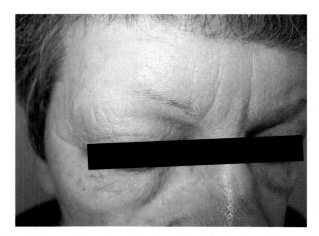

FIG. 19-15. Queen Anne sign of hypothyroidism; lateral third of the eyebrow is missing.

hormone replacement for hypothyroidism is key. When thyroid hormone levels stabilize, a large majority of the symptoms resolve. Since thyroid regulation occurs in a slow negative feedback loop, it can take several weeks for the thyroid levels to normalize once appropriate therapy has been instituted. TSH levels should be checked every 2 to 3 months until it normalizes and after any changes in dosage. In hyperthyroidism, ablation with radioactive therapy or surgical thyroidectomy is the most common treatment.

Prognosis and Complication

Prognosis is good for individuals with thyroid dysfunction. Once corrected, symptoms usually resolve but may be dependent on the severity, chronicity, comorbidities, and treatment. Hyperthyroid patients undergoing thyroid ablation should be monitored for hypothyroidism. Half of the patients with Graves disease have ocular symptoms, with about 5% having severe ophthalmopathy.

Referral and Consultation

Thyroid disease is often managed by a PCP but may necessitate referral to an endocrinologist for complex cases. A dermatologist may be consulted for specific cutaneous manifestations and an OB/GYN for women with fertility problems. Graves disease requires management by an endocrinologist and often an ophthalmologist.

Patient Education and Follow-up

It is not uncommon for resolution of symptoms of hypo- and hyperthyroidism to lag behind normalization of thyroid levels. Patients can become frustrated when their thyroid level is normal but symptoms have not resolved. Educating patients on palliative treatment of the symptoms while the evaluation and treatment is ongoing can be helpful. Patients should know the signs and symptoms of abnormal thyroid function and report them immediately. Regular monitoring of serum levels should occur, more often when there is a change in dose or for changes in symptoms.

INTERNAL MALIGNANCIES

Involvement of the skin by visceral tumors may be either direct or indirect. There are a multitude of syndromes, tumors, and dermatoses that are manifestations of internal malignancy. There are some very characteristic cutaneous signs of specific internal malignancies that should be a "red flag" to clinicians (Table 19-4). These associations are not always based on evidence but are empiric. A keen awareness of these associations may aid the clinician in earlier recognition and a diagnosis that may improve the patient outcomes or prognosis.

Carcinoid Syndrome

Carcinoid syndrome manifests as episodes of flushing (without sweating) lasting 10 to 30 minutes involving only the upper half of the body. It is associated with a neuroendocrine tumor. The flushing may be followed by a serpiginous (snake-like)-patterned rash. Attacks may become more progressive and take on a cyanotic quality. A rosacea-like rash with permanent facial cyanosis and

TABLE 19-4 Cutaneous Lesions and Internal Malignancy—Paraneoplastic Syndromes

SYNDROME	CLINICAL PRESENTATION	MALIGNANCY
Carcinoid flushing or syndrome	Episodes of flushing (face, neck, chest)	Serotonin containing tumor of body parts such as appendix, small intestine, bronchus
	Dyspnea	
	Asthma	
	Diarrhea	
	Murmur (pulmonary)	
Erythroderma or exfoliative dermatitis (see chapter 5)	Extensive erythema & scaling involving 80%–90% of the body	Internal malignancy
	Body surface becomes dull scarlet with small scales that exfoliate	Mycosis fungoides (MF), a form of cutaneous T-cell lymphoma
	Extreme pruritus	Sézary syndrome (the leukemic phase of MF)
Paraneoplastic pemphigus (see chapter 15)	Painful, intractable, erosive ulcerative stomatitis, and polymorphic cutaneous eruption (erythema, papules, iris lesions, bullae, erosions)	Non-Hodgkin lymphoma (80%)
		Chronic lymphocytic leukemia
		Castleman disease
		Thymoma
		Waldenström macroglobulinemia
Sign of Leser–Trélat (see chapter 11)	Sudden onset, increased size and number of seborrheic keratoses	Adenocarcinomas of GI, lungs, and breast chemotherapeutics agents
Dermatomyositis (see chapter 15)	Heliotrope of eyelids, Gottron papules	Ovarian and cervical lung, prostate, and pancreatic, gastric carcinomas, non-Hodgkin lymphoma
	Scaly erythematous patches or plaques, especially over the back/shoulders (Shawl sign)	
	Dilated capillary loops proximal to nail folds	
	Weakness usually in distal extremities	
Sister Mary Joseph nodule	Palpable nodule protruding into the umbilicus	Metastasis from malignancy of the pelvis and abdomen (including pancreatic)

TABLE 19-4	Cutaneous Lesions and Internal Malignancy—Paraneoplastic Syndromes *(continued)*	
SYNDROME	**CLINICAL PRESENTATION**	**MALIGNANCY**
Vasculitis (see chapter 16)	Large variation of symptoms and presentations depending on vessels affected Can have cutaneous and systemic symptoms (including major organs and airway involvement) Clinical presentations range from petechial hemorrhages, palpable purpura, painful subcutaneous nodules, ulcerations	Leukocytoclastic vasculitis Henoch–Schönlein purpura, adult Polyarteritis nodosa, Wegener granulomatosis Microscopic polyangiitis
Coagulopathies	Tender subcutaneous, red nodules or cords fat over trunk and extremities	Trousseau syndrome (acquired hypercoagulopathy with recurrent superficial thrombophlebitis) 50% of cases associated with cancer, usually lung and pancreatic

Adapted from Habif, T. P. (2010). *Clinical dermatology: A color guide to diagnosis and therapy* (5th ed.). St. Louis, MO: Mosby-Elsevier.

telangiectasias may develop. The flushing may be accompanied with abdominal pain with watery diarrhea, bronchospasm, dyspnea, hypotension, murmur of pulmonary stenosis, and tachycardia. Patients should be evaluated for possible carcinoid tumors.

Exfoliative Erythroderma

Exfoliative erythroderma (ED), also called generalized exfoliative dermatitis, is a dermatitis covering about 90% of an individual's BSA. It begins as erythema and scaling, progressing into a dull scarlet color with extensive exfoliation of the skin—often called the "red man" syndrome (Figure 19-16). Patients have marked palmar-plantar keratoderma (thickened scale of palms and soles) and extreme pruritus. ED can be a true dermatologic emergency due to the vasodilation, hypothermia, hypotension, and electrolyte imbalances.

ED can be caused by psoriasis, medications, pityriasis rubra pilaris, HIV infections, or idiopathic. It can occur secondarily to underlying lymphoproliferative disorder, cutaneous T-cell lymphoma (especially Sézary syndrome). Patients should be immediately sent to a dermatologist for further evaluation, diagnosis, and management. Patients with severe ED may need to be sent to the emergency department for stabilization and hospitalization.

Sign of Leser–Trélat

Seborrheic keratoses (SKs) are considered to be a benign finding on the skin. Yet the sudden appearance of numerous SKs has been empirically noted to precede or occur with an internal malignancy (Figure 19-17). There is no evidence to support this association, but practitioners still consider its clinical presentation as a red flag (see chapter 11).

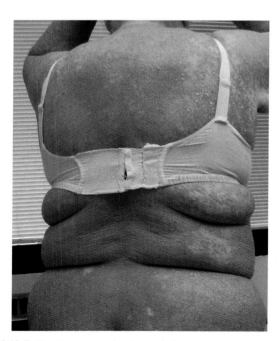

FIG. 19-16. Erythroderma secondary to psoriasis.

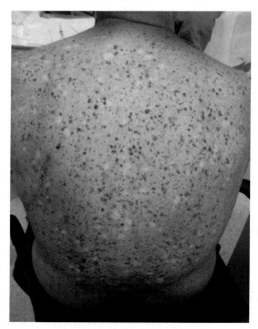

FIG. 19-17. Sign of Leser–Trélat, or sudden onset of numerous seborrheic keratoses, may be associated with an underlying malignancy.

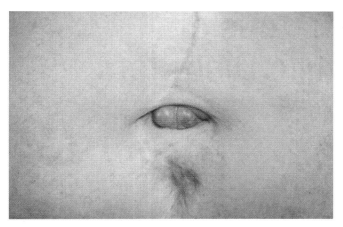

FIG. 19-18. Sister Mary Joseph nodule.

Sister Mary Joseph Nodule

The Sister Mary Joseph nodule is a palpable, easily visualized nodule that protrudes into the umbilicus (Figure 19-18). It is formed due to localization of metastatic tumors to the umbilicus. The primary sites of the malignancy are the stomach, large bowel, ovaries, and pancreas. Usually the primary malignancy has been diagnosed prior to the presentation of the nodule.

BILLING CODES ICD-10

Acanthosis nigricans	L83
Hyperthyroidism, NOS	E05.9
Hypothyroidism, NOS	E03.9
Neurotic excoriation	L98.1
Other phakomatosis, including Peutz–Jeghers syndrome	Q85.8
Other porphyria	E809.2
Other specified diabetes mellitus with other skin complication	E13.628
Disorder of skin or subcutaneous tissue, unspecified	L98.9
Porphyria cutanea tarda	E80.0
Pruritus, unspecified	L 29.9
Psychogenic pruritus	F45.8
Unspecified diabetes mellitus with other specified complication	E14.69

READINGS

Artantas, S., Gül, U., Kılıç, A., & Güler, S. (2008). Skin findings in thyroid diseases. *European Journal of Internal Medicine, 20*(2), 158–161. doi:10.1016/j.ejim.2007.09.021 orhttp://www.aai.org.tr/managete/UploadedFiles/2009-01/012% 202009-1.%20Sayi.pdf

Balwani, M., & Desnick, R. J. (2012). The porphyrias: Advances in diagnosis and treatments. *Hematology,* 19–27. doi: 10.1182/asheducation-2012.1.19.

Calva, D., & Howe, J. R. (2008). Harmatomatous polyposis syndromes. *Surgical Clinics of North America, 88*(4), 779–817. doi:10.1016/j.suc.2008.05.002.

Cordova, K. B., Oberg, T. J., Malik, M., & Robinson-Bostom, L. (2009). Dermatologic conditions seen in end-stage renal disease. *Seminars in Dialysis, 22*(1), 45–55.

Ferringer, T., & Miller, F. (2002). Cutaneous manifestations of diabetes mellitus. *Dermatologic Clinics, 20,* 483–492.

James, W. D., Berger, T. G., & Elston, D. M. (Eds.). (2011). *Andrews' diseases of the skin: Clinical dermatology* (11th ed.). Elsevier Saunders.

Stander, S., Weisshaar, E., Mettang, T., Szepietowski, J. C., Carstens, E., Ikoma, A., ... Bernhard, D. (2007). Clinical classification of itch: A position paper of the International Forum for the Study of Itch. *Acta Dermato-Vernereologica, 87,* 291–294.

Steinhoff, M., Cevikbas, F., Ikoma, A., & Berger, T. G. (2011). Pruritus: Management algorithms and experimental therapies. *Seminars in Cutaneous Medicine and Surgery, 30,* 127–137. doi:10.1016/j.sder.2011.05.001

Thiers, B. H., Sahn, R. E., & Callen, J. P. (2009). Cutaneous manifestations of internal malignancy. *CA: A Cancer Journal for Clinicians, 59*(2), 73–98.

Yosipovitch, G., & Bernhard, J. D. (2013). Clinical practice: Chronic pruritus. *New England Journal of Medicine, 368*(17), 1625–1634.

CHAPTER 20

Granulomatous and Neutrophilic Disorders

Pamela Fletcher and Diane Solderitsch

In dermatology, many disorders have similar histologic findings of cutaneous inflammation, but the clinical presentations are dissimilar and causes are often unknown. These disorders are grouped histologically into categories of granulomatous and neutrophilic dermatoses. This chapter will deal with the most common conditions found in each of these categories, defining clinical presentations, diagnosis, and management.

NONINFECTIOUS GRANULOMATOUS DISORDERS

Skin conditions in this category are disorders of Langerhans cells and macrophages. Histiocytes are a type of macrophage and play an important role in the body's immune system. In response to inflammation or infection, these histiocytes aggregate and form granulomas in the skin.

Granuloma Annulare

Granuloma annulare (GA) is a common, self-limiting inflammatory process affecting the dermis, with females affected twice as often as males. The localized form of GA is most common in patients under the age of 30 years. Although it has been linked with diabetes mellitus (DM), there is no evidence to support it. However, there is a correlation between DM and generalized or disseminated GA, occurring often in 30- to 60-year-olds. Patients with HIV commonly present with generalized GA. Atypical forms of GA have been associated with paraneoplastic granulomatous reactions to Hodgkin disease, non-Hodgkin lymphoma, solid organ tumors, and mycosis fungoides.

Pathophysiology

The cause of GA is unknown but may be related to vasculitis, trauma, monocyte activation, or delayed hypersensitivity reaction in the skin. There is a degeneration of collagen and accumulation of mucin. Histiocytes are palisaded (elongated and perpendicular in the superficial and mid-dermis).

Clinical presentation

The clinical presentation of GA varies widely. The term *annulare* refers to the round or arciform shape of the lesions, which are often erythematous, dome-shaped papules that form a circle with central clearing (hence its frequent diagnosis as ringworm) or faintly erythematous depression at the center. Lesions may be asymptomatic or pruritic.

Localized

The localized form usually starts as a small ring of skin color or lightly erythematous papules favoring the dorsal surfaces of hands, feet, or extensor surfaces of the arms (especially the elbows) or legs (Figure 20-1). Over several weeks, lesions coalesce and evolve into annular plaques, which undergo central involution and increase in diameter from 0.5 to 5 cm over several months. It may also present

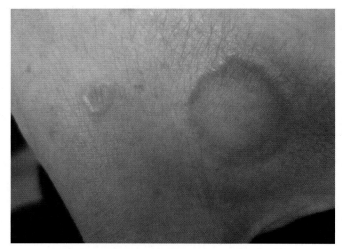

FIG. 20-1. Localized GA on the dorsal hand with the classic plaques with a raised border and central clearing.

as brownish-red plaques and papules that can be difficult to detect on dark skin.

Generalized

The generalized form of GA (15% of cases), typically presenting on the trunk and extremities of middle-aged Caucasian women, can be cosmetically distressing. Lesions are usually red to violaceous macules, patches, or flat, slightly elevated papules, which may be either pruritic or asymptomatic (Figure 20-2).

DIFFERENTIAL DIAGNOSIS Granuloma annulare
• Tinea corporis
• Lichen planus
• Necrobiosis lipoidica (NL)
• Sarcoidosis
• Secondary syphilis

Diagnostics

Diagnosis is usually made based on clinical presentation but can be confirmed with a punch biopsy if there is any doubt. Histologically, there are two patterns of GA, palisading and interstitial (such as interstitial GA). The latter should not be confused with interstitial granulomatous dermatitis. A KOH slide can help differentiate GA from tinea corporis, which has scale. Serologies can be ordered if syphilis is considered.

Management

Localized GA is usually not treated unless it concerns the patient due to appearance. Treatment is provided mainly for cosmetic purposes

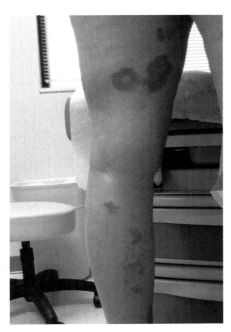

FIG. 20-2. The generalized form of GA presents as chronic lesions, as on legs of this 62-year-old woman with diabetes.

and often with less than optimal results. First-line treatment includes high-potency topical corticosteroids (TCS) with or without occlusion, intralesional (IL) corticosteroid injections into the elevated portions of the lesions with triamcinolone acetonide (depending on location), or cryotherapy. Risks from these treatments include atrophy and scarring. Off-label use of tacrolimus, pimecrolimus, and imiquimod has been reported to have some efficacy. Second-line treatment that may be used in dermatology for severe localized GA includes systemic agents such as isotretinoin, antimalarials, cyclosporine or dapsone.

Treatment for *generalized GA* is difficult and the patient should be referred to a dermatologist for photochemotherapy using oral psoralen and ultraviolet light A (PUVA), CO_2 laser, or systemic agents.

Special considerations

Lesions in children aged 2 to 5 years may present as deep, painless, skin-colored papules near joints, on the palms, soles, or buttocks. The generalized form in older patients may present as hundreds to thousands of small, flesh-colored papules in symmetric distribution on the trunk and extremities.

Prognosis and complications

Most lesions resolve spontaneously after several months to several years (50%–75% clear within 2 years) but may recur. The generalized form may last for an extended period of time. GA does not typically result in scarring but may occur secondary to treatments.

Referral and consultation

Refer to dermatology if the diagnosis is unclear or when lesions are unresponsive to first-line treatment. Clinicians providing IL triamcinolone should be experienced to minimize side effects.

Patient education and follow-up

Educate patients about the disease; provide anticipatory guidance and reassurance. They should be alert for side effects to medications and treatments, seeking appropriate intervention if they occur.

Patients may become anxious if they develop multiple lesions, the lesions involve several areas, and/or lesions expand.

Patients are often evaluated by a dermatologist and may be monitored occasionally since GA is benign and self-limiting. Patients with generalized GA should have regular checkups and be monitored for side effects of immune-modifying medications. Any signs or symptoms of infection should be evaluated immediately and care coordinated with a dermatologist.

Actinic Granuloma (of O'Brien)

A granulomatous skin disease first described by Dr. O'Brien in 1975, actinic granuloma is also called annular elastolytic giant cell granuloma. There is some controversy as to whether it is a variant of GA. Actinic granuloma is uncommon and occurs more frequently in middle-aged individuals with a history of excessive sun exposure. A typical patient is a fair-skinned female aged 40 to 50 years and living in a sunny area.

Pathophysiology

The pathophysiology of actinic granuloma is unknown, but it is thought to be an inflammatory response to sun exposure.

Clinical presentation

As the name implies, lesions present as asymptomatic annular plaques on sun-exposed areas. Lesions may be flesh or pink color with classic GA morphology (Figure 20-3).

DIFFERENTIAL DIAGNOSIS Actinic granuloma
• Tinea corporis or capitis
• Granuloma annulare
• Necrobiosis lipoidica
• Discoid lupus

Diagnostics

As with GA, diagnostic tests are usually not indicated but may be necessary to confirm the diagnosis.

Management

First-line treatments for actinic granulomas are similar to GA, but the response is usually poor. Other treatments, such as phototherapy and antimalarials, have been reported. Sun protection is important to prevent new lesions.

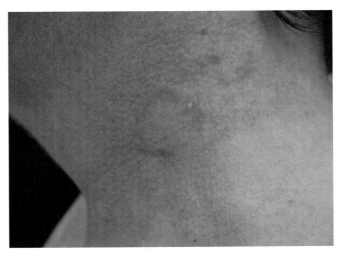

FIG. 20-3. Actinic granuloma occurs in areas with heavy photodamage.

Prognosis and complications

Most lesions resolve spontaneously after several months to several years. Lesions may recur or spread secondary to sun exposure. Actinic granuloma does not usually cause scarring. Secondary scarring may occur with atrophy from IL corticosteroid injections.

Referral and consultation

Refer to dermatology if the diagnosis is unclear, lesions are atypical, or for second-line therapy. Patients may desire consultative care for cosmetic treatment.

Patient education and follow-up

Follow-up care of patients with actinic granuloma is same as GA. Emphasis should be placed on patient education for sun protection to avoid the development of new lesions.

Foreign-Body Granuloma

Foreign-body granulomas are common skin reactions that can occur from exogenous or endogenous sources. They can occur in any age group, but exogenous sources are more common during working years since occupational injury is the most common cause.

Pathophysiology

Initially, foreign-body granulomas are caused by trauma that develops into granulomas, from either allergic or nonallergic inflammation. It is a chronic process of granulomatous changes. Any *exogenous* source such as glass, metal, wood, ink from tattoos, collagen injections, suture material, or inorganic materials that enter the body (either accidentally or by insertion) can cause a foreign-body granuloma. The increasing use of dermal fillers for cosmetic enhancements has also been associated with foreign-body granulomatous reactions (see chapter 23). *Endogenous* or biologic sources, such as ruptured hair follicles or cysts, are the most common internal causes of foreign-body granulomas. Although the body is the source of the material, the immune system responds as though it is foreign.

Clinical presentation

Foreign-body granulomas usually present as an inflamed nodule or plaque usually accompanied by tenderness. In the early stage, there can be purulence. In time, the chronic lesion may become firm, sclerotic, or scarred (chronic stage) (Figure 20-4).

DIFFERENTIAL DIAGNOSIS Foreign-body granuloma

- Pyogenic granuloma
- Basal cell carcinoma
- Contact dermatitis
- Pseudofolliculitis barbae
- Acne keloidalis nuchae
- Cellulitis
- Osteomyelitis
- Cyst

Diagnostics

Accurate diagnosis depends on history taking. Biopsy may be helpful, and an x-ray may identify the foreign body if it is substantial in size and radiopaque. A punch biopsy may be curative.

Management

Management depends on symptoms and patient preference. Surgery may be necessary for removal of the foreign body. Lasers have been used for tattoo removal with variable results.

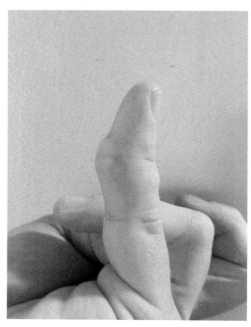

FIG. 20-4. Foreign-body granuloma from broken glass embedded in the fifth digit of a bartender.

Prognosis and complications

A foreign-body granuloma is not life- or limb-threatening but may limit function, create annoyance, or be cosmetically displeasing. Complications from surgical removal include risk of infection and scarring.

Referral and consultation

Foreign-body granulomas of the hands, feet, or digits may require consultation with a specialist such as a hand surgeon or orthopedic surgeon. Cosmetically sensitive areas may require consultation with a plastic surgeon or dermatologist.

Patient education and follow-up

Emphasis should be placed on prevention of new lesions from repeated exposure. Follow-up with their primary care provider (PCP) or specialist should be as needed.

Necrobiosis Lipoidica

NL is a granulomatous skin disease that is commonly associated with DM, hence the previous nomenclature *NL diabeticorum.* Nearly 75% of those with NL have or will develop DM, with skin lesions that may appear years in advance of the diagnosis. Conversely, only a very small percentage of diabetics develop NL. The onset is highest during the third or fourth decade, with female predominance of 3:1.

Pathophysiology

The pathophysiology of NL is unknown, as with other noninfectious granulomatous diseases. Histologic analysis shows a degeneration of collagen (necrobiosis) and granulomatous inflammation.

Clinical presentation

Skin lesions start as small, violaceous, round or oval, sharply defined patches or thin plaques favoring the anterior lower legs (Figure 20-5). Then slowly, the lesion expands in size, with the borders remaining red and center evolving into a waxy yellow/brown color. The surface is often shiny with telangiectasias present (Figure 20-6). Lesions may

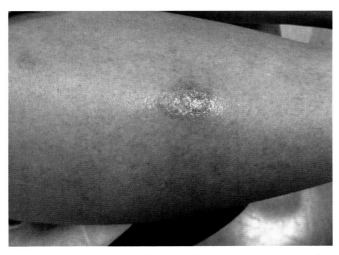

FIG. 20-5. Early necrobiosis lipoidica can begin as a violaceous plaque, often found on the anterior lower legs.

be asymptomatic or can have tenderness, pruritus, itching, paresthesias, or numbness. Trauma in the area frequently leads to nonhealing ulcers.

DIFFERENTIAL DIAGNOSIS Necrobiosis lipoidica
• Granuloma annulare
• Diabetic dermopathy
• Stasis dermatitis
• Erythema nodosum (early)
• Infectious granulomas
• Cutaneous sarcoidosis
• Nonmelanoma Skin cancer
• Morphea
• Lichen sclerosis
• Pretibial myxedema
• Xanthomas

Management

Lesions of NL are often very resistant to treatment. The focus of therapy should be to prevent leg ulcers and to heal them quickly should they develop. Corticosteroids are the mainstay of treatment for NL. Potent TCS used daily for 2 to 4 weeks is recommended for active areas (usually borders) of large, thick plaques. It provides little improvement and may even cause a worsening of atrophy in "burnt-out" lesions of NL. IL triamcinolone acetonide (10 mg/mL), which can be diluted with lidocaine or sodium chloride to reduce risk for atrophy, may be used for smaller lesions or injected into their erythematous border. Oral corticosteroids can be effective in healing ulcerations. The benefits and risk of this systemic therapy should carefully be considered in diabetic patients. Ulcerations from NL have been reported to respond to off-label treatment with pentoxifylline, as well as aspirin and dipyridamole. Other medications include cyclosporine, tacrolimus ointment 0.1%, PUVA, and hydroxychloroquine. Skin grafting may be necessary for extensive, nonhealing ulcers.

Special considerations

The clinical presentation of NL is distinctive, so a biopsy is usually not needed and may result in additional nonhealing ulcers, especially in diabetic patients.

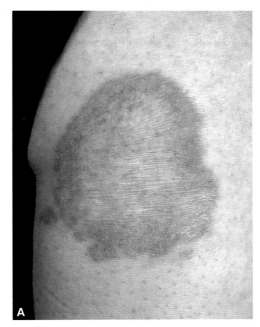

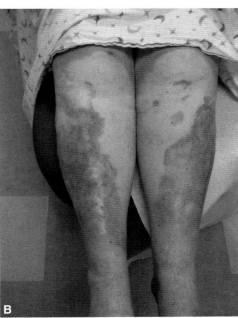

FIG. 20-6. **A:** Necrobiosis lipoidica can expand with waxy, yellow centers and erythematous borders. **B:** Larger lesions may become shiny and atrophic with telangiectasias.

CLINICAL PEARL
Sarcoidosis and NL may exist in the same patient. Therefore, if atypical lesions occur, a biopsy and full assessment of the patient for cutaneous and systemic sarcoidosis may be indicated.

Prognosis and complications

Treatment with topical, IL, or systemic corticosteroids means discussing the side effects of the medication and the benefits of wound healing or halting the progression of an ulceration. The course of the disease is usually benign, and spontaneous remission occurs in about 20% of cases.

Referral and consultation

Refer to a dermatologist for diagnosis, initiation of treatment, and systemic therapy when indicated. If DM or other metabolic disorders are suspected, an endocrinologist may be consulted. Wound care specialists may be consulted for nonhealing ulcers and plastic surgeons if skin grafts are required.

Patient education and follow-up

Patients should be educated about the disease along with the signs and symptoms of DM. Emphasis should be placed on preventative health and skin protection, and avoidance of trauma to the lower extremities, which could cause ulcers, is important. The unpredictable course of the disease and side effects of chronic TCS should be discussed.

Nondiabetic patients should be followed up by a PCP and screened regularly for potential development of DM. Patients with active NL should be followed up every 2 weeks until the lesions are stabilized or resolved. If treated with corticosteroids, close monitoring should be continued until the appropriate taper from the medication is completed.

Cutaneous Sarcoidosis

Sarcoidosis is an uncommon granulomatous disease that can affect the skin, lungs, lymph nodes, liver, spleen, parotid glands, and eyes. Cutaneous sarcoidosis occurs in 25% of patients with systemic disease and may be the first presenting symptom, or it may be the only organ involved. There are several variants, including subcutaneous, lupus pernio, and ulcerative sarcoidosis.

Sarcoidosis can occur at any age but peaks in individuals 25 to 35 years of age and in females 45 to 65 years. In the United States, sarcoidosis is both more common and more severe in African American women 40 years of age, with a rate over 10 times that of Caucasians. In general, individuals with dark skin tones are affected more than Caucasians by 14:1. Reports of cases seem to follow a seasonal pattern, with a higher number of cases in the winter, and a clustering of cases with erythema nodosum in early spring. This raises the possibility of an environmental etiology.

Pathophysiology

The pathophysiology of sarcoidosis is unknown, but autoimmune and infectious factors, as well as genetic susceptibility, have been implicated. The hallmark histology of cutaneous sarcoidosis shows noncaseating epithelioid granulomas without lymphocytic infiltration. A cardinal feature of sarcoidosis is the presence of CD4 positive T cells, interacting with antigen-presenting cells to initiate and maintain the formation of granulomas.

Clinical presentation

Cutaneous sarcoidosis mimics other diseases. It typically presents as superficial red-brown to violaceous papules and plaques appearing most often on the face (Figure 20-7), around the eyes, lips (frequent), neck, upper back, and extremities (Figure 20-8). Some lesions may have a distinctive yellowish-brown color that looks like apple jelly. Diascopy (applying pressure to the lesion with a clear microscope slide) of the papules reveals the unique color or "apple jelly sign," considered a diagnostic clue for granulomatous disease, especially sarcoidosis (Figure 20-9). A scaly, ichthyosiform (quadrangular or "fish scale" pattern of skin) presentation is less common. Lesions tend to favor scars or sites of previous trauma (a great diagnostic clue) to the skin or can develop a central clearing giving them an annular appearance.

Acute subcutaneous sarcoidosis may be accompanied by erythema nodosum (up 20% of patients) and may be the harbinger of systemic sarcoidosis. It presents with tender red/brown nodules on the extremities, especially the lower legs. Cutaneous involvement of

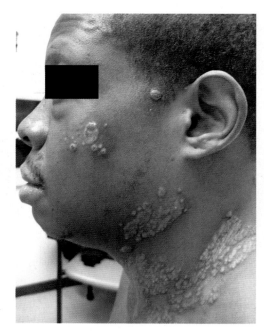

FIG. 20-7. Reddish-brown plaques and nodules of cutaneous sarcoidosis frequently occur on the head, face, and neck.

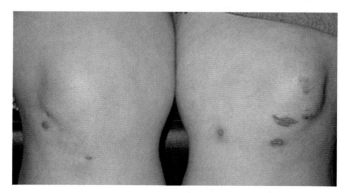

FIG. 20-8. Persistent nodules on the legs of a patient with systemic sarcoidosis.

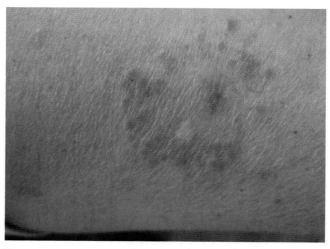

FIG. 20-9. Small brown-red-yellow papules with "apple jelly" appearance characteristic of cutaneous sarcoidosis. This patient does not have systemic involvement.

sarcoidosis may be classified as specific (granulomas) or nonspecific (reactive) disease.

Subtypes

Lupus pernio is a distinct variant of sarcoidosis and should not be confused with *lupus erythematosus* or *perniosis*, diseases that sound similar but are unrelated. Purplish-brown papules and plaques develop around the nose, ears, lips, face, and fingers (Figure 20-10). Early diagnosis of lupus pernio is important because of its high association with pulmonary or respiratory tract involvement, which causes scarring, fibrosis, and deformity. Rarely does it remit spontaneously. It is also associated with a higher incidence of systemic disease with bony involvement.

Other cutaneous variants include *ulcerative sarcoidosis,* a rare type characterized by ulcerations on the lower extremities or in other sarcoidal skin lesions. It is more common in young African American women.

Löfgren syndrome consists of bilateral hilar adenopathy, fever, arthralgia, erythema nodosum, and uveitis. It usually resolves spontaneously and does not require systemic corticosteroids.

Heerfordt syndrome is a variant that presents with uveitis, facial nerve palsy, fever, and parotid gland swelling.

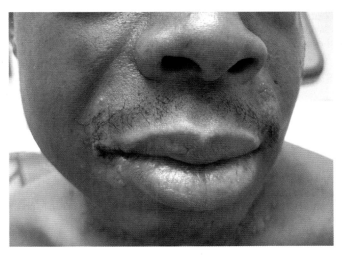

FIG. 20-10. Lupus pernio are violaceous papules and plaques located around the nose, mouth, and cheeks. They are associated with systemic sarcoidosis and a higher prevalence of lung and respiratory tract involvement.

> **DIFFERENTIAL DIAGNOSIS** Cutaneous sarcoidosis
>
> - Other granulomatous diseases
> - Drug reaction
> - Cutaneous lupus erythematosus
> - Cutaneous T cell lymphoma
> - Hodgkin disease
> - Metastatic cancer
> - Hypertrophic lichen planus
> - Secondary syphilis
> - Cutaneous tuberculosis

Diagnostics

Cutaneous sarcoidosis is a diagnosis of exclusion which can be challenging as it mimics other serious diseases. A biopsy should be performed to rule out other granulomatous diseases. If histology shows noncaseating granuloma, then further evaluation and documentation are warranted to search for the presence (or absence) of systemic sarcoidosis. The initial workup usually includes a complete blood count with differential, comprehensive chemistry panel, chest x-ray, and sometimes a pulmonary function study. A serum angiotensin-converting enzyme (ACE) level should be measured as it is elevated in 60% of patients with systemic involvement, especially if there is hilar adenopathy, pulmonary infiltration, or extrathoracic disease.

Management

In the absence of systemic sarcoidosis, cutaneous symptoms do not require treatment. Watchful waiting may be the best approach for possible spontaneous resolution for the majority of mild cutaneous cases. For plaques that are symptomatic, high-potency TCS or IL triamcinolone acetate can be used. Thick plaques, however, may be recalcitrant. Cutaneous sarcoidosis which affects the cosmetic areas or the ulcerative type is an indication for systemic therapy with oral corticosteroids or corticosteroid-sparing agents. Doxycycline and minocycline have been reported to be effective. Surgical excision with grafting may be required to treat ulcerative sarcoidosis.

Special considerations

Sarcoidosis is rare in childhood but should be in the differential for any child diagnosed with arthritis that also has symptoms of uveitis.

Prognosis and complications

Cutaneous sarcoidosis has a good prognosis, while systemic disease depends on the progression of organ involvement. Most cases resolve without treatment in a few years, especially for those with Löfgren syndrome. The main concern for complications with skin lesions is scarring. Patients with lupus pernio form of sarcoidosis also have a low risk of developing destruction of facial bone or cartilage. If the patients also have systemic sarcoidosis, they are at increased risk for malignancies, especially lung cancer. Sarcoidosis with cardiac involvement has a poor prognosis.

Referral and consultation

Patients suspected of cutaneous sarcoidosis should be referred to a dermatologist for definitive diagnosis, workup, and treatment. Signs or symptoms of systemic disease will likely require collaboration of a multidisciplinary team, including a rheumatologist, pulmonologist, cardiologist, ophthalmologist, and other specialists as indicated.

Patient education and follow-up

Patients should be educated about sarcoidosis, as well as the signs and symptoms of progressing disease. Health promotion and disease prevention are important. Smoking cessation, diet, and exercise should be discussed and reinforced at office visits.

Although cutaneous sarcoidosis is benign, regular patient monitoring should occur as symptoms may worsen or systemic disease may develop without the patient's awareness. Patients with systemic sarcoidosis require management with specialists depending on their organ involvement. The PCP is key to providing the coordination of care between the specialties, ongoing health screenings, and monitoring for control or progression of the disease.

NEUTROPHILIC DERMATOSES

Neutrophilic dermatoses (NDs) are a category of skin diseases that vary in clinical appearance but have a characteristic histology of noninfectious, inflammatory infiltrates of neutrophils. They may manifest in the epidermis, dermis, or subcutaneous fat. NDs can resolve spontaneously after months or years, or require intensive treatment for disease control. The ability to correctly diagnose these diseases is dependent on the clinician's ability to recognize or suspect the presenting pattern and constellation of symptoms.

Sweet Syndrome

Sweet syndrome, first described by Dr. Sweet in 1964, is also known as acute febrile neutrophilic dermatosis. It is a rare disease that has been associated with inflammatory bowel diseases (IBD) such as ulcerative colitis and Crohn disease. However, there is a higher incidence of IBD patients developing pyoderma gangrenosum (another type of neutrophilic skin disease) compared to Sweet syndrome. Autoimmune diseases, such as Hashimoto thyroiditis and Sjörgren syndrome, as well as streptococcal infection, have been associated with Sweet syndrome. Intestinal bypass surgery may precede onset of Sweet syndrome.

Pathophysiology

The pathophysiology of Sweet syndrome is not known, but it is thought to be a hypersensitivity reaction to infection, a tumor antigen, or cetain drugs. Lesions are located within the upper dermis, giving them a vesicular or bullous appearance.

Subtypes

Three subtypes of Sweet syndrome have been identified: idiopathic, malignancy-associated, and drug-induced.

The *idiopathic* or *classical* form of the disease occurs most often in women between the ages of 30 and 60, but can occur in younger patients. Classical Sweet syndrome is usually associated with an upper respiratory tract or gastrointestinal tract infection, IBD, or pregnancy. These patients will often appear to be systemically ill, with fever and a significant level of physical distress.

Malignancy-associated Sweet syndrome occurs equally in men and women and is most often associated with myelogenous leukemia but can occur with solid tumor malignancies of the breast and genitourinary or gastrointestinal systems.

Drug-induced Sweet syndrome has been associated with granulocyte colony-stimulating factor (G-CSF), although other drugs have been implicated (Box 20-1).

Clinical presentation

Sweet syndrome is characterized by the sudden occurrence of painful, edematous, erythematous or purple, "juicy" papules and plaques. There may be vesicles and bullae or a surface with mammilated (nipple-like) appearance. Sweet syndrome favors the dorsum of the hands (Figure 20-11) but may also occur on the face, neck, and trunk (Figure 20-12). Clinicians should have a high index of suspicion when patients present with characteristic lesions and the

| BOX 20-1 | Drugs That May Be Associated with Sweet Syndrome* |

- Granulocyte colony-stimulating factor
- Oral isotretinoin
- Oral contraceptives
- Trimethoprim/sulfamethoxazole
- Hydralazine
- Furosemide
- Minocycline, doxycycline

*Suspect drug-induced Sweet syndrome if lesions occur within 1 week to 1 month after administration of one of these drugs and resolve after the drug is discontinued.

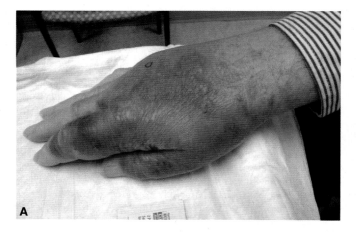

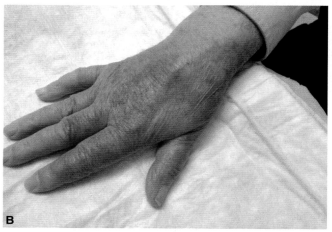

FIG. 20-11. **A:** Sweet syndrome. Painful, violaceous, and "juicy" plaque with pseudovesicles commonly occur on the back of the hand. **B:** One month later, after treatment with dapsone.

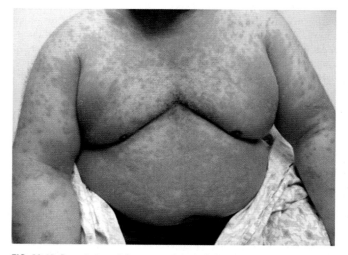

FIG. 20-12. Drug-induced Sweet syndrome. A 54-year-old man developed this pruritic eruption 1 month after being started on doxycycline for hidradenitis suppurativa. Note the dusky erythematous papules and plaques with sloughing vesicles in the axillary folds. WBCs were 11.6 million/mcL biopsy showed the neutrophilic infiltrate characteristic of Sweet syndrome.

sudden onset of fever, abdominal pain, malaise, joint pain, headache, conjunctivitis, or pregnancy. A recent history of upper respiratory or gastrointestinal tract infection may be noted. A few patients may not have constitutional symptoms or appear acutely ill.

DIFFERENTIAL DIAGNOSIS Sweet syndrome

- Pyoderma gangrenosum (PG)
- Bullous diseases
- Erythema multiforme
- Bowel-associated dermatosis-arthritis syndrome
- Behçet disease
- Erythema nodosum
- Drug eruption
- Urticaria
- Cellulitis
- Paraneoplastic syndrome

Diagnostics

A punch biopsy from a lesion suspicious for Sweet syndrome may show a dense neutrophilic infiltrate in the dermis without evidence of leukocytoclastic vasculitis. The biopsy alone is not diagnostic. Major and minor criteria have been proposed and outline the clinicopathologic features of the condition (Box 20-2).

Laboratory studies should include a CBC with differential, which may show elevated WBCs, specifically neutrophilia (except in drug-induced Sweet syndrome). Serum erythrocyte sedimentation rate (ESR) and alkaline phosphatase are usually elevated. Additional diagnostics may be indicated for the evaluation of possible underlying malignancy, especially hematologic malignancies.

Management

Patients with Sweet syndrome are referred to a dermatology for co-management of lesions. Once the diagnosis of Sweet syndrome is

confirmed, the first-line treatment is systemic corticosteroids and should be initiated after assessing the patient for contraindications. Antibiotics with anti-inflammatory effects (tetracycline class) may also prove useful. Severe or recalcitrant cases may be treated with off-label use of dapsone (corticosteroid-sparing agent), which is favored by dermatology clinicians for NDs. Potassium iodine has also been used.

Sweet syndrome can occur secondary to a drug, which should be discontinued immediately. Any suspected metabolic condition or neoplastic etiology should be evaluated and treated.

Prognosis and complications

Sweet syndrome responds quickly to systemic corticosteroids, with laboratory values often returning to normal within 72 hours and skin lesions clearing within 1 to 2 weeks. Approximately 15% of patients have relapses occurring for several years. Systemic diseases associated with Sweet's include Crohn disease, ulcerative colitis, and myeloproliferative disorders (acute myelocytic leukemia, chronic myelogenous leukemia, lymphoma) and warrant close monitoring. In 15% to 20% of patients, Sweet syndrome may precede the malignancy by up to 6 years.

Referral and consultation

Patients suspected of Sweet syndrome should be referred immediately to a dermatologist for evaluation and management. A hematologist/oncologist should also be consulted if associated malignancy is suspected.

Patient education and follow-up

Educate the patient about Sweet syndrome and the importance of prompt treatment for any symptoms of infection or illness. Emphasis should be placed on age-appropriate routine health screenings.

Patients should be followed up closely while undergoing treatment for Sweet syndrome. After resolution of cutaneous symptoms, PCPs should follow up with routine and symptomatic health screenings.

Pyoderma Gangrenosum

PG is a neutrophilic dermatosis that produces nonhealing ulcers often misdiagnosed as a severe skin infection. The average age of onset is 40 to 60 years, but it can occur in any age group, including children. PG is more predominate in females. Its name is a misnomer as PG is neither infectious nor gangrenous. There is a higher incidence in patients with IBD, such as Crohn's and ulcerative colitis, hematologic disorders, rheumatoid arthritis, vasculitis, and other autoimmune diseases.

Pathophysiology

The pathophysiology of PG, like other NDs, is mostly unknown. Its association with other conditions suggests that it may be an altered immune response to infection, trauma, and systemic disease. Lesions may occur secondary to *pathergy* where minor trauma such as an abrasion, insect bite, needle stick, or hematoma results in an expanding papule, pustule, or nodule.

Clinical presentation

Classic or *ulcerative* PG is the most common and destructive type of PG. Lesions begin suddenly as small pustules, papules, or nodules that slowly evolve into erythematous/violaceous ulcers (Figure 20-13A). The borders are typically raised with rolled edges that are underminded (overhanging edges). PG ulcerations often

---

BOX 20-2 **Diagnostic Criteria for Sweet Syndrome***

Major Criteria
1. Sudden onset of pathognomonic skin lesions
2. Histopathology of skin biopsy neutrophilic infiltrates of the dermis without signs of leukocytoclastic vasculitis

Minor Criteria
1. Preceding respiratory tract infection, gastrointestinal infection, or vaccination; or associated inflammatory disease, pregnancy, hemoproliferative disorder, or malignancy
2. Constitutional symptoms, including fever (>38°C), arthralgia, or malaise
3. Good response to systemic corticosteroids or potassium iodide
4. Elevated erythrocyte sedimentation rate (ESR) >20 mm/h; positive C-reactive protein; CBC with leukocyte count > 8,000; and peripheral blood smear with >70% consisting of segmented-nuclear neutrophils (mature) and stabs/bands (immature). *Must have 3 out of 4 of these.*

---
*Diagnosis requires both major criteria and 2 of the 4 minor criteria.

Modified from von den Driesch, P. (1994). Sweet's syndrome (acute febrile neutrophilic dermatosis). *Journal of the American Academy of Dermatology, 31*(4), 535–556.

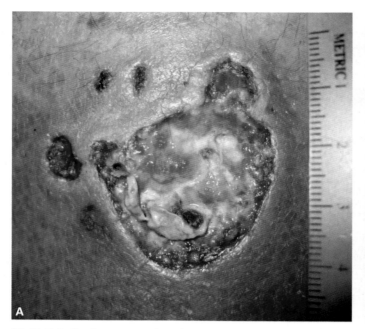
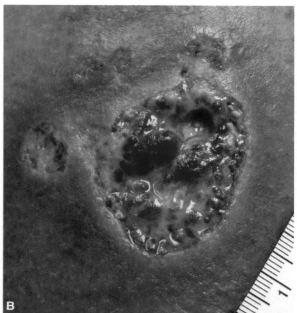

FIG. 20-13. A: Classic cutaneous ulceration of PG located on the lower legs, with rolled borders and underminded edges. **B:** Healing with good response to cyclosporine after 2 weeks.

have a necrotic base with some purulent drainage and are exquisitely painful. Lesions may be solitary or multiple, coalescing into larger crater-like ulcers and small fistulas. These sinus tracks are characteristic of PG. The most common location for PG is on the lower legs, but atypical lesions can occur on the scalp, trunk, genitals, buttocks, and upper extremities. Ulcerations around the site of a stoma (peristomal PG) can create terrible wounds for ostomy patients. Healed ulcers result in atrophic cribriform scars.

Other atypical forms include *vegetative* PG, seen in patients with IBD and characterized by a verrucous surface without underminded borders. It affects the buccal and labial mucosa. *Pustular* PG forms vesicles and pustules at the border of the lesion and is often seen with IBD. The *bullous* form of PG has a juicy appearance and thus often mistaken for Sweet syndrome. This variant is usually more superficial and less destructive, resulting in less scarring.

PG patients may exhibit constitutional symptoms that may or may not be associated with organ involvement. A detailed history and physical examination are essential for an accurate diagnosis of underlying disease or coexisting conditions.

Diagnostics

PG is a diagnosis of exclusion. In addition to clinical appearance and history of pathergy, clinicians must consider other ulcerative or inflammatory skin diseases. A punch biopsy for histology, as well as tissue cultures to rule out bacterial, fungal, or mycobacterial infection, should be performed. Histology of PG will reveal a classic dense neutrophilic infiltration of the dermis. Diagnostic studies for venous or arterial insufficiency will be normal. About half of the patients with PG have an underlying systemic disease. Therefore, an extensive workup may be indicated for possible organ involvement or comorbid conditions.

Management

Patients with nonhealing ulcers should be referred promptly to a dermatologist or wound care specialist as PG can progress very rapidly. Management depends on the type, number, severity, and location of the ulcerations. The initial treatment goal of PG is to stop the progression of the lesion and formation of new ulcers. PG ulcers are slow healing and may take 6 or more weeks. Patients with one or two small lesions may be treated with IL corticosteroids. TCS or off-label use of tacrolimus 0.3% ointment can also be effective in small superficial lesions. Dakin's solution (diluted sodium hypochlorite) can help optimize healing and reduce the risk for secondary infection. A barrier such as white petrolatum can be used to protect the surrounding skin.

Surgical treatment or debridement is usually not indicated and should be avoided as it can expand the wound. Areas with PG ulcers should be protected from trauma or friction due to pathergy. For more extensive PG, dermatologists or wound care specialists may use high-dose corticosteroids, cyclosporine, and other systemic agents which have been effective (Figure 20-13B). In patients with Crohn disease, infliximab may treat both the cutaneous lesions of PG and gastrointestinal symptoms.

DIFFERENTIAL DIAGNOSIS   Pyoderma gangrenosum

- Venous or arterial ulcers
- Squamous cell carcinoma
- Necrobiosis lipoidica
- Sweet syndrome
- Brown recluse spider bite
- Vasculitis
- Progressive synergistic gangrene
- Ecthyma and ecthyma gangrenosum
- Pyoderma (including atypical mycobacteria and mycosis)
- Pemphigus vegetans
- Antiphospholipid antibody syndrome

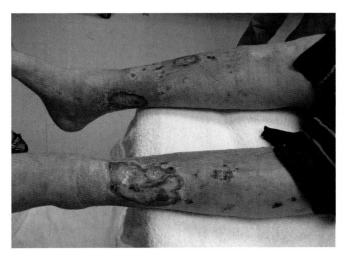

FIG. 20-14. The characteristic rapidly expanding and necrotic ulcerations of PG should prompt an immediate referral to a dermatologist.

Prognosis and complications

Spontaneous healing of PG has been known to occur; however, if untreated, it can last for months or years. Healing ulcers typically take months to heal, and new ulcers may appear as older ones resolve. With treatment, more than 50% of patients heal completely within 1 year but relapses occur. Severe disease requiring aggressive immunosuppressive therapy has a higher risk of morbidity and mortality. Even with successful treatment and resolution, the disfigurement, scarring, and pain with PG can be devastating.

Referral and consultation

Although very mild lesions may be managed by PCPs, it is highly recommended that all patients with PG be referred to experienced dermatologists or wound care specialists due to its rapid (and unpredictable) destructive nature (Figure 20-14). Treatment of underlying or comorbid diseases should be identified and referred to the appropriate specialists like gastroenterologists for possible IBD. Consultation with pain management may be indicated for relief from severe and chronic pain from the disease.

Patient education and follow-up

Patients should be educated about the disease and essential diagnostics not only for PG but also for possible associated systemic disease. Treatment options, along with risks and side effects, must be discussed in detail. Patients must be cautioned to avoid any trauma or friction near the ulcerations. Realistic expectations are important as ulcers may take weeks or months to heal and have scarring. The formation of any new papules or blisters should immediately be reported to their specialist.

Patients with PG must be followed up closely by a dermatologist, especially during the healing phase or during use of immunosuppression therapy. Regular follow-up visits with primary care for comorbdities, side effects, or complications are vitally important.

Behçet Disease

First described by Hippocrates, Behçet disease (BD) or Adamantiades-BD is a rare, potentially fatal, systemic vasculitis. The onset occurs in young adults (20 to 30 years old) and rarely in infants and the elderly. BD is more prevalent in women from Asia, northern Europe, and the United States, whereas men from Middle Eastern countries are more affected. Patients with the gene HLA-B51 are at higher risk.

Pathophysiology

The pathophysiology of BD is unknown but is thought to be a combination of genetic, environmental, hematologic, and infectious factors triggering an immunologic dysfunction of the innate immune system. The autoimmune response is characterized by a neutrophilic vascular response resulting in inflammation and damage to the endothelium of arteries and veins. BD can affect vessels of any size but is predominant in small and medium-sized vessels. In addition to cutaneous manifestations, BD can affect any organ in the body.

Clinical presentation

BD is chronic, unpredictable, and relapsing. The onset of cutaneous symptoms may be sudden or insidious. The characteristic triad of skin lesions includes the eyes (iritis and uveitis), oral mucosa and tongue (ulcers), and genitals (ulcers). Almost all patients with BD experience painful oral apthae that begin as erythematous round macules, developing a yellow pseudomembrane evolving into painful ulcerations (Figure 20-15).

Mucocutaneous symptoms, along with arthritis, are usually the first symptoms of BD. Other cutaneous symptoms include acneiform lesions, pseudofolliculitis, and erythema nodosum–like plaques. Systemic symptoms may vary according to organ involvement and can manifest as arthritis, gastrointestinal ulcers, thrombophlebitis, endocarditis and valvular disease, and meningitis.

DIFFERENTIAL DIAGNOSIS Behçet disease

- Idiopathic oral aphthae
- Ocular or oral mucous membrane syndromes
- Autoimmune blistering diseases
- Uveitis
- Viral infection (herpes, etc.)
- Syphilis
- Systemic lupus erythematosus

Diagnostics

BD is a diagnosis of exclusion, requiring an experienced clinician with a high index of suspicion. Thus, the diagnosis of BD may take

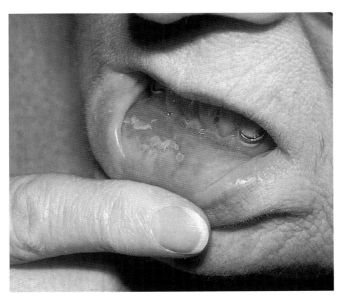

FIG. 20-15. Recurrent oral aphthae are the most common clinical findings in patients with Behçet disease.

years after the initial onset of symptoms. Several versions of diagnostic criteria have been proposed but have not been agreed upon. A punch biopsy may show neutrophilic infiltrates in the dermis and sometimes vasculitis. A positive pathergy test (a pinprick evolves into a papule, then a sterile pustule) is usually present but is seen in other diseases such as Sweet syndrome, PG, and erythema elevatum diutinum. Bacterial and viral cultures can help rule out underlying infections. A serum HLA-B51 may be positive and a marker for severe disease prognosis. Radiologic, cardiac, and pulmonary testing may be appropriate depending on organ involvement.

Management
Aggressive systemic treatment by an experienced dermatologist is usually required. Oral corticosteroids, azathioprine, colchicine, cyclophosphamide, chlorambucil, mycophenolate mofetil, cyclosporine, IV immunoglobulin, and TNF-α inhibitors have been effective.

Special consideration
Oral corticosteroids are the treatment of choice in patients who are pregnant.

Prognosis and complications
The clinical course of BD varies significantly and prognosis depends on early diagnosis. Prompt treatment can minimize organ damage, especially in the presence of central nervous system and large artery or vein involvement. Ten percent of patients suffer from severe disease that can result in death from organ failure or complications. BD with central nervous system, gastrointestinal, or vascular involvement has the highest risk of mortality. Spontaneous remission of some or all of the disease manifestations has been known to occur. BD in children has a good prognosis. Young male patients with early signs of systemic involvement have a worse prognosis.

Referral and consultation
Patients suspected of BD disease should be immediately referred to a dermatologist. Multiple specialists may be needed, including ophthalmologists, otolaryngologists, rheumatologists, gastroenterologists, vascular specialists, neurologists, and others.

Patient education and follow-up
Patients should be educated concerning the disease, symptoms, prognosis, and treatments. The purpose and side effects of the potent immunosuppressive agents should be discussed with patients in great detail. They should also be cautioned that abrupt cessation of systemic treatment could cause severe relapse.

Patients with severe disease will probably need to follow many specialists depending on the organ and cutaneous involvement. PCPs should coordinate specialty care and routinely monitor the patient's health.

BILLING CODES ICD-10

Actinic granuloma	L57.5
Behçet disease	M35.2
Foreign-body granuloma	L92.3
Granuloma annulare	L92.0
Necrobiosis lipoidica	L92.1
Pyoderma gangrenosum	L88.0
Sarcoidosis, unspecified	D86.9
Sweet syndrome	L98.2

READINGS

Baldessari, E. M., Garcia, N., & Villarroel, A. M. (2012). Sweet's syndrome. *Internal Medicine Journal, 42*(1), 103–104. doi:10.1111/j.1445-5994.2011.02632

Cohen, P. R., Hönigsmann, H., & Kurzrock, R. (2008). Acute febrile neutrophilic dermatosis (sweet syndrome). In L. A. Goldsmith, S. I. Katz, B. A. Gilchrest, A. S. Paller, D. J. Leffell, & K. Wolff (Eds.), *Fitzpatrick's dermatology in general medicine* (7th ed., pp. 289–295). New York, NY: McGraw Hill.

Moschella, S. L. & Davis, M. D. (2012). Neutrophilic dermatoses. In J. L. Bolognia, J. L. Jorizzo, J. V. Schaffer (Eds.), *Dermatology* (3rd. ed., pp. 423–439). Philadelphia, PA: Mosby.

Jamet, A., Lagarce, L., Le Clec'h, C., Croue, A., Hoareau, F., Diquet, B., & Laine-Cessac, P. (2008). Doxycycline-induced Sweet's syndrome. *European Journal of Dermatology, 18*(5), 595–596. doi:10.1684/ejd.2008.0482; 10.1684/ejd.2008.0482

Merola, J. (2013). Sweet syndrome (acute febrile neutrophilic dermatosis): Pathogenesis, clinical manifestations, and diagnosis. Retrieved from http://www.uptodate.com/contents/sweet-syndrome-acute-febrile-neutrophilic-dermatosis-pathogenesis-clinical-manifestations-and-diagnosis?source=preview&anchor=H1950361&selectedTitle=1~150#H1950361

Rapini, R. P. (2012). Actinic granuloma of O'Brien. Retrieved from http://www.expertconsultbook.com/expertconsult/ob/book.do?method=display&type=bookPage&decorator=none&eid=4-u1.0-B978-0-323-06658-7.00007-5--s0045&isbn=978-0-323-06658-7

Rochet, N. M., Rahul, B. S., Chavan, N., Cappel, M. A., Wada, D. A., & Gibson, L. E. (2013). Sweet syndrome: Clinical presentation, associations, and response to treatment in 77 patients. *Journal of the American Academy of Dermatology, 69*(4), 557–563.

von den Driesch, P. (1994). Sweet's syndrome (acute febrile neutrophilic dermatosis. *Journal of the American Academy of Dermatology, 31*(4), 535–556.

Wolverton, S. E. (2012). *Comprehensive dermatologic drug therapy* (3rd ed.). Philadelphia, PA: Saunders Elsevier.

Zouboulis, C. C. (2008). Adamantiades-behçet's disease. In K. Wolff, L. A. Goldsmith, S. I. Katz, B. A. Gilchrest, A. S. Paller, & D. J. Leffell (Eds.), *Fitzpatrick's dermatology in general medicine* (7th ed., pp. 1620–1626). New York, NY: McGraw Hill.

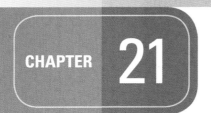

CHAPTER 21 Genital Dermatoses

Linda Hansen-Rodier

Numerous skin conditions can affect the genitalia of men and women and can be common manifestations of disorders involving other areas of the body. Often, genital dermatoses go untreated because of embarrassment, shame, and physical or emotional discomfort in treating these problems. Disease and infection involving the genitalia may be painful, affect sexual function and relationships, impact self-esteem, and alter the quality of life. Genital dermatoses may be related to infection, inflammation, and sometimes skin cancer.

GENITALIA

Skin in the genital area is a combination of keratinized, modified mucous membrane and membranous skin which makes the clinical presentation unique and challenging to diagnose disease. Knowledge of the normal male and female genital anatomy is paramount to correctly identifying abnormal signs and symptoms. The secretory glands on the glans penis and the vulva, as well as cervical and vaginal mucous secretions, can alter the appearance of the genitalia, especially when inflammation is present. For example, the typical scaly plaques of a papulosquamous disease on the trunk may lack defined borders, erythema, and scale when it involves the genitalia. Inflammatory dermatoses on the genitalia may be difficult to appreciate and appear hyperpigmented instead of red. The normal rugation of the labia majora and the scrotum may mask lichenification. Normal papillae on the vulva or pearly papules on the corona of the glans penis may be mistaken for verrucal papules.

Female

The skin on the mons pubis which extends to the lateral aspect of the labia majora is dry, keratinized, and usually hair bearing. Medial aspects of the labia majora, and including the labia minora, are partially keratinized and partially modified mucous membrane which is generally moist and hair bearing (Figure 21-1A).

Male

The male genitalia include the pubis, scrotum, and penis. The pubis and part of the shaft of the penis and scrotum have dry, keratinized skin that may have hair. The penile shaft is modified mucosa and most often contains no hair, as well as the glans of the penis and the border of the glans or corona. The urethra is located on the tip of the glans and composed of mucous membrane. For uncircumcised males, the glans and corona are covered by the prepuce (foreskin). Careful examination of this otherwise obstructed area is important because of the increased incidence of psoriasis, lichen planus, lichen sclerosus, balanitis, and squamous cell carcinoma (Figure 21-1B).

Hygiene

With the variation of skin of the genitalia in mind, we must also consider personal hygiene practices and how they can affect the skin barrier and clinical presentation. Many people wash frequently or apply multiple products to the genitals in an effort to "clean" the area. Over cleansing may contribute to a compromised skin barrier, making it more susceptible to infectious organisms or inflammation. Likewise, urine and feces left on the skin can result in chronic irritation. Adult incontinence products are widely utilized and may be tight or occlusive resulting in friction and increased moisture, all of which may affect the skin barrier of the genitalia.

GENITAL HERPES VIRUS

Genital herpes, one of the most common sexually transmitted diseases (STDs), has increased by 30% in the United States over the past two decades and affects more than 50 million people aged 12 and older. There are 500,000 new cases each year, many of which have no symptoms and are unaware that they have been infected. The incidence of herpes simplex virus (HSV) is higher in individuals with decreased access to health care and is an increased risk for other STDs. Individuals who are immunocompromised (HIV

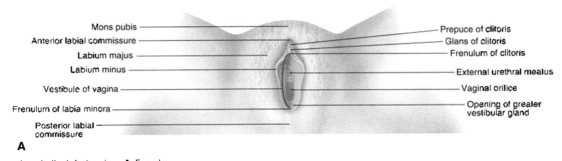

Mons pubis — ⎯⎯⎯⎯⎯⎯⎯⎯⎯⎯⎯⎯
Anterior labial commissure — ⎯⎯⎯⎯⎯⎯⎯⎯
Labium majus — ⎯⎯⎯⎯⎯⎯⎯⎯⎯⎯
Labium minus — ⎯⎯⎯⎯⎯⎯⎯⎯⎯⎯
Vestibule of vagina — ⎯⎯⎯⎯⎯⎯⎯⎯
Frenulum of labia minora — ⎯⎯⎯⎯⎯⎯
Posterior labial commissure —

— Prepuce of clitoris
— Glans of clitoris
— Frenulum of clitoris
— External urethral meatus
— Vaginal orifice
— Opening of greater vestibular gland

A

FIG. 21-1. External genitalia, inferior view. **A:** Female.

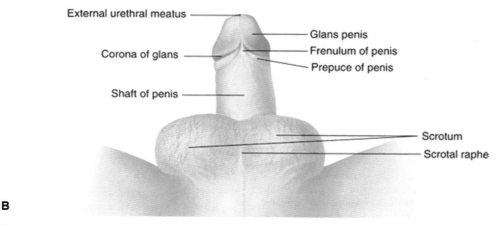

External urethral meatus — Glans penis
— Frenulum of penis
Corona of glans — — Prepuce of penis

Shaft of penis —

Scrotum
Scrotal raphe

B

FIG. 21-1. *(continued)* External genitalia, inferior view. **B:** Male.

infection, immunosuppressive therapy, organ transplant recipients, and immunologic disorders) are at greater risk for a severe HSV outbreak and often struggle with nonhealing ulcers and superinfections.

Pathophysiology

Genital herpes is most often caused by HSV type 2, but HSV type 1 may also be the causative agent most likely from orogenital contact. The pathogenesis of HSV is discussed in chapter 10 along with nongenital HSV infections. A *primary infection* occurs after exposure to the virus in an individual who has no antibodies to HSV1 or HSV2, whereas *recurrent infection* occurs when there is a reactivation of the virus after a period of latency. A *nonprimary* initial infection is an individual with antibodies to one HSV type and then acquires a new infection to the other HSV type. This is most often the case when an HSV2 infection develops in the presence of HSV1 antibodies, usually transmitted during orogenital contact. People with a known history of HSV1 are three times more likely to develop an asymptomatic HSV2 infection. These patients usually have fewer recurrences and milder symptoms.

Transmission

HSV is transmitted through direct skin contact, which includes vaginal intercourse, orogenital contact, and anal sexual contact. HSV can also be acquired by autoinoculation or contact with infected saliva. It can be spread in the presence of active lesions or in the absence of visible sores or symptoms (silent shedding). There is a higher concentration of viral shedding after a primary outbreak and for the following 3 months, compared to a recurrent or nonprimary episode. Transmission often occurs when an individual or even both partners are unaware that they are infected. Asymptomatic infection can be in the cervix, prostate, or urethra. This may occur due to antibody acquisition to HSV2 without a history of or active disease. Thus, decreasing the number of lifetime partners also decreases the chance of transmission.

It can be a disconcerting situation for a couple in a long-term relationship when one individual develops a new genital herpes outbreak after years of monogamy. Hasty assumptions and accusations of infidelity may ensue unless both individuals are educated about the virus. There may have been a "silent" first outbreak with no lesions, and due to some change in the person's immune function, a symptomatic outbreak occurs.

Transmission to a fetus can occur during pregnancy, delivery, or postpartum. The greatest risk for neonatal infection occurs when the mother develops a primary HSV2 infection within the last 3 months of pregnancy. Women who have had a previous infection develop IgG antibodies that cross the placenta and may offer protection to the fetus. Neonatal infection is rare but can be serious and possibly fatal to the newborn. Prevention is the primary goal, especially in the last weeks of pregnancy.

Clinical Presentation

Primary infection

The first outbreak of genital herpes may occur between 2 and 20 hours after exposure but may be delayed for up to 2 weeks. The infection may begin with constitutional symptoms, including fever, nausea and vomiting, muscle aches, sore throat, and lymphadenopathy, but no overt skin lesions. Then, cutaneous symptoms of HSV may present initially as erythematous papules that develop into a cluster of vesicles and coalesce into "punched out," irregularly bordered ulcerations. Erosions on the mucous membranes or intertriginous areas may appear macerated or as linear fissures due to the moist environment. There may be itching, tingling, or intense burning pain at the site of the outbreak. Lymphadenopathy is often present. Symptoms, beginning with a prodrome, may last from 1 to 3 weeks.

In women, the HSV lesions are found primarily on the labia, fourchette, cervix, buttocks, thighs, and occasionally the nipples (Figure 21-2A). An accompanying discharge from the cervix or vagina can mislead the clinician to believe that there is a vaginitis or cervicitis. Ulcerations near the urethra can result in dysuria and even urinary retention (Figure 21-2B). Males with HSV can report ulcerations on the penis, buttocks, or thighs (Figure 21-3A). Urethral discharge may also be noted along with urinary retention. Erosive balanitis can occur, especially in immunosuppressed patients.

Generally, immunosuppressed individuals may experience larger ulcers or ulcers at multiple sites. It should be noted that patients with systemic symptoms, severe mucocutaneous disease, and at-risk individuals should be carefully evaluated for disseminated herpes, which can lead to organ failure and death. These patients warrant hospitalization, evaluation for viremia, IV antiviral therapy, and supportive care.

First nonprimary infection

In a first, nonprimary episode, both cutaneous and constitutional symptoms may be very mild or asymptomatic. This is attributed to

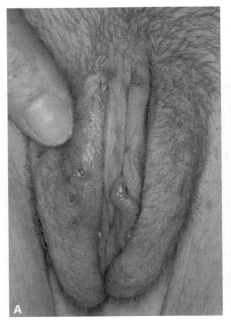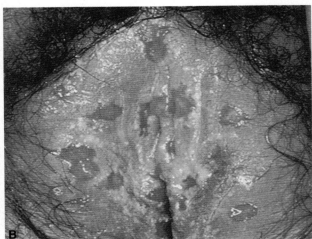

FIG. 21-2. **A&B:** HSV2. Note the punched-out quality to the erosions.

the antibodies that the patient already has to one type of HSV. The lesions in a first, nonprimary HSV infection are the same as primary HSV infection except the number and severity of the ulcerations are milder. Vesicles heal faster, and there are usually fewer recurrences.

Recurrent infection

Prodromal symptoms with recurrent HSV outbreaks may last hours to 3 days on average. In a recurrence, the outbreak is usually in the same site or unilateral location. There may be tender lymph glands but usually no vaginal discharge or urinary symptoms. Recurrences may occur four to seven times per year and are thought to be triggered by illness, stress, tight clothing, abrasion, or friction from the lack of lubrication with sexual contact.

DIFFERENTIAL DIAGNOSIS Herpes simplex virus

- Genital aphthae
- Syphilis, primary (chancre)
- Behçet disease
- Lymphogranuloma venereum

Diagnostics

A common but frequently overlooked diagnosis of HSV should be based on clinical and laboratory findings. The CDC recommends laboratory confirmation of suspected HSV infections and clinical correlation regarding the diagnostic method used. Since lesions may be subclinical, accurate diagnosis can be difficult even to the most trained eye. There may be pertinent positives/negatives in the history and physical that can aid clinicians in differentiating HSV from other diseases and infection. Chancroid usually presents as a deep solitary and nonpainful ulcer compared to the multiple shallow and painful ulcers of HSV (Figure 21-3B). The chancre of primary syphilis and the lesions of lymphogranuloma venereum both have tender lymphadenopathy.

Viral culture is the most commonly used and commercially available diagnostic tool, but not the most accurate, for the diagnoses of HSV. Culture should be performed within 7 days of the first

episode and within 2 days of a recurrence. To obtain the best specimen, unroof a vesicle and sample the exudate at the base by rolling the culturette across the wound base. Viral culture has a 50% to 75% rate of sensitivity and requires a newer lesion. If the first culture is negative, repeating the culture during a recurrence is important to confirm diagnosis.

Although viral culture is the standard for the diagnosis of HSV, a polymerase chain reaction or PCR assays have the highest sensitivity and specificity. PCR is especially advantageous during asymptomatic shedding, Cerebrospinal fluid (CSF) infection, neonates, and for monitory antiviral suppression therapy. Specimens are collected from serum, CSF, vesicle fluid, tissue, or endocervical sampling (thin prep). The use of PCR can be limited due to the cost and its availability in laboratories. In the absence of a lesion, serologic testing for HSV antibodies can also be performed and will detect evidence of past or recent infection of (IgG and IgM) HSV1 and HSV2.

Tzanck prep can be done to identify multinucleate giant cells. It is necessary to scrape the contents of a freshly opened vesicle, place on a slide and fix with methanol and Wright or Giemsa stain. If this can be done in the office, it will provide an immediate answer. Most clinicians will send to their laboratory, which will delay results.

Management

Supportive care

Comfort measures are important for patients with HSV outbreaks. Tepid baths soothe the perineal area which can become inflamed when urine passes over ulcerations. Urinary retention secondary to dysuria may be relieved with sitz bath. Personal hygiene will help to keep the area free of irritants and reduce the risk for secondary infection.

Tight or occlusive clothing should be avoided in an effort to reduce irritation and promote healing. Patients should be advised to abstain from sexual contact not only to reduce transmission of HSV but to reduce friction that can be painful. An emollient-like white petrolatum can provide a soothing barrier and reduce friction that causes pain. Cool packs or compresses can really help to reduce pain and itching.

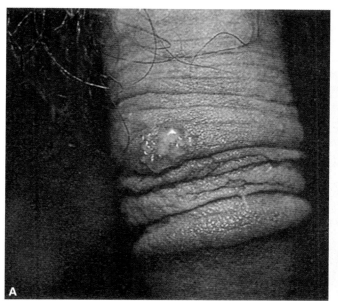 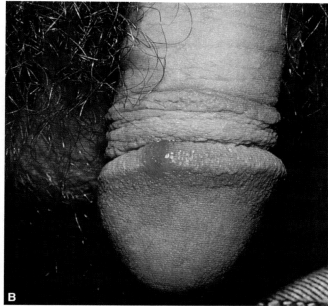

FIG. 21-3. HSV is a clinical diagnosis that should be confirmed with laboratory testing. An accurate diagnosis can be difficult even to the most trained eye. **A:** HSV2 presenting as a painful vesicle on an erythematous base on the shaft of a penis. **B:** A chancre of primary syphilis can have a similar presentation as a painless, solitary ulcer with erythema on the corona of the glans.

Medications

When treating the patient with HSV, consider their immune status, systemic symptoms, frequency of outbreaks, duration of the outbreaks, and asymptomatic shedding. Antiviral therapy is the gold standard and should be initiated in the early onset of the outbreak (ideally 72 hours after lesions erupt), can short the duration and reduce the severity. Chapter 10 discusses recommended antivirals and dosing based on the type of infection (primary vs. recurrence), episodic or suppressive, and immune status of the patient. Parenteral therapy is reserved for complex HSV, and oral therapy is more efficacious than topical antivirals. Acyclovir is a pregnancy category B drug and is also available as an intravenous therapy.

Prognosis and Complications

Most infections with HSV, whether they are primary or recurrent, resolve eventually without treatment. Complications occur with severe infection, secondary infection, systemic symptoms, or immunosuppression. The patient at risk can develop encephalitis, meningitis, or sepsis. The risk for neonatal infection is possible but rare.

Patient Education and Follow-up

The diagnosis of genital herpes and the knowledge that it can recur during one's lifetime can be devastating. Patients and their partners may struggle with a new diagnosis and all of the patient education that is important, so a follow-up office visit to repeat the information and ask questions is vitally important. Patients require additional time to talk or voice their feelings about the infection. It may be important to discuss the health issue with the patients partner, but only if the patient requests. Provider can try to correct any misconceptions and alleviate fears. STD education and testing should be offered. Encourage the use of latex condoms with sexual contact (even if asymptomatic) and lubricants to reduce friction that may cause pain or trigger a recurrence. Have patients avoid direct contact when an active lesion appears,

emphasize good hand washing, and discourage the use of shared personal items.

Disease prevention through stress reduction and healthy living is recommended. Patients should return if more than six outbreaks occur a year or if other circumstances prevail.

Referral and Consultation

Patients with an atypical presentation, severe constitutional symptoms, history of immunosuppression, or those not improving with treatment should be referred without delay to an infectious disease specialist or the emergency department. Consult obstetrics if the patient is pregnant.

GENITAL HUMAN PAPILLOMAVIRUS

At least 5.5 million cases of human papillomavirus (HPV), presenting as *genital warts* and *condyloma accuminata*, are diagnosed annually. Epidemiologists think that the number is higher because of the large number of subclinical cases that go undiagnosed. There are almost 100 serotypes of HPV affecting mucocutaneous surfaces.

HPV types 6 and 11 are associated with benign condyloma, while HPV types 16, 18, 31, and 33 are associated with genital dysplasia. Squamous cell carcinoma in situ (SCCIS), Bowenoid papulosa, erythroplasia of Queyrat, cervical dysplasia, and cervical cancers have been associated with HPV. Oropharyngeal cancer has been linked to HPV, with some studies suggesting transmission through orogenital sex. Smoking, parity, immunity, hormonal levels and nutritional status, and environmental influences increase the risk of transformation into malignancy. Nongenital HPV is discussed in chapter 10.

Transmission

The most common path of transmission is through sexual contact or direct skin to skin contact. It takes only one sexual contact with a

partner who does not know that he or she has HPV to transmit the virus. Sexual contact with a new partner who has a different strain of HPV can trigger an outbreak of warts. Nongenital warts can also be spread to the genital area. Condoms are often limited in preventing transmission because they cover only the shaft of the penis. Risk for infection includes a high number of sexual partners or a partner who had multiple contacts previously. The frequency of sexual intercourse also increases risk.

Pathophysiology

HPV is a double-stranded circular DNA genome. Some viral types, such as types 16, 18, and 31, can cause the p53 protein and RB proteins to be inactivated and can cause a normal cell to become a cancerous one. HPV type 16 is thought to be the most oncogenic and can result in cancers of the vulva, vagina, cervix, penis, and anal area. The virus infects the squamous cells and creates characteristic koilocytes within the cell. They initially enter the skin or mucous membrane through tiny tears or abrasions that may be created through trauma or friction during sexual contact. The virus enters the basaloid epithelium and is able to evade immune surveillance. It takes days, months, or years to develop the condyloma, if at all. Often the body is able to clear the virus in time through cell-mediated immunity and antibodies induced by the viral infection itself.

Clinical Presentation

Genital warts may present with pruritus and pain or be asymptomatic depending on the size and extent of the lesions. The number of presenting lesions depends upon an individual's immune response to the virus. Genital warts have varied presentations, including small, smooth papules that are red, brown, or flesh color (Figure 21-4A). They can look similar to pearly penile papules that are a normal variant (Figure 21-4B). Others may appear rough on the surface (verrucal), filiform, pointed, or flat. They may be solitary, pedunculated like a skin tag, or a verrucous plaque of coalescing papules (Figure 21-5). On moist mucosal surfaces, they may be white and keratotic (Figure 21-6B). The warts that develop on the cervix are usually flat and may not be visible without the aid of colposcopy. On male genitalia, warts can erupt on the pubis, shaft of the penis, scrotum, foreskin, meatus, urethra, or perianal area (Figure 21-7). Genital warts in females may involve the pubis, vulva, vagina, urethra, or anal area. They may bleed easily and cause dyspareunia. They can be mistaken for normal vestibular papillae (Figure 21-6A). *Oral warts* may result from orogenital contact and may not be easily visible. The tongue is the most common site (Figure 21-8).

DIFFERENTIAL DIAGNOSIS Human papillomavirus
• Condyloma lata
• Molluscum contagiosum
• Pearly penile papules
• Vestibular papillae
• Vulvar papillomatosis
• Fox–Fordyce
• Lichen nitidus
• Bowenoid papulosis

Diagnostics

Diagnosis is based on clinical presentation and symptoms. Any persistent lesion that does not appear typical, does not respond to treatment, or does not heal should be biopsied. Histopathology that reveals koilocytosis can help the clinician eliminate many of the differential diagnoses.

Condyloma lata are large flat-topped lesions associated with secondary syphilis, so serologic screening may be necessary. It can be very challenging to determine whether the papules are molluscum contagiosum, which are usually isolated to the mons pubis, but may be on the scrotum, penis, and/or groin and appear as shiny papules with central delling. Curettage of a lesion and KOH prep revealing Henderson–Patterson bodies can differentiate it from HPV (see chapter 10). Some clinicians perform acetic acid whitening test for diagnosis of genital warts; however, it is not recommended as it is neither specific nor sensitive for HPV.

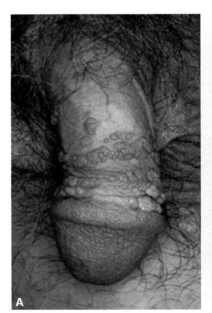
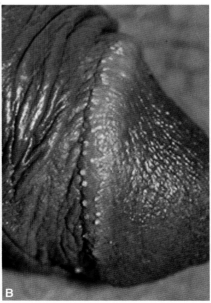

FIG. 21-4. A: Penile warts; verrucal papules of HPV on the penis. These skin-colored, brown, and slightly hypopigmented, lobular papules on the penis are a very common morphology of genital warts. **B:** Pearly penile papules (*arrow*) can be differentiated from genital warts by the monomorphous, symmetric appearance and by the finding that each is discrete. These papules are most often located on the corona in circumferential, parallel rows.

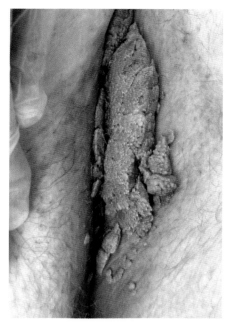

FIG. 21-5. HPV starts as verrucal papules before coalescing into plaque. Giant condyloma acuminatum (Buschke and Löwenstein) is at risk for transformation into a malignancy.

Management

No treatment offers a 100% cure rate; prevention is the best approach. Treatment should be aimed at eliminating the visible condyloma and discomfort that may be associated with the wart lesions. Treating visible lesions also reduces the chance of transmission of the virus. However, a subclinical infection exists in the surrounding tissue that leads to the high rate of recurrence even after treatment. Selection of treatment should consider cost to the patient, potential discomfort and scarring, recurrence rate, and effectiveness.

Vaccination

The CDC's Advisory Committee on Immunization Practices now recommends Merck's HPV vaccine, Gardasil, for males as well as females between the ages of 11 and 26 years, to aid in the prevention of HPV types 6, 11, 16, and 18. Patients in this age group should be encouraged to do so if they haven't already. It is given in three doses at 0, 2, and 6 months. It is not recommended in pregnancy, but if a pregnancy occurs after a dose is given, the remaining doses would be postponed until after delivery. Cervarix, a newer HPV vaccine with the same guideline recommendation, only vaccinates against HPV types 16, 18, and possibly other HPV types.

Destructive Therapies

Physical destruction

Cryotherapy with the use of liquid nitrogen can be useful if there are a limited number of warts, particularly on the penile shaft and vulva. This should not be done for lesions in the vagina or vaginal mucosa. Liquid nitrogen should be applied with a cotton-tipped applicator or a cryogen. The lesions should be frozen including a small rim of normal tissue around the border lasting for at least 10 seconds and then allowed to thaw. Some clinicians will repeat the cycle after the lesion thaws. Blisters and small erosions begin to develop in 1 to 3 days and heal completely in 1 to 2 weeks. Side effects include discomfort, blistering, dyspigmentation, and scarring with a very small risk for infection and paresthesias.

Electrocautery includes electrodessication and the loop electrosurgical excision procedure (LEEP). Destruction of the lesions by electrocautery should only be performed by a dermatologist or gynecologist and requires local anesthesia. LEEP uses a high-frequency current to cut and cauterize tissue and is generally used for cervical treatment and performed by urology and gynecologic specialists.

Laser therapy with a YAG or CO_2 laser can be used to treat a group of lesions. This should be done by someone experienced in laser surgery, usually a dermatologist. Special care must be taken to control the plume from laser treatment, which can aerosolize the virus and pose a potential hazard for patients and staff.

Surgery is generally reserved for large lesions and may be done as a debulking process performed under general anesthesia. Smaller lesions may be surgically removed under local anesthesia. The postoperative pain may be significant, and it may recur. Scarring and hypo- or hyperpigmentation can occur with any of the physical destruction methods and should be discussed with the patient beforehand.

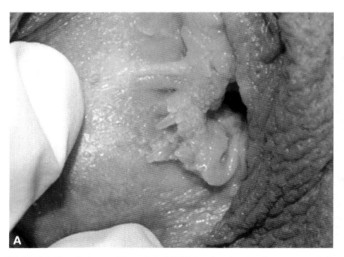
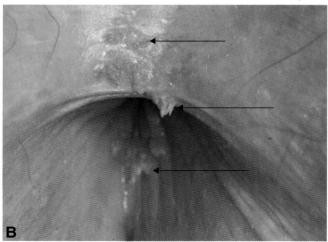

FIG. 21-6. **A:** Vestibular papillae mimic HPV infection, but the tips are rounded, and individual papillae are discrete to the base. **B:** Some genital warts are spiky, or acuminate, leading to the term *condylomata accuminata*. There are small lobular warts just above these acuminate lesions.

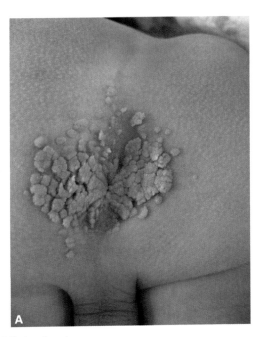

FIG. 21-7. Perianal warts.

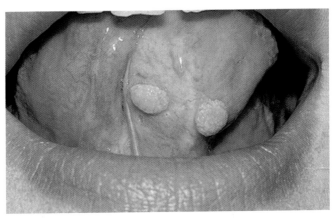

FIG. 21-8. HPV can be transmitted through orogenital contact, increasing risk for oropharyngeal SCC.

Chemical destruction

Trichloroacetic acid (TCA) and bichloracetic acid (BCA) are strong topical keratolytics that result in chemical cauterization (similar to cryotherapy or electrodessication) of the skin and destruction of the lesion. Vaseline should be applied to the surrounding tissue to protect it from the burning chemical. TCA and BCA are applied with the wooden end of the cotton-tipped applicator. The lesion turns white upon application, and sodium bicarbonate powder is used to remove any excess acid. The most common side effect is burning at the sites. It may be used in pregnancy on external lesions. Treatment requires weekly applications for 4 to 6 weeks and has a high recurrence.

Podophyllin may be used in the office, but it must be used in small areas and normal tissue should be avoided. It can be absorbed systemically, especially when used in the perianal area, with potential neurotoxic effects, and therefore it is contraindicated for use in pregnancy. The patient is generally advised to wash it off in 1 to 4 hours depending on the individual circumstances and should be repeated every 2 to 3 weeks.

Podofilox (Condylox 0.5%) solution or gel is an antimitotic agent FDA approved for the treatment of genital warts. It is prescribed for at-home use and applied to the lesion by the patient, twice daily, 3 days per week for 4 weeks. If the lesion is located on the perianal area, the application is once daily for 3 days a week, repeated for 4 weeks. This treatment can be very irritating and must be allowed to dry well and is not indicated for moist areas. The surrounding skin should be protected with petrolatum to prevent extensive irritation to normal skin.

No more than 0.5 g of the gel should be used each day. This agent should not be used in pregnancy.

Immune-based therapy

Imiquimod is a topical immune enhancer that uses the body's immune defense system to induce cell-mediated activity against HPV and is not a destructive method. It is applied three times per week at night for 16 weeks. This treatment has shown to have the lowest recurrence rate. It causes mild-to-moderate irritation and may cause hypopigmentation.

Sinecatechins 15% (Veregen) is a topical treatment for external warts approved for use in patients 18 years and older. It is produced from green tea leaves, and the mode of action is not known. Apply no more than 0.5 cm of ointment to the warts, three times daily for up to 16 weeks. Do not use on the genital mucosa (urethra, vagina, or rectum) or open wounds. Caution the patient that use of sinecatechins can decrease the effectiveness of condoms and diaphragms. A backup contraceptive method should be used, even though abstinence is advised to reduce the risk of transmission. Be sure patients wash their hands after applying and do not touch eyes, nose, or mucous membranes with this ointment. Side effects include burning, pruritus, erythema, vesicular lesions, and discomfort at the treatment site.

Special Considerations

Pregnancy. Warts tend to grow during pregnancy because of the hormonal changes and immune suppression. Visible warts should be treated but after the first trimester, and liquid nitrogen is the treatment of choice for genital warts. An obstetrician/gynecologist should be consulted before treating the patient. Interferon, 5-fluorouracil, podophyllin, and TCA are contraindicated in pregnancy. Imiquimod is a pregnancy category C drug.

High-risk populations. Men having sex with men and anal sexual contact may increase the risk of developing anal cancers from HPV.

Children. Autoinoculation resulting in genital warts in children is not uncommon; however, 50% of cases occur as a result of sexual abuse.

Immunosuppression. Patients who are immunocompromised are at greater risk for persistent infection and transformation into carcinoma, especially SCC. Patients who have extensive or atypical infections, or are recalcitrant to treatment, should be screened for HIV and immunosuppression.

Prognosis and Complications

In pregnancy, transmission of HPV to the newborn can occur during vaginal delivery. The greatest of HPV in general, complication is transformation into malignancy, as discussed previously (Figure 21-9).

Referral and Consultation

For suspected atypical lesions or carcinomas of the external genitalia, refer appropriately to a dermatology specialist, obstetrician and gynecologist, or urologist for evaluation and treatment.

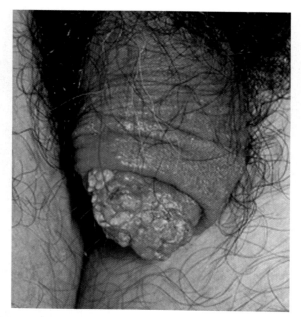

FIG. 21-9. This SCC is the color of the patient's skin, verrucous, and precipitated by HPV.

A gastroenterologist or colorectal surgeon should be consulted for the evaluation of anal warts or suspected anal carcinomas.

Patient Education and Follow-up

Transmission of HPV involves sexual contact, and behaviors that promote transmission include an increase in the number of partners, the presence of warts in either partner, and the frequency of sexual activity. Patients must be educated about the risk factors for contracting the infection, risk for cancer, and preventative behaviors. Patients should be advised to notify their sexual contacts to be evaluated for HPV and other STDs. Condoms should be used while warts are visible or are being treated; otherwise abstinence should be advised.

Patients undergoing treatment for HPV, regardless of the type, should be followed every 2 to 4 weeks until there is no clinical evidence of infection. After eradication of the HPV, patients should be followed up in 3 months and 6 months for evaluation of possible recurrence. If they remain free of any condyloma after 6 months, annual visits are indicated. Follow-up Pap smears and STD tests should be completed based on their test results and recommendations of their obstetrician/gynecologist. Women who have a negative Pap smear but are older than 30 years and have positive HPV should have both tests repeated in 1 year.

GENITAL PRURITUS

Pruritus or itching is a symptom associated with a desire to scratch and can be generalized or localized to a specific region of the body.

Chapter 19 discusses the pathophysiology of generalized pruritus, along with the careful evaluation, diagnosis, and management of symptoms. Although pruritus may be localized in the genitalia, clinicians should not exclude a careful assessment of the patient's entire body which might provide important diagnostic clues. For this reason, a good medical history and physical examination are essential. Is there a rash elsewhere, if so, what is the presentation of this rash or lesions located on another region

of the body and what is the associated history of this other rash in other areas? These clues may assist in the diagnosis of the rash in the genital area.

It is important to provide an environment of comfort and acceptance in your professional approach to a patient with genital concerns. Patients with genital pruritus can experience great anxiety because of the location of the itch coupled with a possible sense of embarrassment and loss of personal privacy associated with the location. Be sure to ask if they have seen another provider or attempted self-treatment in an attempt to resolve the problem.

Eczema

Eczema is a common inflammatory skin condition and common cause of chronic pruritus in the genital area. Eczematous dermatitis encompasses atopic dermatitis (AD), seborrheic dermatitis, irritant contact dermatitis, and allergic contact dermatitis (ACD). These dermatoses may affect other areas of the body outside of the genital area and are discussed in detail in chapter 3.

Atopic Dermatitis

AD is an inflammatory disorder usually associated with atopy, which includes a possible family or personal history of seasonal allergies, medication allergies, skin allergies, and/or asthma. It is the itch that induces scratching, resulting in the changes seen in the genital area. People with AD usually have a sensation of itch in response to irritation of the skin, rather than soreness. For AD patients, scratching offers a sense of relief and feels good, which in turn keeps the itch/scratch cycle active and produces a secondary rash. It is referred to as the eczema that "itches and rashes" and may be localized to one area but usually involves other areas of the body. Patients with AD should have a full skin examination.

Pathophysiology

The exact cause of AD is unknown but is believed to be multifactorial, resulting in a defect in the epidermal barrier. Environmental variables, including normal skin flora, can activate inflammatory mediators along with increased IgE (see chapter 3). Eosinophils activate mast cells, and chronic inflammation is the result of the interaction of the allergen and the immune system. It is often difficult to determine the initial causative agent.

Clinical presentation

In AD, flexor surfaces of the body are often affected with erythematous scaling plaques or patches. However, adults can have a flare involving the genitalia and sparing other regions of the body. The clinical presentation of AD on the genitalia can appear different than AD on the arms or legs. Often what is seen on the genitalia after prolonged pruritus and scratching is a thickening of the tissue with accentuated skin lines known as lichen simplex chronicus (Figure 21-10). This is the part of AD that is chronic.

For men, it usually involves the scrotum, where skin lines may blend with the normal rugae or the skin may appear somewhat shiny (Figure 21-11). Occasionally, the shaft of the penis is also included. Women will often be affected on the labia majora, which may appear smooth with a wrinkled appearance, hyperpigmented and excoriated (Figure 21-12). There is hyperkeratosis of the stratum corneum and thickening of the epidermis analogous to a callus. It is possible to see a similar appearance for both men and women. Fissuring in these areas may occur, and candida may be found in the fissures. If there is crusting, pustules, or moist scale, there may be a bacterial infection. The erythema and scaling may also affect the thighs and perianal area but spare other extensor surfaces.

DIFFERENTIAL DIAGNOSIS Atopic dermatitis

- Psoriasis
- Irritant contact dermatitis (ICD)
- Allergic contact dermatitis
- Scabies
- Pediculosis
- Candida
- Dermatophyte infection

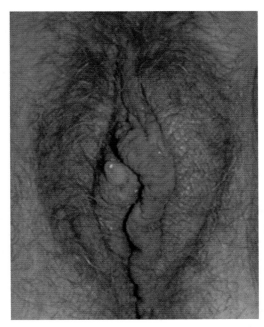

FIG. 21-12. Even patients who are not naturally dark sometimes exhibit hyperpigmentation that obscures the inflammation of lichen simplex chronicus, as seen on this left labium majus.

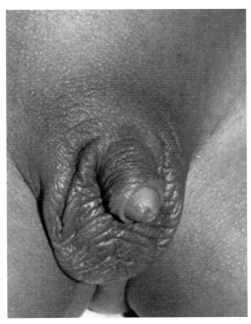

FIG. 21-10. Lichenified AD of the scrotum and penis in a young boy who has extragenital eczema as well. Shiny, monomorphous papules of papular AD can be seen on the proximal thighs.

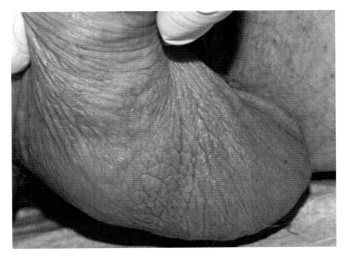

FIG. 21-11. Accentuated skin lines of lichen simplex of the scrotum.

Diagnostics

The diagnosis may be made by clinical appearance; a KOH test may be helpful to rule out candida or dermatophyte as a source of the itch. Careful history of the patient's hygiene practices and use of

cleansing products will be helpful. A biopsy is rarely needed unless the patient does not respond to standard treatment.

Management

The treatment goal is to eliminate the itch and subsequent rash. Management begins with identifying and removing any triggers or treating infections that are present. Daily use of emollients (petrolatum or zinc oxide) should be used to restore the skin barrier. Patients should be warned against overcleansing and use of any potential irritants or allergens. Recommended skin care and algorithmic approach, including topical corticosteroid (TCS) as the mainstay of treatment for AD, are discussed in detail in chapter 2.

A mid-potency TCS (class IV or V) such as triamcinolone 0.1% ointment may be used b.i.d. for 1 to 2 weeks. If the area is lichenified, use of a more potent TCS (class II or III) such as fluocinonide 0.05% or clobetasol 0.05% ointment may be needed initially. When the inflammation is more intertriginous, a less potent corticosteroid such as aclometasone 0.05% or desonide 0.05% ointment (class VI or VII) is used to decrease the potential for atrophy of the skin. TCS creams may cause stinging or irritation but are not occlusive, whereas ointments cause irritation and are lubricating. Patient preference may determine the vehicle. A limited amount of TCS should be prescribed for 1 to 2 weeks and then the patient should return for reevaluation. If the dermatitis is improved, the clinician should taper the TCS and promote healing with emollients. AD that worsens should prompt a change in the TCS or the vehicle.

First-generation antihistamines such as hydroxyzine can be more sedating but may help with nighttime scratching. The second-generation, nonsedating antihistamines may be needed for daytime pruritus and at higher doses.

Prognosis and complications

AD is a chronic condition that may not be cured, so the ideal goal is control. Genital pruritus caused by AD can affect the quality of life for individuals, and certainly impacts the patient's body image and sexual intimacy. Complications can include bacterial and viral infections secondary to a break in the skin barrier.

Referral and consultation

AD that is severe or recalcitrant may require consultation with dermatology and collaboration with the patient's obstetrician/gynecologist.

Patient education and follow-up

It is important that patients are followed every 2 to 4 weeks to monitor improvement and worsening symptoms. Once resolved, patient should be educated about triggers and advised to restart therapy at the earliest signs of recurring symptoms.

Irritant Dermatitis

Irritant contact dermatitis (ICD) is an inflammatory skin condition that is not immunologically mediated and may be acute or chronic. Patients with a history of eczema or AD may be at greater risk for ICD. Diaper dermatitis is discussed in detail in chapter 6.

Pathophysiology

The etiology of ICD is related to direct or indirect irritation of the skin in the genitalia. The offending agent can be water, moisture, and humidity, or chemicals from soaps, detergents, and personal hygiene products (Box 21-1). Moisture and humidity in the genital area can lead to a change in the pH and increase microbial growth. Irritation can also occur from exposure to a strong irritant, or it may take repeated exposures to weaker agents. Exposure time to any irritant may increase the severity of the dermatitis. ICD may be exacerbated by continuous cleansing, which breaks down the skin barrier, causing an increase in the inflammation and irritation. Some evidence shows that diabetic women have an increased incidence for vulvar itching.

Clinical presentation

Patients with genital ICD may complain of soreness, burning, stinging, and a feeling of being "raw" or tender. Conversely, the symptoms may be mild and go unnoticed initially. The genitalia may be erythematous, shiny, edematous, and with secondary erosions from scratching (Figure 21-13). In the acute stages, vesicles may be present but easily ruptured (and unnoticed) because the skin is thin, not well keratinized on the glans, vulva, and inner prepuce. Erosions may be left in their place (Figure 21-14). When the irritation is chronic, hypo- or hyperpigmentation with lichenification may be present. Patients who wear incontinence garments, both infants and adults, may already have alterations in the epidermal barrier from continuous moisture, ammonia from urine, and friction from undergarment or pad.

DIFFERENTIAL DIAGNOSIS Irritant dermatitis

- Allergic contact dermatitis
- Psoriasis
- Candidiasis
- Tinea cruris

Diagnostics

The diagnosis of ICD can be made based on history, symptoms, clinical presentation, and exclusion of other conditions. ICD in the genitalia is usually localized to the area of contact, which may spare the intertriginous areas, compared to allergic contact dermatitis

---

BOX 21-1 | **Common Irritants to Genital Areas**

Frequent cleansing with soap/water
Perfumed products
Douches
Fragrances
Sprays
Nylon underwear
Feminine hygiene pads (brands can vary)
Tampon strings
Alcohols
Spermicides
Prescribe vaginal medications
Personal lubricants
Trichloroacetic acid for treatment of HPV

(ACD), which may include the folds of the skin and multifocal areas. Biopsy is not generally indicated, but histology would show spongiosis, dermal inflammatory infiltrate, and possible vesicles. It can help to exclude other differential diagnoses such as tinea and psoriasis. A KOH scraping can identify candidiasis.

Management

Identification and elimination of the offending irritant will usually alleviate the symptoms. Reducing moisture to the area is important and can be improved by avoiding occlusive clothing and undergarments. If a woman develops ICD from a specific brand of feminine hygiene pads, she may try another brand. If it is persistent across the brands, she may have to try tampons during menses. For immediate relief, cool packs or sitz baths can decrease the pruritus. Antihistamines may be helpful, and a short course of TCS can be prescribed, as mentioned previously in AD management. Continued warm baths or sitz baths daily for 5 to 10 minutes followed by a thin layer of petrolatum or zinc oxide preparation help repair and restore the epidermal barrier of the genitalia.

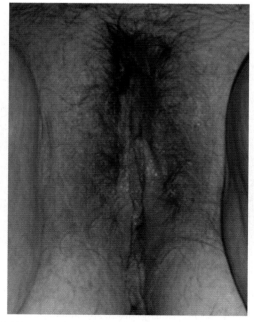

FIG. 21-13. This acute ICD produced by a reaction to an azole cream exhibits erythema and edema sufficient to produce an exudate.

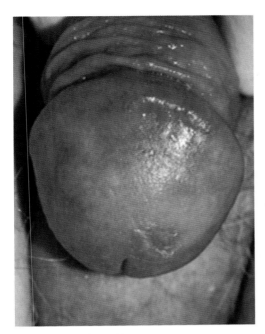

FIG. 21-14. Irritant contact dermatitis.

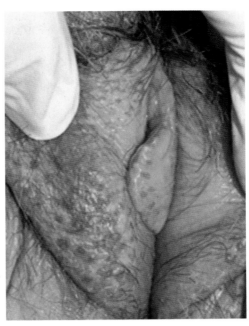

FIG. 21-15. Allergic contact dermatitis from an over-the-counter anti-itch medication containing benzocaine and resorcinol, characterized by blisters that have resulted in small round erosions.

Patient education and follow-up

Patients must be educated about common irritants associated with the genitalia (Box 21-1). Emphasis should be on avoiding of known irritants and maintaining a high index of suspicion when new flares occur. A diary of activities and products can help the patient identify their sensitivities.

Allergic Contact Dermatitis

ACD of the genitalia is a cell-mediated or type IV delayed hypersensitivity reaction. This means that it can take hours, months, or years for the skin to react. ACD occurs more frequently from exposures to products applied or transferred to the genitalia and less commonly from personal hygiene pads or undergarments.

Pathophysiology

Chapter 3 discussed the pathophysiology of ACD in detail; however, the common allergens associated with ACD are more product specific.

Clinical presentation

The clinical presentation of ACD in the genitalia is usually localized and with the distribution providing very important clues for diagnosis. Erythema, pruritus, and burning are usually present but may also include swelling, weeping, crusting, and/or vesicular eruption in acute cases (Figure 21-15). Secondary lesions can occur from scratching or infection. The clinical presentation may be confusing as there may be a multifactorial etiology. In women, look for evidence of low estrogen, such as atrophy, dryness, and thinning of the vaginal/ vulvar mucosa as this may be the cause of the itching.

Allergens may be introduced or transferred to the genitalia from touching or rubbing. Chemicals on the patient's, caregiver's, or partner's hands or mouth may be the offending agent. ACD may not have distinct borders or may present with a helpful distribution (i.e., linear) that can provide helpful diagnostic clues about the offending agent.

DIFFERENTIAL DIAGNOSIS Allergic contact dermatitis

- Irritant or atopic dermatitis
- Candidiasis, or balanitis
- Seborrheic dermatitis
- Atrophic vaginitis
- Tinea cruris
- Lichen simplex chronicus
- Inverse psoriasis
- Drug eruption
- Sexually transmitted diseases
- Bacterial vaginosis
- Bowen disease
- Blistering diseases

Diagnostics

A good history and timeline may be helpful. Patients and clinicians can play detective and may identify obvious allergens. Appropriate cultures and serologies may be indicated to rule out other causes of genital dermatitis, including STDs. If the allergen is not identified through a thorough history and physical, patch testing by dermatology specialist can be helpful.

Management

The treatment goals are to relieve symptoms, identify and remove the allergen, and restore the skin barrier. Initially, cleansing with water, sitz baths, or cool soaks followed by petrolatum can calm and protect the genitalia. Consider treatment with oral antimicrobials for possible bacterial, yeast, or viral infections, if indicated. In the absence of infection, TCS such as triamcinolone 0.1% ointment may be applied twice daily to decrease the inflammation and pruritus. For severe ACD, oral prednisone 40 to 60 mg/day for 7 to 10 days may be required. If there is any suspicion of HSV, concurrent use of a systemic antiviral agent is recommended. Oral antihistamines may be added as needed for symptomatic relief. Complete resolution of ACD may take several weeks even when the allergen is identified and eliminated.

Referral and consultation

ACD in the genitalia can be difficult to diagnose. Refer to dermatology for evaluation and patch testing or to an immunologist if the dermatitis is severe or unremitting. Collaboration between the primary care provider, gynecologist, and dermatologist may be necessary for complete resolution.

Patient education and follow-up

Close attention should be given to personal hygiene and avoidance of personal products with known common allergens (Box 21-2). It may be necessary to use plain water for bathing, avoiding soaps, cleansers, and hygiene wipes until the allergen is identified. The patient can record their activities and symptoms in a diary. Have the patient avoid tight, occlusive clothing or those that are newly purchased. Launder in fragrance-free and dye-free detergents before wearing. If there is no improvement in 2 to 3 weeks, consider biopsy for diagnostic confirmation.

CANDIDIASIS

Candidiasis is included here as it is often a concomitant infection that occurs with other genital dermatoses. It can be a primary or secondary infection involving the genitalia.

Pathophysiology

The causative agent in the majority of yeast infections in the genitalia is *C. albicans*, and less commonly from *C. tropicalis* and *Candida glabrata*. It can affect both the vaginal and vulvar areas in females and the glans penis in males. *C. albicans* is part of the normal flora in the vagina and gastrointestinal tract. However, sweating, interruption of the skin barrier (i.e., chronic moisture from urinary incontinence), oral antibiotic therapy, obesity, diabetes, use of oral contraceptives, pregnancy, and immunosuppression can result in an overgrowth of the yeast. It may be transmitted to the neonate through an infected vaginal tract. Coitus with an infected partner may cause candidal balanitis in men, especially uncircumcised males.

BOX 21-2	Common Allergens in Genital Dermatitis

Bacitracin
Latex (found in condoms or contraceptive devices)
Personal lubricants (K-Y jelly contains propylene glycol)
Perfumed hygiene sprays (fluorinated hydrocarbons)
Lipstick (octyl gallate) transferred to genitals
Nail polish from the hand
Balsam of Peru (fragrances)
Panty liners: adhesive (acetyl acetonate or cull-acetyl acetonate) fragrance or blue dye
Candida or semen
Resin in the wax for string instruments (colophony)
Medicated wipes contain methylisothiazolinone and methylchloroisothiazolinone found in Huggies and Cottonelle brands.
Benzocaine or other topical anesthetics
Para-aminobenzoic acid
Hemorrhoidal medication

Clinical Presentation

Candidiasis in the genitals often presents as erythematous and moist plaques that may be macerated, favoring intertriginous areas such as the inframammary, inguinal, and abdominal areas. Acute infections may have violaceous papules or pustules that extend just beyond the border of the plaque (Figure 21-16A). Scale may not be evident (Figure 21-16B). Males typically have ill-defined erythema with itching and burning on the penis. Erythematous pustules or erosions may extend to the glans and/or shaft of the penis. Uncircumcised men can have white plaques or erosions under the prepuce (Figure 21-17). On the female genitalia, there may be swelling and shiny erythema as well as a clumpy white, adherent discharge in the vagina or spreading onto the vulva.

DIFFERENTIAL DIAGNOSIS Candidiasis
• Lichen simplex chronicus
• Atopic dermatitis
• Inverse psoriasis
• Tinea cruris
• Bowen disease

Diagnostics

Candidiasis is usually a clinical diagnosis. Yet a KOH prep is an easy and inexpensive in-office test that can confirm the presence of hyphae, pseudohyphae, and spores. See chapter 24 for instructions on KOH prep. Lichen simplex chronicus, AD, and inverse psoriasis will have negative KOH prep. A full body examination and biopsy may be helpful if the symptoms are severe or not responsive to antiyeast medications. Recurrent candidiases infections should also prompt the clinician to perform a culture and consider screening test for diabetes, HIV, or immunosuppression. Additional STD testing may be indicated.

Management

If there is no other underlying disease or concomitant infections, candidiasis may be treated with oral or topical antifungals. For men and women, topical azole therapy, or imidazole creams applied twice daily for 7 days, is usually effective (see chapter 12). If the infection does not respond, consider changing to terconazole cream 0.4% (effective for all three common candida species) vaginal tablets or cream inserted nightly for 1 week. Topical antiyeast cream can be used in conjunction with oral therapy to achieve symptomatic relief more quickly.

Oral fluconazole 150 mg in a single oral dose treats the external genitalia and vagina, as well as balanitis in men. If the patient has more than four candida infections per year, the clinician should consider a *nonalbicans* species and treat with an alternate medication. It may require a longer treatment period or partner treatment at the same time when one of the partners is the colonizer of the candida.

Referral and Consultation

In cases of frequent recurrence, refer to a gynecologist for further evaluation and treatment. Candidiasis in pregnancy should also be managed by the patient's obstetrician. Long-term therapy or prophylaxis is advisable.

Patient Education and Follow-up

Patients should be advised that frequent intercourse may also be a factor for recurrence. Counsel diabetic patients that control of hyperglycemia may decrease recurrences. Uncircumcised males

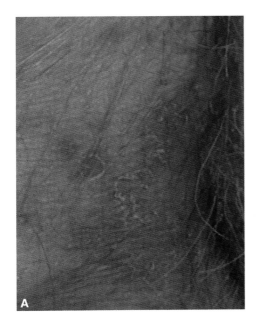

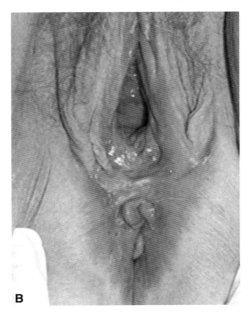

FIG. 21-16. **A:** In acute candidiasis infections, papules and pustules may extend beyond the border of the violaceous plaque. **B:** Vaginal candidiasis frequently infects the vulva with characteristic redness, fissuring, and shiny skin, but it may lack scale.

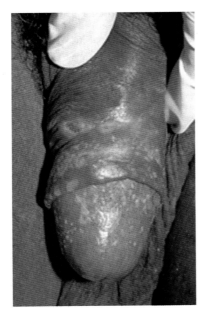

FIG. 21-17. This uncircumcised man with candidiasis also exhibits white papules and erosions.

must be vigilant in retracting the foreskin for thorough cleansing and drying before returning the foreskin.

LICHEN PLANUS

Lichen planus (LP) is a chronic, inflammatory dermatosis with episodes of partial remission and flares. There are several variants of LP, including the classic cutaneous form (skin only), erosive LP involving mucous membranes (oral, anogenital, bladder, conjunctiva, and esophagus), and a variant with both types. Other subtypes exist but are beyond the scope of this text. Characteristic nail findings are present in about 10% of patients with LP. Chapter 5 provides a general overview of the epidemiology and pathophysiology of lichen planus. This section will only focus on the disease as it affects the genitalia.

Clinical Presentation

Genital LP can present as the classic flat, purple papules/plaques of the disease (Wickham striae) localized in the anogenital region. In males, LP involves the genitalia in 25% of cases, with the glans penis the most common location. Nonerosive, annular plaques are located near the coronal rim. An erosive type of LP (ELP) occurs less frequently and reveals erosions and white reticular striae (Figure 21-18).

Women diagnosed with genital LP often have a combination of nonerosive and ELP types. Approximately 50% of females diagnosed with oral LP also have genital lesions that may not be reported by the patient. Nonerosive LP can present as lacey (reticular), white papules on the vulva and vaginal mucosa with surrounding erythema (Figure 21-19). The mucosa may become very thin and shiny, similar to lichen sclerosus. These lesions frequently itch, burn, and cause dyspareunia. Women with ELP can have significantly inflamed (violaceous) erosions anywhere in the vulvovaginal area and often have coexisting lesions present in their buccal mucosa and gingiva. ELP on the genitalia are extremely painful and debilitating, and may cause vaginal discharge or urethral stenosis.

Assessment of patients must go beyond a physical examination and include the psychosocial symptoms.

Another variant of LP is lesions that present as hyperkeratotic, thicker papules, plaques or even nodular lesions.

DIFFERENTIAL DIAGNOSIS Lichen planus
• Drug eruption
• Lichen sclerosus (LS)
• Contact dermatitis
• Herpes simplex virus
• Psoriasis
• Secondary syphilis
• Stevens–Johnson syndrome
• Autoimmune blistering diseases
• Squamous cell carcinoma

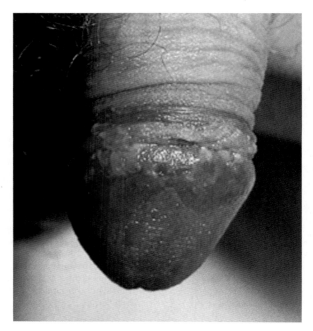

FIG. 21-18. The uncircumcised penis with erosive LP, like the vulva, exhibits nonspecific erosions.

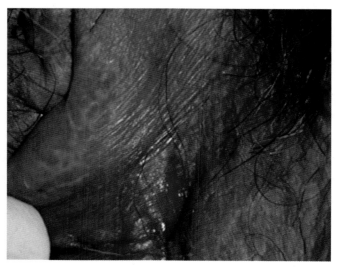

FIG. 21-19. This erosion is pathognomonic for LP because of the surrounding white, reticular papules.

Diagnostics

When evaluating patients for symptoms in the genital area, be sure to examine the rest of the body, including wrists, scalp/hair, nails, and the oral mucosa and gingiva for clues. A diagnosis of genital LP can be a clinical one that is made easier if the patient has classic LP on extragenital areas. Unfortunately, there is often a significant delay in the diagnosis of genital LP and in referral to a specialist for further evaluation. A punch biopsy may be necessary to confirm the diagnosis of LP and rule out diseases or infections. All patients with diagnosed LP should be screened for hepatitis C. Bacterial and viral cultures may be indicated to exclude an infectious etiology or identify a secondary infection.

Management

There is a paucity of evidence to guide care in the treatment of genital LP. Management should be individualized for each patient, with potent TCS as the treatment of choice. Fluocinonide 0.05% or clobetasol 0.05% ointment applied twice daily can be effective. Corticosteroid sparing, tacrolimus ointment 0.1% used for 2 to 4 weeks, has been effective but can cause significant stinging and burning with application (see chapter 3). Viscous lidocaine applied externally can provide some pain relief. Many clinicians report using hydrocortisone 25-mg rectal suppositories inserted into the vagina for symptom relief. The suppositories (kept refrigerated) can be inserted twice daily for up to 2 months and then tapered to twice a week.

ELP involving the vulvovaginal area is extremely difficult to manage, requiring aggressive and collaborative care with gynecology and dermatology. Severe genital LP or ELP may initially need a short course of oral prednisone. The goal would be to gain control of the disease and transition the patient to a nonsteroidal agent such as methotrexate, hydroxychloroquine, retinoids, azathioprine, and mycophenolate mofetil. The aggressive treatment with high-risk medications emphasizes the importance of follow-up and monitoring.

Treatment must also address the chronic pain of genital LP that may be treated with tricyclic antidepressants. Hydroxyzine is helpful for nighttime pruritus and sedation at 10 to 25 mg nightly. Classic lesions of LP lesions in the genital area are not associated with scarring, while adhesions at the vaginal introitus may require surgical removal or regular use of graduated dilators. Ultrapotent TCS may be useful for their thinning side effect.

Skin care for patients with genital LP requires meticulous attention to personal hygiene. A compromised skin barrier, along with TCS, makes patients at risk for secondary infections. Perineal care should include sitz baths, the use of emollients such as petroleum jelly and loose-fitting clothing to reinforce the skin barrier and reduce irritation. Also, uncircumcised males often see improvement after circumcision.

Prognosis and Complications

Sequelae of ELP are more profound than those of nonerosive LP. The intermittent and chronic nature of LP can lead to phimosis, urethral strictures, scarring, alopecia, abnormal pigmentation, vulvar and vaginal adhesions, and fissures. Regardless of the gender, patients with genital LP can experience dysuria, dyspareunia, depression and anxiety, loss of function, and overall altered quality of life. ELP has an increased risk of SCC. Vulvodynia has been associated with extensive or long-term inflammation of the vulva.

Referral and Consultation

Any patients with genital erosions that do not respond to antimicrobial therapies (viral, bacterial, mycologic) should be referred appropriately to gynecology, dermatology or urology for accurate diagnosis and ongoing management. Often, oral and genital LP is concomitant and requires dental care with an experienced provider. If the patient has hepatitis C, follow-up with a gastroenterologist or hepatologist is essential.

Patient Education and Follow-up

Genital LP, especially ELP, requires ongoing monitoring of response to medications and possible side effects. With significant improvement, TCS can be tapered off. In severe disease, patients on prednisone or corticosteroid-sparing agents should be advised not to stop the drug on their own and to report any side effects to their specialist. Routine laboratory monitoring is usually performed during maintenance on high-risk medications. Patient should also be instructed to watch for signs and symptoms of infection and promptly report them.

LICHEN SCLEROSIS

LS is a chronic inflammatory skin disorder that has a predilection for the genital area but can also be found on extragenital sites. LS is no longer referred to as *lichen sclerosus et atrophicus* and *hypoplastic dystrophy*. LS is a different disease entity and should not be confused with scleroderma. It does have a strong association with other autoimmune disorders such as vitiligo, thyroid disorders, alopecia areata, morphea, pernicious anemia, and may be hereditary.

LS affects women more than men and has a bimodal onset. It is prevalent in prepubescent children up to age 13 years and then again in adulthood (postmenopausal) during the fifth or sixth decade of life. When it occurs in young children, there may be resolution by puberty—lending support to the hypothesis that it is hormonally influenced. Most importantly, females with vulvar disease may have increased risk of developing SCC at the sites of the lesions.

Pathophysiology

The etiology and pathogenesis of LS is not completely understood. The current belief is that autoantibodies develop against extracellular matrix protein 1, leading to cell-mediated cytotoxicity and ultimately inflammation and fibrosis in the upper dermis.

Clinical Presentation

Extragenital LS usually develops symmetrically on the upper back, shoulders, and inframammary areas that are exposed more frequently to friction. There are no lesions on the oral mucosa or inside the vagina. Genital LS can vary from mild plaques that go unnoticed to severe lesions which can be smooth or waxy, hypopigmented or white (porcelain), fixed, atrophic plaques (*sclerotic*) with telangiectasias, erythema, and erosions (Figure 21-20). Older lesions may have a thin, tissue paper (some refer to it as "cigarette paper")–like skin that is *shiny* and wrinkled. Plugging may be present from follicular destruction. The affected area may surround the labia major and extend posteriorly to the perianal area, creating a "figure eight" (or key hole) appearance. The perianal area is affected in women but not in men. Involvement into the crural folds may be noted with extension into the intergluteal cleft that may become macerated from thinning and moisture.

Older lesions may take on a different appearance and become thickened and hyperkeratotic, some of which may occur as a result of rubbing or scratching. Architectural changes occur when there is a loss of definition of the structures as they thin. LS can obliterate the labia majora or minora and fuse with the introitus (Figure 21-21). Further stenosis of the introitus can create great discomfort and dyspareunia for a sexually active woman. Postmenopausal women may have further atrophy due to the thinning effects from diminished estrogen.

In males, genital LS is often misdiagnosed as phimosis (foreskin cannot be retracted) or balanitis. Lesions usually involve the glans, prepuce, and frenulum, and less commonly the shaft or scrotum. Sclerotic plaques around the glans may be friable and bleed easily with intercourse, or result in urethral strictures (Figure 21-22). Retracting the foreskin may become impossible, and stenosis of the meatus may be noted. In young males, LS often presents with phimosis or symptoms of balanitis, especially if they are not circumcised. LS may appear as white patches and may not have associated pruritus.

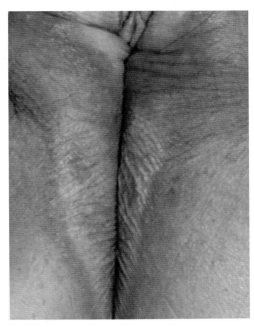

FIG. 21-20. Although hypopigmentation is the most striking abnormality in LS, the texture change is the key to diagnosis including the crinkled or tissue paper-like appearance.

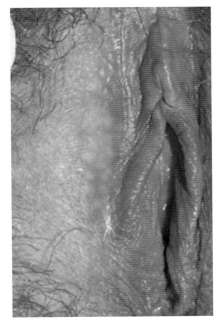

FIG. 21-21. Architectural changes occur as structures thin and fuse together.

Young women and children with LS may initially report pruritus with an eruption of small pink or white papules that coalesce. Papules develop a central dell from follicular plugging forming a figure eight or "key hole" plaque of erythema around the vulvar and perianal areas. This clinical presentation is often misdiagnosed as postinflammatory hypopigmentation or vitiligo (Figure 21-23A). As the disease progresses, agglutination of the labia can occur. There may be pain with defecation or urination, resulting in constipation or urinary retention because it is so painful.

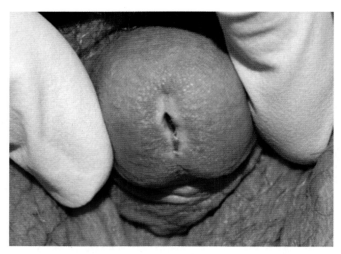

FIG. 21-22. Lichen sclerosus often affects the urethral meatus and can cause strictures.

DIFFERENTIAL DIAGNOSIS Lichen sclerosis

- Lichen planus
- Pinworms (anal pruritus)
- Vitiligo
- Lichen simplex chronicus
- Irritant dermatitis
- Postinflammatory hypopigmentation
- Morphea
- Trauma or sexual abuse
- Candidiasis/balanitis
- Squamous cell carcinoma
- Erythroplasia of Queyrat
- Leukoplakia

Diagnostics

Patients with LS have often seen more than one provider before the correct diagnosis is made. They may have complained of repeated yeast infections, urinary tract infections, dyspareunia, vulvar pain, and pain with defecation. Many of these symptoms can confuse the clinical picture. A diagnosis of genital LS is based on clinical presentation and confirmed with a punch biopsy of the lesion. The selection of the biopsy site is important and will provide the greatest diagnostic information if it is taken from an area of thin, tissue-paper–like skin. Additional biopsies may be necessary to confirm the diagnosis or when changes in a chronic lesion occur, possibly signaling transformation into SCC.

Management

The goal of treatment is to alleviate the symptoms and prevent progression or destruction. Good skin hygiene is fundamental for any genital dermatosis for the promotion of healing and prevention of infection. Potent (class II) and ultrapotent (class I) TCS are the preferred first-line treatment for genital LS. Clobetasol 0.05% or halobetasol 0.05% ointment are recommended as initial therapy twice daily for 4 weeks. Given the side effects of these TCS, the patient should be reevaluated and potency of the TCS reduced with signs of improvement. Do not expect that the LS will be resolved as it can take months. Topical tacrolimus 0.1% has been used with good results and can provide a safer, long-term, nonsteroidal alternative for the disease. Due to the chronicity of the disease, clinicians must be sure to monitor the use of TCS, taper off appropriately, and watch for adverse effects.

Two thirds of children diagnosed with LS will achieve spontaneous remission and require minimal, if any, treatment. One third will continue into adulthood and struggle with the chronic symptoms of the skin disease. Young females can be treated with a high-potency (class II) TCS such as betamethasone 0.05% ointment twice daily for 4 weeks and then follow up for reevaluation (Figure 21-23B). Improving lesions should be treated with tapering potencies of TCS, with reevaluation every 4–6 weeks until the vulva appears normal. It may take up to 6 months to see complete resolution of the lesions, as the

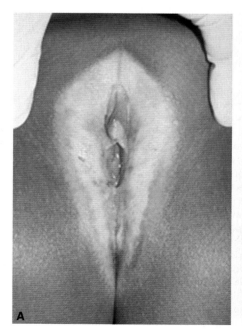
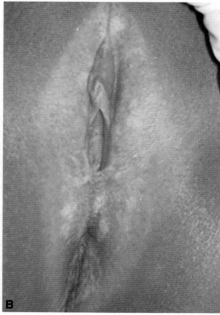

FIG. 21-23. A: Lichen sclerosus before treatment with corticosteroids. **B:** Lichen sclerosus after treatment with corticosteroids.

TCS is tapered down to hydrocortisone 1% ointment once daily for 3 months during that time. Topical tacrolimus 0.1% has also shown to be effective initial and maintenance therapy.

The treatment of choice for young, uncircumcised males is circumcision followed by topical tacrolimus 0.1% postoperatively for 3 weeks. If the patient is circumcised, application of betamethasone 0.1% ointment to the prepuce two times daily for 6 weeks is first line. For severe cases or stenosis of the meatus, referral for advanced surgical or systemic therapy should be considered.

Referral and Consultation

Patients who do not respond to topical therapy should be referred to a specialist for reevaluation to ensure the diagnosis is accurate. Treatment of genital LS often requires a multidisciplinary approach with primary care, dermatology, gynecology and urology (as appropriate). If it is confirmed to be recalcitrant or severe LS, systemic treatment, or surgical or laser therapy may be used for control. Postmenopausal women may benefit from the addition of estrogen creams. Men treated with high-potency TCS for about 8 weeks may be able to avoid circumcision.

Prognosis and Complications

For males, urethral obstruction from LS can interfere with urination. Lesions can also cause pain with erection, interfering with intimate relationships. Women with genital LS are at higher risk for developing SCC (Figure 21-24).

Dyspareunia, urinary retention and constipation, secondary infections, and corticosteroid atrophy are risks associated with the chronic disease and management.

Patient Education and Follow-up

Patients should be examined regularly for the occurrence of flares, side effects from TCS therapy, secondary infections, and possible

transformation into malignancy. In women, the most common site of SCC is near the clitoris or on the labia. The amount of time from diagnosis to the possible development of SCC is unknown. Patients with LS should be followed every 1 to 3 months until the lesions stabilize. Once they are controlled, follow-up is recommended every 6 to 12 months.

Scarring and architectural changes from genital LS are not reversible, emphasizing the importance of prompt diagnosis and treatment. Patients may need counseling about sexual function or dyspareunia. Since genital LS is a chronic disorder, written instruction can be helpful when there is a time lag between flares as patients forget the instructions for applications of TCS. Educating patients about personal hygiene and reducing risk for secondary infection is essential. Self-examination should be taught and encouraged so that patients can report early recognition of new or changing lesions.

BILLING CODES ICD-10

Allergic contact dermatitis, unspecified	L23.9
Anogenital warts	A63.0
Candidiasis, vulvovaginal	B37.3
Candidiasis, other urogenital site	B37.4
HSV, perianal or rectum	A60.01
HSV, urogenital (male or female)	A60.0
Irritant dermatitis, unspecified	L24.9
Lichen planus, unspecified	L43.9
Lichen sclerosus external genitalia, female	N90.4
Lichen sclerosus external genitalia, male	N48.0
Lichen simplex chronicus	L28.0
Pruritus, anogenital	L29.3
Psoriasis	L40.9

READINGS

Bolognia, J. L., Jorizzo, J. L., & Schaeffer, J. V. (2012). *Dermatology* (2nd ed.). China: Elsevier Saunders.

Cheng, S., Kirtschig, G., Cooper, S., Thornhill, M., Leonardi-Bee, J., & Murphy, R. (2012). Interventions for erosive lichen planus affecting mucosal sites. *Cochrane Database of Systematic Reviews, 15*(2), doi: 10.1002/14651858.CD008092.pub2.

Consolmagno, L. (2013). Lichen sclerosus. *Journal of the Dermatology Nurses' Association, 5*(4), 213–216.

Edwards, L., & Lynch, P. (2010). *Genital dermatology atlas* (2nd ed.). Philadelphia, PA: Lippincott Williams & Wilkins.

Habif, T. (2010). *Clinical dermatology: A color guide to diagnosis and therapy* (5th ed.). Philadelphia, PA: Mosby, Elsevier.

Lebwohl, M., & Heymann, W. (2010). *Treatment of skin diseases* (3rd ed.). China: Mosby.

Levinson, W. (2008). *Medical microbiology & immunology* (10th ed.). Lange, New York, NY: McGraw-Hill.

Wolff, K., & Johnson, R. (2013). *Fitzpatrick's color atlas and synopsis of clinical dermatology*. New York, NY: McGraw-Hill.

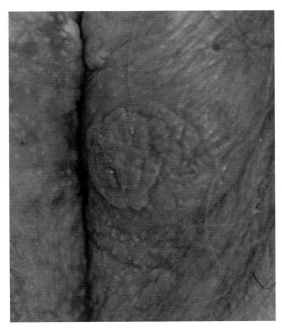

FIG. 21-24. This skin-colored SCC occurred in a setting of LS in an elderly woman.

It has been estimated that the prevalence of chronic, nonhealing wounds (NHWs) is about 2% of the US population. As a point of reference for this number, this estimate of prevalence is very similar to that of heart failure in America. The overall cost burden of NHWs is estimated conservatively at $35 to $50 billion per year. The impact on the health care system can be great, as those with NHWs have an average of at least two comorbid factors, often including diabetes, heart disease, or obesity. In addition, the presence of NHWs takes an emotional toll (including quality of life) on the patient, as well as their family, significant others, and community. NHWs can be life-impairing or life-altering for a short period or can continue for many years. They affect the very young to the very old, and have become a rapidly expanding health issue for our American veterans.

Wounds is a broad term that can encompass a variety of "types" of wounds. On the basis of the wound type, a "wound" may also be referred to as an "ulcer." These terms are used interchangeably, and it is acceptable to do so. There are countless etiologies for wounds, but there are broad and common wound categories, which include (but are not limited to) pressure ulcers (PrUs), thermal injuries (frostbite and burns), venous ulcers, arterial ulcers, traumatic wounds, surgical wounds, infectious wounds (such as from abscesses), skin tears, wounds from systemic and chronic disease, and more. It is imperative that all types of health care providers, regardless of the setting, possess a basic working knowledge of wounds. The purpose of this chapter is to provide a high-level overview of wounds, with specific information that is applicable for the primary care clinicians.

Patients with NHWs are present in every health care setting. Clinicians may find themselves both intimidated and uninformed about just what to do about these health issues. Providers understand that wounds are complex, but often do not understand wound complexities. Unquestionably, the best action to take in providing quality patient care is to acquire the human, material, and equipment resources available for wounded patients in the particular geographical location. Certified wound ostomy continence nurses (CWOCNs) are the gold standard in nursing resources.

WOUND HEALING

A brief review of the phases of wound healing, physiology, and repair is essential to understand the treatment of any wound. Clinicians must address both the etiology and complications of a wound that has not healed. The "normal" timeline of wound healing is considered to be orderly. Wounds that do not progress should be assessed and determined whether they are acute or chronic. Ascertaining a thorough history of the wound is imperative to determining the course of care and cannot be overemphasized (Box 22-1).

Arguably, the most important question in the history surrounds the age of the wound, which automatically determines chronicity. An *acute wound* is considered to be one that passes through the wound healing process and responds to the local treatment within

BOX 22-1	Gathering Wound History

How did the wound occur?
When did the wound occur?
When was the wound noticed? This question is important for neuro-pathic patients.
What treatment was initially given to the wound?
What other wound treatments have been given and when?
Have any home or alternative remedies been used, and if so what?
Has the wound been infected?
Has any medication been prescribed or used on the wound?
Was it prescribed for this wound or left over from another occurrence?
Is there pain, including location, characteristics, occurrence, relievers, triggers?
Does this wound open and close cyclically?

the expected time frame. Acute wounds such as surgical wounds, skin tears, and lacerations respond generally to standard treatment, though any wound can become chronic.

Conversely, a wound that does not respond to treatment within 30 days is considered to be a *chronic wound*. Assumed to be stuck in the inflammatory process, a chronic wound has itself become a chronic response with cellular transaction changes. Because the logical order of healing demands the inflammatory phase give way to proliferation, if the inflammatory phase is in control of the wound environment, healing will not progress. Chronicity can occur with any type of wound, but is most often found in PrUs, leg ulcers, and neuropathic ulcers.

Phases of Wound Healing

As mentioned, wound healing should progress through an orderly process (Figure 22-1). At the time of wounding, there is a disruption of cells, collagen, and tissues, which causes a hemorrhage. This event activates a series of cellular transactions that stop the hemorrhage, and ultimately form a fibrin clot, within minutes of the injury. Within 10 to 15 minutes, this clot is dissolved to allow the next cascade of events to occur, and it is at this point that the inflammatory stage begins.

Inflammatory phase

Initially in the inflammatory phase, the cellular trash is contained and removed as neutrophils and macrophages arrive. There is also a vasodilation process that occurs, which permits plasma and blood cells to pass into the wound bed, bringing growth factors and a host of other cells to the wound. Clinical signs of the inflammatory phase include edema, erythema, and exudate. By days 3 to 5, the inflammatory phase will lead to the proliferative phase.

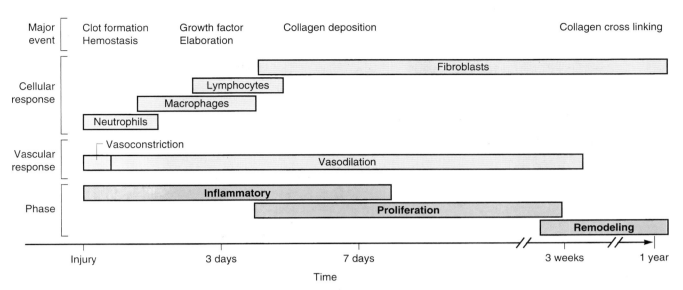

FIG. 22-1. Timeline of phases of wound healing with dominant cell types and major physiologic events.

Proliferative phase

The proliferative phase is the time when the wound surface is restored and connective tissue is deposited. Beefy-red granulation tissue is formed, giving way to wound contraction and epithelial migration. It is in this stage that the growth factors that were released show their results, and new cells are formed to heal the wound, and provide collagen deposition and other transactions to result in tissue healing.

Remodeling phase

The remodeling phase (also called maturation) may begin as early as 1 week postinjury. Proliferation results in collagen deposition, but this deposition is unorganized. The maturation phase consists of collagen and cellular remodeling. This remodeling results in strength of the skin. At the end of proliferation, the skin has about 20% tensile strength, while at the completion of remodeling, the tensile strength approaches 80%.

Complications

Regardless of etiology, wounds are intended to pass through the phases of wound healing without any complication. However, comorbid conditions, chronicity, and confounding factors can impair the velocity and the mechanisms with which repair should occur. Any wound that is older than 1 year deserves a biopsy (including the margin of the wound) to rule out malignancy and transformation of cells that can signal other conditions.

Other variables prompting a workup include a cyclic wound, as the cycle itself is a symptom of some type of impairment in the wound environment at the very least. Cyclical wounds are chronic wounds that open and close; that is, wound closure cannot be sustained. This is the characteristic wound that heals, and reopens in a few days, or almost closes and then opens exponentially. This wound cycle of nonhealing can be due to circulatory conditions and autoimmune conditions that are not detected or controlled, and if the wound is associated with a bone, often signal acute or chronic osteomyelitis.

Infection of wounds, which can often be very subtle, can also lead to chronicity. Certainly, cellulitis, sepsis, and classic signs like purulent exudate and foul odor are indicators that are more evident.

Often, the only sign of wound infection is delay of healing. Exploration and workup of these contributors to chronicity will be discussed later in this chapter.

Understanding the causes of wounds assists with differential diagnosis, leading to appropriate referral and management. Generally, wound healing principles are consistent across wound types. However, because wounds heal when the etiology is also treated, becoming familiar with etiologies is important. The following are common wounds seen in primary care but are certainly not inclusive of all wound types.

PRESSURE ULCERS

PrUs affect about 3 million people per year across all care settings, including at home, and almost $12 billion is spent on PrU treatment in the United States alone. The number of people affected and associated costs are only projected to increase in the coming years. Infection is the most common complication of PrUs. Geriatric patients with PrUs develop bacteremia at the rate of 3.5 per 10,000 hospital discharges, with a mortality rate approaching 50%. Statistics related to morbidity and mortality in relation to human skin wounds have not generally been collected, but the implications of poor life outcomes related to wounds are anecdotally noted (Sen et al., 2009).

PrUs are defined as localized injury to the skin and/or underlying tissue usually over a bony prominence as a result of pressure or in combination with shear and friction. Common locations for PrUs include the sacrum/coccyx, heels, buttocks, and the ischium (often called the sitting bones). The cellular death that can occur with pressure injury can be significant, and the damage incurred by the body can be very rapid and widespread.

Clinical Presentation

The staging and classification of PrUs provide a categorical approach to describing tissue destruction and clinical presentation. There are six stages or categories of injury, and the definitions are standardized (NPUAP, 2007). The staging of PrU can be complex. However, clinicians inexperienced with staging should take the purist approach—abide by the definitions and ensure your documentation of the wound supports the diagnosis (Table 22-1).

TABLE 22-1   Pressure Ulcer Stages (Categories)

Stage I: Nonblanchable erythema

Intact skin with nonblanchable redness of a localized area, usually over a bony prominence. It can be difficult to identify in darkly pigmented skin as they may not have visible blanching; its color may differ from the surrounding area. The area may be painful, firm, soft, warmer, or cooler as compared to adjacent tissue. The presence or development may indicate "at-risk" persons.

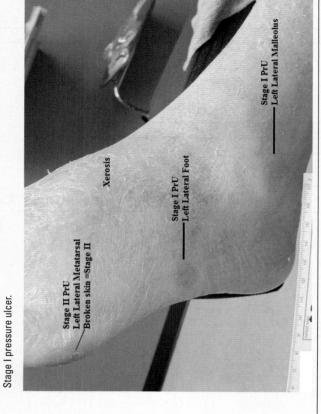

Stage I pressure ulcer.

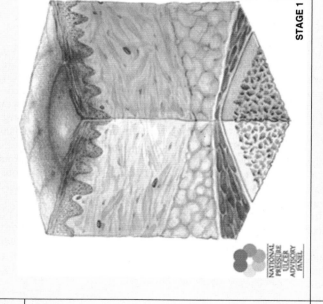

STAGE 1

Stage II: Partial thickness

Partial thickness loss of dermis presenting as a shallow open ulcer with a red pink wound bed, without slough. May also present as an intact or open/ ruptured serum-filled or serosanguineous- filled blister. A shiny or dry, shallow ulcer without slough or bruising indicates deep tissue injury. This category should not be used to describe skin tears, tape burns, incontinence- associated dermatitis, maceration, or excoriation.

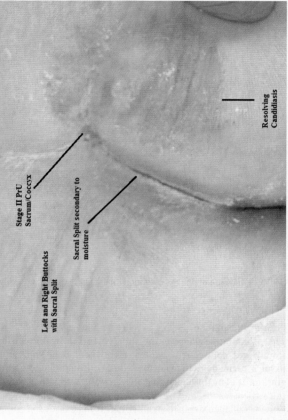

Stage II pressure ulcer.

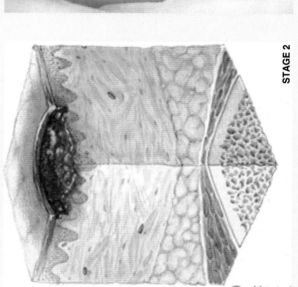

STAGE 2

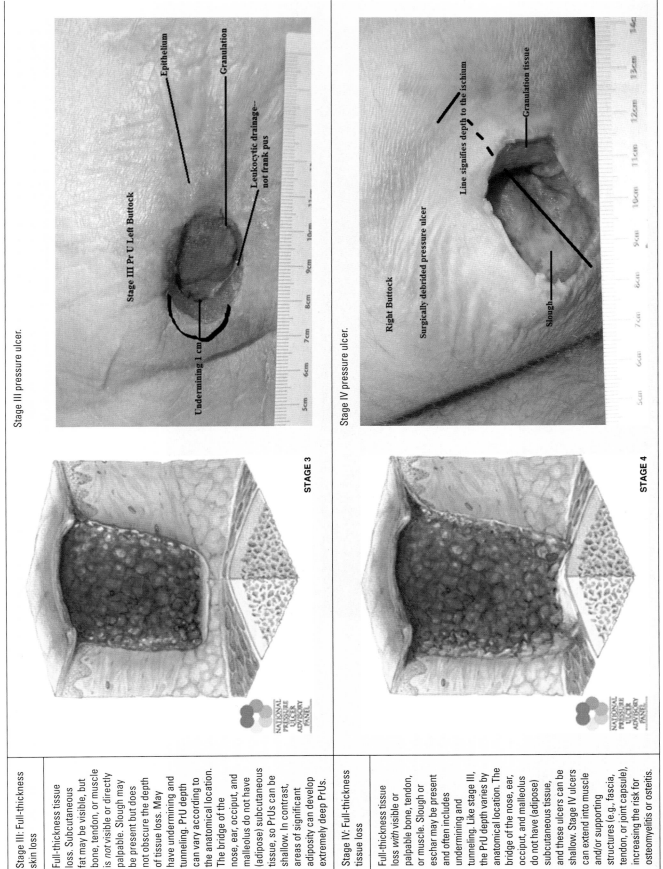

Stage III pressure ulcer.

Stage IV pressure ulcer.

Stage III: Full-thickness skin loss

Full-thickness tissue loss. Subcutaneous fat may be visible, but bone, tendon, or muscle is *not* visible or directly palpable. Slough may be present but does not obscure the depth of tissue loss. May have undermining and tunneling. PrU depth can vary according to the anatomical location. The bridge of the nose, ear, occiput, and malleolus do not have (adipose) subcutaneous tissue, so PrUs can be shallow. In contrast, areas of significant adiposity can develop extremely deep PrUs.

Stage IV: Full-thickness tissue loss

Full-thickness tissue loss *with* visible or palpable bone, tendon, or muscle. Slough or eschar may be present and often includes undermining and tunneling. Like stage III, the PrU depth varies by anatomical location. The bridge of the nose, ear, occiput, and malleolus do not have (adipose) subcutaneous tissue, and these ulcers can be shallow. Stage IV ulcers can extend into muscle and/or supporting structures (e.g., fascia, tendon, or joint capsule), increasing the risk for osteomyelitis or osteitis.

(continued)

Unstageable pressure ulcer.

Site: Left medial knee

Wound base filled with slough—Unstageable PrU

Unstageable pressure ulcer with eschar on the heel.

Red hue could signify sDTI component

Necrotic tissue

Opened blister

UNSTAGEABLE

NATIONAL PRESSURE ULCER ADVISORY PANEL

Unstageable: Full-thickness skin or tissue loss—depth unknown

Full-thickness tissue loss in which actual depth of the ulcer is completely obscured by slough (yellow, tan, gray, green, or brown) and/or eschar (tan, brown, or black) in the wound bed. Until enough slough and eschar are removed to expose the base of the wound, the true depth cannot be determined. Stable (dry, adherent, intact without erythema, or fluctuance).

Eschar on the heels serves as "the body's natural (biological) cover" and should not be removed.

| Suspected deep tissue injury—depth unknown (sDTI) |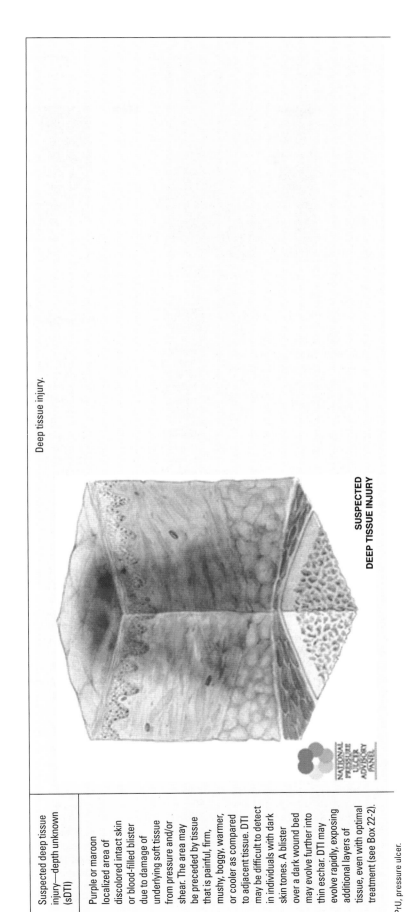

Deep tissue injury.

SUSPECTED DEEP TISSUE INJURY |
|---|---|
| Purple or maroon localized area of discolored intact skin or blood-filled blister due to damage of underlying soft tissue from pressure and/or shear. The area may be preceded by tissue that is painful, firm, mushy, boggy, warmer, or cooler as compared to adjacent tissue. DTI may be difficult to detect in individuals with dark skin tones. A blister over a dark wound bed may evolve further into thin eschar. DTI may evolve rapidly, exposing additional layers of tissue, even with optimal treatment (see Box 22-2). | |

PrU, pressure ulcer.

BOX 22-2 | **Progression of Suspected Deep Tissue Injury**

Day 1   Day 3   Day 10

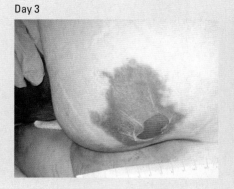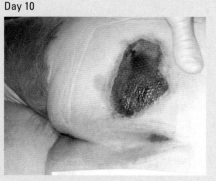

It is important to note that PrUs, while classified into stages, could present to the provider at any stage in the continuum. While the physiology and risk factors of PrUs are the same for any stage, clinicians may not see a stage I PrU prior to its advancement to a stage II PrU. Likewise, a PrU that presents as a sore and red area today could change and have a significantly different clinical presentation the next day. While there are limitations with the staging process, it can be very helpful in recognizing and guiding the management of a PrUs and sDTIs.

Management

Stage I pressure ulcers

When stage I PrUs are identified, it is important to consider the etiology—namely unrelieved pressure. Since individuals with one PrU are at increased risk to develop more, it's important to consider pressure reduction both locally and globally. Optimal care of patients with a stage I PrU would include referral to a wound specialist/center. Yet primary care clinicians should develop management goals to reduce progression of the PrU, the development of new ulcers, and complications during the healing process.

The first and most important step in medical management is reducing/relieving the pressure (called "offloading") to promote wound healing and prevention of new PrUs. *Global* pressure relief measures for PrUs can be ordered by the primary care clinician (e.g., a pressure-reducing mattress and/or chair cushion if they sit upright). Federal guidelines identify "group" surface for patients with staged PrUs (Box 22-3). Durable medical equipment (DME) companies are well versed and can help procure the necessary equipment to offload the patient. Patients may be eligible for a pressure-reducing mattress/hospital bed at home.

Whether lying in bed or sitting in the chair, frequent repositioning, definitely no less than at least every 2 hours, is essential. If the ulcer is on the dorsal surface of the body, consider side-to-side positioning rather than back-lying. If the ulcer has pressure on it when sitting, even with a pressure-reducing chair cushion, the patient's sit time should be monitored. Consider a sitting restriction of no more than 2 hours up, and 2 hours in bed, as a rotation during awake hours.

Localized pressure relief measures for stage I PrUs are pressure reduction of the affected area (Figure 22-2). Consider practical measures such as elevation of heels. Try to avoid foam rings or doughnuts as pressure-reducing devices, because they concentrate the pressure to surrounding tissues rather than redistributing/reducing the pressure interface for the area. Positioning aids such as pillows or wedges or commercial heel offloading boots/devices might be useful.

BOX 22-3 | **Group Surfaces Criteria**

Group 1
Support surfaces are designed to either replace a standard hospital or home mattress or as an overlay placed on top of a standard hospital or home mattress. Products in this category include mattresses, pressure pads, and mattress overlays (foam, air, water, or gel).

Group 2
In addition to above, these powered air flotation beds, powered pressure-reducing air mattresses, and nonpowered advanced pressure-reducing mattresses

Group 3
Complete bed systems, known as air-fluidized beds, which use the circulation of filtered air through silicone beads

Topical therapies are not necessary for stage I PrUs. In fact, it was once thought that massage of the affected area would help to reestablish blood supply to the area. However, the current thinking is that massage to the area directly can actually cause more damage to occur and is no longer recommended. If the skin is scaly, a common problem with heel PrUs, for example, gentle application of a moisturizer may be warranted. In general, petrolatum is an effective moisturizer, but multiple compounds are on the market, including mixes of petrolatum and dimethicone, petrolatum and lanolin, and various natural moisturizers, which work as well.

Advanced pressure ulcers (stages II–IV)

The initial management of stages II, III, and IV PrUs is the same as that for stage I, in relation to offloading the pressure with surfaces and repositioning. Management decisions should be based on ulcer presentation. For example, a wound with cellulitis, bad odor, or frank pus may require a local or systemic anti-infective treatment. Advanced-stage PrUs require consultation and continuous care from a wound specialist, unless there is limited access.

Selection of dressings is based on the goal of care, and not on wound etiology. Palliative care goals involve comfort, while active care goals strive for wound healing. Stages III and stage IV PrUs may require packing to fill the void or "dead space" left from tissue destruction. Packing deep wounds is important to prevent infection and abscess formation. Presence of frank pus and odorous exudate demand microbiologic analysis. If palliation is the goal, less frequent

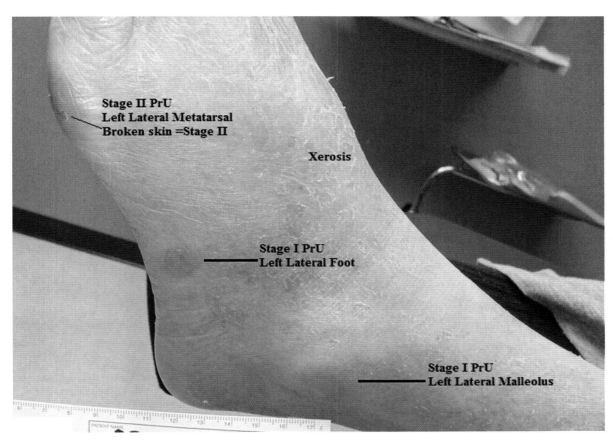

FIG. 22-2. Stage I pressure ulcer.

dressing changes are preferred, in general. There are a variety of other complex treatment modalities available that would be best employed by the wound care specialist.

Nutritional screening should be performed on all patients with a stage II, III, or IV PrUs in addition to wound treatment. While visual examination of the patient may indicate general nutritional deficiencies, a thorough dietary assessment, as well as serum testing, is used to analyze the patient's nutritional status. Patients with PrUs can have significant and undetected nutritional issues that impact their wound healing. It is considered a standard of care to assess the patient's nutritional status, and it is imperative to incorporate this aspect of care into the wound treatment process. This is addressed at the end of this chapter.

Unstageable pressure ulcers

It is certainly possible to presume the depth of tissue injury, but technically, no classifiable stage can be determined until the wound base is visible. Treatment for unstageable PrUs should follow the same pathway as any advanced PrU, assuming the worst-case scenario of tissue destruction.

Suspected deep tissue injuries

Outpatient care to halt the progression of a suspected deep tissue injury (sDTI) is limited to simple pressure reduction (discussed above in PrUs) and protection of the area, using a "watch and wait" approach. Hospitalized patients and some wound care centers can offer low-frequency ultrasound therapy (LFUS), which can be beneficial in the treatment of sDTIs. Nutrition and overall health status must be assessed, and steps to intervene with comorbid factors should be implemented.

Topical ointments that contain trypsin and balsam of Peru may increase perfusion to the area applied but carry the risk contact dermatitis. These ointments act as a wound cover and protect the wound. Otherwise, protecting the wound with a soft dressing and changing one to two times per day would be indicated and may provide some relief to the patient. Systemic treatment for a sDTI is not indicated. However, primary care clinicians should address any and all confounding or comorbid conditions that may contribute to the delayed wound healing.

Referral and Consultation

Patients with an advanced PrU should be referred to the nearest wound care specialist. If the wound has necrotic tissue or exposed structures, consider surgical consult for debridement and potential skin graft/muscle flap. Some general and plastic surgeons can offer these services. Surgical consult should be sought as early as possible to prevent further complications such as sepsis, osteomyelitis (if not already present), and other complications. Optimal care of patient with an sDTI would include referral to a wound specialist or center who can provide other treatment modalities such as ultrasound.

Patient Education and Follow-up

Patients and caregivers should be educated and instructed about the importance of pressure redistribution and offloading. Follow-up visits for a stage I PrU highly depend on general patient condition. Patients at high risk to develop more PrUs warrant a follow-up in 1 to 2 weeks. However, changes in the patient's condition should necessitate a call to you by the caregiver. Important changes include a break in the skin or the development of a blister in the area (both would upgrade the wound to stage II) or development of new PrUs, even if only stage I. These changes should prompt a patient referral for a wound specialist.

Advanced PrU patients living at home will need nursing care and possibly other services providing therapy. Facilitating this support is important for the patient, family, and caregivers, who may be overwhelmed in caring for their loved one. Feelings of guilt may arise if a loved one develops a PrU at home. Reassurance and education to caregivers may be needed, and should involve information regarding debility and its relationship to skin integrity failure.

As mentioned, patients with sDTIs are best managed and followed up by wound specialists. However, if none are available, the primary care clinician should monitor the patient weekly until the wound has stabilized and has declared to its fullest extent (meaning that the tissue destruction has stopped, and the wound now presents in the truest destructive form) and then every 1 to 2 weeks with coordinated care and support from home care and durable medical equipment resources.

VENOUS ULCERS

It is estimated that 500,000 to 600,000 people deal with venous leg ulcers (VLUs) each year in the United States. VLUs are the most common lower extremity ulcer, accounting for 80% to 90% of leg ulcers and frequently encountered in primary care practice. There are multiple causes of leg ulcers. Systemic diseases and conditions may present with cutaneous manifestations on the legs, including leukemias, syndromes, carcinomas, hematologic aberrancies, lymphatic abnormalities, and circulatory disorders (both venous and arterial). Often, leg ulcers have mixed etiologies, which makes for complex evaluation and management. For this chapter, focus will be on venous and arterial insufficiency.

Pathophysiology

VLUs are the result of venous insufficiency which is an impairment of the valves in the veins of the lower extremities. Insufficiency in the veins leads to pooling of blood in the lower extremities referred to as "stasis" or "venous stasis." This malfunction causes tired, achy legs, dry skin, skin discolorations, skin texture changes, and ulcerations. Venous insufficiency is common in those who stand for long periods of time, are obese, have hypertension, and have vein varicosities and/or a history of superficial or deep vein thrombosis. Venous insufficiency can lead to chronic venous disease, commonly referred to as chronic venous insufficiency (CVI) or more recently as lower extremity venous disease (LEVD).

The presenting history of a patient with LEVD may include hypertension, deep or superficial thrombosis, history of tired or heavy legs, obesity, leg edema, and nicotine use. Varicosities are frequently present (Figure 22-3). Often, the patients report that in the morning their legs are not swollen and feel fine but that at the end of the day they have a "sock line" and "aching" (not a pain) in their legs. Elevation of their legs is soothing. Work history could include jobs that require prolonged standing.

Clinical Presentation

Assessment of the lower extremity in the patient with CVI/LEVD should include both physical assessment and diagnostics tests. Venous duplex imaging or ultrasound is indicated in the workup for LEVD, but experienced clinicians may certainly be able to make diagnosis based on clinical presentation (Box 22-4). Still an ankle-brachial index (ABI) should be completed at the office visit in order to complete the assessment and determine an appropriate plan of care (Box 22-5).

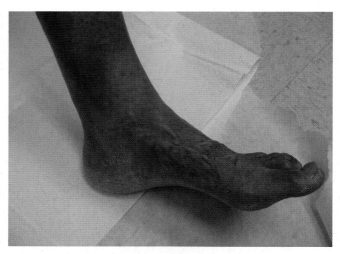

FIG. 22-3. Varicose veins.

BOX 22-4	Characteristics of Lower Extremity Venous Disease

Edema
Inverted champagne bottle-shaped leg
Hemosiderosis/hemosiderin staining—red/brown discoloration in gaiter area leg, resulting in increased pigmentation
Lipodermatosclerosis—leathery or woody skin change result of subcutaneous fat inflammation
Stasis dermatitis resulting in itchy red patches and plaques on anterior lower legs
Atrophie blanche—white spots with evident red capillaries and hyperpigmented borders
Varicosities or knotty/bulging veins

BOX 22-5	Ankle-Brachial Index Testing

Equipment needed: stethoscope, sphygmomanometer, doppler (portable/hand held)
The patient should be supine for this procedure.
Obtain brachial pressures in both arms, unless contraindicated.
Place the sphygmomanometer cuff on the leg, just above the ankle.
Locate the dorsalis pedis or posterior tibial pulse—each will be tested.
Apply ultrasound gel to the area of pulse.
Apply a doppler to pulse area, then inflate cuff until the pulse sound disappears.
Deflate the cuff slowly, and listen for the pulse sound to return.
The higher of the two ankle pressures number reading is used in the calculation.
Calculate the ABI—highest ankle pressure/brachial pressure = ABI
Example: brachial 120, ankle 114, 114/120 = 0.95

Interpretation of ABI	
>1	Within normal limits
≤0.9	Mild LEAD
≤0.6–0.8	Moderate LEAD
<0.5	Critical limb ischemia
Noncompressible	Get arterial doppler

VLU classic characteristics would include a lesion on the lower extremity, typically in the gaiter area (the lower leg just below the calf, extending to and including the ankle area). The most common site is just above the medial malleolus. The lesion is usually irregular in shape, shallow, and weepy. The surrounding skin, especially over varicosities, may be warm. The base of the wound is usually red and can have a thin layer of fibrin cover. In addition, there can be chronic skin changes such as hyperpigmentation (also called hemosiderin staining) and lipodermatosclerosis, thickening of the skin with the appearance of an upside-down champagne bottle (Figure 22-4). VLUs are not staged in the same manner as PrUs. Instead they are described as partial- or full-thickness wounds, based on level of tissue destruction.

Management

Treatment of LEVD, even when accompanied by VLU, should include compression of the legs. Control of the leg edema is equally as important as treatment of the ulcer. Therapeutic compression is thought to be achieved at the 30 to 40 mm Hg range. This can be applied with compression devices, compression stockings, and if an ulcer is present, probably best managed with a compression wrap. The patient with LEVD who does not have a leg ulcer also needs compression to prevent complications of the disease, such as ulceration. Clinicians should use caution as there are contraindications to compression (Box 22-6).

Knee high compression hose at 20 to 30 mm Hg are frequently recommended if there has been no history of ulceration. If an ulceration history exists, 30 to 40 mm Hg compression must be

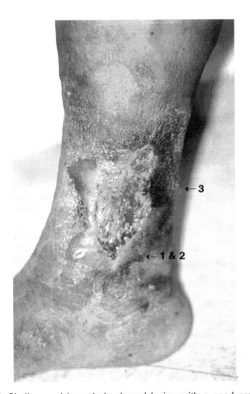

FIG. 22-4. Shallow and irregularly shaped lesion with a good granulating base. The associated physical signs of chronic venous insufficiency, such as hyperpigmentation, chronic scarring, and skin contraction in the ankle region, are readily identified. Note the classic characteristics of venous disease: (1) irregular edges, (2) shallow ulcer, (3) evidence of hyperpigmentation (hemosiderosis), and (4) location above the medial malleolus.

BOX 22-6	Contraindications and Caution for Lower Extremity Compression

If ABI <0.7, obtain arterial doppler to rule out the presence of PAD.
If the ABI is moderate to normal (≥0.6–1.0) with clinical signs of PAD, obtain an arterial doppler study to assess the presence/severity of PAD.
Presence of uncompensated or uncontrolled congestive heart failure (compression of the lower extremities could lead to pulmonary edema or respiratory compromise)

---

considered, and in severe cases of LEVD even higher compression, thigh-high stockings or custom-fitted garments. Compression hose can be obtained online, as well as through local DME providers. Be cautioned that the compression hose sold at many retail stores are not to be used for therapeutic compression—they are usually 0 to less than 20 mm Hg compression. "Diabetic socks" are not compression hose, which is a common misconception.

Referral and Consultation

Consider referral of the patient with VLU to a wound specialist for ongoing management and treatment of the VLU. The wound specialist will likely continue compression wraps until wound closure, and then recommend transition in compression hose as a permanent lifestyle change, for the treatment of LEVD or edema control. Collaboration between primary and wound care providers is essential for the patient with LEVD and VLU. Patient may have additional consultation with a dermatologist for stasis dermatitis and cardiovascular specialist for evaluation and treatment of varicosities.

Patient Education and Follow-up

Education for the patient should include not only the importance and purpose of compression, but also should stress control of hypertension, smoking cessation, and even weight loss, if indicated. Be sure to ask your patients about the age of their compression hose (their average life is 6 months) and if they have had any ulcers or other problems. Individuals with VLU should be urged to elevate legs to promote venous return and to avoid extended positions with lower leg dependency as this works against the calf muscle pump.

Educate and reinforce the use of compression hose. Instruct patients how to apply them each morning within 1 hour of getting out of bed and removing at night before going to bed. Emphasize that skipping compression for even just a few days can lead to uncontrolled edema and ulceration.

ARTERIAL ULCERS

The second most common type of leg ulcer (10%–20% of lower extremity ulcers) is arterial ulcers, more prevalent in those older than 65 years. Peripheral arterial disease (PAD) is the major contributor to lower extremity arterial disease (LEAD) that can lead to arterial ulcers (also called "ischemic ulcers") development. Arterial ulcers can ultimately represent limb threat, and without reperfusion of the area, the ulcer cannot heal. PAD affects 8 to 12 million Americans with multiple issues related to morbidity and mortality. Patients with PAD may have other cardiovascular diseases such as hypertension, myocardial infarction, TIA, stroke, and even coronary artery bypass surgery. Often, other surgical procedures may have occurred, such as a femoral-popliteal bypass, or even arterial grafting site. Ascertaining a careful and thorough cardiac history is very important.

Pathophysiology

Risk factors for PAD include nicotine use, obesity, hyperlipidemia diabetes, and age. In addition, thrombotic-type events due to emboli from aneurysms, hypercoagulation states, and/or vascular plaques, as well as a host of other causes, can induce local ischemic events that can result in ulceration. Ischemia can affect large or small vessels, including micro vessels. Arterial ulcers can ultimately represent limb threat, and without reperfusion of the area, the ulcer cannot heal.

Clinical Presentation

The presenting history of the patient with LEAD and ulceration is very important. Patients may report pain at the site of ulceration, in their leg, especially with walking or other activity (claudication). Pain that can occur with arterial ulcers can be intense. Pain at rest may be present, and described as a constant ache. More advanced LEAD pain can mimic neuropathic pain, often described as tingling, like electric shocks, or burning. LEAD pain differs from VLU discomfort. The VLU patient often describes legs feeling "heavy" at the end of the day, whereas the LEAD patient may not be able to keep their legs still from the intensity of the pain experience.

In addition to the presenting history, it is important to always consider LEAD as a confounding factor, especially in any leg or foot ulcer. For example, someone may fall and suffer a skin tear on their leg which does not respond to treatment. A lower extremity workup may reveal poor ABI, which can indicate the presence of LEAD. This condition may not be allowing enough perfusion to the skin to allow wound healing. Arterial ulcers may be present because of the arterial disease, or it may contribute to their chronicity. LEAD can be silent and undetected unless really sought out, especially in the early stages. Many people think that the pain they experience in the lower extremities is a normal and expected aging change. Many times an ulcer of another origin with this confounding factor is present, and may lead the provider down an unexpected path of intervention to preserve a limb, with the healing of the wound being a second priority.

Assessment of patients with LEAD may reveal a restless leg, though in reality, the leg is moving secondary to the pain response. The greater the level of ischemia, the greater pain sensation the patient will have. Other findings could include sparse hair or hairless leg, and the skin may be shiny. Often, when the leg is dependent, it can be rubrous, but elevation of the extremity can produce pallor. Pulses may be present, diminished, absent, or a combination of these findings in the femoral, popliteal, posterior tibial, and dorsalis pedis. It is also possible to see cyanosis or mottling, and this would require immediate referral to a vascular specialist. Clinical characteristics for the patient with LEAD are detailed in Box 22-7.

Arterial ulcer characteristics differ from venous ulcers. Arterial ulcers generally are punched out in appearance and are very dry. The skin surrounding the wound (periwound) can be pale and shiny and cool. Often, there is necrotic tissue present in the wound base, since

---

| BOX 22-7 | **Characteristics of Lower Extremity Arterial Disease** |

Legs cool, painful, thin, and shiny with hair loss
Hypertrophic toenails, usually yellow
Diminished or absent leg/foot pulses
Feet cool/cold
Disparity in temperature between thigh and lower extremity
Leg ruborous in dependent position; pallorous with elevation of leg
Delayed capillary refill of toenails

---

tissue death is a natural result of poor perfusion (Figure 22-5). When a true wound base is seen, it is often pale red or pale pink. Arterial ulcers are often, but not always, located on lateral ankle, toes, tips of toes, and distal lower leg. The more distal sites are more likely to manifest arterial insufficiency. Arterial ulcers are not staged, but are classified as either partial- or full-thickness ulcers.

Management

Ischemic ulcers should be regarded as an urgent health issue and a hallmark of underlying cardiovascular disease. Screening for arterial disease in a limb can easily be performed with the ABI test. If the ABI is questionable or there is clinical suspicion for arterial disease, a noninvasive arterial doppler study of the lower extremities should be obtained. Concurrently, if an arterial ulcer is suspected, referral to a vascular provider and a wound specialist is imperative to try to preserve the limb. Compression for this affected leg is dangerous and can result in further ischemia and should be avoided.

Arterial ulcers can be limb threatening, and even life threatening. Wound treatment selection should focus on keeping the wound as infection free as possible, while workup is being completed for possible vascular intervention. Management by a wound specialist is highly recommended. Arterial ulcers are very dry, and if there is not any necrotic tissue present, gentle donation of moisture, such as with a petrolatum-impregnated gauze, may be appropriate. Consider betadine painted on and around the wound edges and cover with gauze. Betadine will keep the immediate wound environment dry, which is an important strategy to try and prevent wet gangrene. However, in the presence of black eschar, cellulitis, odor, and fluctuance, emergent evaluation is necessary.

Referral and Consultation

Arterial ulcers should prompt immediate consult with a vascular specialist to ascertain the level and site of the LEAD. A variety of treatment options, including revascularization procedures and medications impacting wound healing, may be offered by the vascular specialist. Wound specialists are optimal for healing and prevention of complications.

Patient Education and Follow-up

Patients with arterial ulcers will need to be reevaluated at least weekly. Primary care clinicians should stay well-informed by specialists regarding the frequency of wound evaluation and treatment goals. Patients should be educated about cardiovascular health promotion and smoking cessation, if needed.

MIXED INSUFFICIENCY

It is possible for a patient to have impairment in both the arterial and venous systems, and have both LEVD and LEAD (Figure 22-6). It is also possible for these patients to develop leg ulcerations. It is very challenging to treat these patients, and the priority of care must be dictated by the degree of arterial insufficiency, since poor limb ischemia precludes the compression therapy that is required to combat the insufficient venous system. Follow the LEAD guidelines and get a vascular opinion before proceeding with an active treatment plan to ensure the best outcome for the patient.

NEUROPATHIC ULCERS

Neuropathy affects about 26 million Americans, causing motor, sensory, and autonomic damage to the nervous system, thus altering

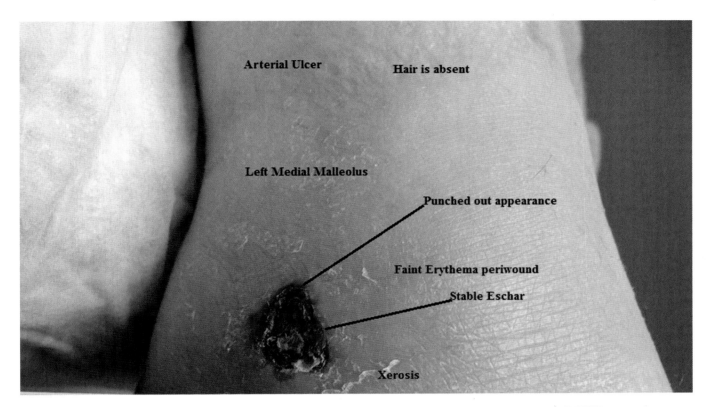

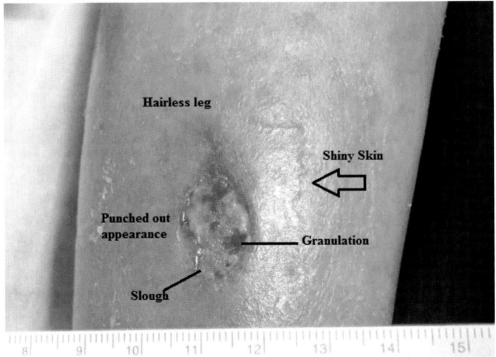

FIG. 22-5. Arterial ulcers.

protective mechanisms that relate to sensation, such as pain, temperature, and touch. Diabetic peripheral neuropathy (DPN) is probably the most well known and studied in the literature and affects 15 to 18 million people.

While neuropathy is not solely associated with diabetes, it is estimated that 10% to 100% of diabetics will deal with DPN in their lifetime. Diabetics with foot problems occupy more hospital beds than diabetics with any other complications, leading to lower

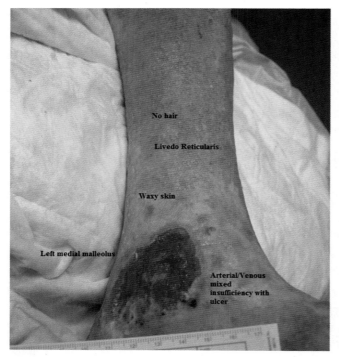

FIG. 22-6. Mixed insufficiency ulcer.

extremity complications such as amputation, ulceration, and other injuries.

Pathophysiology

Neuropathy is nerve damage to peripheral nerves, which can be caused by disease, drugs, or may be idiopathic. Neuropathy can lead to complications with skin, particularly due to the loss of protective sensation (LOPS; insensate). A common mistake is the interchange of "diabetic" ulcer with "neuropathic" ulcer, probably because a good percentage of these patients also have diabetes. In addition to neuropathy, ulcer formation is probable due to multiple etiologies, including abnormal microvascular circulation, arterial insufficiency, poor glycemic control, and mechanical forces (friction and pressure) (Box 22-8).

Clinical Presentation

The presenting history of the patient with lower extremity neuropathic disease (LEND) will most likely include the burning, electric

BOX 22-8	Common Causes of Neuropathy

Diabetes and other metabolic disorders
Infectious disease (Lyme disease, HIV/AIDS)
Autoimmune dysfunction
Chemotherapy/cancer
Hereditary
Idiopathy
Nerve entrapment/trauma
Toxins
Nutritional deficiencies
Gastrointestinal disorders

shock–like sensation in the legs, numbness, and weakness. Pressure secondary to ill-fitting shoes can cause red, dry ulcerations anywhere on the foot where there is a pressure point or friction; it favors the plantar, heels, and metatarsal areas (Figures 22-7 and 22-8). There is typically very little edema or exudate. Clinical presentation may vary depending on whether the patient is aware of the lesion and has been treating it. Neuropathic ulcers are not staged, but are classified as either partial- or full-thickness ulcers.

Management

Immediate care of the patient with LEND accompanied by a neuropathic (or other etiology) ulcer will center on immediate referral to a wound or diabetic foot specialist, who often is a podiatrist. If the wound has a draining exudate, a culture should be obtained, and a dressing that will pack the wound is indicated. Offloading of the area is important, even if it is only accomplished through manipulation of dressings. Addressing systemic causes or factors like glycemic control of the diabetic patient is vital. Primary care clinicians must assess and monitor the patient's diabetes to promote healing and prevent the occurrence of new wounds.

Referral and Consultation

It is highly recommended that patients with LEND and a neuropathic ulcer be referred for comprehensive care. Clinicians may include a vascular specialist, dietician, wound care specialist, podiatrist, and medical providers who specialize in wound care, to prevent ulceration and further complications.

Pedorthists can help provide fitted shoes and orthotics for patients. Routine dermatologic follow-up is as needed, but foot inspection at every encounter cannot be overemphasized. If the LEND patient is diabetic, emphasis on good glycemic control should always be discussed at each encounter.

Patient Education and Follow-up

For those patients who present with known LEND, asking them to remove their shoes and socks for foot inspection is a great idea. Because of the LOPS, any encounter with a care provider should yield not only foot inspection, but also reinforcement of the practice of daily foot inspections by the patient. Feet should be kept clean and dry, without adhesive, medicaments (including foot powders), or chemicals.

Consider a referral to a pedorthotist or podiatrist in your area to assist them with shoe selection which can include wider toe boxes. The patient's shoe should be monitored for dirty or uneven wear patterns or bulges. Orthotics inserted into shoes can adjust for balance deformities and reduce weight-bearing forces. A diabetes diagnosis will qualify the patient for special shoes and does not require an ulceration for coverage. However, the presence of an ulcer or other major foot deformity may help them qualify for other special shoe benefits. Arming your patients with this information is essential to maintaining proper foot health.

WOUND ENVIRONMENT

Globally, no matter what type of wound is present, there are obstacles that can prevent wound healing and favorable response to even the best topical care. Often, practitioners want to culture a wound and give an antibiotic, thinking that since the wound is open it must be infected. Other practitioners skip the culture, and just prescribe an antibiotic with full spectrum capabilities for the same

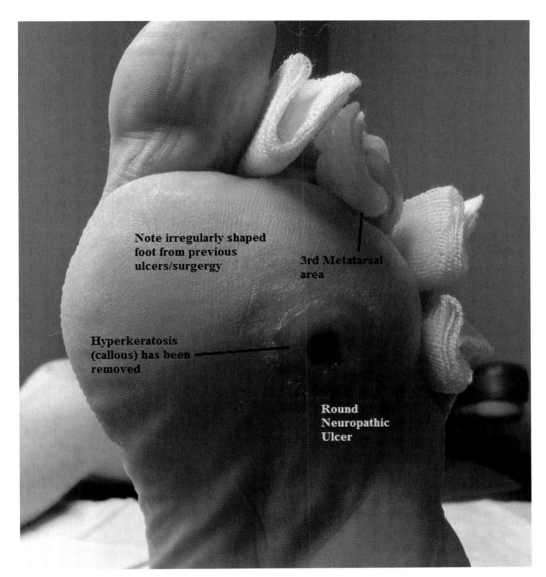

FIG. 22-7. Neuropathic ulcer, plantar foot.

reason. However, the notion that all wounds are infected is untrue. Most wounds are colonized to some extent with microorganisms. Some experts believe that the concentration and type of flora have a role in both healing and occurrence of infection. Therefore, careful consideration should be given when treating patients with systemic and topical antibiotics if patients are without symptoms of infection and do not have a culture and sensitivity from the wound exudate or tissue. Knowing when and how to treat, whether to culture, and how to determine the influence of bacteria on the wound is key considerations in antimicrobial stewardship and management of the patient.

Bioburden

Bioburden is the degree of microbial contamination or microbial load and is thought to be one of the *most* important barriers to wound healing and currently the focus of many researchers. The bioburden is the type and concentration of bacteria present in the wound (Box 22-9). *Biofilm* is the organization of the microorganisms that are found in the bioburden. Biofilm is not traditional

organization of bacteria, but is instead composed of "free floaters" called planktonic organisms. This community of microorganisms is phenotypically and genetically different from other bacteria. These microorganisms attach to each other or to a surface encased in an extracellular polymeric substance also known as "slime." The slime provides increased resistance to cellular and chemical attack. These microorganisms replicate outside the host on the wound surface (contamination). They can also utilize nutrients on the wound surface (colonization). If proliferation of these bacteria continues, host invasion occurs, resulting in infected tissues (infection).

Wound Culture

To culture or not, that is the question. The answer is not black and white. While indeed all wounds do have some bioburden, its presence may not be influencing the wound healing mechanics. However, eventually a culture may be indicated because the biofilm replicates and can become resistant to topical remedies such as

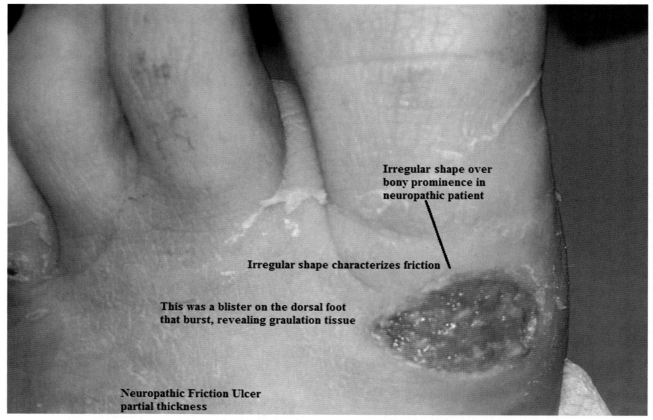

Irregular shape over bony prominence in neuropathic patient

Irregular shape characterizes friction

This was a blister on the dorsal foot that burst, revealing graulation tissue

Neuropathic Friction Ulcer partial thickness

FIG. 22-8. Neuropathic ulcer, dorsal foot.

antimicrobials and dressing modes of action. Culturing accurately, however, is not simply swabbing the top of the wound, for that will only yield surface contaminants. Culturing for accurate results in an outpatient clinic really calls for collection of fluid of some type or tissue.

BOX 22-9 | **Bioburden Continuum**

Bioburden
A measure of the degree of microbial contamination or microbial load

Biofilm
Organization of the microorganisms found in the bioburden

Contamination
Presence of nonreplicating microorganisms on a wound surface which do not incite a clinical response

Colonization
Presence of replicating microorganisms attached to the wound surface without host injury, allowing wound healing to continue predictably

Critical Colonization
Involves replication of microbial burden in the wound surface compartment, without signs of wound injury or delayed healing

Wound Infection
Proliferation of microorganisms within a deep compartment of the wound with signs and symptoms of an infection detectable.

Culturing the wound, then, has more to do with assessing the bioburden inside the wound versus what is occurring superficially on the outside of the wound. A wound culture is indicated when there are signs and symptoms of infection present, including periwound redness, purulent exudate, increased, new, or persistent pain, periwound warmth, swelling, and odor. It is at this point that a wound culture is valuable for the selection of the appropriate systemic antibiotic to combat the culprit(s) that is monopolizing the wound environment. If the patient is already on an antibiotic, culturing the wound may not be valuable, and may not yield good results.

There are three ways to culture wounds. The clinician's choice in culture technique may be dependent on the lab company and capabilities, the availability of equipment, or other practical limitations. No matter the technique, proper collection will yield better results.

Tissue biopsy, or *tissue culture,* is considered to be the gold standard for wound culturing. This can be completed with a scalpel or a punch, after cleansing with a nonantiseptic solution, such as saline. Use of antimicrobial solutions may provide some kill action, which would influence the culture result. This technique may be employed in the office setting, without any problem, as long as hemostasis can be achieved.

Needle aspiration of tissue fluid is another way to collect media for culture. With this technique, there could be opportunity to aspirate exudate directly into a syringe, which could then be sent to the lab for analysis. With this technique, it is permissible to prep the skin with an antimicrobial cleanser, because the aspirate would not be in contact with the antiseptic.

Swab collection is the last type of culture. This is the most popular type of culture, because of access to laboratory analysis and ease of collection by a nursing technologist/medical assistant, nurse, advanced provider, or physician. When using the swab, it is important to not cleanse the wound for methods already outlined. It is important that the swab remain sterile and that the dry tip be moistened with sterile normal saline in order to enhance the capture of microbes present. The swab should be firmly placed into the wound, using a "Z" technique, using enough pressure to cause exudation from the wound. Once the exudate is collected on the swab, it is placed in the swab tube and sent to the lab.

When ordering the culture, keep in mind that wounds may have aerobic or anaerobic organisms present. For example, if obtaining a tissue or aspirate culture, ordering both aerobic and anaerobic studies is important. But when obtaining a swab culture, anaerobic study is indicated in any diabetic who has a wound, or if there is undermining or tracking occurring in the wound. Take caution that even if the diabetic patient has a wound without a tract or tunnel, because of the diabetes, both types of culture are warranted.

Nutrition

Another obstacle to wound healing is nutrition. Nutrition impairment can prolong the inflammatory phase of wound healing, and cause cellular transactions to be impaired, delayed, or absent. Not all wounded patients have nutrition issues, but a nutritional assessment is warranted, especially in people with PrUs, or those who have multiple wounds of any type. There is a proven strong correlation between malnourishment and PrU development, for example. There is also an association between a weight loss of 5% or greater from usual body weight with the development of PrUs. Therefore, a quick visual assessment is not adequate to ascertain the level of nutritional reserves, because both thin and obese people can have nutritional inadequacies not detected with stand-alone visual assessment. Serum testing, diet analysis, and interview are all necessary to determine nutritional status. Assessment of nutritional status should be completed on initial visits for those with a single or multiple PrUs and for anyone who has multiple ulcers of any type.

What comprises a general nutritional assessment? Visual inspection of the patient, body mass index (BMI), biochemical data, and interview of the patient are the components of a general nutritional assessment (Box 22-10). There are tools available online for nutrition screening, and availability of a registered dietician to help counsel an undernourished individual certainly would be optimum. Where this resource is not available, guidelines do exist for treating undernourished patients (Figure 22-9). Often, the nutrition guides are related to PrUs, but the principles can be applied for any nutritionally compromised wound patient.

Biochemical data such as serum albumin and prealbumin levels have been widely accepted as important nutritional markers. The idea is that the prealbumin is most accurate, as it is a liver protein with a half-life of 2 to 3 days. The albumin marker has a half-life of 12 to 23 days. These markers now are thought to be less accurate as a solitary nutritional assessment, and should not be interpreted as a gold standard type testing. There is evidence that perhaps these biochemical analyses instead measure inflammation and metabolic stress than nutrient storage and availability. Obtaining these lab data is perfectly acceptable, but clinical correlation with appearance and condition of the patient must also occur to make any final diagnosis relating to undernutrition, malnutrition, or nutritional status within normal limits.

Many practitioners believe that nutritional supplementation should be given across the board to wounded patients. Some providers give certain vitamins or supplements routinely. However, a patient specific approach is best. Confounding factors such as chronic kidney disease make nutritional supplement difficult, especially in relation to protein and fluid. Approaching nutrition with patient goals and treatment goals in mind is the most logical approach to supplement nutrition.

One of the most debated issues surrounding nutritional requirements for wound healing surrounds the utilization of ascorbic acid (vitamin C), zinc, and copper. There is no clear marker for their

BOX 22-10	Nutritional Assessment Components

Visual Assessment—General Appearance
Frail, thin, obese, pale
Poor dentition/no teeth/poor-fitting dentures
Muscle wasting
Flaky skin
Thin, dry, brittle broken hair
Brittle nails
Cracked lips

Body Mass Index
<19 is risk for increased mortality, pressure ulcer development, undernutrition.
>30 is obese, but not necessarily nutritionally healthy.

Patient Interview
Recent unplanned weight loss
Swallowing/chewing difficulties
Inability to tolerate fluids
Presence of wounds
Medications (can influence appetite)

Biochemical Data
Prealbumin level—normal limits, 28–38 mg/dL
Albumin level—3.5–5 g/dL
Serum transferrin—204–360 mg/dL (not widely used)

Assessment of Weight Loss
Formula: current body weight/usual body weight $\times$ 100
Example: current weight: 137 lbs; usual body weight: 145 lbs
137/145 $\times$ 100 = 94.5% or weight loss of 5.5%, which could be significant

utilization. Current best practice, as recommended by the National Pressure Ulcer Advisory Panel, is to offer a vitamin or mineral supplement when dietary intake is poor, or if deficiencies are confirmed or suspected. The dosage of each nutrient is also highly variable, with no clear research-based recommendations for any extra amount needed for wound healing. See Box 22-11 for information on vitamin C, zinc, and copper.

Blood glucose control in the patient who is diabetic is important. It is a balance between allowing extra calories and protein (and inevitably carbohydrates) and the insulin uptake in the body. Blood glucose levels definitely influence healing in the diabetic patient. Blood glucose levels that are consistently at 140 mg/dL or below characterize better healing, while levels consistently above 150 mg/dL indicate slower and diminished wound healing. Obtaining a current Hgb A_{1c} (glycated hemoglobin) is important to determine the average blood glucose that the patient experiences, in order the primary provider to adjust or add any glycemia-regulating medications to the medication profile. Blood glucose control, even if obtained with the addition of insulin or other hypoglycemic medications, must be achieved for wound healing to occur.

Lastly, if a patient is malnourished in any way, a referral to a registered dietician is the most prudent approach. Once skin becomes impaired and comorbidities abound, the nutritional status of the patient becomes a separate complex problem.

WOUND DOCUMENTATION

Standardized documentation for open wounds provides consistency in care, facilitates safe hand-off and collaboration, and can provide a very clear clinical scenario. Aside from naming the appropriate wound etiology, using a set of standard descriptors is very useful. For example, wounds should be measured in centimeters, where often

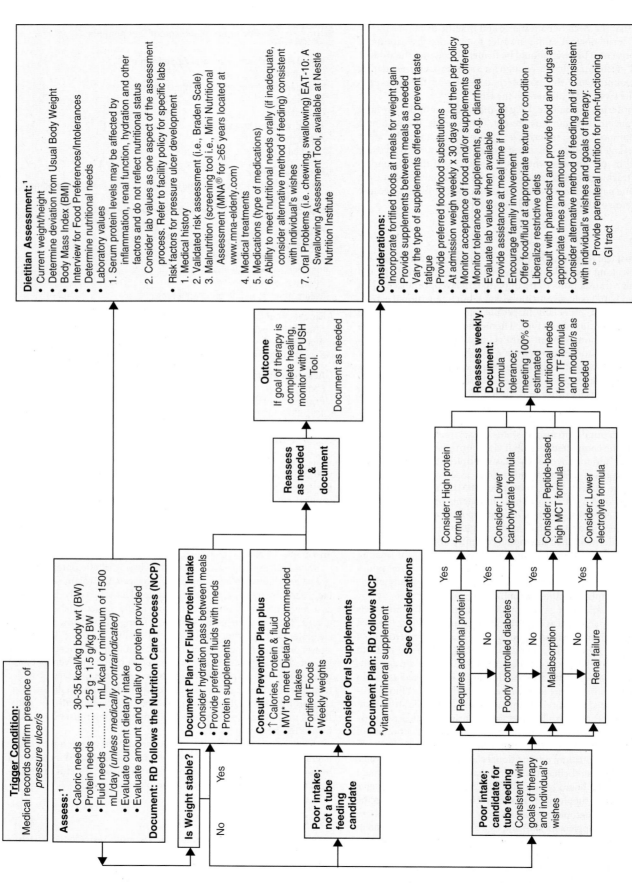

FIG. 22-9. Algorithm for treatment of pressure ulcers: nutrition guidelines.

Trigger Condition:
Medical records confirm presence of *pressure ulcer/s*

Assess:[1]
- Caloric needs .... 30-35 kcal/kg body wt (BW)
- Protein needs .... 1.25 g - 1.5 g/kg BW
- Fluid needs .... 1 mL/kcal or minimum of 1500 mL/day *(unless medically contraindicated)*
- Evaluate current dietary intake
- Evaluate amount and quality of protein provided

Document: RD follows the Nutrition Care Process (NCP)

Is Weight stable? No Yes

Document Plan for Fluid/Protein Intake
- Consider hydration pass between meals
- Provide preferred fluids with meds
- Protein supplements

Consult Prevention Plan plus
- ↑Calories, Protein & fluid
- MVI* to meet Dietary Recommended Intakes
- Fortified Foods
- Weekly weights

Consider Oral Supplements

Document Plan: RD follows NCP
*vitamin/mineral supplement

See Considerations

Poor intake; not a tube feeding candidate

Poor intake; candidate for tube feeding
Consistent with goals of therapy and individual's wishes

Reassess as needed & document

Outcome
If goal of therapy is complete healing, monitor with PUSH Tool.

Document as needed

Requires additional protein — Yes — Consider: High protein formula
No

Poorly controlled diabetes — Yes — Consider: Lower carbohydrate formula
No

Malabsorption — Yes — Consider: Peptide-based, high MCT formula
No

Renal failure — Yes — Consider: Lower electrolyte formula

Reassess weekly. Document:
Formula tolerance; meeting 100% of estimated nutritional needs from TF formula and modular/s as needed

Dietitian Assessment:[1]
- Current weight/height
- Determine deviation from Usual Body Weight
- Body Mass Index (BMI)
- Interview for Food Preferences/Intolerances
- Determine nutritional needs
- Laboratory values
  1. Serum protein levels may be affected by inflammation, renal function, hydration and other factors and do not reflect nutritional status
  2. Consider lab values as one aspect of the assessment process. Refer to facility policy for specific labs
- Risk factors for pressure ulcer development
  1. Medical history
  2. Validated risk assessment (i.e., Braden Scale)
  3. Malnutrition (screening tool i.e., Mini Nutritional Assessment (MNA® for ≥65 years located at www.mna-elderly.com)
  4. Medical treatments
  5. Medications (type of medications)
  6. Ability to meet nutritional needs orally (if inadequate, consider alternative method of feeding) consistent with individual's wishes
  7. Oral Problems (i.e. chewing, swallowing) EAT-10: A Swallowing Assessment Tool, available at Nestlé Nutrition Institute

Considerations:
- Incorporate fortified foods at meals for weight gain
- Provide supplements between meals as needed
- Vary the type of supplements offered to prevent taste fatigue
- Provide preferred food/food substitutions
- At admission weigh weekly x 30 days and then per policy
- Monitor acceptance of food and/or supplements offered
- Monitor tolerance of supplements, e.g. diarrhea
- Evaluate lab values when available
- Provide assistance at meal time if needed
- Encourage family involvement
- Offer food/fluid at appropriate texture for condition
- Liberalize restrictive diets
- Consult with pharmacist and provide food and drugs at appropriate times and amounts
- Consider alternative method of feeding and if consistent with individual's wishes and goals of therapy:
  - Provide parenteral nutrition for non-functioning GI tract

Vitamin C (ascorbic acid)
Essential for collagen synthesis
Boosts immune system function

Zinc
A cofactor for collagen formation
Assists in immune function
Metabolizes protein
Deficiency may occur with increased drainage, long-standing inadequate diet

Copper
Helps with new blood cell formation
Responsible for collagen cross-linking

other dermatologic issues are discussed in millimeters. Wounds can be consistently measured with the standard parameters of length, width, and depth. Wound tissue destruction can be described by PrU staging, or with the terms *partial* or *full* thickness for any other type of wound.

Other wound characteristics include the presence of undermining (tissue destruction under the skin around the perimeter of the wound) or tunneling ("sinus tract" or pathway extending the wound further through subcutaneous or muscle tissue. Wound edges may be open or closed. The base of the wound may be described in percentages of red (granulation), yellow (slough), or black (eschar) tissue that is present. Blisters or bullae should be noted along with size and fluid color (clear, yellow, sanguine, or serosanguineous). The general shape of the wound is important and should be recorded (round, oval, irregular), and so is the condition of the periwound. See Table 22-2 for guidance.

BASIC DRESSING CONCEPTS

Treatment guidelines for wounds always include identification of the causes, management of any infection, and correcting nutritional issues. Practical advice on *what* to treat the wound with is also important, and relies on a few guiding principles. Dressing categories abound, and the number of wound treatment products and modalities number into the thousands. Wound specialists are expert in the selection and management of these wound care systems which is beyond the scope of this textbook. It should be noted that these wound treatment principles can be used, based on the changing wound environment. The basic tenets of wound care are as follows:

- If the wound is dry, moisten it.
- If the wound is wet, dry it.
- If the wound is shallow, cover it.
- If the wound is deep, pack it.

The dressings listed in Table 22-3 provide a basic foundation for dressing selection for the primary care clinician to achieve these principles.

TABLE 22-2 Selected Wound Assessment Parameters

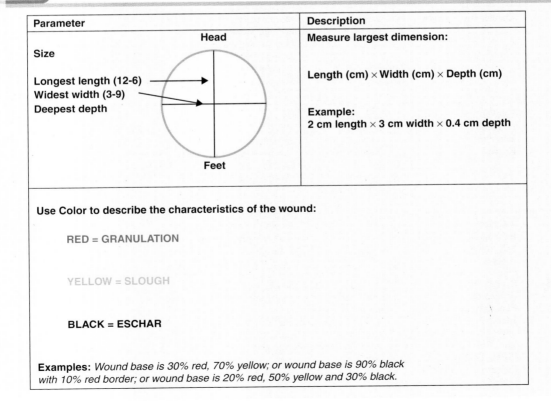

Parameter	Description
Size Longest length (12-6) Widest width (3-9) Deepest depth *(diagram: Head, Feet)*	Measure largest dimension: Length (cm) × Width (cm) × Depth (cm) Example: 2 cm length × 3 cm width × 0.4 cm depth
Use Color to describe the characteristics of the wound: RED = GRANULATION YELLOW = SLOUGH BLACK = ESCHAR **Examples:** *Wound base is 30% red, 70% yellow; or wound base is 90% black with 10% red border; or wound base is 20% red, 50% yellow and 30% black.*	

TABLE 22-3 Dressing Categories

DRESSING TYPE	TRADE NAMES*	WOUND TYPE	GENERAL INFORMATION	CAUTIONS/CONTRAINDICATIONS
Alginate Absorber	Algicel Kalginate Kaltostat Maxsorb	Wet	Needs secondary dressing Can be left in place 1–5 days based on manufacturer's instructions† Change when secondary dressing appears soiled Some alginates turn into a moist substance when saturated, and will not appear in the wound base when changing the dressing	Do not pack the rope form into blind cavities Irrigate the wound to ensure total dressing removal Do not use for 3rd-degree burns
Film Donator	Dermaview Tegaderm Opsite Polyskin	Dry Can be used to prevent friction on some bony prominences	Does not require secondary dressing Can be used to promote autolytic debridement in selected candidates Can be left in place up to 7 days based on manufacturer's instructions† Can be used as a secondary dressing	Caution with fragile skin, as removal can promote skin trauma Remove dressing by stretching it horizontally to break the adhesive, do not pull upwards, as this may cause stripping of skin layers Caution in use on lower extremities and foot in diabetics, or in patients with vascular compromise, as they are more prone to anaerobic proliferation
Foam Absorber	Biatain Polymem Optifoam Mepilex	Wet May also be used as a prevention dressing for high-risk bony prominences	May require a secondary dressing if there is not a waterproof backing on the foam Change every 3–7 days per manufacturer's instructions† Often promote more painless dressing changes due to coating on the foam to aid in nonsticking Change when saturated Can also be used as a protectant, such as on elbows or heels Can be used with other dressings as a secondary dressing	Essentially none
Gauze Neutral	Multiple manufacturers	Wet Dry	May be moistened with saline or hydrogel to donate moisture May be used alone to absorb Good to use for mechanical debridement May be used as a secondary dressing Change at least daily	Often promotes pain during dressing changes when used as a primary dressing Considered "cheap" but actually is more expensive due to frequency and intensity of dressing change
Hydrocolloid Moisture donor	Comfeel Duoderm Exuderm Flexicol	Dry Promotes autolytic debridement in some patients	No secondary dressing required May be left in place up to 7 days based on manufacturer's instructions† May be used as a secondary dressing Change if dressing begins to leak or become saturated	Do not apply to stable eschar on heels Caution in use on lower extremities and foot in diabetics, or in patients with vascular compromise, as they are more prone to anaerobic proliferation Do not use in infected wounds
Hydrogel Moisture donor	Amerigel Dermagran Skintegrity Solosite	Dry	Requires a secondary dressing Change every 1–3 days depending on the form of dressing, per manufacturer's instructions†	Monitor wound and wound environment for maceration
Antimicrobials Depends upon dressing form	Cadexomer-iodine (Iodosorb) Honey (Medihoney, Therahoney) Silver (Acticoat, Aquacel Ag+, SSD Cream) PHMB (Kendall AMD, Suprasorb X+ PHMB)	Used to treat infection/bioburden These compounds are available in ointments, creams, as well as the dressing types mentioned above and more. Utilize all per manufacturer's instructions† Apply these all as primary dressings for therapeutic effect Contraindications are allergies to the compounds, as well as any general cautions/contraindications listed		

*Trade names are not all inclusive or exhaustive, and no money was exchanged for inclusion of names in this table.

†Dressings should always be used per manufacturer's instructions, which may vary by dressing type and function.

WOUND CARE SPECIALISTS

Many communities now have facility based or stand-alone wound centers. These centers are often composed of nurses, physicians, physical therapists, dieticians, vascular specialists, surgeons, podiatrists, and infectious disease specialists. The most successful wound clinics utilize a multi- or transdisciplinary model of care to treat the wounded patient. Many of these providers have obtained more education, specific to wounds, and many of them choose to become certified in wound care. A wound care center can offer aggressive treatment in a setting that allows multiple services at once, which can be very convenient and therapeutic for the wounded patient.

READINGS

Baranoski, S., & Ayello, E. A. (2012). *Wound care essentials* (3rd ed.). Philadelphia, PA: Wolters Kluwer.

Bryant, R. A., & Nix, D. P. (2012). *Acute & chronic wounds: Current management concepts* (4th ed.). St. Louis, MO: Mosby.

Cioroiu, M., & Levine, M. (2013). Peripheral arterial disease: Giving appreciation to an often overlooked cause of poor wound healing. *Today's Wound Clinic, 7*(5), 16–18. doi:10.2337/dc12-2625.

Emory University. (2000). *Wound Ostomy Continence Education Program: Wound module.*

Fife, C. E., Carter, M. J., Walker, D., & Thomson, D. W. (2012). Wound care outcomes and associated cost among patients treated in US outpatient wound centers: Data from the US wound registry. *Wounds, 24*(1), 10–17.

Miller, D. R., Enoch, S., Williams, D. T., Price, P. E., & Harding, K. G. (2004). Value of wound biopsy in chronic venous ulceration. *Phlebology, 19,* 65–68. doi:10.1258/026835504323080326.

National Pressure Ulcer Advisory Panel (NPUAP). (2007). *Pressure ulcer stages/categories.* Retrieved from http://www.npuap.org/resources/educational-and-clinical-resources/npuap-pressure-ulcer-stagescategories/.

Posthauer, M. E. (2012). Nutrition strategies for wound healing. *Journal of Legal Nurse Consulting, 23*(1), 15–23.

Salcido, R., & Popescu, A. (2012). Pressure ulcers and wound care. *Medscape Reference.* Retrieved from http://emedicine.medscape.com/article/319284-overview.

Sen, C. K., Gordillon, G. M. Saswati, R., Kirsner, R., Lambert, L., Hunt, T. K., . . . & Longaker, M. T. (2009). Human skin wounds: A major and snowballing threat to public health and the economy. *Wound Repair and Regeneration, (17)*6, 763–771. doi:10.1111/j.1524-475X.2009.00543.x.

Sussman, C., & Bates-Jensen, B. (2012). *Wound care: A collaborative practice manual for health professionals.* Baltimore, MD: Lippincott Williams & Wilkins.

Wound, Ostomy and Continence Nurses Society (WOCN). (2008). *Guideline for management of wounds in patients with lower-extremity arterial disease.* Mount Laurel, NJ: WOCN. NGC:006521.

Wound, Ostomy and Continence Nurses Society (WOCN). (2010). *Guideline for prevention and management of pressure ulcers.* Mount Laurel, NJ: WOCN. NGC:007973.

Wound, Ostomy and Continence Nurses Society (WOCN). (2011). *Guideline for management of wounds in patients with lower-extremity venous disease.* Mount Laurel, NJ: WOCN. NGC:009276.

Wound, Ostomy and Continence Nurses Society (WOCN). (2012). *Guideline for management of wounds in patients with lower-extremity neuropathic disease.* Mount Laurel, NJ: WOCN. NGC:009275.

CHAPTER 23

Aging Skin: Diagnosis, Prevention, and Treatment

Diane Hanna

This chapter reviews key concepts that contribute to the aging process of the skin, steps to avoid future skin damage, basic treatment options for over the counter, and prescribed therapeutic options in the nondermatology setting.

BEAUTY AT A GLANCE

In the past decade, the aesthetic dermatology marketplace has undergone an explosive expansion. Despite recent and increasingly difficult economic times, the demand for cosmetic procedures to enhance, rejuvenate, or maintain beauty standards continues to grow. Since 2000, the Food and Drug Administration (FDA) has approved three neurotoxins and over twenty dermal filler devices, which are indicated for the treatment of soft tissue augmentation and temporary improvement of wrinkles associated with muscle movement and volume loss. The American Society of Plastic Surgeons (ASPS) reported that 1.1 billion dollars was spent on cosmetic procedures in 2012, which is a 5.5% increase from 2011, and office procedures performed by plastic surgeons grew by 10%. According to the ASPS, an estimated 14.6 million cosmetic procedures were performed in the United States in a medical office setting. Of the total estimated procedures, 1.6 million were defined as cosmetic surgical procedures, 13 million as cosmetic minimally invasive procedures (Table 23-1), and 5.6 million reconstructive procedures. Men and women, 40 to 54 years of age, are the largest demographic groups of the minimally invasive procedures, accounting for 48% of the cosmetic procedures. A 3% increase from 2011 was noted in minimally invasive procedures in females from the ages of 13 to 39. Females represent 91% of the paying consumers seeking cosmetic procedures, and males represent 9% of cosmetic procedures.

The accelerated growth of the overall beauty industry and the recent increase in the FDA approval of medical devices, dermal fillers, and neurotoxins have blurred the lines between traditional medical interventions, elective procedures, and beauty services. The brisk influx of products and services to the marketplace and the ever-increasing use of off-label indications of approved devices and therapies present a unique educational dilemma to establish competency for providers of aesthetic products and services.

The Dermatology Landscape

The specialty of dermatology has undergone a dramatic evolution over the past decade, including the introduction of aesthetic medicine. It is common for medical and surgical specialties, as well as individual providers, to claim expertise and ownership of lucrative cash-based aesthetic procedures and services. While there is no question that the demand for these services is present and the financial gains are obvious, it is imperative to have formal training, core competencies, and credentialing for providers to ensure safe and efficacious practice. Regardless of the clinician's educational pedigree, the lack of competency specific to aesthetic services equates to an increased risk for poor outcomes and decreased safety for patients.

The science and art of aesthetics goes beyond the knowledge and skills of procedures and requires that clinicians assess and discern patients who are at risk for, or are suffering from, a psychiatric disorder. Patients seeking multiple aesthetic procedures have the highest risk for depression, anxiety, mood disorders, personality disorders, and body dysmorphia (BDD).

BDD is characterized by preoccupation with perceived appearance defect(s), with excessive concern over any slight physical anomaly, as well as significant distress or impairment in functioning that is not accounted for by a diagnosis such as anorexia nervosa. Because these patients have unyielding negative perceptions about their appearance, they are at risk for poly-procedures from multiple providers. When the clinician does not perceive the same defect or severity as the patient, it is a hallmark warning for BDD. Patients' intrusive obsessions about their physical appearance can occupy an inordinate amount of their time and focus. The pervasive distortion can magnify poor self-image, esteem, avoidance, and interference with daily living. This can lead to extreme behaviors where they seek

TABLE 23-1	Cosmetic Minimally Invasive Procedures Performed in the United States	
PROCEDURE	**NO. OF PROCEDURES IN 2012**	**CHANGE FROM 2011 (%)**
Botulinum Toxin Type A	6.1 Million	8
Soft Tissue Filler	2 Million	5
Chemical Peel	1.1 Million	2
Laser Hair Removal	1.1 Million	4
Microdermabrasion	947,000	8

Adapted from American Society of Plastic Surgeons (2012).

multiple procedures from different specialists. It can also include suicidal ideation.

When assessing a patient at risk for BDD, remember that he or she will engage in camouflaging behaviors such as body position and use of hats, hair, makeup, glasses, etc. Patients will often be distracted during an examination to gaze at themselves in reflective surfaces such as spoons, mirrors, or windows. Other patients may avoid mirrors as their reflection is so disturbing to them. Other obsessive compulsive behaviors, including skin picking, excessive exercising, and changing clothes repeatedly throughout the day, may be reported.

Clinicians must establish safe and strong boundaries with patients who have BDD by limiting their procedures. Be aware that patients may seek drastic alternatives such as buying products from the black market in an attempt to self-treat (Figure 23-1). Hence, a safe and successful aesthetic practice begins with a careful assessment of the patient's motivation to enhance or modify their appearance long before the initiation of any procedure. Depression and anxiety screening tools can be incorporated into an assessment if there is any suspicion for BDD. A collaborative approach, including psychiatry and counseling, is recommended.

Clinicians practicing aesthetics should take note that despite high quality education, training, and good patient screening, aesthetic patients are known to be high risk for litigious actions. The result is increased premiums for professional malpractice insurance for clinicians providing cosmetic services.

FDA Intervention in Aesthetic Devices

In 2008, the device arm of the FDA convened a panel of dermatology experts to examine the increasing trends of adverse events (AEs) and serious adverse events (SAEs) reported as a result of soft tissue augmentation devices. Most of the AEs and SAEs reported were from off-label use of products (Dang, Francis, Durfor, Mirsaidi, & Shoaibi, 2008). The FDA advisory panel has recommended changes in the

clinical trials process of products and the AEs reporting system. It also acknowledged that dermatology, as a specialty, had been scrutinized when in reality these devices were being used by many non-dermatology physicians, nurse practitioners, physician assistants, and nurses. One of the panel's recommendations was that manufacturers restrict the sale of their products to dermatologists and plastic surgeons. Many manufacturers require that a clinician have a valid Drug Enforcement Agency number and a state medical license to purchase their products.

FDA Labeling

The reality of aesthetic services is that most procedures for soft tissue augmentation and neurotoxins are performed off label and lack the data or evidence required by the FDA to approve the product or device for both safety and efficacy. Although manufacturers may have clinical data that have been gathered and studied outside of the FDA approval processes, use of the product or device is still considered off label. It is both cost prohibitive and time sensitive for manufacturers to submit every indication to the FDA for approval. Accordingly, one must carefully weigh the risk versus benefits before deciding to perform procedures outside of FDA-labeled indications. This includes black-box warnings, contraindications, other warnings, and precautions. In the event of an adverse outcome, the assumption of legal risk is compounded.

ANATOMIC AND PHYSIOLOGIC IMPACTS ON THE AGING PROCESS

The skin ages in two distinct and biologically different processes. The *intrinsic* process refers to slow tissue degeneration that is uniquely influenced by an individual's genetics and the process of time. This natural concept accounts for the differences in how individuals age. It usually begins during our mid-20s and continues throughout the life span (Figure 23-2).

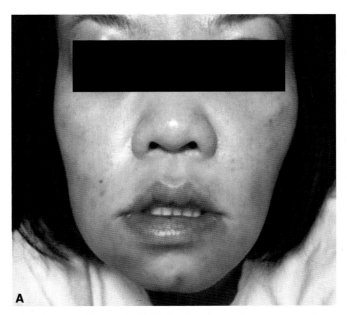
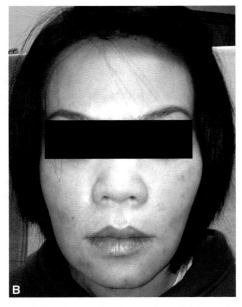

FIG. 23-1. This patient was diagnosed with BDD and under a written agreement for treatment with both her treating dermatology clinician and psychologist. **A:** She presented with complications after purchasing 1 mL of dermal filler from the internet black market and self-injecting. The patient had an acute foreign body reaction to the unknown substance. **B:** Four weeks later, the swelling and inflammation have subsided but resulted in residual post inflammatory hyperpigmentation.

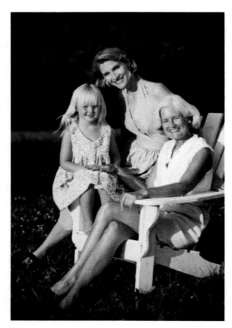

FIG. 23-2. Wrinkles, gray hair, and "age spots" result from changes to the integumentary system that occur with aging, as shown across three generations of a family. Genetics, time, and extrinsic factors are key elements that influence an individual's aging process. Although there is little ability to change the intrinsic factors, the impact of ultraviolet radiation on the skin can be reduced.

Intrinsic aging is characterized by several features (Table 23-2). Fibroblasts are the connective tissue cells that produce and secrete collagen (commonly referred to the scaffolding of our skin) and elastin fibers present in the dermis. Aging means changes in fibroblasts that result in the degeneration of elastin, which affects the skin's ability to "stretch and recoil," as well as maintains and repairs healthy cells. Decreased collagen synthesis and fragmentation cause dermal atrophy and loss of structure and elasticity. These changes are realized as wrinkles and textural changes in aging skin.

The loss of hydration also contributes to the process of aging skin. Hyaluronic acid, touted as a valuable ingredient in many commercially available moisturizers, is a large molecule in the dermis that has the ability to attract and hold water. It is described as being akin to a sponge that is able to hold over a thousand times its weight in water. Decreased levels of hyaluronic acid account for the changes in texture and elasticity and the wrinkles that come with age.

Extrinsic aging is a result of environmental factors and repeated exposures. The greatest influence on the degree of extrinsic aging is ultraviolet light radiation (UVR), which accounts for the classic appearance of "age spots" (Figure 23-3). Other external factors that prematurely age our skin include repetitive facial expressions (frowning, squinting, smiling, laughing); smoking; and pollution, gravity, and chemical exposures (Figure 23-4).

ULTRAVIOLET RADIATION

Understanding photobiology is essential to appreciating the role of UVR in photoaging, skin cancer, immunosuppression, and cataract formation. The sun emits energy over a wide range of spectrums. Unlike infrared radiation (visible light), UVR is neither seen by the naked eye nor felt. It has a shorter wavelength and possesses more energy than visible light. Other artificial sources of UVR exist and will be discussed.

There are three bands of UV radiation: UVA, UVB, and UVC. The stratospheric layer, or ozone, acts as a layer of protection from most of the sun's UV exposure. UVC is completely absorbed by the ozone layer, while UVB is partially filtered, and UVA is without any filtration (Figure 23-5). Exposure to all types of UVR can have both beneficial and adverse effects on human health (Figure 23-6). This has led to vigorous debate in the scientific community as to the amount of UVR that is considered healthy. The U.S. Department of Health and the World Health Organization have classified UVR emitted from both natural and artificial light (sun and tanning beds) as a human carcinogen. The American Academy of Dermatology and Dermatology Nurses' Association have taken a consistent stand on the harmful effects of tanning beds and are actively advocating for legislative limitations and regulations for the tanning industry.

Tanning is a form of self-defense against UVR. Depending on the individual's skin type, there is an increase in melanin in the skin when exposed to moderate levels of radiation. The function of melanin is to absorb UVR and disperse the energy, minimizing the damaging effects to the skin (Figure 23-7). Yet the common urban myth of getting a base tan to reduce the risk of sunburn before an intense exposure (i.e., vacation) is a fallacy. It is important to note that a tan from UVA, such as tanning beds, will provide a tan by oxidizing that which was already present in the skin and signals the release of additional melanin from surrounding melanocytes. The resulting tan from UVA is cosmetic in nature and does not protect the skin from UVB exposure and sunburn. Unfortunately, the myth of the prevacation tan safety gives individuals a false sense of protection, leading to extended periods of sun exposure and risk.

TABLE 23-2	Classification of Photoaging		
TYPE I MILD PHOTOAGING	**TYPE II MODERATE PHOTOAGING**	**TYPE III ADVANCED PHOTOAGING**	**TYPE IV SEVERE PHOTOAGING**
Mild pigmentary changes	Early solar lentigines	Obvious dyschromia and telangiectasias	Sallow (yellow-gray) color
No keratoses	Rare keratoses, mainly palpable	Visible keratoses	Keratoses and skin malignancies
Minimal or no wrinkles	Wrinkles seen only with facial expression	Wrinkles seen at rest	Wrinkles throughout, little normal skin
Patient age: 20s	Patient age: 30s or 40s	Patient age: 50s	Patient age: 60s or 70s
Minimal or no makeup	Usually wears some foundation	Always wears heavy foundation	Can't wear makeup - 'cakes and cracks'

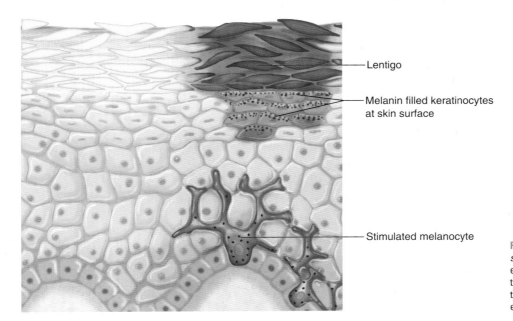

Lentigo

Melanin filled keratinocytes at skin surface

Stimulated melanocyte

FIG. 23-3. Solar lentigos, also known as *liver spots* or *age spots*, typically appear on sun-exposed areas. Although they are characterized as age-associated skin changes, they can develop at a younger age with excessive ultraviolet radiation exposure.

Pathophysiology of Photoaging

Photoaging occurs when UVR activates the elastin promoter, which leads to an acceleration of abnormal elastin biosynthesis and accumulation in the dermis. Repeated UVR exposure impairs the biosynthesis of new collagen and increases the expression of matrix metalloproteinase (MMP) enzymes that break down collagen. UVA and UVB exposure also causes a vitamin A (retinol) deficiency which accelerates the aging process of skin. Histologically, UV-exposed skin reveals thickened and irregularly-shaped collagen bundles in the dermis. The physical manifestations of this change are referred to as *solar* or *actinic* elastosis.

Photoaging occurs over decades. With repeated exposure to the sun, the skin looses the ability to repair itself, and the damage accumulates. The resulting volume loss, skin laxity, fragility, and thinning are evident by the presence of fine lines and wrinkles, thinning skin, loss of underlying fat pads, loss of skin tone, and dry skin (Figure 23-8).

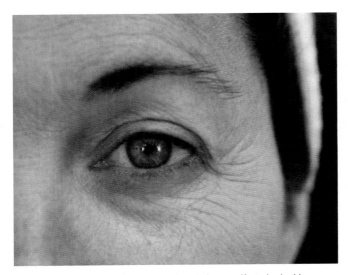

FIG. 23-4. Extrinsic aging from years of squinting manifests in rhytides, commonly called "crow's-feet," which are present at rest.

The patterns of photoaging are predictable, mostly on the sun-exposed areas of the hands, forearms, face, shoulders, chest, and upper back. Other clinical manifestations of photoaging are xerosis (rough and dry skin), mottled or spotty pigmentation, telangiectasias, static and dynamic lines, volume loss, follicular plugging, and the presence of benign or malignant neoplasms (Table 23-3). Altered elastin formation can cause the deposition of abnormal, yellow amorphous material that is incapable of forming functioning elastic fibers in the skin. The amount of photoaging that develops depends on a person's skin color and their history of long-term or intense exposure. Individuals with fair skin that have a history of UV radiation develop more signs of photoaging than those with darker skin coloring. In darker skin, the signs of photoaging are usually limited to fine wrinkles and a mottled complexion.

Sun protection

While halting or arresting chronological aging is not yet scientifically possible, photoaging can be diminished with UV avoidance and sun-protection habits. Currently, there is no accurate way to measure UVA radiation blockage clinically because UVA alone does not cause the presence of erythema in the skin, which is a key component of sun protection factor (SPF) measurements. Despite this, it is important that effective sunscreens are broad spectrum and block both UVA and UVB to reduce the risk of skin cancers and premature aging (discussed in chapters 2 and 8).

Vitamin D synthesis

It is well known that UVB is needed for the synthesis of vitamin D, which is important for our health. However, research has not established the amount of sun exposure necessary to maintain adequate vitamin D levels. Many experts recommend 5 to 30 minutes of sun exposure on unprotected skin twice a week for adequate levels. The risk of carcinogenesis must always be weighed against the benefits of even limited amounts of UVA and UVB exposure.

Other Damaging Effects from UVR

Ocular damage

The most common cause of blindness in the world is due to cataracts. Evidence supports that UVR, especially UVB, is a known risk factor for

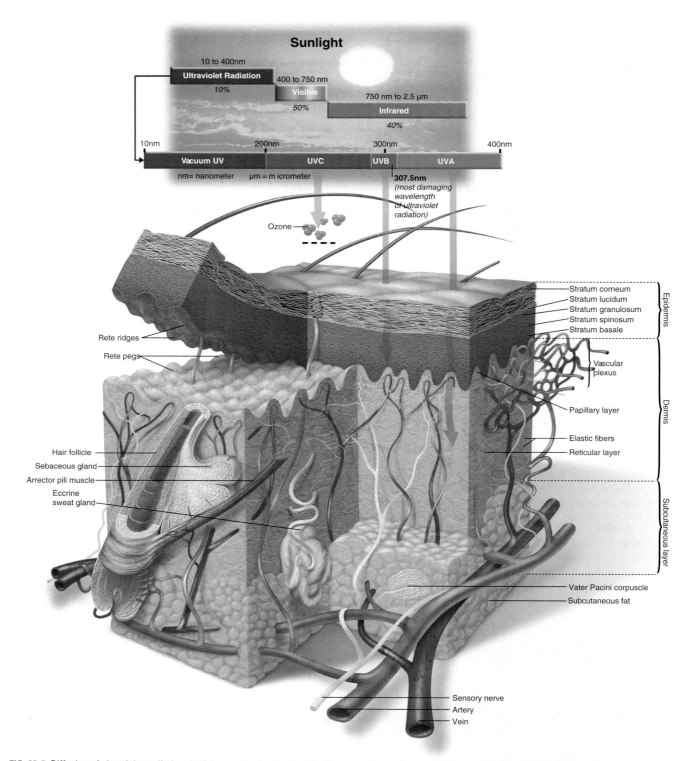

FIG. 23-5. Diffusion of ultraviolet radiation. UVC is completely absorbed by the ozone layer, whereas UVB is partially filtered, and UVA is without any filtration.

developing cataracts. UVR also contributes to formation of pterygiums, skin cancers near the eye, and macular degeneration. The skin on the eyelid is the thinnest skin and is also the most susceptible to the effects of extrinsic aging (Figure 23-9). Public awareness campaigns have been launched to increase awareness and reduce the risk of ocular exposure. Sunglasses or eyewear that provides 99% to 100% protection from UVA and UVB is recommended. Furthermore, lenses with UV 400 protection block UV wavelengths up to 400 nm—offering superior protection.

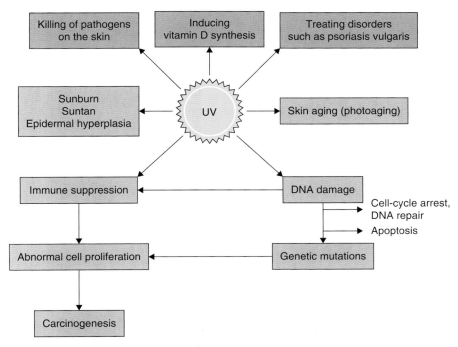

FIG. 23-6. Summary of the effects of ultraviolet radiation on skin.

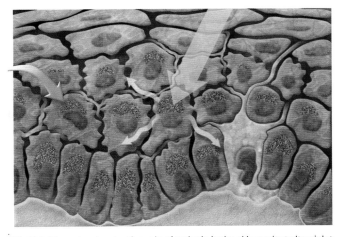

FIG. 23-7. The natural protective role of melanin in the skin against ultraviolet radiation.

Immunosuppression

UVR can have an immunosuppressive effect on skin, preventing the body from fighting infection and protecting itself from cancers. It is known to be mutagenic to basal cell keratinocytes. Conversely, the immunosuppressive properties of UVR can be used for the treatment of various skin diseases such as psoriasis, atopic dermatitis, and cutaneous T-cell lymphoma. In these settings, the risk benefit to the patient is always taken into consideration as part of the treatment plan.

Skin cancer

The most common cancer in the United States is skin cancer with one out of every five Americans developing it in their lifetime. UVR is the greatest risk factor for melanoma and basal cell and squamous cell carcinomas. Chapter 2 highlights photobiology and UVR

protection. Chapters 7 and 8 provide additional information about melanoma and nonmelanoma skin cancers.

THE AGING FACE

Understanding the intrinsic and extrinsic effects of aging on the skin is key to accurately understanding, diagnosing, and managing the aging skin.

Facial Assessment

When assessing the anatomy of the face, it is convenient and practical to divide the face into three distinct parts. The first is the upper third of the face, which consists of the forehead and brows; the second is the midface and nose; and the third is the lower portion consisting of the chin, jaw line, and neck (Figure 23-10). The most widely used terms used to describe the effects of the cumulative facial aging process are static and dynamic wrinkles and folds, volume loss, and facial hollowing.

Wrinkles

In addition to the processes described above, wrinkles can occur from repeated muscle movement over time, or anatomic variations, such as a functioning frontalis. Wrinkles are classified as *static wrinkles* (present without movement; Figure 23-11) or *dynamic wrinkles* (present with movement; Figure 23-12). Superficial and deep wrinkles that are present without facial muscle movement are generally an indicator of severe UV exposure, tobacco use, or secondhand tobacco exposure. In addition to static and dynamic wrinkles, volume loss or lipoatrophy is most notable in the central and lower face. Patients with advanced AIDS commonly have hollowing and loss of central facial fat. This is also seen in long-distance runners with very low levels of body fat (Figure 23-13).

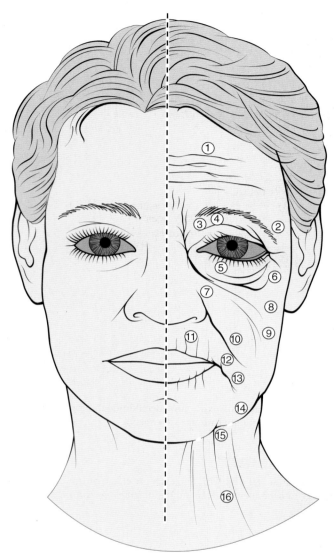

FIG. 23-8. Aging changes in the face. *(1)* forehead and glabella creases; *(2)* ptosis of the lateral brow; *(3)* redundant upper eyelid skin; *(4)* hollowing of the upper orbit; *(5)* lower eyelid laxity and wrinkles; *(6)* lower eyelid bags; *(7)* deepening of the nasojugal groove; *(8)* ptosis of the malar tissues; *(9)* generalized skin laxity; *(10)* deepening of nasolabial folds; *(11)* perioral wrinkles; *(12)* downturn of oral commissures; *(13)* deepening of labiomental crease; *(14)* jowls; *(15)* loss of neck definition and excess fat in neck; *(16)* platysmal bands.

Anatomical variations are individualized and occur on a spectrum. The functioning frontalis is a normal variant of facial anatomy and is illustrated by the presence of wrinkles in the youthful skin of children when they lift the eyebrows. As the aging process continues in adulthood, the functioning frontalis may sag and cause drooping of the eyelids and sagging forehead (Figure 23-14). Understanding the possibilities of anatomical variation is especially important when using neurotoxins and fillers. If the functioning frontalis is missed, it will result in the drooping and sagging of the forehead for several months.

Another aspect of facial aging is the loss of bone formation. This results in the slipping of natural fad pads, loss of the soft tissue. Therefore, understanding the natural landmarks and pitfalls of the anatomy is essential.

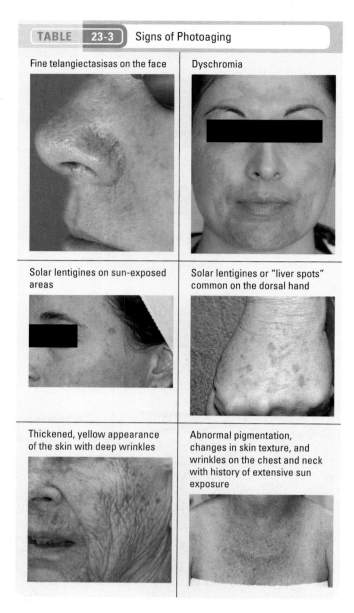

TABLE 23-3	Signs of Photoaging
Fine telangiectasisas on the face	Dyschromia
Solar lentigines on sun-exposed areas	Solar lentigines or "liver spots" common on the dorsal hand
Thickened, yellow appearance of the skin with deep wrinkles	Abnormal pigmentation, changes in skin texture, and wrinkles on the chest and neck with history of extensive sun exposure

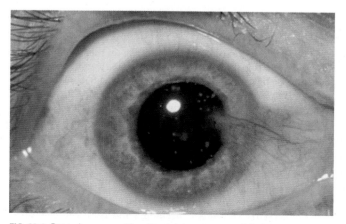

FIG. 23-9. Pterygium caused by ultraviolet exposure and drying.

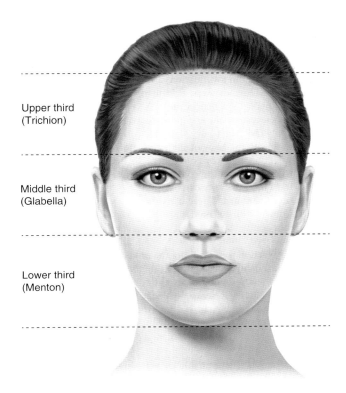

FIG. 23-10. Diagram of the "rule of thirds" facial assessment.

Upper third
(Trichion)

Middle third
(Glabella)

Lower third
(Menton)

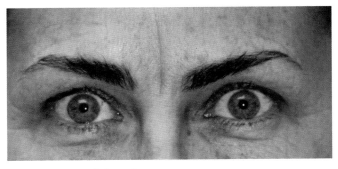

FIG. 23-11. Deep static frown line.

THERAPEUTIC INTERVENTIONS

There is a vast armamentarium of therapeutic interventions, prescriptive and over-the-counter products used to counteract the signs of aging skin. Consumers and providers can be easily confused by the aggressive direct advertising campaigns, home shopping networks, physician-dispensed lines, and illegal Internet distribution of fillers and neurotoxins. Cosmeceuticals, such as makeup, skin care lines, and beauty creams, do not have to gain FDA approval, and the claims surrounding these products can often be completely unsubstantiated.

A clear understanding of the patient's goals, along with the science of aging skin, is essential for selecting the appropriate therapeutic intervention, which will lead to the optimal outcome. It is not uncommon, however, for several modalities to be necessary to achieve the agreed-upon outcomes. Therefore, clinicians who are limited in their aesthetic services must carefully assess the patient's needs. A referral to a cosmetic specialist may be necessary to ensure patient safety and satisfaction.

Topical Retinoids

Retinoic acid

Topical retinoids are considered the gold standard for visibly improving the signs and symptoms of the aging skin. Topical retinoids such as Renova (tretinoin 0.2% and 0.5% emollient cream) have been evaluated for the safety and efficacy of reducing the appearance of fine wrinkles and mottled hyperpigmentation (skin discoloration) and to help improve the texture and appearance of the skin. They have not, however, demonstrated clinical efficacy in reducing the signs of chronic exposure such as the elimination of coarse or deep wrinkles, or the reversal of photodamage. Topical retinoids are most often indicated and used for the treatment of acne and have been commercially available for decades. The secondary benefit of reversing the signs of aging was noted later and then subsequently evaluated.

Clinical Pharmacology

Tretinoin is a metabolite of vitamin A and is available in various formulations and vehicles. The mechanism of action (MOA), as with many drugs, is not clearly understood. The evidence supports that tretinoin modifies abnormal follicular keratinization and modulates the proliferation and differentiation of the epidermal cells. The

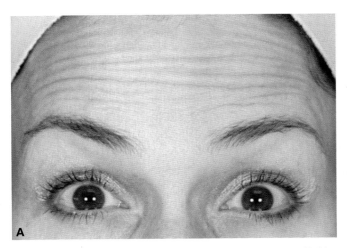

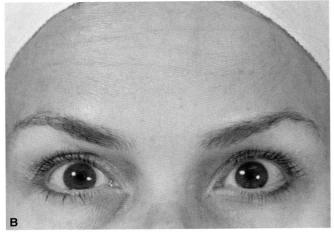

FIG. 23-12. **A:** Dynamic lines on the forehead with muscle movement. **B:** After treatment with botulinum toxin.

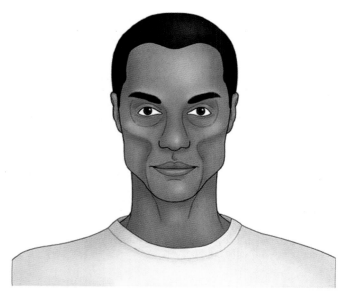

FIG. 23-13. Lipoatrophy.

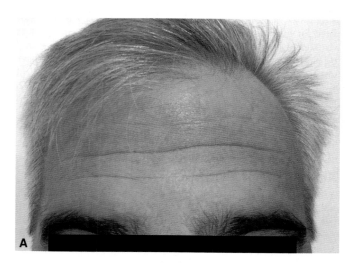

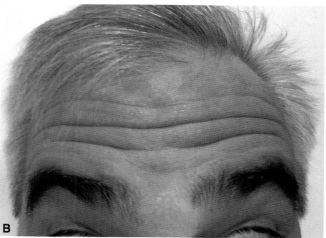

FIG. 23-14. **A:** Forehead at rest and the presence of static lines and the eyelids resting on eyelashes. **B:** There is a dramatic lift in the forehead and eyelid with manual lifting of eyebrows.

molecular weight of tretinoin is small and hence tretinoin is readily absorbed into the skin.

It is important to understand that with topical medicines, concentration does not equal potency. It is well documented that natural and synthetic tretinoin formulations are known to be irritating to the skin, causing redness, dryness, flaking, or peeling (*retinoid-induced dermatitis*). This is expected in the first several weeks of treatment and tends to lessen over time. If individuals are prone to sensitivity, it is best to apply the drug to dry skin. It is common practice to titrate the frequency with the hope of achieving more frequent use.

Sun protection is a key component with retinoid use. The removal of the top layer of the epidermis removes a protective barrier from UVR. Photosensitivity can occur with usage as well as risk for acceleration of sunburn. There is a dose response for both efficacy and AEs known with retinoid class. It is common to use the pea-sized amount analogy with patients. The general rule for application is that a pea-sized amount of most formulations will cover the entire face. Application is by dabbing the medication in the four zones of the face and gently spreading to the affected area, watching out for increased irritation potential in the corner of the eyes, nose, and mouth (Figure 23-15). Refer to the package insert for each formulation recommendations. Artificial tanning while using topical retinoids can result in blistering and burning.

Retinol

Retinol or vitamin A is available in over-the-counter preparations. Unlike tretinoin, retinols are milder and more gentle than tretinoin and therefore more widely accepted when used to improve the signs and symptoms of photoaging.

Azeleic acid

Prescription azelaic acid (FINACEA gel, 15%) is an FDA-approved topical medication indicated for the treatment of inflammatory

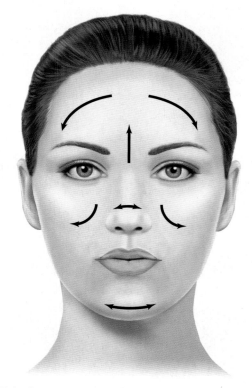

FIG. 23-15. Application of retinoid on the face.

papules and pustules of mild-to-moderate rosacea. Azelex cream 20%, which is no longer available in the United States, was indicated for the use of acne. The proposed MOA is twofold, normalization of keratinization (the process of cellular maturity and eventually shedding) and antimicrobial effect. While not covered by insurance for the use of photoaging, azelaic acid is used off label for mottled pigmentation and erythema. For patients with sensitive skin, the gel can be slightly drying or irritating, especially during the first few weeks of therapy. The side effects typically resolve as the skin becomes acclimated to the therapy.

Alpha-Hydroxy Acids

Alpha-hydroxy acids (AHAs) are a group of organic carboxylic compounds. Common ingredients found in AHA skin products are produced from nature and include glycolic acid (sugar cane), lactic acid (soured milk), malic acid (apples), citric acid (citrus fruits), and tartaric acid (wine grapes). Glycolic acid has a lower molecular weight, making it easier to penetrate the epidermis (compared to the others with higher molecular weights) and is therefore better known and utilized in applications.

AHAs are promoted as an agent that improves the appearance of photoaging. AHAs are used in chemical peels, creams, lotions, and washes and in combination with other antiaging ingredients. The FDA mandates that AHAs used in cosmeceutical products do not exceed 10%. Medical aestheticians can use higher concentrations generally limited to 30%. AHAs are available in physician-dispensed cosmetics lines, over-the-counter preparations, and therapeutic chemical peels. It is important to consider all other current topical therapies, and consider any potential drug-to-drug interactions or potential synergies. While AHAs' effects on the skin have been well documented, many over-the-counter preparations have unfounded claims of exaggerated performance.

AHAs are generally considered safe when used in the recommended dosage. Much like tretinoins, the most common side effects are erythema, flaking, and skin irritation. The range of side affects generally correlates with the pH and concentration of the acid used. The misuse of AHAs and glycolic acid peels can have severe and potentially permanent side effects such as blistering, scarring, and dyschromia. They may also increase photosensitivity and the acceleration of sun burns. A newer hypothesis proposes that the consistent removal of the stratum corneum may accelerate the aging process and photodamage by removing the protective layer of the epidermis.

Chemical Peels

Much like AHAs, chemical peels have the potential to affect all three layers of the skin, depending on the concentration and contact time with the skin. Skin type plays a role in predicting adverse events that could result from an aggressive chemical peel. Most chemical peels that produce destruction of the mid dermal layer, considered a deep peel, should be done with careful consideration and monitoring. Chemical peels and AHAs are not generally covered by insurance as they are cosmetic in nature.

Aesthetic Services

Microdermabrasion

Microdermabrasion is a service that is offered in the medical setting. It is a procedure that uses a mechanical method for light exfoliation of the skin. The units have two parts: the exfoliating crystals or diamond flakes and suction attachment to gently lift the skin during the procedure. Microdermabrasion is considered a noninvasive procedure and should be administered by a licensed professional; however, the units are found in medical spas and salons (Figure 23-16).

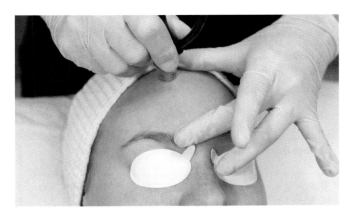

FIG. 23-16. Microdermabrasion performed for light exfoliation of the skin.

Dermabrasion

Dermabrasion is not to be confused with microdermabrasion, and is generally performed in a medically controlled setting most commonly by a dermatologist or a plastic surgeon. The procedure involves controlled removal of the upper to mid layers of the dermis by an abrasive device. Due to the depth of abrasion, the risk for AEs and complications is greater than microdermabrasion. Licensed and specialized training is required in order to provide safe and effective outcomes.

Laser resurfacing

Resurfacing procedures have common characteristics; the results of resurfacing occur very quickly. Side effects and AEs range from mild to severe, and risk of complications such as dyschromia and scarring are real. In order to prevent the ongoing effects of aging, topical treatments are needed postprocedure, which can be very expensive.

Laser resurfacing and ablation to treat signs of photoaging is gaining notoriety and popularity. The level of resurfacing can be superficial, medium, and deep dermis. The amount of destruction is controlled by the depth of light penetration and the number of passes over the given area. Intentional destruction of the epidermis and dermal layers is thought to stimulate collagen reformation, growth, and repair. Depending on the chosen procedure, the risks can include infections, scarring, hyperpigmentation, and hypopigmentation. Clinicians should be expertly trained to select the correct intervention and manage any possible untoward side effects.

Intense pulse light

Intense pulse lights (IPLs) are light sources that are used to treat dyschromia, unwanted hair, and many vascular lesions. They are promoted as having photorejuvenation properties and can be used safely and effectively. They are generally nonablative in nature and have a controlled energy delivery system into the tissue. IPL procedures are generally performed in the medical setting by a licensed personnel or medical aesthetician.

SOFT TISSUE AUGMENTION

Soft tissue augmentation is a valued procedure that allows patients to have an immediate softening or correction of the signs and symptoms of aging. It is performed using a variety of medical filler substances. Clinicians providing these aesthetic services should understand the pharmacodynamics of each product, approved FDA indications, and any contraindications or warnings. Table 23-4 lists

TABLE 23-4 FDA-Approved Soft Tissue Augmentation Devices

BRANDED NAME	MATERIAL	MANUFACTURER	APPROVAL DATE	INDICATION
Juvederm Volumna XC	Hyaluronic acid with lidocaine	Allergan	10/22/2013	Indicated for deep (subcutaneous and/or supraperiosteal) injection for cheek augmentation to correct age-related volume deficit in the midface in adults over the age of 21 years
Restylane-L injectable gel	Hyaluronic acid with lidocaine	Medicis Aesthetics Holdings, Inc.	8/30/2012	Injection into the mid-to-deep dermis for correction of moderate-to-severe facial wrinkles/folds (such as nasolabial folds) and for lip augmentation in those over the age of 21 years
Belotero Balance	Hyaluronic acid	Merz Pharmaceuticals	11/14/2011	Injection into facial tissue to smooth wrinkles and folds, especially around the nose and mouth (nasolabial folds).
Restylane injectable gel	Hyaluronic acid	Medicis Aesthetics Holdings, Inc.	10/11/2011	Lip augmentation in those over the age of 21 years
Sculptra Aesthetic	Poly-l-lactic acid (PLLA)	Sanofi Aventis U.S.	7/28/2009	Use in shallow-to-deep nasolabial fold contour deficiencies and other facial wrinkles
Radiesse 1.3cc and 0.3cc	Hydroxyapatite	Bioform Medical, Inc.	12/22/2006	Restoration and/or correction of the signs of facial fat loss (lipoatrophy) in people with HIV
Radiesse 1.3cc and 0.3cc	Hydroxyapatite	Bioform Medical, Inc.	12/22/2006	Subdermal implantation for correction of moderate-to-severe facial wrinkles and folds (such as nasolabial folds)
Elevess	Hyaluronic acid with lidocaine	Anika Therapeutics	12/20/2006	Use in mid-to-deep dermis for correction of moderate-to-severe facial wrinkles and folds (such as nasolabial folds)
Artefill	Polymethylmethacrylate beads, collagen and lidocaine	Suneva Medical, Inc.	10/27/2006	Use in facial tissue around the mouth (i.e., nasolabial folds)
Juvederm 24 HC, Juvederm 3	Hyaluronic acid	Allergan	6/2/2006	Use in mid-to-deep dermis for correction of moderate-to-severe facial wrinkles and folds (such as nasolabial folds)
Restylane injectable gel	Hyaluronic acid	Medicis Aesthetics Holdings, Inc.	3/25/2005	Injection into the mid-to-deep dermis for correction of moderate-to-severe facial wrinkles and folds (such as nasolabial folds)
Sculptra	Poly-l-lactic acid (PLLA)	Sanofi Aventis U.S.	8/3/2004	Restoration and/or correction of the signs of facial fat loss (facial lipoatrophy) in people with HIV
Hylaform (hylan B gel)	Modified hyaluronic acid derived from a bird (avian) source	Genzyme Biosurgery	4/22/2004	Injection into the mid-to-deep dermis for correction of moderate-to-severe facial wrinkles and folds (such as nasolabial folds)
Restylane injectable gel	Hyaluronic acid	Q-med Ab	12/12/2003	Injection into the mid-to-deep dermis for correction of moderate-to-severe facial wrinkles and folds (such as nasolabial folds)
No Longer Commercially Available in the United States				
Evolence collagen filler	Collagen	Colbar Lifescience ltd.	6/27/2008	The correction of moderate-to-deep facial wrinkles and folds (such as nasolabial folds)
Prevelle Silk	Hyaluronic acid with lidocaine	Genzyme Biosurgery	2/26/2008	Injection into the mid-to-deep dermis for correction of moderate-to-severe facial wrinkles and folds (such as nasolabial folds)
Captique injectable gel	Hyaluronic acid	Genzyme Biosurgery	11/12/2004	Injection into the mid-to-deep dermis for correction of moderate-to-severe facial wrinkles and folds (such as nasolabial folds)
Cosmoderm 1 Human-Based C	Collagen	Inamed Corp	3/11/2003	Injection into the superficial papillary dermis for correction of soft tissue contour deficiencies, such as wrinkles and acne scars
Fibrel	Collagen	Serono Laboratories	2/26/1988	The correction of depressed cutaneous scars which are distendable by manual stretching of the scar borders
Zyplast	Collagen	Collagen Corp	6/24/1985	Use in mid-to-deep dermal tissues for correction of contour deficiencies
Zyderm collagen implant	Collagen	Allergan	9/18/1981	Use in the dermis for correction of contour deficiencies

HIV, human immunodeficiency virus.

all soft tissue augmentation devices that have been approved by the FDA. The first device gained FDA approval in 1981; however, there are no longer any collagen-based fillers that are commercially available. While the list looks extensive, it is important to recognize that Canada and Europe have more than 150 fillers approved for use. An extensive black market exists, and in order to ensure that counterfeit products do not infiltrate the United States distribution channels, manufactures have developed extensive security measures and holograms for their products.

It is currently illegal in the United States for providers to access dermal fillers or neurotoxins outside of the FDA-approved distribution channels. The FDA stamp of approval on manufacturering plants ensures that the ingredients and processes are standardized, and the safety and efficacy requirements are met. Outside the United States, the same standards are not taken, even within the same global organization. When obtaining a patient history, again it is key to ask if they have received any treatments or tissue augmentation outside of the United States. Several case reports of severe allergic or foreign body reactions have been published in patients that have previously received fillers from outside of the United States and then had additional procedures with FDA-approved products.

The devices that are currently FDA approved and commercially available include hylarouinc acid-based fillers, calcium hydroxyapatite polymethylmethacrylate (PMMA) microspheres, and polylactic acid (PLLA). PMMA and PLLA are considered semipermanent or permanent fillers and have higher reported AEs, and are restricted to dermatologists and plastic surgeons. The following are the FDA product information and use recommendations regarding approved dermal fillers.

Most injectable wrinkle fillers have a temporary effect, because over time they are absorbed by the body. The FDA has only approved one product made from a material that remains in the body and is not absorbed. Some wrinkle fillers contain lidocaine, which is intended to decrease pain or discomfort related to the injection. The FDA (FDA Medical Devices) identifies materials used as injectable wrinkle fillers as either absorbable (temporary) or nonabsorbable (permanent), as listed in Box 23-1.

Avoiding Adverse Events

Necrosis (Figures 23-17 to 23-20) is one of the SAEs. It can result from injection of the dermal filler into the vascular system, compression of an artery or vein from the swelling, or manual deposition of dermal fillers. Far too often, when a serious adverse event occurs, it is a frightening time for both provider and patient. The perceived shame of a patient error can cloud the judgment of the provider and set the patient up for the risk of partial or incorrect treatment of the tissue death. Vascular occlusion can occur during the procedure and is noted by immediate blanching of the skin. Early intervention is a priority. If necrosis does occur, time is of the essence and collaboration with a vascular specialist, plastic surgeon, or competent aesthetic provider is key.

Patient Education and Follow-up

Patient education and discussion of treatment goals are very important prior to any procedure. It is important to document the counseling that identifies appropriate expectations for both the patient and provider, preprocedure workup, a copy of informed consent and photography consent, documentation of the procedure and postprocedure instructions, and plan for follow-up care. Informed consent varies from practice to practice; however, the FDA (2012) recommends that patients be made fully aware of both the risks and known adverse effects listed in Box 23-1.

NEUROTOXINS

Botulinum toxin (BTX) is a protein and known neurotoxin produced by the bacterium *Clostridium botulinum*. The estimated median human lethal dose is in the range of 1.3 to 2.1 ng per kg when administered intravenously or intramuscularly. BTX from uncontrolled sources can cause botulism, a serious and life-threatening illness in humans and animals. Three forms of botulinum toxin type A (BTX-A) are FDA approved with cosmetic indications in the United States. They are known by their brand names as Botox, Dysport, and Xeomin. One form of botulinum toxin type B (BTX-B), Myobloc, is available commercially for various cosmetic and medical procedures in the United States.

The cosmetic applications of BTX-A were observed in the late 1990s by Dr. Caruthers in Canada. While treating patients for the approved indication for blepharospasms, Dr. Caruthers noted that the crow's-feet or lines, associated with the repeated movement of the orbicularis oculi, were diminished. This spurred research and development to examine the safety and efficacy BTX-A for use on glabellar lines commonly known as "elevens". BTX- A was approved by the FDA in 2002 for the temporary treatment of moderate-to-severe dynamic glabellar lines in adults. Prior to that, BTX-A had been approved in the United States for the treatment of strabismus (1989), blepharospasm (1989), and in patients over 12 years (1989), upper motor neuron syndrome (2000), and cervical dystonia (2000). Approval for the temporary treatment of primal axillary hyperhidrosis (2004) and migraine headaches (2010) came later. New and novel uses are constantly evolving in aesthetic medicine as well as general medicine. It is important to know that the clinical trials were in the glabellar muscles, with the appropriate dosing that is noted in each of the package inserts.

While the safety of BTX-A has been well established across indications, the greatest risk for AEs falls on the hands of the provider. Because the MOA is the temporary induction of paralysis, a solid command of head and neck anatomy is required. Once the neurotoxin is injected, there is currently no way to reverse the effects outside of the passage of time. As previously discussed, the majority of BTX-A usage is off label. Incorrect placement can lead to unwanted drooping, muscle laxity, and sagging. In the treatment of neck lines, the risk of laryngeal paralysis as well as decreased ability to suck on a straw or form certain sounds is real.

The recommended dosing for BTX-A is based on the inclusion criteria for each approved toxin. As a general rule, men with stronger muscle mass, and adults with severe lines, will require a stronger dosage to achieve the temporary arrest of wrinkles associated with movement. There are basic and advanced procedures that are utilized. Soft tissue replaces volume associated with the aging process, and neurotoxins diminish the appearance of fine lines and wrinkles associated with repeated muscle movement. It is common to use both dermal fillers and neurotoxins at the same time, in order to enhance the outcome. The effects of the treatment can last between 3 and 6 months depending on the reconstitution and dosage per patient.

In summary, there is a large available armamentarium for the improvement of the signs and symptoms of aging, both over the counter and approved by the FDA. Prevention is still the strongest defense against the unwanted effects of photoaging. The pipe-line for devices and neurotoxins is rich and will continue to expand in order to meet the marketplace demand. To effectively provide an excellent level of care, it is imperative to understand all the options that are available, their indications and usage, and most importantly, the prevention and management of AEs.

BOX 23-1 **U.S. Food and Drug Administration Description of Injectable Wrinkle Fillers**

Absorbable Materials (temporary)

Collagen is a type of protein that is a major part of skin and other tissues in the body. Sources of purified collagen used in wrinkle fillers can be from cow (bovine) or human cells. The effects of collagen fillers generally lasts for 3 to 4 months. They are the shortest lasting of injectable filler material. Bovine collagen had a high incident for allergic reaction, and skin testing a month prior to injection was required. The short duration of bovine collagen and the added burden of skin testing provided significant hurdles for the product to overcome. Porcine collagen did not require skin testing and had a longer duration, extending for a year, prior to its withdrawal from the market.

Hyaluronic acid is a type of sugar (polysaccharide) that is present in body tissues, such as in skin and cartilage. It is able to combine with water and swell when in gel form, causing a wrinkle smoothing effect. Sources of hyaluronic acid used in wrinkle fillers can be from bacteria or rooster combs (avian). In some cases, hyaluronic acid used in wrinkle fillers is chemically modified (crosslinked) to make it last longer in the body. The effects of this material last approximately 6 to 12 months depending on the different manufacturers. No skin testing is needed prior to injecting.

Calcium hydroxyapatite is a type of mineral that is commonly found in human teeth and bones. For wrinkle filling, calcium hydroxyapatite particles are suspended in a gel-like solution and then injected into the wrinkle. The effects of this material last approximately 18 months. No skin testing is needed prior to injection.

Poly-L-lactic acid (PLLA) is a biodegradable, biocompatible man-made polymer. This material has wide uses in absorbable stitches and bone screws. PLLA is a long-lasting filler material that is given in a series of injections over a period of several months. The effects of PLLA generally become increasingly apparent over time (over a period of several weeks), and its effects may last up to 2 years.

Nonabsorbable Materials (permanent)

Polymethylmethacrylate beads (PMMA microspheres) are a non-biodegradable, biocompatible, man-made polymer. This material is used in other medical devices, such as bone cement and intraocular lenses. PMMA beads are tiny, round, smooth particles that are not absorbed by the body. For wrinkle filling, PMMA beads are suspended in a gel-like solution that contains cow (bovine) collagen and injected into the wrinkle.

Indications

The absorbable (temporary) injectable wrinkle fillers are FDA approved for the correction of moderate-to-severe facial wrinkles and skin folds, such as nasolabial folds. Nasolabial folds are the wrinkles on the sides of your mouth that extend toward the nose.

While these products are often used off label in other areas of the face, nonabsorbable (permanent) injectable wrinkle filler is FDA approved *only* for the correction of nasolabial folds. There are some injectable wrinkle fillers approved for the restoration and/or correction of the signs of facial fat loss (lipoatrophy) in people with human immunodeficiency virus (HIV). The FDA has approved two absorbable injectable wrinkle fillers for lip augmentation in patients over the age of 21.

Patients may need more than one injection to get the desirable wrinkle smoothing effect. Successful results will depend on the health of the skin, the skill of the injector, and the type of filler used. The time that the smoothing effect lasts depends on the filler material used.

Injection Techniques

There are many widely used and accepted injection techniques for soft tissue augmentation. The most common are serial function, linear threading, cross-hatching, and bolus deposition. Ultimately, preference and technique is unique to each injector and are an expert skill developed over time.

Risks and Side Effects

As in any medical procedure, there are risks involved with the use of injectable wrinkle fillers. It is imperative that clinicians understand their limits and possible risks. Most side effects associated with wrinkle fillers happen shortly after injection and most go away after several days. In other cases, side effects may appear weeks, months, or years after injection, and be a permanent or long-term. Common side effects include bruising, redness, swelling, pain, tenderness, itching, and rash. Less common side effects may be nodules or granulomas, infection, open or draining wounds, allergic reaction, and necrosis. Allergy testing is required for particular types of filler materials, such as those taken from cows (bovine). Severe allergic reaction (anaphylactic shock) that requires immediate emergency medical assistance can occur.

The following side effects have also been reported to the FDA:

- Migration/movement of filler material from the site of injection
- Leakage or rupture of the filler material at the injection site or through the skin (which may result from tissue reaction or infection)
- Blurred vision and flu-like symptoms

If you choose to have these fillers removed through surgery, you may experience the same risks typically associated with surgery. You should be aware that it may be difficult to remove the filler material. Wrinkle fillers should not be injected into blood vessels, because they may obstruct blood flow.

Off-label Uses

The FDA has approved injectable wrinkle fillers for treatment of moderate-to-severe wrinkles and localized fat loss (lipoatrophy) in the face. The FDA has approved two absorbable injectable wrinkle fillers for lip augmentation in patients over the age 21.

The FDA has *not* approved injectable wrinkle fillers to augment (increase volume of) or alter the shape of facial features; increase breast size (breast augmentation); increase size of the buttocks; rejuvenate the hands or feet; or implant into bone, tendon, ligament, or muscle. The FDA has *not* approved liquid silicone or silicone gel for injection to fill wrinkles or augment tissues anywhere in the body.

Additionally, patients should be aware that:

- FDA approval for these devices is based on controlled, clinical study of these products when used in the face, most commonly the nasal labial folds or, more recently, the midface.
- The safe use of these products (filler devices) with Botox or other wrinkle therapies has not been evaluated in a controlled, clinical study. This means that there is no safety and efficacy data for multiple procedures or products approved by the FDA.
- The safe use of these products repeatedly over a long period of time has not been evaluated in a controlled, clinical study. This standard language means that long-term data at the time of the approval have not been captured after the approval date. However, data are continually gathered via FDA MedWatch by both industry and self-report via injectors. After published FDA approval, data are continually assessed as well as an ongoing commitment to safety monitoring.
- Health insurance does not typically cover elective surgical procedures such as wrinkle correction.
- The safety of these products is unknown when used during pregnancy, while breastfeeding or in patients under 18 years. This means that the FDA did not study the safety or efficacy of these devices in adults under 18 or any pregnant females during their trials.

Modified from U.S. Food and Drug Administration. (2012). *Wrinkle fillers*. http://www.fda.gov/medicaldevices/productsandmedicalprocedures/cosmeticdevices/wrinklefillers/default.htm.

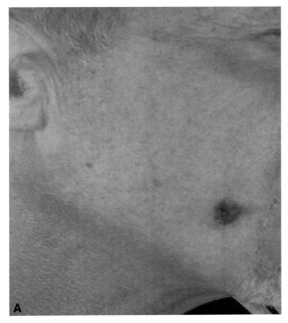

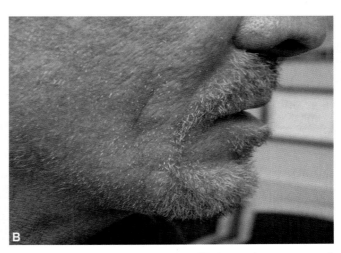

FIG. 23-17. **A:** Necrosis on day 2 postinjection of a dermal filler. Patient called reporting that the "bruise is not healing." **B:** Two weeks posttreatment for tissue necrosis with complete healing.

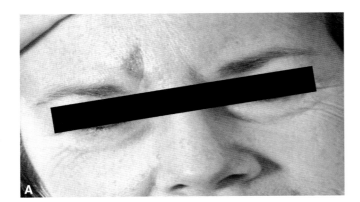

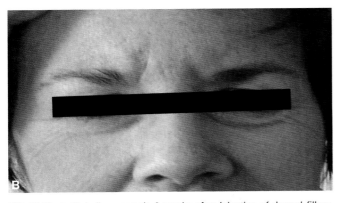

FIG. 23-18. **A:** Glabellar necrosis 2 weeks after injection of dermal fillers. **B:** Two more weeks later, there was significant improvement.

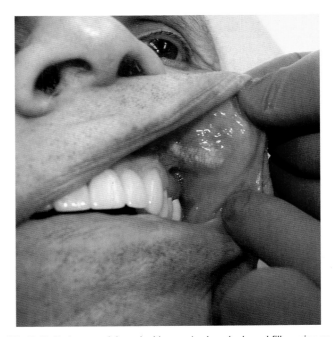

FIG. 23-19. Patient was injected with a nonhyaluronic dermal filler using an unapproved technique and location (through the buccal mucosa for cheek augmentation). A bolus of product was misplaced and resulted in referral for surgical excision.

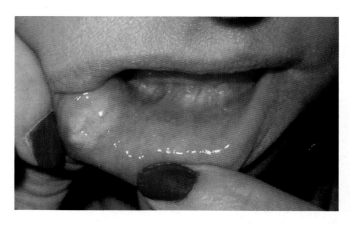

FIG. 23-20. Patient was injected with a collagen-based product, which resulted in a large deposit of filler in the oral mucosa.

READINGS

American Board of Dermatology, Inc. (n.d.). *Subspecialty certification*. http://www.abderm.org/subspecialties/qualification.html.

American Society of Plastic Surgeons. (2012). *2012 Plastic surgery procedural statistics*. http://www.plasticsurgery.org/news/plastic-surgery-statistics/2012-plastic-surgery-statistics.html

APRN Consensus Work Group & the National Council of State Boards of Nursing APRN Advisory Committee. (2008, July 7). *Consensus model for APRN regulation: Licensure, accreditation, certification and education*. www.ana.org.

Cheng, C. E., Kimball, A. B., & VanCott, A. (2010). A survey of dermatology nurse practitioners: Work setting, training, and job satisfaction. *Journal of the Dermatology Nurses' Association*, 2(1), 19–23.

Dang, J. M., Francis, J., Durfor, C. N., Mirsaidi, N., & Shoaibi, A. (2008). Executive summary dermal filler devices. *Food and Drug Administration Center for Devices and Radiological Health, Office of Device Evaluation, General and Plastic Surgery Devices Panel Public Advisory Committee Meeting*. 2–41.

Dermatology Nurses Association. (2011). *About DNA: Membership*. http://www.dnanurse.org/about/about-dna.

From Novice to Expert. (2012). *Nursing theories: A companion to nursing theories and models*. http://currentnursing.com/nursing_theory

Food and Drug Administration USA Medical Devices. (2014). *Wrinkle fillers*. http://www.fda.gov/MedicalDevices/ProductsandMedicalProcedures/CosmeticDevices/WrinkleFillers/default.htm

Kimball, A. B., & Resneck, J. S. (2008). The US dermatology workforce: A specialty remains in shortage. *Journal of the American Academy of Dermatology*, 59, 741–745.

Resneck, J. S., Lipton, S., & Pletcher, M. J. (2007). Short wait times for patients seeking cosmetic botulinum toxin appointments with dermatologist. *Journal of the American Academy of Dermatology*, 57(6), 985–989.

Resneck, J. S. & Kimball, A. B. (2004). The dermatology workforce shortage. *Journal of the American Academy of Dermatology*, 50(1), 50–54.

Resneck, J. S., & Kimball, A. B. (2008). Who else is providing care in dermatology practices? Trends in the use of nonphysician clinicians. *Journal of the American Academy of Dermatology*, 58(2), 211–216.

Wesley, N. O., & Dover, J. S. (2009). The filler revolution: A six-year retrospective. *Journal of Drugs in Dermatology*, 8(10), 903–907.

The following discussion presents some of the common dermatologic procedures performed in the office setting by advanced practice clinicians. Content is provided to serve as a guideline that is incorporated into the clinical judgment. Performing these, or any, procedural skills requires the development of competency to optimize patient safety and outcomes. Therefore, it is recommended that clinicians should:

- Acquire essential knowledge of the procedure, indications, and complications. However, knowledge alone does not confer competency.
- Obtain basic instruction for the skill, including observation.
- Demonstrate the skill under the supervision of a trainer or experienced clinician until it can be performed in its entirety without any mistakes or concerns. This should be done in a variety of settings that simulate real patient care.
- Perform continuous self-assessment, with patient and peer feedback and educational updates.
- Document competency of skills, which is both valuable and required in some health care settings or by regulatory boards.

PUNCH BIOPSY
Author:
Theodore D. Scott, RN, MSN, FNP-C, DCNP

Description
Punch biopsy is a nonsterile procedure by which sampling of an endophytic skin lesion or full thickness of skin is performed for the purpose of histopathologic examination.

Indications
- Small pigmented lesions of the skin (nevi or small melanomas)
- Benign skin tumors (i.e., dermatofibroma, neurofibroma)
- Vascular disease of the skin or subcutaneous fat
- Superficial inflammatory or granulomatous diseases
- Papulosquamous disease (i.e., psoriasis)
- Connective tissue disorders (i.e., systemic lupus erythematosus, discoid lupus erythematosus)

Contraindications
- Infection at the biopsy site
- Superficial artery or nerve (i.e., Erb's point) at biopsy site
- Pigmented lesion larger than available punches

Equipment
- Alcohol or chlorhexidine prep pads
- Examination gloves and sterile gloves
- Syringe, usually 3 mL or 5 mL
- 25G to 31G needle depending on site; 31G insulin syringes are helpful for noses and ears.
- Lidocaine 1% or 2%, with or without epinephrine, depending on site
- Sterile 4 × 4 or 2 × 2 gauge sponges
- Baker-type biopsy punch or equivalent, commercially available in sizes 2 to 12 mm
- Pickup forceps
- Iris scissors or scalpel
- Needle drivers
- Monofilament nonabsorbable suture appropriate for the thickness of skin; 4-0 black nylon on a P-12 needle is useful for most punches.
- Absorbable suture for larger punches (8 to 12 mm)
- Formalin in normal saline specimen containers of appropriate size for the specimen prelabeled with the patient's name and medical record number—never label after the fact. A biopsy for direct immunofluorescence should be placed in a container with Michel's transport medium.
- Hyfrecator for control of bleeding
- Petrolatum-based ointment (like Vaseline or Aquaphor)
- Adhesive dressing of appropriate size (check for allergy)

Preparation
- Procedure details, risks, and alternatives are discussed with the patient. All questions are answered and informed consent is given by the patient.
- All specimen containers to be used and histology requisitions are labeled and information is verified by patient.
- After gloving, the area to be sampled is cleaned with alcohol or chlorhexidine.
- Lidocaine is injected intradermally below the lesion to be sampled; if done correctly, the lesion will be raised on a wheal (Figure 24-1).

Procedure
- Sterile gloves are preferred for closure with sutures.
- With the nondominant hand, stretch the skin perpendicular to the relaxed skin lines. This will result in an elliptical defect when the tension is released making for a much more cosmetically acceptable closure.
- With the dominant hand, place the biopsy punch over the lesion and gently apply downward pressure while twisting the punch until you *feel* a slight pop and the punch goes through the dermis (Figure 24-2A and B).
- Retract the punch from the defect. *Gently* lift the freed skin specimen with the pickups and cut or snip the bottom attachment with the subcutaneous fat (Figure 24-2C).
- Place the specimen into a container and seal.

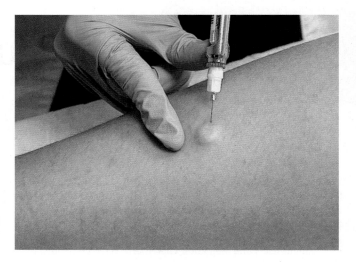

FIG. 24-1. Intradermal injection of local anesthetic using a 30G needle that produces a wheal under the lesion for biopsy. Localized blanching will occur when lidocaine with epinephrine is used as anesthetic.

- Blot biopsy site with gauze square and apply direct pressure to the site. Electrocautery with a hyfrecator may be used with caution. Proceed when hemostasis is complete.
- Suture the defect closed with interrupted sutures; larger defects may also require an absorbable deep cuticular suture to prevent a dead space at the wound base (Figure 24-3).
- Apply petrolatum ointment to wound after hemostasis is achieved.
- Apply adhesive dressing.
- Give patient both verbal and printed aftercare instructions in their preferred language.

Anticipated Outcomes

- Mild pain at biopsy site
- Possible infection
- Possible bleeding
- Possible separation of the wound edges of punch biopsy
- Scar at the biopsy site. Be sure to emphasize this point when you obtain informed consent.

Aftercare

- Initial bandage may be left in place for 24 hours unless saturated with blood.
- After 24 hours, bathe as normal and wash the biopsy site with gentle soap and water only.
- After drying, apply petrolatum ointment to the suture line and bandage.
- Stay out of oceans, lakes, and swimming pools until after the sutures are removed.

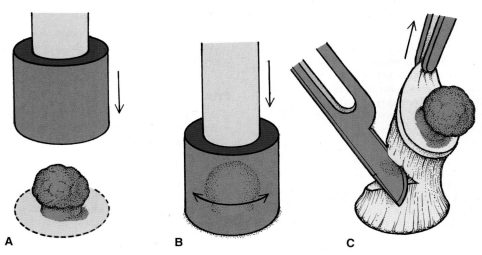

A   B   C

FIG. 24-2. Punch biopsy.

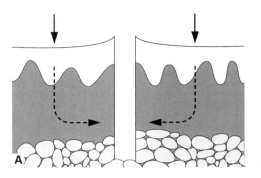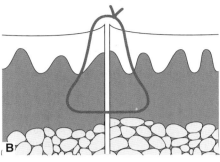

FIG. 24-3. Simple interrupted suture. **A:** Closure for punch biopsy with equal amounts of tissue on both sides of the defect. **B:** Eversion of the wound edges for optimal healing.

- Return for suture removal as indicated
  - Face and neck in 3 to 7 days
  - Arms in 7 to 10 days
  - Trunk and legs in 10 to 14 days
- Keep wound moist with petrolatum and covered for 1 to 2 weeks for optimal healing and best cosmetic results.
- The patient should be educated about the signs and symptoms of infection, including redness, warmth, tenderness, and discharge. Contact information should be given in the event that this should occur.
- Inform patient when and how they will receive the results of their biopsy.
- Arrange for suture removal.

SHAVE BIOPSY

Author:

Theodore D. Scott, RN, MSN, FNP-C, DCNP

Description

Shave biopsy is a nonsterile procedure by which sampling of an exophytic or shallow endophytic skin lesion is performed for the purpose of histopathologic examination.

Indications

- Raised lesions
- Dome-shaped nevi and benign tumors
- Nonmelanoma skin cancers

Contraindications

- Infection at the biopsy site
- Vascular lesion of unknown extent for depth (cavernous hemangioma)
- Deep melanocytic lesions suspected for melanoma (only punch, excisional, or deep saucerization are indicated for these deep lesions).

Equipment

- Alcohol or chlorhexidine prep pads
- Examination gloves
- Syringe, size as required (usually 3 cc or 5 cc)

- 25G to 31G needle depending on site. 31G insulin syringes are helpful for noses and ears.
- Lidocaine 1% or 2%, with or without epinephrine, depending on site
- Sterile 4 × 4 or 2 × 2 gauge sponges
- DermaBlade or scalpel blade (no. 15)
- Formalin in normal saline specimen containers of appropriate size for the specimen prelabeled with the patient's name and medical record number—never label after the fact.
- Aluminum chloride 20% solution (Drysol), Monsel's solution, or hyfrecator
- Cotton-tipped applicators
- Petrolatum-based ointment (Vaseline or Aquaphor)
- Adhesive dressing of appropriate size

Preparation

- Same as for Punch Biopsy

Procedure

- Using the DermaBlade or scalpel blade, tangentially shave the lesion off the skin with a gentle side-to-side movement (Figure 24-4).
- Place the specimen into a container and seal.

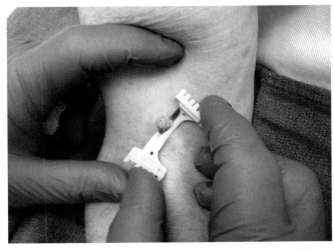

FIG. 24-4. Shave biopsy. Holding the DermaBlade tangentially to the skin surface, the blade can remove a sample of the epidermis and dermis. A deeper saucerization requires a sharper angle to the skin, allowing the blade to scoop deep into the dermis.

- Blot biopsy site with gauze square and apply cotton-tip applicator saturated (not dripping) with the aluminum chloride or Monsel's solution. Light electrocautery with a hyfrecator may be needed.
- Apply petrolatum ointment to wound after hemostasis is achieved.
- Apply adhesive dressing.
- Give patients both verbal and printed aftercare instructions in their preferred language.

Anticipated Outcomes

- Same as with punch biopsy

Aftercare

- Same as for punch biopsy, except for suture removal

CLINICAL PEARLS

- Avoid epinephrine on fingertips and penile tip.
- Punch biopsies ≤4 mm can be left open to heal by secondary intention.
- Alcohol and hydrogen peroxide are no longer used for routine wound care as they are toxic to the keratinocytes.
- Neomycin, polymyxin, and bacitracin ointments (Neosporin) are not recommended as they are potential sensitizers and may provide little protection.
- For all skin diseases other than pigmented lesions, a 4-mm punch will give the pathologist adequate material to make a diagnosis.
- For pigmented lesions, select a punch that will completely sample the lesion and a slim margin of clear skin.
- Never perform a shallow shave biopsy of a pigmented skin lesion to avoid the risk of transecting the pigmented lesion. The most predictive factor in the clinical course of melanoma treatment is the depth of invasion on initial biopsy. This information would be lost.
- Never take a small punch or several small punches of a large pigmented lesion. A small punch of a large lesion will not provide the most accurate measurement of the depth.
- If a pigmented lesion is too large to sample comfortably in your clinic, arrange expedient referral to a provider skilled in dermatology or surgery.
- Avoid Monsel's solution and silver nitrate in cosmetically sensitive areas as they can leave a permanent pigmentation.

SKIN TAG REMOVAL

Author:

Kathleen E. Dunbar Haycraft, DNP, FNP/PNP-BC, DCNP, FAANP

Description

- Procedure to remove benign skin tags by various methods

Indications

- Symptomatic (tender, bleeding, or itching)
- Cosmetic concerns

Equipment

Depending on the method used:

- Alcohol swabs
- Gauze 4 × 4
- Lidocaine, or topical anesthetic
- Small sharp scissors (gradle)
- Forceps (optional)
- Liquid nitrogen
- Hyfrecator

Preparation

- Procedure details, risks, alternatives, and recurrence are discussed with the patient. All questions are answered and informed consent is given by the patient.
- Advise patients that this may be considered a cosmetic procedure and *not* covered by insurance.
- If you have any doubt as to the benign nature of the lesion, *send it for biopsy.*
- Cleanse the area with antiseptic preparation and allow it to dry.
- Consider anesthesia options: ice for 1 minute prior to removal; a brief spray of liquid nitrogen (LN$_2$); topical anesthetic; lidocaine injection (more painful than the actual removal); and no anesthesia, which is very common for clipping, hyfrecation, and cryotherapy.

Procedures

Several techniques, including snip removal, shave removal, hyfrecation, and cryosurgery.

Scissor removal

- Grasp the skin tag and slightly extend it upward. Make sure to use sharp tissue scissors to assure a quick and accurate snip at the base of the lesion (Figure 24-5). Bleeding should be controlled with pressure, as it is the least likely method to result in scarring. Ammonium chloride (Drysol) is irritating but can be used if the pressure is ineffective. If bleeding continues, electrocautery/hyfrecation may be used after assurance of anesthesia. Before using cautery, remove all alcohol and ammonium chloride (flammable) that may be left on the skin.

Shave removal

- Perform the procedure by gently grasping the acrochordon with forceps, slightly extending the lesion upward. Using a DermaBlade or scalpel, shave the lesion at the base (similar

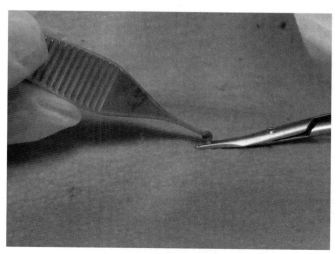

FIG. 24-5. Snip skin tag.

technique as shave biopsy). This is the preferred technique for a larger acrochordon or fibroepithelial polyps. Control bleeding as above.

Hyfrecation

- Touch the base of the skin tag with the tip of the hyfrecator (high-frequency eradicator) set at lowest frequency. Contact the skin at a few second intervals until the base turns white/gray. Limit the contacts to three for each skin tag if possible.

Liquid nitrogen

- Place the LN_2 spray gun nozzle about 1.5 cm from the lesion and aim at the center. Spray until a minimal ice ball encompasses the skin tag. Do up to three freeze and thaw cycles. Freeze times that exceed 30 seconds or are performed at very close range may result in significant tissue damage and hyperpigmentation.
- To minimize the risk of spray to the surrounding tissue, cold forceps can be used to apply the therapy. Place the tip of a small needle holder or mosquito forceps into a styrofoam cup of LN_2 for 30 seconds, allowing the temperature of the metal instrument to drop. Then grasp the papule, and the cold will transfer to the lesion, creating an ice ball. The effect of cryotherapy can be controlled so that surrounding skin is not damaged. This method is also used for warts (Figure 24-6).

Anticipated Outcomes

Minimal discomfort
Small blister formation or crust for 5 to 7 days
Scarring and recurrence

Aftercare

Postprocedure care will depend on the type of technique you use.

- Advise the patient what to expect postprocedure, as the skin tag usually doesn't fall off immediately with cryotherapy or hyfrecation. It usually takes a week.
- With snip or shave method, advise wound care with daily cleansing with soap and water, petrolatum, and small bandage as needed.
- Warn patients that the skin tag may darken or turn black before it falls off.

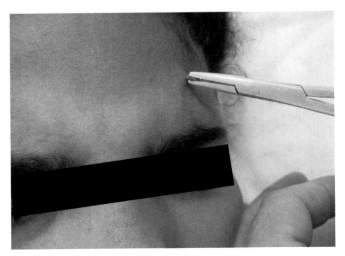

FIG. 24-6. Cryotherapy with needle holder.

- Educate patients on the signs of infection and report any promptly.
- Patient should understand that skin tags can recur and new ones develop.

CLINICAL PEARLS

- Skin tags are a clinical diagnosis. Therefore, the clinician must be confident in their diagnosis when treating with cryotherapy or hyfrecation because there is no tissue sample for histologic analysis.
- If you are unsure of the diagnosis, biopsy the lesion!
- There is no consensus about the histologic testing on removed skin tags. Some clinicians believe that it is an unnecessary expense to send skin tags to pathology, while others harbor a concern that there is the possibility that a malignancy could arise in a skin tag–appearing lesion.

LIQUID NITROGEN CRYOTHERAPY

Author:

Kelly Noska, RN, MSN, ANP-BC

Description

LN_2 (–198 °C) applied directly to warts or other epidermal lesions induces a localized form of frostbite, causing tissue damage to keratinocytes. A blister develops at the dermal–epidermal junction. When the blister dries and erodes, the affected area will slough part or all of the epidermis.

Indications

- Verruca (warts), molluscum contagiosum, actinic keratoses, seborrheic keratoses, solar lentigines, keloids, and other benign cutaneous lesions
- *Cryosurgery* performed on some nonmelanoma skin cancers by experienced dermatologists is not the same as *cryotherapy*.

Contraindications

- Patients with Raynaud's, cold urticaria, cryoglobulinemia

Equipment

- LN_2
- Cryogun (Brymill or Cry-Ac spray)
- Insulated storage container (or one-time-use styrofoam cup) with cotton-tipped applicators
- Disposable otoscope tips

Procedure

- Explain the procedure risks, alternatives, and expected course of treatment.
- Using a cryogun or cotton-tipped applicator, LN_2 is applied to the lesion (Figure 24-7A&B).
- The visibly frozen area (ice ball) will turn white and should be maintained for 5 to 10 seconds depending on the type of lesion and location. A 2-mm border surrounding the perimeter of the lesion should be included (Figure 24-8).
- Placing a disposable otoscope tip directly over the lesion before treating will allow you to confine the freeze to the specific lesion without treating too much surrounding tissue (useful in children).

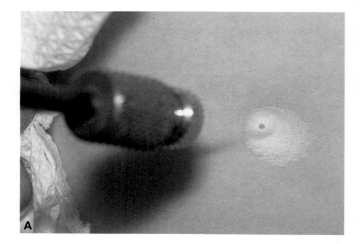

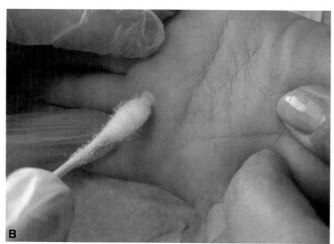

FIG. 24-7. Cryotherapy. **A:** Spray gun. **B:** Cotton applicator.

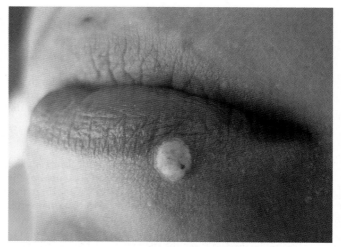

FIG. 24-8. Ice ball.

- Cryotherapy is painful during procedure and in the immediate few minutes postprocedure.
- Cryotherapy can result in hypo-, hyper-, or depigmentation, especially in darkly-skinned individuals.
- Scarring can occur with intense or extensive cryotherapy treatment.

Aftercare

- Blisters commonly form within days. Plain petrolatum should be applied.
- Warn patients that they may develop blood blister (especially on the fingers/toes and with repeated freeze–thaw cycles).
- Try to keep blister intact. If necessary, rupture with sterile pin but don't unroof.

- The ice ball should thaw in 30 to 60 seconds. The cycle may be repeated up to three cycles, which may lead to a better treatment response in thicker warts.

Actinic keratosis

- Chapter 8 defined actinic keratoses (AKs) as precancerous lesions, and therefore special awareness is necessary when treating with LN_2.
- AKs are technically confined to the epidermis and should respond nicely to cryotherapy (Figure 24-9).
- However, thicker or hypertrophic lesions may represent squamous cell carcinoma in situ, especially on the scalp. Patients should be advised to return for follow-up if the lesion does not completely resolve (Figure 24-10).
- Watch for increasing size, induration, or erosion.
- If a lesion has been treated with LN_2 more than once without resolution, it should be biopsied.

Anticipated Outcomes

- Patient response can vary from minimal erythema to hemorrhagic blistering.

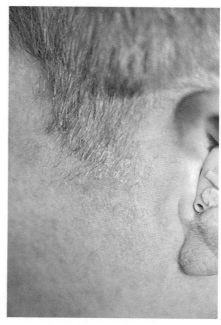

FIG. 24-9. Actinic keratosis.

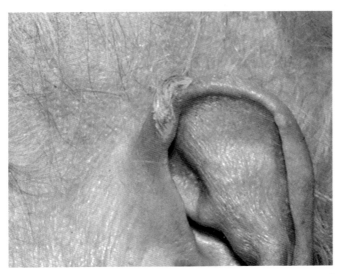

FIG. 24-10. Hypertrophic actinic keratosis, which should be treated and followed carefully if not resolved.

CLINICAL PEARLS

It is better to undertreat a lesion and retreat at a later date than to overtreat.

- Use of liquid nitrogen around the nail may cause damage to the nail plate.
- Over-the-counter (OTC) freeze sprays (dimethyl ether) are available but much less effective than liquid nitrogen.
- If a margin beyond the border of the verruca is not treated, the patient could develop a "doughnut"-shaped lesion that has cleared in the middle.
- Cotton-tipped applicator should be used on only one patient, then discarded. The applicator should not be dipped into the storage container and cause contamination.
- A pulsing spray or intermittent contact with the applicator maintains the ice ball without causing a spread to healthy tissue.
- Thinner lesions require a shorter treatment time, while thicker lesions should have a longer ice ball and repeated treatment may be needed.
- A fast freeze and slow thaw is the most effective cryotherapy treatment.

CANTHARIDIN
Author:
Kelly Noska, RN, MSN, ANP-BC

Description
- This is a liquid derived from a blistering insect and causes acantholysis (loss of adhesion between keratinocytes). The result is a blister that develops between the epidermal and dermal layers of skin.
- Cantharidin is not FDA approved in the United States, but was placed on the FDA's proposed bulk substances list and may only be used in the professional setting. It cannot be prescribed or applied by patients.

Indications
- Molluscum contagiosum and verruca vulgaris (except mosaic warts)

Contraindications
- Use with caution on the digits and genital mucosa.

Equipment
- Cantharidin 0.7%, Cantharone
- Canthacur PS (combination of Cantharone plus podophyllin 5% and salicylic acid [SA] 30%)
- Wooden-tipped applicator or toothpicks (flat end)
- Clear tape

Procedure
- The clinician should carefully apply the liquid directly to the lesion and avoid any contact with the surrounding healthy tissue.
- The wooden end of a cotton-tipped applicator or flat tooth pick is helpful in applying minute amounts to 1- to 2-mm lesions. Each applicator is discarded after touching the lesion (Figure 24-11).
- As the liquid dries, it forms a clear film (Canthacur PS produces a white film) over the area. Cover with a nonporous tape.
- There is a large variation in practice regarding the amount of treatment time that cantharidin is left on the skin. Some suggest removing the tape and washing off the film in 4 hours after application. Others recommend leaving it in place for 24 hours.
- Variation also depends on the location. Thicker skin (plantar surface) may require longer application time.
- Petrolatum should be applied twice daily for comfort and to promote healing.

Anticipated Outcome
- A blister can form within hours after application. At that time, the tape should be removed, and the area washed with soap and water to remove any residual medication.
- Severe blistering can result even with correct application.

Aftercare
- Treat the blister with plain petrolatum twice daily.
- Try to keep blister intact. If necessary, rupture with sterile pin but do not unroof.
- When treating warts, salicylic acid may be reapplied when blisters heal, if wart tissue remains.

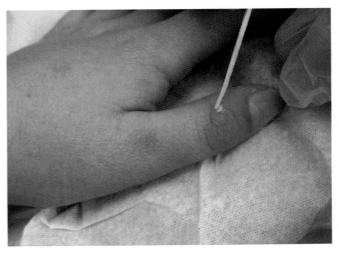

FIG. 24-11. Cantharidin applicator.

CLINICAL PEARLS

- At the first visit, treat only a few lesions to assess the patient's response and tolerance.
- A hypersensitivity reaction is rare but possible.
- Severe blistering can occur if cantharidin is applied incorrectly.
- Avoid contact with opposing skin (axillae, thighs, gluteal folds, etc.).
- Use a new toothpick for *each application* to prevent contamination of multidose bottles.
- Repeated treatments every 3 to 4weeks are often required.
- Patient application of topical salicylic acid on warts between visits can accelerate the treatment process.

TOPICAL SALICYLIC ACID

Author:

Kelly Noska, RN, MSN, ANP-BC

Description

SA is a keratolytic agent which is intended to soften and thin excess skin which can build up over and around warts, callus, and other benign growths.

Indications (for Use at Home)

- Warts, calluses, and corns

Contraindications

- Pregnancy
- Peripheral neuropathy (diabetes)
- Peripheral artery disease
- Nonintact skin or erosions

Equipment

- SA is available in liquid or plaster forms and with various applicators: Duofilm, Duoplant, Compound W, Wart-off, Occlusal-HP, Trans-Ver-Sal, Virasal, and Mediplast
- Most OTC preparations are 17% SA. OTC plasters with 40% SA are more effective and may shorten treatment.

Procedure

- Soak the affected area in warm water for 10 to 20 minutes prior to treatment.
- Rub the surface with a nail or foot file to remove loosened skin. There may be some pinpoint bleeding.
- Apply liquid or plaster to the affected area and only a few millimeter border of normal skin.
- Leave in place for 12 to 24 hours, and then remove.
- Repeat daily until lesions resolve.
- If discomfort develops, discontinue for several days until better, then resume for shorter intervals.

Anticipated Outcomes

- *Gradual* destruction and peeling of skin will occur in the treated area.
- It can take weeks or months to eradicate a wart using this method, especially on the plantar surface, but reduction of callus will relieve discomfort.

- Skin may become white and macerated.
- Swelling, tenderness, and secondary infection can occur from overuse.

Aftercare

- Pare down (exfoliate) hyperkeratotic skin with nail file or pumice stone in between treatments to ensure that medication penetrates the affected area.

CLINICAL PEARLS

Salicylic acid will destroy all skin it comes in contact with; so careful application is advised.

- Plain petrolatum can be applied to the normal skin surrounding the wart prior to treatment to prevent damage to normal skin.
- Disposable emery boards may be used for exfoliating the lesion. Discard after use.
- A pumice stone can harbor the virus and recontaminate any surface it may be used on.
- Duct tape or a Band-Aid can be used to keep the SA in place.

POTASSIUM HYDROXIDE PREPARATION

Author:

Janice T. Chussil, MSN, ANP-C, DCNP

Description

Potassium hydroxide (KOH) prep allows the immediate examination of scale or debris to determine the presence or absence of superficial fungal elements or other organisms.

Indications

- Any scaling, vesicular or pustular eruption that could represent a dermatophyte or yeast infection
- Identification of molluscum bodies
- Demodex (mites) infestations

Contraindications

- None

Equipment

- Microscope, glass slides, and coverslip
- #10 or 15 blade or curette
- Solution: 10% to 20% KOH; 20% KOH with added dimethylsulfoxide (DMSO); Swartz–Lamkin stain (SLS) or chlorazol black E counterstain containing KOH plus dye (makes the fungal elements more visible)
- Alcohol lamp or disposable lighter as heating source (not needed with DMSO)

Procedure

Skin, nails, and hair

- For skin, scrape the active scaly border of the lesion (area of highest yield) and place scale on a glass slide.
- For blisters or pustules, the fungus is in the roof of the vesicle. Gently dissect the vesicle and scrape the underside with no. 15 blade and smear on the glass slide.

- For nails, collect subungual debris from the distal lateral edge of the nail or the white scale from the underside of the nail surface.
- For hair, pull hairs from affected site ensuring that the root or bulb is present. Gently scrape the scalp or use a sterile toothbrush to collect the scale. Place on a glass slide.
- Add a drop or two of KOH or SLS to the specimen and place a coverslip over the specimen (Figure 24-12A and B).
- Heat *gently,* but not to boiling, for 3 to 5 seconds. If using KOH with DMSO, heating is not necessary. KOH obliterates the cellular components, making fungal elements easier to visualize (Figure 24-12C).
- SLS prep can be examined immediately but KOH slides or thicker specimens may need to sit for 10 minutes.
- Place slide on microscope with low to medium light. Focus with the low-power objective (4x or 10x) and scan the slide until possible hyphae or spores are identified. Then switch to a higher power (10x or 40x) for a closer examination.

- Dermatophytes will be seen as long, segmented hyphal elements which will be bluish/green if stained with SLS (Figure 24-13A).
- For tinea versicolor or pityrosporum folliculitis, you will see both hyphae and spores, the classic "spaghetti and meatballs" sign (Figure 24-13B).
- *Candida* will show mainly budding yeast cells (Figure 24-13C).
- Molluscum is seen as spheric bodies within the keratinocytes.

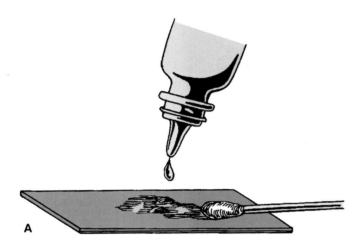

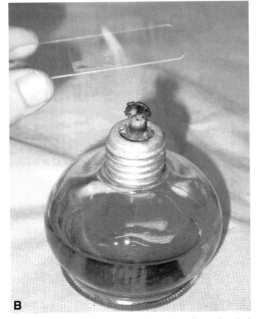

FIG. 24-12. KOH preparations. **A:** The specimen is collected and placed onto a glass slide. A drop of 10% to 20% KOH is also placed on the slide. The preparations are then covered with a cover slide for microscopic viewing. **B:** Gentle heating of a small amount of scale with KOH prep over an alcohol lamp is the key for a useful fungal preparation.

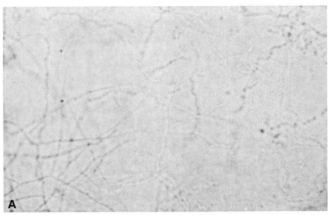

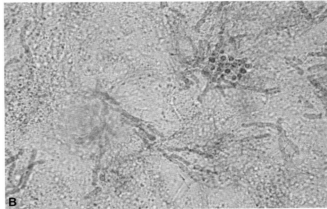

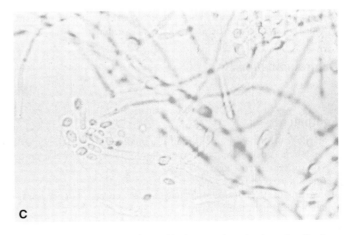

FIG. 24-13. **A:** KOH preparation, with dermatophyte hyphae visualized on microscopic examination. **B:** Tinea versicolor on KOH preparation. Note the short, stubby hyphae ("spaghetti") and the clusters of spores ("meatballs"). **C:** Budding yeast cells of *Candida.*

Anticipated Outcome

- This procedure causes minimal discomfort to the patient.
- Confirmation of the presence or absence of spores or hyphae or molluscum bodies helps develop a differential diagnosis.
- If the KOH prep is negative but there is strong clinical suspicion, repeat the KOH prep and/or perform a fungal culture.

Aftercare

- None

CLINICAL PEARLS

- ■ Microscope skills take time to develop. A counterstain such as Swartz–Lamkin can be helpful for novices to identify hyphae.
- ■ Allowing the KOH slide to sit for 30 minutes can make visualization of fungal elements much easier. So be patient!
- ■ Remember, hyphae and spores must be present within the epithelial cells. Elements present outside the cells are artifacts.
- ■ If the patient has been using an antifungal preparation, the KOH prep may be negative despite inadequate clearing of the infection. If possible, ask the patient to discontinue any topical medication at least several days prior to procedure.
- ■ The examination of hair for fungal elements on KOH prep is very difficult.

FUNGAL CULTURE

Author:

Janice T. Chussil, MSN, ANP-C, DCNP

Description

Fungal culture of a skin, nail or hair specimen is performed to detect the presence of superficial fungal elements

This is *not* the appropriate laboratory testing for deep fungal infections.

Indications

- Specimens should be tested for fungus if you are unable to perform a KOH prep; still suspect a fungus even with a negative KOH prep; or need to identify the specific causative fungal organism. Sensitivities may also be ordered and performed.

Contraindications

- None

Equipment

- Sterile transport container or culture media relative to the type of test, such as dermatophyte test medium (DTM), Mycosel agar, or Sabouraud dextrose agar
- Alcohol prep pads
- Instruments to collect sample: nail clippers, curette, #10 or 15 scalpel blade, brush (toothbrush)

Procedure

- These are general guidelines for most fungal specimen collection. Fungi can remain viable for days in scale and hair; so no medium

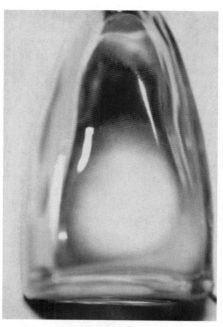

FIG. 24-14. Fungal culture using the DTM. Note the positive result indicated by the color change from yellow to red.

is required, and the specimen is sent directly to the laboratory in a sterile culture container.
- If there is a specific test such as DTM or laboratory analysis being used, follow the recommended procedures for collection according to the company (Figure 24-14).

Skin specimens

- Collect specimens from areas that are clean and dry. Avoid collecting skin that has topical moisturizers or medications.
- Using a #10 or 15 scalpel blade, gently scrape the leading edge of the scaly patch or plaque. Allow the scale to fall into the sterile container or culture medium.

Nail specimens

- Prior to collection, clean the nail and surrounding skin with warm, soapy water. Let dry. Then wipe the area with alcohol prep pad and air dry.
- Use sterile instruments to trim the free edge of the nail and expose debris.
- Discard the nail.
- Gently wipe with a new alcohol pad and air dry (again).
- Use a sterile curette to remove subungual debris and collect in a sterile specimen container or specific container requested by the laboratory.
- Label appropriately and complete requisition.

Hair specimens

- Avoid collection of hair with hair care products.
- Identify the area and trim hairs close to the scalp. Pluck hairs with a tweezer, forceps, or brush and place in sterile container or on specified culture medium.

Scalp specimens

- Use a sterile scalpel/blade and/or toothbrush-like tool to scrape over the affected area and transfer scale into collection container. The brush may also be submitted.

Anticipated Outcome

- Minimal discomfort
- Confirmed diagnosis

Aftercare

- None unless there is bleeding and then small bandage is sufficient.

WOOD LAMP EXAMINATION

Author:

Katie Brouillard O'Brien, MSN, ANP-BC

Description

The Wood lamp is a safe and inexpensive office tool which is useful to diagnose infections of the skin and disorders of pigmentation.

The Wood lamp emits black light (long-wave UVR) produced by a high-pressure mercury arc fitted with a compound filter, known as the "Wood filter." Fluorescence of skin occurs when the Wood light is absorbed and radiation of a longer wavelength, usually visible light, is emitted.

Indications

- Bacterial skin infections, fungal skin infections, hypopigmentation or depigmentation, hyperpigmentation, melasma, and porphyria

Equipment

- Wood lamp

Procedure

- Allow Wood lamp to warm up for about 1 minute.
- The examination room should be completely darkened.
- Topical medications, lint, deodorant, and soap residue should be wiped off from the site being examined as these can fluoresce under Wood light.
- Hold the Wood lamp 4 to 5 inches away from the skin. Beginning at the scalp, you can gradually pass the light over the entire surface of the skin in a "windshield wiper" type of motion. Be sure to look at axilla and genital areas, especially if you suspect vitiligo.

Anticipated Outcome

- Fluorescence of normal skin is faint or absent.
- Vitiligo: Lesions are well demarcated and fluorescent under Wood's lamp examination. A blue-white color is noted and varies in intensity depending on decreased or absent melanin (Figure 24-15).

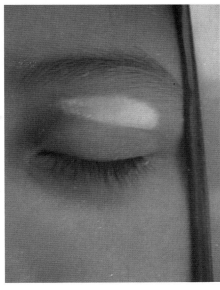

FIG. 24-15. Wood light examination. Note the enhanced coloration of the depigmented area.

- Hyperpigmentation: Lesions show an increased border contrast under Wood lamp.
- Pseudomonas fluoresces green in folliculitis and infected wounds.
- Erythrasma fluoresces coral red because of the *Corynebacterium*.
- Propionibacterium acnes show orange-red in comedones.
- Tinea versicolor: *Malassezia furfur* fluoresces yellowish-white or copper-orange.
- Tinea capitis: blue-green (most *Microsporum* species), sometimes dull yellow (*Microsporum gypseum*) and dull blue (*Trichophyton schoenleinii*)
- Porphyria: Urine, teeth, and feces may fluoresce pink-red.

Aftercare

- None

MINERAL OIL PREP

Author:

Melissa E. Cyr, MSN, ANP-BC, FNP-BC

Description

Mineral oil mount for microscopic analysis to identify mites, eggs, or scybala (feces)

Indications

- Scabies (*Sarcoptes scabiei*)

Equipment

- Mineral oil
- Glass microscope slide
- No. 15 surgical blade (nonsterile)
- Slide coverslip
- Microscope

Procedure

- Identify new, nonexcoriated burrow (typically linear) or vesicle. Look for a black dot at one end, which may represent the mite, and scrape at that location.
- Apply a drop of mineral oil onto the center of a glass microscope slide. Dip the edge of a no. 15 surgical blade also in the oil (or apply a drop of oil to the blade).
- Utilizing the lateral edge of the scalpel blade, at a 45° angle, scrape the skin to attain several wide superficial skin scrapings. There may be some pinpoint bleeding.
- After scraping, mix the accumulated debris on the blade into the mineral oil on the slide, and apply a coverslip.
- Scan the slide at low power (4x or 10x) before switching to high power (40x), to look for scabiei mites.
- Eggs may be present as discrete and ovoid-shaped figures, either containing a larval mite or the empty remains of a hatched egg. Scybala, or fecal pellets, will appear as brownish-black, poorly-defined globules (Figure 24-16).

Anticipated Outcome

- Slight discomfort and minimal bleeding are expected with scraping.

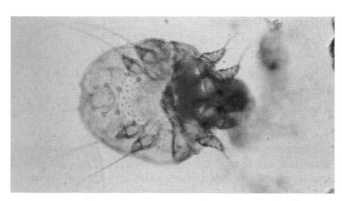

FIG. 24-16. Scabies mite.

Aftercare

- None

CLINICAL PEARL

- Scabies mites are often few in numbers (except in the case of crusted scabies). The diagnosis can be confirmed with the presence of eggs or scybala alone.

READINGS

Usatine, R. (1998). *Skin surgery: A practical guide.* St. Louis, MO: Mosby.

Micromedix. (2014). Micromedex Medication, Disease and Toxicology Management. (Micromedix 2.0). Greewood Village, CO: Truven Health Analytics.

Scott, T. D. (2011). Procedure primer: The potassium hydroxide preparation. *The Journal of the Dermatology Nurses' Association, 3*(5), 304–305.

Sterry, W., Paus, R., & Burgdorf, W. (2006). *Thieme clinical companions: Dermatology* (5th ed.). New York, NY: Thieme.

INTERNET RESOURCES

American Academy of Allergy, Asthma & Immunology, www.aaaai.org

American Academy of Dermatology, www.aad.org

American Board of Wound Management, www.aawm.org

American Cancer Society: melanoma skin cancer overview, http://www.cancer.org/acs/groups/cid/documents/webcontent/003063-pdf.pdf

American Diabetes Association, www.diabetes.org

American Lyme Disease Foundation, www.aldf.com

Association of Cancer Online Resources: Peutz–Jeghers syndrome, http://listserv.acor.org/scripts/wa-ACOR.exe?A0=PJS

Centers for Disease Control and Prevention, www.cdc.gov

Dermatology Nurses'Association, www.dnanurse.org

DermNet NZ, www.dermnetnz.org

Food Allergy Research and Education (FARE), www.foodallergy.org

National Institutes of Health: granuloma annulare, http://rarediseases.info.nih.gov/gard/6546/granuloma-annulare/resources/1

International Psoriasis Council, www.psoriasiscouncil.org

Mayo Clinic: diseases and conditions, www.mayoclinic.com/health/Diseases Index/DiseasesIndex

Medscape: dermatology, http://emedicine.medscape.com/dermatology

National Eczema Association, www.nationaleczema.org

National Institute of Diabetes and Digestive and Kidney Diseases, www2.niddk.nih.gov

National Institutes of Health, Office of Rare Diseases Research, http://rarediseases.info.nih.gov

National Kidney Foundation, www.kidney.org

National Library of Medicine, www.nlm.nih.gov

National Organization for Rare Diseases, www.rarediseases.org

National Psoriasis Foundation, www.psoriasis.org

National Rosacea Society, www.rosacea.org

National Vitiligo Foundation, www.mynvfi.org

Nestlé Nutrition Institute Mini Nutritional Assessment, www.mna-elderly.com

Rush University Medical Center: Vasculitis Clinic Resources, www.rush.edu/rumc/page-1298328986581.html

Sarcoidosis Network Foundation, www.sarcoid-network.org

The Acne and Rosacea Society, www.acneandrosacea.org

The American Porphyria Foundation, www.porphyriafoundation.com

The Skin Cancer Foundation, www.skincancer.org

Tuberous Sclerosis Alliance, www.tsalliance.org

Tuberous Sclerosis Association, www.tuberous-sclerosis.org

U.S. Environmental Protection Agency Sunwise Program, www.epa.gov/sunwise/doc/uvradiation.html

UNC Healthcare Kidney Center: ANCA vasculitis, www.unckidneycenter.org/kidneyhealthlibrary/anca.html#ancapath

Wound Ostomy and Continence Nurses Society, www.wocn.org

Wound Ostomy and Continence Nursing Certification Board, www.wocncb.org

ART CREDITS

The editors and publisher thank the following individuals and publications for permission to use copyrighted images in this work.

CHAPTER 1

Figure 1-4 (photographs only), Figures 1-5A, 1-5B, 1-5D, 1-5E, 1-5G–K, 1-5N, 1-5P, 1-5T, 1-5V, 1-5X. ©Margaret Bobonich

Figure 1-5L. Fleisher, G. R., Ludwig, S., & Baskin, M. N. (2004). *Atlas of pediatric emergency medicine*. Philadelphia, PA: Wolters Kluwer Health| Lippincott Williams & Wilkins.

CHAPTER 2

Figure 2-1. ©Thomas P. Habif
Figure 2-2. ©Gail Lenahan

CHAPTER 3

Figures 3-2, 3-3C, 3-5D, 3-6, 3-10B, 3-12 to 3-14, 3-16, 3-17. ©Margaret Bobonich

Figures 3-3A and B, 3-4, 3-5A and B, 3-7, 3-8B, 3-9, 3-10A, 3-11. ©Susan Tofte

Figure 3-5C. Ilona J. Frieden

Figures 3-8A and 3-15. Stedman's

CHAPTER 4

Figure 4-1. Rubin, R., Strayer, D. S., & Rubin, E. (Ed.). (2011). *Rubin's pathology: Clinicopathologic foundations of medicine* (6th ed.). Philadelphia, PA: Wolters Kluwer Health| Lippincott Williams & Wilkins.

Figures 4-2 to 4-6, 4-7B. ©Margaret Bobonich

Figure 4-9. Goodheart, H. P. (2003). *Goodheart's photoguide of common skin disorders* (2nd ed.). Philadelphia, PA: Wolters Kluwer Health| Lippincott Williams & Wilkins.

Figure 4-10. Stedman's

CHAPTER 5

Figures 5-1, 5-2, 5-4, 5-5, 5-6B. ©Margaret Bobonich
Figure 5-12A. ©Victoria Lazareth
Figures 5-6A, 5-10, 5-12B, 5-17. International Psoriasis Council

CHAPTER 6

Figures 6-2 and 6-19. ©Victoria Garcia-Albea
Figures 6-6, 6-9, and 6-21. ©Margaret Bobonich
Figures 6-7 and 6-8. Jessica Galvin
Figure 6-11. W. Elliot Love
Figure 6-14. George A. Datto III
Figures 6-17 and 6-18. Fleisher, G. R., Ludwig, W., & Baskin, M. N. (2004). *Atlas of pediatric emergency medicine*. Philadelphia, PA: Wolters Kluwer Health| Lippincott Williams & Wilkins.
Figures 6-20, 6-22, and 6-23. Samuel Moschella

CHAPTER 7

Box 7-4. Images copyright © 2013 *American Academy of Dermatology*. Used with permission.

Figure 7-1. Premkumar, K. (2004). *The massage connection: Anatomy and physiology*. Baltimore, MD: Wolters Kluwer Health| Lippincott Williams & Wilkins.

Figures 7-2, 7-9, 7-13B, 7-18, 7-19, 7-23B, 7-24A, 7-25. ©Theodore Scott

Figure 7-3. McConnell, T. H. (2007). *The nature of disease pathology for the health professions*. Philadelphia, PA: Wolters Kluwer Health| Lippincott Williams & Wilkins.

Figures 7-4 to 7-8, 7-10 to 7-13A, 7-14 to 7-17, 7-20, 7-22, 7-23A, 7-24B, 7-27. ©Margaret Bobonich

Figure 7-21. DeVita, V. T., Lawrence, T. S., & Rosenberg, S. A. (2008). *DeVita, Hellman, and Rosenberg's Cancer: Principles & practice of oncology* (8th ed.). Philadelphia, PA: Wolters Kluwer Health| Lippincott Williams & Wilkins.

Figure 7-26. Miller, C., Goodheart, H. P. (2009). *Goodheart's photoguide to common skin disorders: Diagnosis and management* (3rd ed.). Philadelphia, PA: Wolters Kluwer Health| Lippincott Williams & Wilkins.

Figure 7-28. Goodheart, H. P. (2003). *Goodheart's photoguide of common skin disorders* (2nd ed.). Philadelphia, PA: Wolters Kluwer Health| Lippincott Williams & Wilkins.

Figure 7-29. Rubin, R., Strayer, D. S., & Rubin, E. (Ed.). (2011). *Rubin's pathology: Clinicopathologic foundations of medicine* (6th ed.). Philadelphia, PA: Wolters Kluwer Health| Lippincott Williams & Wilkins.

Table 7-2. ©Margaret Bobonich, and assets provided by Anatomical Chart Co.

CHAPTER 8

Figures 8-2 to 8-5, 8-7 to 8-33. ©Victoria Lazareth
Figure 8-6. ©Margaret Bobonich

CHAPTER 9

Figures 9-1 ©Margaret Bobonich

Figure 9-4A. Fleisher, G. R., Ludwig, W., & Baskin, M. N. (2004). *Atlas of pediatric emergency medicine*. Philadelphia, PA: Wolters Kluwer Health| Lippincott Williams & Wilkins.

Figure 9-4B. Berg, D., & Worzala, K. (2006). *Atlas of adult physical diagnosis*. Philadelphia, PA: Wolters Kluwer Health| Lippincott Williams & Wilkins.

Figure 9-5. McConnell, T. H. (2007). *The nature of disease pathology for the health professions*. Philadelphia, PA: Wolters Kluwer Health| Lippincott Williams & Wilkins.

Figures 9-7, 9-10, 9-11, and 9-16. ©Thomas P. Habif

Figure 9-9. Anatomical Chart Co.

Figure 9-15A. Berg, D., & Worzala, K. (2006). *Atlas of adult physical diagnosis*. Philadelphia, PA: Wolters Kluwer Health| Lippincott Williams & Wilkins.

CHAPTER 10

Figures 10-2, 10-3, and 10-8, 10-22B. ©Margaret Bobonich

Figures 10-4 10-8, to 10-10, 10-20, 10-21. Goodheart, H. P. (2003). *Goodheart's photoguide of common skin disorders* (2nd ed.). Philadelphia, PA: Wolters Kluwer Health| Lippincott Williams & Wilkins.

Figure 10-11. Neville, B. et al. (1991). *Color atlas of clinical oral pathology*. Philadelphia PA: Lea & Febiger.

Figure 10-13. Fleisher, G. R., Ludwig, W., & Baskin, M. N. (2004). *Atlas of pediatric emergency medicine*. Philadelphia, PA: Wolters Kluwer Health| Lippincott Williams & Wilkins.

Figure 10-16. ©Thomas P. Habif

Figure 10-17. Herbert A. Hochman

Figure 10-18B. Clemente, C. D. (2010). *Anatomy: A regional atlas of the human body* (6th ed.). Philadelphia, PA: Wolters Kluwer Health| Lippincott Williams & Wilkins. Illustration used with permission of Elsevier.

Figure 10-19. National Institute of Allergy and Infectious Diseases

Figure 10-22A. Weber, J., & Kelley, J. (2003). *Health assessment in nursing* (2nd ed.). Philadelphia, PA: Wolters Kluwer Health| Lippincott Williams & Wilkins.

CHAPTER 11

Figures 11-1 ©Kathleen Haycraft and Margaret Bobonich.

Figures 11-3, 11-4, 11-6, 11-7, 11-9, 11-10, 11-12, 11-13 to 11-18, 11-20 to 11-23. ©Margaret Bobonich

Figures 11-2, 11-5, 11-8, 11-11, 11-19. ©Kathleen Haycraft

CHAPTER 12

Figures 12-1, 12-2, 12-4, 12-6 to 12-10, 12-12, 12-14, 12-16, 12-19 to 12-21. ©Margaret Bobonich

Figures 12-3, 12-5, 12-11, 12-13, 12-15, 12-17, 12-18, 12-23, 12-24. Goodheart, H. P. (2003). *Goodheart's photoguide of common skin disorders* (2nd ed.). Philadelphia, PA: Wolters Kluwer Health| Lippincott Williams & Wilkins.

Figure 12-22. ©Janice T. Chussil

CHAPTER 13

Figures 13-1, 13-2, 13-4. Goodheart, H. P. (2003). *Goodheart's photoguide of common skin disorders* (2nd ed.). Philadelphia, PA: Wolters Kluwer Health| Lippincott Williams & Wilkins.

Figure 13-3. ©Melissa Cyr

Figures 13-5, 13-12, 13-18, 13-22. ©Thomas P. Habif

Figure 13-6. Hans B. Kersten

Figure 13-7. Sweet, R. L., & Gibbs, R. S. (2005). *Atlas of infectious diseases of the female genital tract*. Philadelphia, PA: Wolters Kluwer Health| Lippincott Williams & Wilkins.

Figure 13-8. Bauer, S. (2009). The Agricultural Research Service, The Research Agency of the United States Department of Agriculture.

Figure 13-9. Adapted with permission from the American Lyme Disease Foundation

Figure 13-13. Centers for Disease Control and Prevention

Figures 13-11, 13-17, 13-19. ©Margaret Bobonich

Figure 13-14. Thomas, J., Zuber, E. J., & Mayeaux, J. R. (2004). *Atlas of primary care procedures*. Philadelphia, PA: Wolters Kluwer Health| Lippincott Williams & Wilkins.

Figure 13-15. Gathany, J. (2008). Centers for Disease Control and Prevention.

Figure 13-16. Starr, S. (2011). The Children's Hospital of Philadelphia. Philadelphia, PA.

CHAPTER 14

Figures 14-1 and 14-2. Anatomical Chart Co.

Figure 14-3. Adapted from *Endocrinology Metabolism Clinics of North America*. (2007). (36), 381. ©2007 Elsevier Inc.

Figure 14-5. LifeART image copyright (c) 2014 Wolters Kluwer Health| Lippincott Williams & Wilkins. All rights reserved.

Figures 14-6, 14-7B, 14-8, 14-9, 14-11, 14-14. ©Margaret Bobonich

Figure 14-10. Carrie Ann Cusack

Table 14-3. Habif, T. P. (1990). *Clinical dermatology: A color guide to diagnosis and therapy* (2nd ed.). St. Louis, MO: CV Mosby; ©Margaret Bobonich; Sams, W. M. Jr, & Lynch, P. J. (1990). *Principles and practice of dermatology*. New York, NY: Churchill Livingstone; Goodheart, H. P. (2003). *Goodheart's photoguide of common skin disorders* (2nd ed.). Philadelphia, PA: Wolters Kluwer Health| Lippincott Williams; & Image provided by Stedman's.

CHAPTER 15

Figure 15-1. Modified from Sontheimer, R. D., & Provost, T. T. (2004). *Cutaneous manifestations of rheumatic diseases* (2nd ed.). Philadelphia, PA: Wolters Kluwer Health| Lippincott Williams & Wilkins.

Figures 15-3 and 15-4. Sontheimer, R. D., & Provost, T. T. (2004). *Cutaneous manifestations of rheumatic diseases* (2nd ed.). Philadelphia, PA: Wolters Kluwer Health| Lippincott Williams & Wilkins.

Figures 15-5 to 15-8, 15-9A and B, 15-10, 15-11, 15-13 to 15-15, 15-18, 15-20 to 15-28. ©Margaret Bobonich

Figure 15-19. ©Jesse Keller

CHAPTER 16

Figure 16-1. ©Margaret Bobonich and Cathleen Case

Figure 16-2. ©Lauren Alberta-Wzolek

Figure 16-3A. McConnell, T. H. (2007). *The nature of disease pathology for the health professions*. Philadelphia, PA: Wolters Kluwer Health| Lippincott Williams & Wilkins.

Figures 16-4, 16-6, 16-11, 16-12, 16-14, and 16-22. ©Margaret Bobonich

Figures 16-5, 16-13, and 16-26. ©Cathleen Case

Figures 16-7 to 16-10, 16-15, 16-25. Fleisher, G. R., Ludwig, W., & Baskin, M. N. (2004). *Atlas of pediatric emergency medicine*. Philadelphia, PA: Wolters Kluwer Health| Lippincott Williams & Wilkins.

Figure 16-21. Neville, B. et al. (1991). *Color atlas of clinical oral pathology*. Philadelphia, PA: Lea & Febiger.

Figure 16-23. Callen, J. P.

Figure 16-27. Mayra Ianhez

Figure 16-28. George A. Datto III

CHAPTER 17

Figure 17-1. ©Thomas P. Habif

Figures 17-2, 17-7, and 17-10. ©Margaret Bobonich

Figure 17-3A. © Basil Mahmoud

Figure 17-3C. ©Jessica Galvin

Figure 17-4. Courtesy of Melissa Cyr

Figures 17-5A and 17-6. Goodheart, H. P. (2003). *Goodheart's photoguide of common skin disorders* (2nd ed.). Philadelphia, PA: Wolters Kluwer Health| Lippincott Williams & Wilkins.

Figure 17-5B. Fleisher, G. R., Ludwig, W., & Baskin, M. N. (2004). *Atlas of pediatric emergency medicine*. Philadelphia, PA: Wolters Kluwer Health| Lippincott Williams & Wilkins.

Figure 17-8. Courtesy Global SkinAtlas

CHAPTER 18

Figures 18-1 to 18-3, 18-5, 18-7, 18-8, 18-9, 18-10. ©Margaret Bobonich

Figure 18-4A. George A. Datto III

Figures 18-6B and 18-13. Stedman's

CHAPTER 19

Figure 19-3. Stedman's

Figures 19-10, 19-12. Goodheart, H. P. (2003). *Goodheart's photoguide of common skin disorders* (2nd ed.). Philadelphia, PA: Wolters Kluwer Health| Lippincott Williams & Wilkins.

Figures 19-12, 19-16, and 19-17. ©Margaret Bobonich

CHAPTER 20

Figures 20-1, 20-2, 20-5 to 20-7, 20-9 to 20-11, 20-13, 20-14. ©Margaret Bobonich

Figures 20-4 and 20-12. ©Pamela Fletcher

Figure 20-15. Goodheart, H. P. (2003). *Goodheart's photoguide of common skin disorders* (2nd ed.). Philadelphia, PA: Wolters Kluwer Health| Lippincott Williams & Wilkins.

CHAPTER 21

Figure 21-2A. ©Thomas P. Habif

Figure 21-2B. Willis, M. C. (2002). *Medical terminology: A programmed learning approach to the language of health care*. Baltimore, MD: Wolters Kluwer Health| Lippincott Williams & Wilkins.

Figures 21-5 and 21-7. ©Margaret Bobonich

CHAPTER 22

Figures 22-2, 22-5 to 22-8. ©Dea Kent

Figure 22-4. C. Donayre

Table 22-1. Illustrations copyright © National Pressure Ulcer Advisory Panel, 2007

Table 22-1. Photographs ©Dea Kent

Box 22-2. Jeremy Honaker

CHAPTER 23

Figures 23-1, 23-14, 23-17 to 23-20. ©Diane Hanna

Figure 23-3. ©Margaret Bobonich

Figure 23-4. ©R. Small

CHAPTER 24

Figure 24-2. Neil O. Hardy, Westpoint, CT

Figure 24-3. Zuber, T. J., & Mayeaux, E. J. Jr. (2004). *Atlas of primary care procedures*. Philadelphia, PA: Wolters Kluwer Health| Lippincott Williams & Wilkins.

Figure 24-4. ©Theodore Scott

Figures 24-5, 24-6, 24-7B, 24-8, 24-11, 24-15. ©Margaret Bobonich

Figures 24-7A, 24-13B, 24-14, 24-14, 24-16. Goodheart, H. P. (2003). *Goodheart's photoguide of common skin disorders* (2nd ed.). Philadelphia, PA: Wolters Kluwer Health| Lippincott Williams & Wilkins.

Figure 24-9. Sauer, G. C. (1985). *Manual of skin diseases* (5th ed.). Philadelphia, PA: JB Lippincott.

Figure 24-12. Beckmann, C. R. B., Frank W, et al. (2006). *Obstetrics and gynecology* (5th ed.). Philadelphia, PA: Wolters Kluwer Health| Lippincott Williams & Wilkins.

Figure 24-13A. Victor Newcomer, MD, Santa Monica, CA.

INDEX

Note: Page numbers followed by "*f*", "*t*", and "*b*" denote figures, tables, and boxes, respectively.